Planning, Implementing, and Evaluating Health Promotion Programs

A Primer

SEVENTH EDITION

James F. McKenzie, Ph.D., M.P.H., M.C.H.E.S.
Ball State University

Brad L. Neiger, Ph.D., M.C.H.E.S.
Brigham Young University

Rosemary Thackeray, Ph.D., M.P.H.
Brigham Young University

PEARSON

Senior Acquisitions Editor: *Michelle Cadden*
Project Manager: *Lauren Beebe*
Program Manager: *Susan Malloy*
Editorial Assistant: *Heidi Arndt*
Program Management Team Lead: *Mike Early*
Project Management Team Lead: *Nancy Tabor*
Production Management: *Charles Fisher, Integra*
Compositor: *Integra*

Design Manager: *Marilyn Perry*
Cover Designer: *Yvo Riezebos, Tandem Creative, Inc.*
Rights & Permissions Project Manager: *William Opaluch*
Rights & Permissions Management: *Rachel Youdelman*
Senior Procurement Specialist: *Stacey J. Weinberger*
Executive Product Marketing Manager: *Neena Bali*
Senior Field Marketing Manager: *Mary Salzman*
Cover Photo Credit: *Edhar Shvets / Shutterstock*

Library of Congress Cataloging-in-Publication Data

McKenzie, James F.
  Planning, implementing, and evaluating health promotion programs: a primer/
James F. McKenzie, Brad L. Neiger, Rosemary Thackeray.—7th ed.
    p. ; cm.
  Includes bibliographical references.
  ISBN 978-0-13-421992-9—ISBN 0-13-421992-9
I. Neiger, Brad L. II. Thackeray, Rosemary. III. Title.
  [DNLM: 1. Health Promotion—United States. 2. Health Education—United States.
3. Health Planning—United States. 4. Program Evaluation—United States. WA 590]
  613.0973—dc23
                                                            2015044450

2 16

www.pearsonhighered.com

ISBN-10:   0-13-421992-9
ISBN-13: 978-0-13-421992-9

This book is dedicated to seven special people—

Bonnie, Anne, Greg, Mitchell, Julia, Sherry,
and Callie Rose

and to our teachers and mentors—

Marshall H. Becker (deceased), Mary K. Beyer, Noreen Clark (deceased),
Enrico A. Leopardi, Brad L. Neiger, Lynne Nilson, Terry W. Parsons,
Glenn E. Richardson, Irwin M. Rosenstock (deceased),
Yuzuru Takeshita, and Doug Vilnius

CONTENTS

Chapter 4 Assessing Needs   67

Chapter 5 Measurement, Measures, Measurement Instruments, and Sampling 105

T his book is written for students who are enrolled in a professional course in health promotion program planning. It is designed to help them understand and develop the skills necessary to carry out program planning regardless of the setting. The book is unique among the health promotion planning textbooks on the market in that it provides readers with both theoretical and practical information. A straightforward, step-by-step format is used to make concepts clear and the full process of health promotion planning understandable. This book provides, under a single cover, material on all three areas of program development: planning, implementing, and evaluating.

▷ Learning Aids

Each chapter includes chapter objectives, a list of key terms, presentation of content, chapter summary, review questions, activities, and Weblinks. In addition, many of the key concepts are further explained with information presented in boxes, figures, and tables. There are also two appendixes: *Code of Ethics for the Health Education Profession* and *Health Education Specialist Practice Analysis 2015—Responsibilities, Competencies, and Sub-competencies;* an extensive list of references; and a Glossary.

Chapter Objectives

The chapter objectives identify the content and skills that should be mastered after reading the chapter, answering the review questions, completing the activities, and using the Weblinks. Most of the objectives are written using the cognitive and psychomotor (behavior) educational domains. For most effective use of the objectives, we suggest that they be reviewed before reading the chapter. This will help readers focus on the major points in each chapter and facilitate answering the questions and completing the activities at the end.

Key Terms

Key terms are introduced in each chapter and are important to the understanding of the content. The terms are presented in a list at the beginning of each chapter and are printed in boldface at the appropriate points within the chapter. In addition, all the key terms are presented in the Glossary. Again, as with the chapter objectives, we suggest that readers skim the key terms list before reading the chapter. Then, as the chapter is read, particular attention should be paid to the definition of each term.

Presentation of Content

Although each chapter could be expanded—in some cases, entire books have been written on topics we have covered in a chapter or less—we believe that each chapter contains the necessary information to help students understand and develop many of the skills required to be successful health promotion planners, implementers, and evaluators.

Responsibilities and Competencies Boxes

Within the first few pages of all except the first chapter, readers will find a box that contains the responsibilities and competencies for health education specialists that are applicable to the content of the chapter. The responsibilities and competencies presented in each chapter are the result of the most recent practice analysis—the *Health Education Specialist Practice Analysis 2015* (HESPA 2015), which is published in *A Competency-Based Framework for Health Education Specialists—2015* (NCHEC & SOPHE, 2015). These boxes will help readers understand how the chapter content applies to the responsibilities and competencies required of health education specialists. In addition, these boxes should help guide candidates as they prepare to take either the Certified Health Education Specialist (CHES) or Master Certified Health Education Specialist (MCHES) exam. A complete listing of the Responsibilities, Competencies, and Sub-competencies are presented in Appendix B.

Chapter Summary

At the end of each chapter, readers will find a one- or two-paragraph review of the major concepts covered in the chapter.

Review Questions

The questions at the end of each chapter provide readers with some feedback regarding their mastery of the content. These questions also reinforce the objectives and key terms presented in each chapter.

Activities

Each chapter includes several activities that allow students to use their new knowledge and skills. The activities are presented in several different formats for the sake of variety and to appeal to the different learning styles of students. It should be noted that, depending on the ones selected for completion, the activities in one chapter can build on those in a previous chapter and lead to the final product of a completely developed health promotion program plan.

Weblinks

The final portion of each chapter consists of a list of updated links on the World Wide Web. These links encourage students to explore a number of different Websites that are available to support planning, implementing, and evaluating programs.

▷ New to This Edition

In revising this textbook, we incorporated as many suggestions from reviewers, colleagues, and former students as possible. In addition to updating material throughout the text, the following points reflect the major changes in this new edition:

- Chapter 1 has been updated to include information about the revised areas of responsibility, competencies, and subcompetencies based on the *Health Education Specialist Practice Analysis* (HESPA 2015) (NCHEC & SOPHE, 2015), and the implications of HESPA 2015 for the Health Education Profession.

- Chapter 2 has been expanded to include additional information on sources of evidence to support a program rationale, additional information on determining the financial burden of ill health, a new example of a written program rationale, and information on the importance of partnering with others when creating a program.

- Chapter 3 has been restructured to place more emphasis on the prominent planning models used in health promotion. The chapter also now includes the Evidence-Based Planning Framework in Public Health, the CHANGE tool used to plan healthy community initiatives, and more evidence-based examples of how planning models are used in practice.

- Chapter 4 has new information on the importance of needs assessment in the accreditation of health departments and the IRS requirement for not-for-profit hospitals, new information on using technology while conducting a needs assessment, and a new section on organizational health assessments.

- Chapter 5 includes new information on wording questions for different levels of measurement, how to present data in charts and graphs, how to write questions and response items for data collection instruments, and guidelines for the layout and visual presentation of data collection instruments.

- Chapter 6 now includes a new section on short-term, intermediate, and long-term objectives, and a new SMART objective checklist.

- Chapter 7 includes additional information on the expansion of the socio-ecological approach, additional information on the constructs of the social cognitive theory, the inclusion of the diffusion of innovations theory which was previously found in Chapter 11, and a new section on the limitations of theory.

- Chapter 8 features new information on motivational interviewing, new content on the built environment, new content on behavioral economics, information on the Affordable Care Act and its impact on incentives, and new content on the limitations of interventions.

- Chapter 9 includes new information on the renaming of community organizing strategies and updated figures on community organizing and community building typology and on mapping community capacity.

- Chapter 10 now includes expanded information on using volunteers as a program resource, and program funding by governmental agencies.

- Chapter 11 has been reworked and now has several new boxes and tables that include a social marketing planning sheet, factors to consider when selecting pre-testing methods, a 4Ps marketing mix example, types of questions to ask for formative research, and examples of segmentation.

- Chapter 12 content includes expanded information on logic models, new content on professional development including a template for a professional development plan, new content on monitoring implementation, and new content on the implementation of an evidence-based intervention.

- Chapter 13 now includes updated information on CDC's Framework for Program Evaluation and new information on CDC's characteristics of a good evaluator. In addition, new information has been added to support the importance of evaluation and the use of evaluation standards.

- Chapter 14 includes updated terminology and context for internal and external validity, and updated context for experimental, quasi-experimental, and non-experimental evaluation designs.

- Chapter 15 includes updated information for data management, data cleaning, and the transition to data analysis. In addition, new information is presented to show the relationship between levels of measurement and the selection of statistical tests including parametric and non-parametric tests.

- All chapters include more practical planning examples and, where appropriate, new application boxes have been added to chapters.

- A new appendix has been added that contains all of the Responsibilities, Competencies, and Sub-competencies that resulted from the Health Education Specialist Practice Analysis 2015.

- To assist students, the Companion Website (https://media.pearsoncmg.com/bc/bc_mckenzie_health_7) has been updated and includes chapter objectives, practice quizzes, Responsibilities and Competencies boxes, Weblinks, a new example program plan, the Glossary, and flashcards.

- To assist instructors, all of the teaching resources have been updated by Michelle LaClair, Pennsylvania State College of Medicine. These resources are available for download on the Pearson Instructor Resource Center. Go to http://www.pearsonhighered.com and search for the title to access and download the PowerPoint® presentations, electronic *Instructor Manual* and Test Bank, and TestGen Computerized Test Bank.

Students will find this book easy to understand and use. We are confident that if the chapters are carefully read and an honest effort is put into completing the activities and visiting the Weblinks, students will gain the essential knowledge and skills for program planning, implementation, and evaluation.

ACKNOWLEDGMENTS

A project of this nature could not have been completed without the assistance and understanding of many individuals. First, we thank all our past and present students, who have had to put up with our working drafts of the manuscript.

Second, we are grateful to those professionals who took the time and effort to review and comment on various editions of this book. For the first edition, they included Vicki Keanz, Eastern Kentucky University; Susan Cross Lipnickey, Miami University; Fred Pearson, Ricks College; Kerry Redican, Virginia Tech; John Sciacca, Northern Arizona University; and William K. Spath, Montana Tech. For the second edition, reviewers included Gordon James, Weber State; John Sciacca, Northern Arizona University; and Mark Wilson, University of Georgia. For the third edition, reviewers included Joanna Hayden, William Paterson University; Raffy Luquis, Southern Connecticut State University; Teresa Shattuck, University of Maryland; Thomas Syre, James Madison University; and Esther Weekes, Texas Women's University. For the fourth edition, reviewers included Robert G. LaChausse, California State University, San Bernardino; Julie Shepard, Director of Health Promotion, Adams County Health Department; Sherm Sowby, California State University, Fresno; and William Kane, University of New Mexico. For the fifth edition, the reviewers included Sally Black, St. Joseph's University; Denise Colaianni, Western Connecticut State University; Sue Forster-Cox, New Mexico State University; Julie Gast, Utah State University; Ray Manes, York College CUNY; and Lois Ritter, California State University East Bay. For the sixth edition, reviewers included Jacquie Rainey, University of Central Arkansas; Bridget Melton, Georgia Southern University; Marylen Rimando, University of Iowa; Beth Orsega-Smith, University of Delaware; Aimee Richardson, American University; Heather Diaz, California State University, Sacramento; Steve McKenzie, Purdue University; Aly Williams, Indiana Wesleyan University; Jennifer Banas, Northeastern Illinois University; and Heidi Fowler, Georgia College and State University. For this edition, reviewers included Kimberly A. Parker, Texas Woman's University; Steven A. Branstetter, Pennsylvania State University; Jennifer Marshall, University of South Florida; Jordana Harshman, George Mason University; Tara Tietjen-Smith, Texas A & M University, Commerce; Amy L. Versnik Nowak, University of Minnesota, Duluth; Amanda Tanner, University of North Carolina, Greensboro; Deric R. Kenne, Kent State University; and Deborah J. Gibson, University of Tennessee, Martin.

Third, we thank our friends for providing valuable feedback on various editions of this book: Robert J. Yonker, Ph.D., Professor Emeritus in the Department of Educational Foundations and Inquiry, Bowling Green State University; Lawrence W. Green, Dr. P. H., Professor, Department of Epidemiology and Biostatistics, School of Medicine, University of California, San Francisco (UCSF); Bruce G. Simons-Morton, Ed.D., M.P.H., Senior Investigator, *Eunice Kennedy Shriver* National Institute of Child Health and Human Development, National Institutes of Health; and Jerome E. Kotecki, H.S.D., Professor, Department of Physiology and Health Science, Ball State University. We would also like to thank Jan L. Smeltzer, Ph.D., coauthor, for her contributions to the first four editions of the book.

Fourth, we appreciate the work of the Pearson employees Michelle Cadden, Senior Acquisitions Editor for Health, Kinesiology, and Nutrition who has been very supportive of our work, and Susan Malloy, Program Manager, whose hard work and encouragement ensured we created a quality product. We also appreciate the careful work of Allison Campbell and Charles Fisher from Integra–Chicago.

Finally, we express our deepest appreciation to our families for their support, encouragement, and understanding of the time that writing takes away from our family activities.

J. F. M.

B. L. N.

R. T.

Chapter 1

Health Education, Health Promotion, Health Education Specialists, and Program Planning

<table>
<tr><td colspan="2">

Chapter Objectives

After reading this chapter and answering the questions at the end, you should be able to:

- Explain the relationship among good health behavior, health education, and health promotion.
- Explain the difference between health education and health promotion.
- Write your own definition of health education.
- Explain the role of the health educator as defined by the Role Delineation Project.
- Explain how a person becomes a Certified Health Education Specialist or a Master Certified Health Education Specialist.
- Explain what the Competencies Update Project (CUP), Health Educators Job Analysis (HEJA-2010), and Health Education Specialists Practice Analysis (HESPA-2015) have in common.
- Explain how the Competency-Based Framework for Health Education Specialist is used by colleges and universities, the National Commission for Health Education Credentialing, Inc. (NCHEC), Council for the Accreditation of Educator Preparation (CAEP), and the Council on Education for Public Health (CEPH)
- Identify the assumptions upon which health education is based.
- Define the term *pre-planning*.

</td><td colspan="2">

Key Terms

Advanced level 1-health education specialist
Advanced level-2 health education specialist
community
decision makers
entry-level health education specialist
Framework
health behavior
health education

health education specialist
health promotion
Healthy People
pre-planning
primary prevention
priority population
Role Delineation Project
secondary prevention
stakeholders
tertiary prevention

</td></tr>
</table>

History has shown that much progress was made in the health and life expectancy of Americans since 1900. During these 116+ years, we have seen a sharp drop in infant mortality (NCHS, 2015); the eradication of smallpox; the elimination of poliomyelitis in the Americas; the control of measles, rubella, tetanus, diphtheria, Haemophilus influenzae type b, and other infectious diseases; better family planning (CDC, 2001); and an increase of 31.5 years in the average life span of a person in the United States (CDC, 2015e). Over this same time, we have witnessed disease prevention change "from focusing on reducing environmental exposures over which the individual had little control, such as providing potable water, to emphasizing behaviors such as avoiding use of tobacco, fatty foods, and a sedentary lifestyle" (Breslow, 1999, p. 1030). Yet, even with this change in focus we, as a society, have done little to encourage health community design, and as individuals, most Americans have not changed their lifestyle enough to reduce their risk of illness, disability, and premature death. As a result, unhealthy lifestyle characteristics have lead to the United States ranking 94th (out of 225 countries) in crude death rate; 42nd (out of 224 countries) in life expectancy at birth; and 1st in health care spending (CIA, 2015).

Today in the United States, much of the death and disability of Americans is associated with chronic diseases. Seven out of every 10 deaths among Americans each year are from chronic diseases, while heart disease, cancer, and stroke account for approximately 50% of deaths each year (CDC, 2015b). In addition, more than 86% of all health care spending in the United States is on people with chronic conditions (CDC, 2015b). Chronic diseases are not only the most common, deadly, and costly, they are also the most preventable of all health problems in the United States (CDC, 2105b). They are the most preventable because four modifiable risk behaviors—lack of exercise or physical activity, poor nutrition, tobacco use, and excessive alcohol use—are responsible for much of the illness, suffering, and early death related to chronic diseases (CDC, 2015b) (see **Table 1.1**). In fact, one study estimates that all causes of mortality could be cut by 55% by never smoking, engaging in regular physical activity, eating a healthy diet, and avoiding being overweight (van Dam, Li, Spiegelman, Franco, & Hu, 2008).

TABLE 1.1 **Comparison of Most Common Causes of Death and Actual Causes of Death**

Most Common Causes of Death, United States, 2013*	Actual Causes of Death, United States, 2000**
1. Heart disease	1. Tobacco
2. Cancer	2. Poor diet and physical inactivity
3. Chronic lower respiratory diseases	3. Alcohol consumption
4. Unintentional injuries	4. Microbial agents
5. Stroke	5. Toxic agents
6. Alzheimer's disease	6. Motor vehicles
7. Diabetes	7. Firearms
8. Influenza and pneumonia	8. Sexual behavior
9. Kidney disease	9. Illicit drug use
10. Suicide	

*Kochanek, Murphy, Xu, & Arias (2014).

**Mokdad, Marks, Stroup, & Greberding (2004, 2005).

But modifying risk behaviors does not come easy to Americans. One study (Reeves & Rafferty, 2005) has shown that only 3% of U.S. adults adhere to four healthy lifestyle characteristics (not smoking, engaging in regular physical activity, maintaining a healthy weight, and eating five fruits and vegetables a day). If moderate alcohol use were included in the healthy lifestyle characteristics the percentage would be even lower (King, Mainous, Carnemolla, & Everett, 2009). Now in the second decade of the twenty-first century, behavior patterns continue to "represent the single most prominent domain of influence over health prospects in the United States" (McGinnis, Williams-Russo, & Knickman, 2002, p. 82).

Though the focus on good health, wellness, and **health behavior** (those behaviors that impact a person's health) seem commonplace in our lives today, it was not until the last fourth of the twentieth century that health promotion was recognized for its potential to help control injury and disease and to promote health.

> Most scholars, policymakers, and practitioners in health promotion would pick 1974 as the turning point that marks the beginning of health promotion as a significant component of national health policy in the twentieth century. That year Canada published its landmark policy statement, *A New Perspective on the Health of Canadians* (Lalonde, 1974). In the United States, Congress passed PL 94-317, the Health Information and Health Promotion Act, which created the Office of Health Information and Health Promotion, later renamed the Office of Disease Prevention and Health Promotion (Green 1999, p. 69).

This paved the way for the U.S. government's *Healthy People: The Surgeon General's Report on Health Promotion and Disease Prevention* (USDHEW, 1979), which brought together much of what was known about the relationship of personal behavior and health status. The document also presented a "personal responsibility" model that provided Americans with a prescription for reducing their health risks and increasing their chances for good health.

It may not have been the content of ***Healthy People*** that made the publication so significant, because several publications written before it provided a similar message. Rather, *Healthy People* was important because it summarized the research available up to that point, presented it in a very readable format, and made the information available to the general public. *Healthy People* was followed by the release of the first set of health goals and objectives for the nation, titled *Promoting Health/Preventing Disease: Objectives for the Nation* (USDHHS, 1980).

These goals and objectives, now in their fourth generation (USDHHS, 2015c), have defined the nation's health agenda and guided its health policy since their inception. And, in part, they have kept the importance of good health visible to all Americans.

This focus on good health has given many people in the United States a desire to do something about their health. This desire, in turn, has increased the need for good health information that can be easily understood by the average person. One need only look at the Internet, current best-seller list, read the daily newspaper, observe the health advertisements delivered via electronic mass media, or consider the increase in the number of health-promoting facilities (not illness or sickness facilities) to verify the interest that American consumers have in health. Because of the increased interest in health and changing health behavior, health professionals are now faced with providing the public with information. However, obtaining good information does not mean that those who receive it will make healthy decisions and then act on those decisions. Good health education and health promotion programs are needed to assist people in reducing their health risks in order to obtain and maintain good health.

▷ Health Education and Health Promotion

There is more to health education than simply disseminating health information (Auld et al., 2011). Health education is a much more involved process. Two formal definitions of health education have been frequently cited in the literature. The first comes from the *Report of the 2011 Joint Committee on Health Education and Promotion Terminology* (Joint Committee on Health Education and Promotion Terminology [known hereafter as the Joint Committee on Terminology], 2012). The committee defined **health education** as "[a]ny combination of planned learning experiences using evidence-based practices and/or sound theories that provide the opportunity to acquire knowledge, attitudes, and skills needed to adopt and maintain healthy behaviors" (Joint Committee on Terminology, 2012, p. S17). The second definition was presented by Green and Kreuter (2005), who defined health education as "any planned combination of learning experiences designed to predispose, enable, and reinforce voluntary behavior conducive to health in individuals, groups, or communities" (p. G-4).

Another term that is closely related to health education, and sometimes incorrectly used in its place, is health promotion. *Health promotion* is a broader term than *health education*. In the *Report of the 2011 Joint Committee on Health Education and Promotion Terminology* (Joint Committee on Terminology, 2012, p. S19) **health promotion** is defined as "[a]ny planned combination of educational, political, environmental, regulatory, or organizational mechanisms that support actions and conditions of living conducive to the health of individuals, groups, and communities." Green and Kreuter (2005) offered a slightly different definition of *health promotion*, calling it "any planned combination of educational, political, regulatory and organizational supports for actions and conditions of living conducive to the health of individuals, groups, and communities" (p. G-4).

To help us further understand and operationalize the term *health promotion*, Breslow (1999) has stated, "Each person has a certain degree of health that may be expressed as a place in a spectrum. From that perspective, promoting health must focus on enhancing people's capacities for living. That means moving them toward the health end of the spectrum, just as prevention is aimed at avoiding disease that can move people toward the opposite end of the spectrum" (p. 1031). According to these definitions of health promotion, health education is an important component of health promotion and firmly implanted in it (see **Figure 1.1**). "Health promotion takes into account that human behavior is not only governed by personal factors (e.g., knowledge, expectancies, competencies, and well-being), but also by structural aspects of the environment" (Vogele, 2005, p. 272). However, "without health education, health promotion would be a manipulative social engineering enterprise" (Green & Kreuter, 1999, p. 19).

The effectiveness of health promotion programs can vary greatly. However, the success of a program can usually be linked to the planning that takes place before implementation of the program. Programs that have undergone a thorough planning process are usually the most successful. As the old saying goes, "If you fail to plan, your plan will fail."

▷ Health Education Specialists

The individuals best qualified to plan health promotion programs are health education specialists. A **health education specialist** has been defined as "[a]n individual who has met, at a minimum, baccalaureate-level required health education academic preparation qualifications,

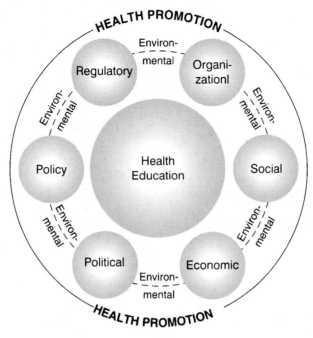

▲ **Figure 1.1** Relationship of Health Education and Health Promotion

who serves in a variety of settings, and is able to use appropriate educational strategies and methods to facilitate the development of policies, procedures, interventions, and systems conducive to the health of individuals, groups, and communities" (Joint Committee on Terminology, 2012, p. S18). Today, health education specialists can be found working in a variety of settings, including schools (K–12, colleges, and universities), community health agencies (governmental and nongovernmental), worksites (business, industry, and other work settings), and health care settings (e.g., clinics, hospitals, and managed care organizations). (Note: Prior to the term *health education specialists* being used by the health education profession, health education specialists were referred to as *health educators*. Throughout the remainder of this book the term *health education specialist* will be used except when the term *health educator* is part of a title or when the term carries historical relevance.)

The role of the health education specialist in the United States as we know it today is one that has evolved over time based on the need to provide people with educational interventions to enhance their health. The earliest signs of the role of the health education specialist appeared in the mid-1800s with school hygiene education, which was closely associated with physical activity. By the early 1900s, the need for health education spread to the public health arena, but it was the writers, journalists, social workers, and visiting nurses who were doing the educating—not health education specialists as we know them today (Deeds, 1992). As we gained more knowledge about the relationship between health, disease, and health behavior, it was obvious that the writers, journalists, social workers, visiting nurses, and primary caregivers—mainly physicians, dentists, other independent practitioners, and nurses—were unable to provide the needed health

TABLE 1.2 **Levels of Prevention**

Level of Prevention	Health Status	Example Interventions
Primary prevention – measures that forestall the onset of a disease, illness, or injury	Healthy, without signs and symptoms of disease, illness or injury	Activities directed at improving well-being while preventing specific health problems, e.g., legislation to mandate safe practices, exercise programs, immunizations, fluoride treatments
Secondary prevention – measures that lead to early diagnosis and prompt treatment of a disease, illness, or injury to minimize progression of health problem	Presence of disease, illness, or injury	Activities directed at early diagnosis, referral, and prompt treatment, e.g., mammograms, self-testicular exam, laboratory tests to diagnosis diabetes, hypercholesterolemia, hypothyroidism, programs to prevent reinjury
Tertiary prevention – measures aimed at rehabilitation following significant disease, illness, or injury	Disability, impairment, or dependency	Activities directed at rehabilitation to return a person to maximum usefulness, e.g., disease management programs, support groups, cardiac rehabilitation programs

education. The combination of the heavy workload of the primary caregivers, the lack of formal training in the process of educating others, and the need for education at all levels of prevention—**primary**, **secondary**, and **tertiary**—(see **Table 1.2**) created a need for health education specialists.

As the role of the health educator grew over the years, there was a movement by those in the discipline to clearly define their role so that people inside and outside the profession would have a better understanding of what the health education specialist did. In January 1979, the **Role Delineation Project** began (National Task Force on the Preparation and Practice of Health Educators, 1985). Through a comprehensive process, this project yielded a generic role for the **entry-level health educator**—that is, responsibilities for health education specialists taking their first job regardless of their work setting. Once the role of the entry-level health educator was delineated, the task became to translate the role into a structure that professional preparation programs in health education could use to design competency-based curricula. The resulting document, *A Framework for the Development of Competency-Based Curricula for Entry Level Health Educators* (NCHEC, 1985), and its revised version, *A Competency-Based Framework for the Professional Development of Certified Health Education Specialists* (NCHEC, 1996), provided such a structure. These documents, simply referred to as the **Framework** were comprised of the seven major areas of responsibility, which defined the scope of practice, and several different competencies and subcompetencies, which further delineated the responsibilities.

Even though the seven areas of responsibility defined the role of the entry-level health educator, they did not fully express the work of the health education specialist with an advanced degree. Thus, over a four-year period beginning in 1992, the profession worked to define the role of an advanced-level practitioner. By July 1997, the governing boards of the National Commission for Health Education Credentialing, Inc. (NCHEC), the American Association of Health Education (AAHE), and the Society for Public Health Education (SOPHE) had endorsed three additional responsibilities for the advanced-level health educator. Those responsibilities revolved around research, administration, and the advancement of the profession (AAHE, NCHEC, & SOPHE, 1999).

The seven entry-level and three additional advanced-level responsibilities served the profession well, but during the mid- to late-1990s it became obvious that there was a need to revisit the responsibilities and competencies and to make sure that they still defined the role of the health educator. Thus in 1998, the profession launched a six-year multi-phase research study known as the *National Health Educator Competencies Update Project* (CUP) to reverify the entry-level health educator responsibilities, competencies, and subcompetencies and to verify the advanced-level competencies and subcompetencies (Airhihenbuwa et al., 2005).

What became obvious from the analysis of the CUP data was that the seven responsibilities and many of the competencies and subcompetencies identified in the earlier Role Delineation Project were still valid. However, the wording of the responsibilities was changed slightly, some competencies and subcompetencies were dropped, and a few new ones were added. Also, certain subcompetencies were reported as more important and performed more regularly by health education specialists who had both more work experience and academic degrees beyond the baccalaureate level. Thus, the CUP model that emerged included responsibilities, competencies, and subcompetencies and the development of a three-tiered (i.e., Entry, **Advanced Level-1**, and **Advanced Level-2**) hierarchical model reflecting the role of the health educator. The results of the CUP, which were published approximately 20 years after the initial role delineation project, lead to the creation of a revised framework titled *A Competency-Based Framework for Health Educators* (NCHEC, SOPHE, & AAHE, 2006).

To keep the role of the health education specialist contemporary and to meet best practice guidelines of the National Commission for Certifying Agencies (NCCA), a third national research study known as the *Health Educator Job Analysis* (HEJA-2010) was conducted. The results of this study generated a new *Framework* titled *A Competency-Based Framework for Health Education Specialist-2010* (NCHEC, SOPHE, AAHE, 2010). The NCCA, the agency that accredits the Certified Health Education Specialist (CHES) and the Master Certified Health Education Specialist (MCHES) exam programs, has a standard that requires periodic updates of a job/practice analysis to keep the practice of the profession contemporary.

The most recent edition of the *Framework* titled *A Competency-Based Framework for Health Education Specialist-2015* (NCHEC & SOPHE, 2015) is the result of the *Health Education Specialist Practice Analysis* (HESPA-2015). Over the years, the number of Areas of Responsibility outlined in the *Framework* have remained fairly consistent (see **Box 1.1**). What has changed over the years is the wording of the Areas of Responsibilities and the number and wording

---

BOX

1.1

Areas of Responsibility for Health Education Specialists

AREA OF RESPONSIBILITY I:	Assess Needs, Resources, and Capacity for Health Education/Promotion
AREA OF RESPONSIBILITY II:	Plan Health Education/Promotion
AREA OF RESPONSIBILITY III:	Implement Health Education/Promotion
AREA OF RESPONSIBILITY IV:	Conduct Evaluation and Research Related to Health Education/Promotion
AREA OF RESPONSIBILITY V:	Administer and Manage Health Education/Promotion
AREA OF RESPONSIBILITY VI:	Serve as a Health Education/Promotion Resource Person
AREA OF RESPONSIBILITY VII:	Communicate, Promote, and Advocate for Health, Health Education/Promotion, and the Profession

Source: *A Competency-Based Framework for Health Education Specialists—2015*. Whitehall, PA: National Commission for Health Education Credentialing, Inc. (NCHEC) and the Society for Public Health Education (SOPHE). Reprinted by permission of the National Commission for Health Education Credentialing, Inc. (NCHEC) and the Society for Public Health Education (SOPHE).

---

of the competencies and subcompetencies found under the Areas of Responsibility. In the 2015 *Framework*, there are 36 competencies and 258 subcompetencies (141 Entry-level, 76 Advanced 1-level, and 41 Advanced 2-level) (NCHEC & SOPHE, 2015).

In reviewing the current seven areas of responsibility, it is obvious that four of the seven are directly related to program planning, implementation, and evaluation and that the other three could be associated with these processes, depending on the type of program being planned. In effect, these responsibilities distinguish health education specialists from other professionals who try to provide health education experiences.

The importance of the defined role of the health education specialist is becoming greater as the profession of health promotion continues to mature. This is exhibited by its use in several major professional activities. First, the *Framework* has provided a guide for all colleges and universities to use when designing and revising their curricula in health education to prepare future health education specialists. Second, the *Framework* was used by the National Commission for Health Education Credentialing, Inc. (NCHEC) to develop the core criteria for certifying individuals as health education specialists (Certified Health Education Specialists, or CHES). The first group of individuals (N=1,558) to receive the CHES credential did so between October 1988 and December 1989, during the charter certification period. "Charter certification allows qualified individuals to be certified based on their academic training, work experience, and references without taking the exam" (Cottrell, Girvan, McKenzie & Seabert, 2015, p. 171). In 1990, using a criterion-referenced examination based on the *Framework,* the nationwide testing program to certify health education specialists was begun by NCHEC, Inc.

In 2011, again using a criterion-referenced examination based on the *Framework*, NCHEC began offering an examination to certify advanced-level health education specialists. Those who passed the examination were awarded the Master Certified Health Education Specialist (MCHES) credential. Prior to the first MCHES examination, this new certification was made available to those who had held active CHES status since 2005 and who could demonstrate that they were practicing health education at an advanced-level. This process was known as the Experience Documentation Opportunity (EDO). All those who successfully completed the EDO were granted the MCHES credential in April 2011. Currently, both the CHES and MCHES examinations are given twice a year—once in April and once in October—at approximately 130 college-campus locations around the United States. Both examinations are composed of 165 questions (150 are scored and 15 are pilot questions) and are offered in a paper-and-pencil format (NCHEC, 2015). Information about eligibility for the examinations and the percentage of questions from each Area of Responsibility are available on the NCHEC Website (see the link for the Website in the Weblinks section at the end of the chapter).

Third, the *Framework* is used by program accrediting bodies to review college and university academic programs in health education. Both the Council for the Accreditation of Educator Preparation (CAEP), which accredits teacher education programs, and the Council on Education for Public Health (CEPH), which accredits public health programs, use components of the *Framework* when accrediting programs that have a focus on health education. The accrediting processes used by both CAEP and CEPH are based on programs conducting a self-study by comparing components of their program to accrediting body criteria or standards. After the self-study is completed, peer external reviewers visit the campus of the college or university seeking accreditation to verify the contents of the self-study. The governing boards of CAEP and CEPH review the findings of the self-study and external reviewers report and vote on awarding accreditation.

The use of the *Framework* by the profession to guide academic curricula, provide the core criteria for the health education specialist examinations, and form the basis of program accreditation processes has done much to advance the health education profession. "In 1998 the U.S. Department of Commerce and Labor formally acknowledged 'health educator' as a distinct occupation. Such recognition was justified, based to a large extent, on the ability of the profession to specify its unique skills" (AAHE, NCHEC, & SOPHE, 1999, p. 9). In 2010, in its most recent update, the U.S. Department of Labor Bureau of Labor Statistics (BLS) described the work of health educators (Standard Occupation Classification [SOC] 21-1091) using the following language:

> Provide and manage health education programs that help individuals, families, and their communities maximize and maintain healthy lifestyles. Collect and analyze data to identify community needs prior to planning, implementing, monitoring, and evaluating programs designed to encourage healthy lifestyles, policies, and environments. May serve as resource to assist individuals, other health professionals, or the community, and may administer fiscal resources for health education programs (USDOL, BLS, 2015, para. 1).

▷ Assumptions of Health Promotion

So far, we have discussed the need for health, what health education and health promotion are, and the role health education specialists play in delivering successful health promotion programs. We have not yet discussed the assumptions that underlie health promotion—all the things that must be in place before the whole process of health promotion begins. In the mid-1980s, Bates and Winder (1984) outlined what they saw as four critical assumptions of health education. Their list has been modified by adding several items, rewording others, and referring to them as "assumptions of health promotion." This expanded list of assumptions is critical to understanding what we can expect from health promotion programs.

Health promotion is by no means the sole answer to the nation's health problems or, for that matter, the sole means of getting a smoker to stop smoking or a nonexerciser to exercise. Health promotion is an important part of the health system, but it does have limitations. Here are the assumptions:

1. Health status can be changed.

2. "Health and disease are determined by dynamic interactions among biological, psychological, behavioral, and social factors" (Pellmar, Brandt, & Baird, 2002, p. 217).

3. "Behavior can be changed and those changes can influence health" (IOM, 2001, p. 333).

4. "Individual behavior, family interactions, community and workplace relationships and resources, and public policy all contribute to health and influence behavior change" (Pellmar et al., 2002, p. 217).

5. "Interventions can successfully teach health-promoting behaviors or attenuate risky behaviors" (IOM, 2001, p. 333).

6. Before health behavior is changed, the determinants of behavior, the nature of the behavior, and the motivation for the behavior must be understood (DiClemente, Salazar, & Crosby, 2013).

7. "Initiating and maintaining a behavior change is difficult" (Pellmar et al., 2002, p. 217).

8. Individual responsibility should not be viewed as victim blaming, yet the importance of health behavior to health status must be understood.

9. For health behavior change to be permanent, an individual must be motivated and ready to change.

The importance of these assumptions is made clearer if we refer to the definitions of health education and health promotion presented earlier in the chapter. Implicit in those definitions is the goal of having program participants voluntarily adopt actions conducive to health. To achieve such a goal, the assumptions must indeed be in place. We cannot expect people to adopt lifelong health-enhancing behavior if we force them into such change. Nor can we expect people to change their behavior just because they have been exposed to a health promotion program. Health behavior change is very complex, and health education specialists should not expect to change every person with whom they come in contact. However, the greatest chance for success will come to those who have the knowledge and skills to plan, implement, and evaluate appropriate programs.

▷ Program Planning

Because many of health education specialists' responsibilities are involved in some way with program planning, implementation, and evaluation, health education specialists need to become well versed in these processes. "Planning an effective program is more difficult than implementing it. Planning, implementing, and evaluating programs are all interrelated, but good planning skills are prerequisite to programs worthy of evaluation" (Minelli & Breckon, 2009, p. 137). All three processes are very involved, and much time, effort, practice, and on-the-job training are required to do them well. Even the most experienced health education specialists find program planning challenging because of the constant changes in settings, resources, and priority populations.

Hunnicutt (2007) offered four reasons why systematic planning is important. The first is that planning forces planners to think through details in advance. Detailed plans can help to avoid future problems. Second, planning helps to make a program transparent. Good planning keeps the program **stakeholders** (any person, community, or organization with a vested interest in a program; e.g., decision makers, partners, clients) informed. The planning process should not be mysterious or secretive. Third, planning is empowering. Once **decision makers** (those who have the authority to approve a plan; e.g., administrator of an organization, governing board, chief executive officer) give approval to the resulting comprehensive program plan, planners and facilitators are empowered to implement the program. Without an approved plan, planners will spend a great deal of time waiting for the "next step" to be approved and risk losing program momentum. And fourth, planning creates alignment. Once the decision makers have approved the program, all organization members have a better understanding of where it "fits" in the organization and the importance that the plan carries.

A general understanding of all that is involved in creating a health promotion program can be obtained by reviewing the Generalized Model (see **Figure 1.2**). (A more in-depth explanation of this model can be found in Chapter 3.) This model includes the five major steps involved in planning a program. However, prior to undertaking the first step in the Generalized Model, it is important to do some pre-planning. **Pre-planning** allows a core group of people (or steering committee) to gather answers to key questions (see **Box 1.2**) that are critical to the planning process before the actual planning process begins. It also helps to clarify and give direction to planning, and helps stakeholders avoid confusion as the planning progresses.

Also prior to starting the actual planning process, planners need to have a very good understanding of the "community" where the program will be implemented. When we say community, do not think of just a geographic area with specific boundaries like a neighborhood, city, county, or state. **Community** should be defined as "a collective body of individuals identified by common characteristics such as geography, interests, experiences, concerns, or values" (Joint Committee on Terminology, 2012, p. S15). For example, a community could be a religious community, a cancer-survivor community, a workplace community, or even a cyber community. Understanding the community means finding out as much as possible about the **priority population** (those for whom the program is intended to serve) and the environment in which it exists. Each setting and group is unique with its own nuances, resources, and culture. These are important to know at the beginning of the process. Planners should never assume they "know" a community. The more background information that planners secure, the better the resulting program can be. However, it is not enough to understand the community, planners also need to engage members of the priority population. Engaging the priority population means involving

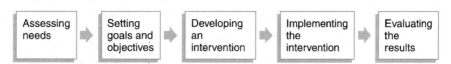

▲ **Figure 1.2** Generalized Model

BOX

1.2

Example Key Questions to Be Answered in the Pre-Planning Process

Purpose of program

- How is the community defined?
- What are the desired health outcomes?
- Does the community have the capacity and infrastructure to address the problem?
- Is a policy change needed?

Scope of the planning process

- Is it intra- or inter-organizational?
- What is the time frame for completing the project?

Planning process outcomes (deliverables)

- Written plan?
- Program proposal?
- Program documentation or justification?

Leadership and structure

- What authority, if any, will the planners have?
- How will the planners be organized?
- What is expected of those who participate in the planning process?

Identifying and engaging partners

- How will the partners be selected?
- Will the planning process use a top-down or bottom-up approach?

Identifying and securing resources

- How will the budget be determined?
- Will a written agreement (i.e., MOA—memorandum of agreement) outlining responsibilities be needed?
- If MOA is needed, what will it include?
- Will external funding (i.e., grants or contracts) be needed?
- Are there community resources (e.g., volunteers, space, donations) to support the planned program?
- How will the resources be obtained?

---

those in the priority population or a representative group from the priority population in the planning process.

Finally, before the actual planning begins thought must be given to "when the best time is to plan such a program, what data are needed, where the planning should occur, what resistance can be expected, and generally, what will enhance the success of the project" (Minelli & Breckon, 2009, p. 138).

The remaining chapters of this book present a process that health education specialists can use to plan, implement, and evaluate successful health promotion programs and will introduce you to the necessary knowledge and skills to carry out these tasks.

Summary

The increased interest in personal health and behavior change, and the flood of new health information have expanded the need for quality health promotion programs. Individuals are seeking guidance to enable them to make sound decisions about behavior that is conducive to their health. Those best prepared to help these people are health education specialists who complete a curriculum based upon the role defined by the profession. Properly trained health education specialists are aware of the limitations of the discipline and understand the assumptions on which health promotion is based. They also know that good planning does not happen by accident. Much time, effort, practice, and on-the-job training are needed to plan an effective program. The planning process begins with pre-planning.

Review Questions

1. Explain the role *Healthy People* played in the relationship between the American people and health.

2. How is *health education* defined by the Joint Committee on Terminology (2012)?

3. What are the key phrases in the definition of health education presented by Green and Kreuter (2005)?

4. What is the relationship between health education and health promotion?

5. Why is there a need for health education specialists?

6. What is the Role Delineation Project?

7. How is the *Competency-Based Framework for Health Education Specialists* used by colleges and universities? By NCHEC? By CAEP? By CEPH?

8. How does one become a Certified Health Education Specialist (CHES)?

9. How does one become a Master Certified Health Specialist (MCHES)?

10. What are the seven Areas of Responsibilities of health education specialists?

11. What is the National Health Educator Competencies Update Project (CUP)?

12. What is the Health Educator Job Analysis – 2010 (HEJA-2010)?

13. What is the Health Education Specialist Practice Analysis – 2015 (HESPA-2015)?

14. What assumptions are critical to health promotion?

15. What are the steps in the Generalized Model?

16. What is meant by the term *pre-planning*? Why is it important? What are some questions that should be answered during the pre-planning process?

17. How have stakeholders, decision makers, and community been defined in this chapter?

Activities

1. Based on what you have read in this chapter and your knowledge of the profession of health education, write your own definitions for *health, health education, health promotion,* and *health promotion program.*

2. Write a response indicating what you see as the importance of each of the nine assumptions presented in the chapter. Write no more than one paragraph per assumption.

3. With your knowledge of health promotion, what other assumptions would you add to the list presented in this chapter? Provide a one-paragraph rationale for each.

4. If you have not already done so, go online (http://profiles.nlm.nih.gov/ps/access /NNBBGK.pdf) or to the government documents section of the library on your campus and read *Healthy People: The Surgeon General's Report on Health Promotion and Disease Prevention* (USDHEW, 1979).

5. Say you are in your senior year and will graduate next May with a bachelor's degree in health education. What steps would you have to take in order to be able to take the CHES exam in April prior to your graduation? (Hint: Check the Website of the National Commission for Health Education Credentialing, Inc.)

6. In a one-page paper describe the differences and similarities in the two credentials— CHES and MCHES—available to health education specialists. (Hint: Check the Website of the National Commission for Health Education Credentialing, Inc.)

7. In a one-page paper describe what the job outlook is projected to be for health education specialists for the next ten years. (Hint: Check the Website of the Bureau of Labor Statistics *Occupational Outlook Handbook*.)

Weblinks

1. **http://www.healthypeople.gov**
   Healthy People
   This is the Webpage for the U.S. government's Healthy People initiative including a complete presentation of *Healthy People 2020*.

2. **http://www.nchec.org/**
   National Commission for Health Education Credentialing, Inc. (NCHEC)
   The NCHEC, Inc. Website provides the most current information about the CHES and MCHES credentials.

3. **http://www.bls.gov/ooh/community-and-social-service/health-educators.htm**
   Occupational Outlook Handbook
   This is a Webpage provided by the Bureau of Labor Statistics that describes the occupation outlook for health educators and community health workers.

PART I **PLANNING A HEALTH PROMOTION PROGRAM**

The chapters in this section of the book provide the basic information needed to plan a health promotion program. Each chapter presents readers with the information they will need to build the knowledge to develop the skills to create a successful program in a variety of settings.

Chapter

2

Starting the Planning Process

Chapter Objectives

After reading this chapter and answering the questions at the end, you should be able to:

- Develop a rationale for planning and implementing a health promotion program.

- Explain the importance of gaining the support of decision makers.

- Identify the individuals who could make up a planning committee.

- Explain what planning parameters are and the impact they have on program planning.

Key Terms

advisory board
cost-benefit analysis
(CBA)
doers
epidemiology
evidence
evidence-based
practice
*Guide to Community
Preventive Services*
influencers
institutionalized

literature
organizational
culture
planning committee
planning parameters
planning team
program ownership
return on investment
(ROI)
social math
steering committee

A noted earlier (Chapter 1), planning a health promotion program is a multistep process that begins after doing pre-planning. "To plan is to engage in a process or a procedure to develop a method of achieving an end" (Minelli & Breckon, 2009, p. 137). However, because of the many different variables and circumstances of any one setting, the multistep process of planning does not always begin the same way. There are times when the need for a program is obvious and there is recognition that a new program should be put in place. For example, if a community's immunization rate for its children is less than half the national average, a program should be created. There are other times when a program has been successful in the past but needs to be changed or reworked slightly before being implemented again. And, there are situations where planners have been given the independence and authority to create the programs that are needed in a community in order to improve the health and quality of life. However, when the need is not so obvious, or when there has not been successful health promotion programming in the past or decision makers want "proof" (i.e., evidence) that a program is needed and will be successful, the planning process often begins with the planners creating a rationale to gain the support of key people in order to obtain the necessary resources to ensure that the planning process and the eventual implementation proceed as smoothly as possible.

BOX

2.1

Responsibilities and Competencies for Health Education Specialists

The content of this chapter includes information on several tasks that occur early in the program planning process. These tasks are not associated with a single area of responsibility, but rather five areas of responsibility of the health education specialist:

RESPONSIBILITY I: Assess Needs, Resources, and Capacity for Health Education/ Promotion

Competency 1.2: Access existing information and data related to health

Competency 1.6: Examine factors that enhance or impede the process of health education/promotion

RESPONSIBILITY II: Plan Health Education/Promotion

Competency 2.1: Involve priority populations, partners, and other stakeholders in the planning process

RESPONSIBILITY V: Administer and Manage Health Education/Promotion

Competency 5.3: Manage relationships with partners and other stakeholders

Competency 5.4: Gain acceptance and support for health education/ promotion

Competency 5.5: Demonstrate leadership

RESPONSIBILITY VI: Serve as a Health Education/Promotion Resource Person

Competency 6.1: Obtain and disseminate health-related information

Competency 6.3: Provide advice and consultation on health education/ promotion issues

RESPONSIBILITY VII: Communicate, Promote, and Advocate for Health and Health Education/ Promotion, and the Profession

Competency 7.2: Engage in advocacy for health education/promotion

Competency 7.3: Influence policy and/or systems change to promote health and health education/promotion

Source: *A Competency-Based Framework for Health Education Specialists—2015*. Whitehall, PA: National Commission for Health Education Credentialing, Inc. (NCHEC) and the Society for Public Health Education (SOPHE). Reprinted by permission of the National Commission for Health Education Credentialing, Inc. (NCHEC) and the Society for Public Health Education (SOPHE).

This chapter presents the steps of creating a program rationale to obtain the support of decision makers, identifying those who may be interested in helping to plan the program, and establishing the parameters in which the planners must work. **Box 2.1** identifies the responsibilities and competencies for health education specialists that pertain to the material presented in this chapter.

▷ The Need for Creating a Rationale to Gain the Support of Decision Makers

No matter what the setting of a health promotion program—whether a business, an industry, the community, a clinic, a hospital, or a school—it is most important that the program have support from the highest level (e.g., the administration, chief executive officer, church elders, board of health, or board of directors) of the "community" for which the program is being planned (Allen & Hunnicutt, 2007; Chapman, 1997, 2006; Hunnicutt & Leffelman, 2006; Ryan, Chapman, & Rink, 2008). It is the individuals in these top-level decision-making positions who are able to provide the necessary resource support for the program.

> "Resources" usually means money, which can be turned into staff, facilities, materials, supplies, utilities, and all the myriad number of things that enable organized activity to take place over time. "Support" usually means a range of things: congruent organizational policies, program and concept visibility, expressions of priority value, personal involvement of key managers, a place at the table of organizational power, organizational credibility, and a role in integrated functioning (Chapman, 1997, p. 1).

There will be times when the idea for, or the motivating force behind, a program comes from the top-level people. When this happens, it is a real boon for the program planners because they do not have to sell the idea to these people to gain their support. However, this scenario does not occur frequently.

Often, the idea or the big push for a health promotion program comes from someone other than one who is part of the top-level of the "community." The idea could start with an employee, an interested parent, a health education specialist within the organization, a member of the parish or congregation, or a concerned individual or group from within the community. The idea might even be generated by an individual outside the "community," such as one who may have administrative or oversight responsibilities for activities in a community. An example of this arrangement is the employee of a state health department who provides consultative services to a local health department. Or it may be an individual from a regional agency who is partnering with a group within the community to carry out a collaborative project. When the scenario begins at a level below the decision makers, those who want to create a program must "sell" it to the decision makers. In other words, in order for resources and support to flow into health promotion programming, decision makers need to clearly perceive a set of values or benefits associated with the proposed program (Chapman, 2006). Without the support of decision makers, it becomes more difficult, if not impossible, to plan and implement a program. A number of years ago, Behrens (1983) stated that health promotion programs in business and industry have a greater chance for success if all levels of management, including the top, are committed and supportive. This is still true today of health promotion programs in all settings, not just programs in business and industry (see **Box 2.2**).

If they need to gain the support of decision makers, program planners should develop a rationale for the program's existence. Why is it necessary to sell something that everyone knows is worthwhile? After all, does anyone doubt the value of trying to help people gain and maintain good health? The answer to these and similar questions is that few people are motivated by health concerns alone. Decisions by top-level management to develop new programs are based on a variety of factors, including finances, policies, public image, and politics, to name a few. Thus to sell the program to those at the top, planners need to develop a rationale that shows how the new program will help decision makers to meet the organization's goals and, in turn, to carry out its mission. In other words, planners need to position their program rationale politically, in line with the organization.

BOX

2.2

Focus On

Measuring Decision Makers' Support for Health Promotion

Though the importance of decision makers' support to the success of health promotion programs has been known for a number of years, it is only recently that efforts have been put forth to actually measure decision makers' support for health promotion programs. Della, DeJoy, Goetzel, Ozminkowski, and Wilson (2008) created a valid instrument to assess leadership support for health promotion programs in work settings. The measurement tool, referred to as the Leading by Example (LBE) Instrument, is a four-factor scale. The four factors are (1) business assignment with health promotion objectives, (2) awareness of the economics of health and worker productivity, (3) worksite support for health promotion, and (4) leadership support for health promotion (Della et al., 2010). Della and colleagues feel that the LBE could be used in two ways. The first would be through a single administration "to assess specific areas in which the health promotion climate might support/hinder programmatic efforts" (p. 139). The second would be to administer the LBE two different times to monitor change in support for health promotion programs over time.

▷ Steps in Creating a Program Rationale

Planners must understand that gaining the support of decision makers is one of the most important steps in the planning process and it should not be taken lightly. Many program ideas have died at this stage because the planners were not well prepared to sell the program to decision makers. Thus, before making an appeal to decision makers, planners need to have a sound rationale for creating a program that is supported by evidence that the proposed program will benefit those for whom it is planned.

There is no formula or recipe for writing a rationale, but through experience, the authors have found a logical format for putting ideas together to help guide planners (see **Figure 2.1**). Note that Figure 2.1 is presented as an inverted triangle. This inverted triangle is symbolic in design to reflect the flow of a program rationale beginning at the top by identifying a health problem in global terms and moving toward a more focused solution at the bottom of the triangle.

Step 1: Identify Appropriate Background Information

Before planners begin to write a program rationale, they need to identify appropriate sources of information and data that can be used to sell program development. The place to begin the process of identifying appropriate sources of information and data to support the development of a program rationale is to conduct a search of the existing literature. **Literature** includes the articles, books, government publications, and other documents that explain the past and current knowledge about a particular topic. By conducting a search, planners gain a better understanding of the health problem(s) of concern, approaches to reducing or eliminating the health problem, and an understanding of the people for whom the program is intended (remember these individuals are referred to as the priority population). There are a number of different ways that planners can carry out a review of the literature (see Chapter 4 for an explanation of the literature search process).

Title the work "A rationale for the development of . . ." and indicate who is submitting the work.

Identify the health problem in global terms, backing it up with appropriate (international, national, or state) data. If possible, also include the economic costs of the problem.

Narrow the health problem by showing its relationship to the proposed priority population. Create a problem statement. State why it is a problem and why it should be dealt with. Again, back up the statement with appropriate data.

State a proposed solution to the problem (name and purpose of the proposed health promotion program). Provide a general overview of the program.

State what can be gained from such a program in terms of the values and benefits to the decision makers.

State why the program will be successful.

Provide the references used in preparing the rationale.

▲ **Figure 2.1** Creating a Rationale

In general, the types of information and data that are useful in writing a rationale include those that (1) express the needs and wants of the priority population, (2) describe the status of the health problem(s) within a given population, (3) show how the potential outcomes of the proposed program align with what the decision makers feel is important, (4) show compatibility with the health plan of a state or the nation, (5) provide evidence that the proposed program will make a difference, and (6) show how the proposed program will protect and preserve the single biggest asset of most organizations and communities—the people. Though many of these types of information and data are generated through a review of the literature, the first one discussed below—needs and wants of the priority population—is not.

Information and data that express the needs and wants of the priority population can be generated through a needs assessment. A *needs assessment* is the process of identifying, analyzing, and prioritizing the needs of a priority population. Needs assessments are carried out through a multiple-step process in which data are collected and analyzed. The analysis generates a prioritized list of needs of the priority population (see Chapter 4 for a detailed explanation of the needs assessment process). Even though information and data that express the needs and wants of the priority population can be very useful in generating a rationale for a proposed program, more than likely at this point in the planning process, a formal needs assessment will not have been completed. Often, a complete needs assessment does not take place until decision makers give permission for the planning to begin. However, the review of literature may generate information about a needs assessment of another related or similar program. If so, it can provide valuable information and data that can help to develop the rationale.

Information and data that describe the status of a health problem within a population can be obtained by analyzing epidemiological data. Epidemiologic data are those that result from the process of **epidemiology**, which has been defined as "[t]he study of the occurrence and distribution of health-related events, states and processes in specific populations, including the study of determinants influencing such processes, and the application of this knowledge to control relevant health problems" (Porta, 2014, p. 95). Epidemiological data are available from a number of different sources including governmental agencies, governmental health agencies, non-governmental health agencies, and health care systems. **Table 2.1** provides some examples of useful sources of epidemiological data.

TABLE 2.1 **Example Sources of Epidemiological Data**

Source	Example Data
International	
World Health Organization	World Health Statistics Report (http://www.who.int/gho/publications/world_health_statistics/en/)
	Country Statistics (http://www.who.int/gho/countries/en/)
National	
Centers for Disease Control and Prevention	National Health and Nutrition Examination Survey (NHANES) (http://www.cdc.gov/nchs/nhanes.htm)
National Center for Health Statistics	National Health Interview Survey (NHIS) (http://www.cdc.gov/nchs/nhis.htm)
State	
Centers for Disease Control and Prevention	Behavioral Risk Factor Surveillance System (BRFSS) (http://www.cdc.gov/brfss/about/index.htm)
	Youth Risk Behavior Surveillance System (YRBSS) http://www.cdc.gov/healthyyouth/data/yrbs/index.htm
Pennsylvania Department of Health	Health Statistics (http://www.portal.state.pa.us/portal/server.pt/community/health_statistics/14136)
Local	
Robert Wood Johnson Foundation & University of Wisconsin Population Health Institute	County Health Rankings & Roadmaps (http://www.countyhealthrankings.org/)

Epidemiologic data gain additional significance when it can be shown that the described health problem(s) is(are) the result of modifiable health behaviors and that spending money to promote healthy lifestyles and prevent health problems makes good economic sense. Here are a couple examples where modifiable health behaviors and health-related costs have been connected. The first deals with smoking. Approximately 17.8% of U.S. adults 18 years of age and older are cigarette smokers (CDC, 2015g). It has been estimated that the cost of ill effects from smoking in the United States totals approximately $300 billion per year. Almost equal amounts are spent on direct medical care ($170 billion) and productivity losses due to premature death and exposure to secondhand smoke ($156 billion) (CDC, 2015g). The second example deals with diabetes. It has been estimated that annual costs associated with diabetes are approximately $245 billion; $176 billion from direct medical costs and $69 billion indirect costs related to disability, work loss, and premature death (CDC, 2014a). We know that not all cases of diabetes are related to health behavior, but it is known for people with prediabetes, lifestyle changes, including a 5%–7% weight loss and at least 150 minutes of physical activity per week, can reduce the rate of onset of type 2 diabetes by 58% (CDC, 2012b). In addition, we know people with diagnosed diabetes have medical expenditures that are about 2.3 times higher than medical expenditures for people without diabetes (CDC, 2012b). When a rationale includes an economic component it is often reported based on a **cost-benefit analysis (CBA)**. A CBA of a health promotion program will yield the dollar benefit received from the dollars invested in the program. A common way of reporting a CBA is through a metric called **return on investment (ROI)**. ROI "measures the costs of a program (i.e., the investment) versus the financial return realized by that program" (Cavallo, 2006, p. 1) (see **Box 2.3** for formulas to calculate ROI). An example of ROI is a study that examined the economic impact of an investment of $10 per person per year in a proven community-based program to increase physical activity, improve nutrition, and prevent smoking and other tobacco use. The results of the study showed that the nation could save billions of dollars annually and have an ROI in one year of 0.96 to 1, 5.6 to 1 in 5 years, and 6.2 to 1 in 10–20 years (TFAH, 2009).

However, it should be noted that "proving" the economic impact of many health promotion programs is not easy. There are a number of reasons for this including the multiple

---

BOX

2.3

Focus On

Return on Investment

In general, ROI compares the dollars invested in something to the benefits produced by that investment:

$$ROI = \frac{(\text{benefits of investment} - \text{amount invested})}{\text{amount invested}}$$

In the case of an investment in a prevention program, ROI compares the savings produced by the intervention, net cost of the program, to how much the program cost:

$$ROI = \frac{\text{net savings}}{\text{cost of intervention}}$$

When ROI equals 0, the program pays for itself. When ROI is greater than 0, then the program is producing savings that exceed the cost of the program.

Source: Copyright © 2009 by Trust for America's Health. Reprinted with permission.

causes of many health problems, the complex interventions needed to deal with them, and the difficulty of carrying out rigorous research studies. Additionally, McGinnis and colleagues (2002) feel that part of the problem is that health promotion programs are held to a different standard than medical treatment programs when cost-effectiveness is being considered.

> In a vexing example of double standards, public investments in health promotion seem to require evidence that future savings in health and other social costs will offset the investments in prevention. Medical treatments do not need to measure up to the standard; all that is required here is evidence of safety and effectiveness. The cost-effectiveness challenge often is made tougher by a sense that the benefits need to accrue directly and in short term to the payer making investments. Neither of these two conditions applies in many interventions in health promotion (p. 84).

A helpful tool for calculating the financial burden of chronic diseases has been the Chronic Disease Cost Calculator Version 2 created by the Centers for Disease Control and Prevention and RTI International (see the link for the Website in the Weblinks section at the end of the chapter). For those planners interested in using economic impact and cost-effectiveness of health promotion programs as part of a program rationale, we recommend that the work of the following authors be reviewed: Centers for Disease Control and Prevention (CDC, 2015f), Chapman (2012), Cohen, Neumann, and Milton (2008), Goetzel and Ozminkowski (2008), Laine et al. (2014), McKenzie (1986), O'Donnell (2014), and Miller & Hendrie (2008).

Other information and data that are useful in creating a rationale are those that show how the potential outcomes of the proposed program align with what decision makers feel is important. Planners can often get a hint of what decision makers value by reviewing the organization's mission statement, annual report, and/or budget for health-related items. Planners could also survey decision makers to determine what is important to them (Chapman, 1997). **Table 2.2** provides a list of values or benefits that can be derived from health promotion programs, while **Table 2.3** provides a list of sources where information about values or benefits could be found.

TABLE 2.2 **Values or Benefits from Health Promotion Programs**

Value or Benefit for:	Types of Values or Benefits
Community	Establishing good health as norm; improved quality of life; improve the economic well-being of the community; provide model for other communities
Employee/Individual	Improved health status; reduction in health risks; improved health behavior; improved job satisfaction; lower out-of-pocket costs for health care; increased well-being, self-image, and self-esteem
Employer	Increased worker morale; enhanced worker performance/productivity; recruitment and retention tool; reduced absenteeism and presenteeism; reduced disability days/claims, reduced health care costs; enhanced corporate image

Sources: Adapted from ACS (2009); CDC (2014c); and Chapman (1997).

TABLE 2.3 **Selected Sources of Information About Values or Benefits of Health Promotion Programs**

Source	Location of Information
American Heart Association	http://www.heart.org/HEARTORG/GettingHealthy/WorkplaceWellness/Workplace-Wellness_UCM_460416_SubHomePage.jsp
Centers for Disease Control and Prevention	
National Center for Health Statistics	http://www.cdc.gov/nchs/
Worklife	http://www.cdc.gov/niosh/twh/default.html
Workplace Health Promotion	http://www.cdc.gov/workplacehealthpromotion/
The Community Tool Box	http://ctb.ku.edu/en
National Committee for Quality Assurance	http://www.ncqa.org
National Business Group on Health	https://www.businessgrouphealth.org/preventive/businesscase/index.cfm
Prevention Institute	http://www.preventioninstitute.org/
Robert Wood Johnson Foundation	http://www.rwjf.org/en.html
Trust for America's Health (TFAH)	http://healthyamericans.org/reports/
U.S. Department of Health & Human Services	
Office of Assistant Secretary for Planning & Evaluation	http://aspe.hhs.gov
Wellness Council of America (WELCOA)	http://www.welcoa.org/resources/

A fourth source of information for a rationale is a comparison between the proposed program and the health plan for the nation or a state. Comparing the health needs of the priority population with those of other citizens of the state or of all Americans, as outlined in the goals and objectives of the nation (USDHHS, 2015c), should enable planners to show the compatibility between the goals of the proposed program and those of the nation's health plan (see Chapter 6 for a discussion of the *Healthy People 2020* goals and objectives).

A fifth source of information and data is *evidence* that the proposed program will be effective and make a difference if implemented. By **evidence** we mean the body of data that can be used to make decisions when planning a program. Such data can come from needs assessments, knowledge about the causes of a health problem, research that has tested the effectiveness of an intervention, and evaluations conducted on other health promotion programs. When program planners systematically find, appraise, and use evidence as the basis for decision making when planning a health promotion program, it is referred to as **evidence-based practice** (Cottrell & McKenzie, 2011).

Various forms of evidence can be placed on a continuum anchored at one end by *objective evidence* (or science-based evidence) and *subjective evidence* at the other of the continuum (Chambers & Kerner, 2007). Others (Howlett, Rogo, & Shelton, 2014) have organized the various forms of evidence as a hierarchy within an *evidence pyramid* with the objective evidence at the top of the pyramid and the more subjective evidence at the base of the pyramid. Irrespective of format for aligning and presenting the various forms of evidence, "[m]ore objective types of evidence include systematic reviews, whereas more subjective data involve personal experience and observations as well as anecdotes" (Brownson, Diez

Roux, & Swartz, 2014, p. 1). Because it is derived from a scientific process, objective evidence is seen as a higher quality of evidence. Planners should strive to use the *best evidence possible* but also understand that "evidence is usually imperfect" (Brownson, Baker, Leet, Gillespie, & True, 2011, p. 6) and, as planners, they will often be faced with having to use the *best evidence available* (Muir Gray, 1997). Over the years, the number of organizations/agencies that have worked to identify evidence of various types of health-related programs (i.e., health care, disease prevention, health promotion) has increased (see **Box 2.4** for examples). A most useful source for those planning health promotion programs is the ***Guide to Community Preventive Services***, referred to simply as *The Community Guide* (CDC, 2015c). *The Community Guide* summarizes the findings from systematic reviews of public health interventions covering a variety of topics. The systematic reviews are used to answer several questions (CDC, 2015c, para. 1):

* "Which program and policy interventions have been proven effective?
* Are there effective interventions that are right for my community?
* What might effective interventions cost; what is the likely return on investment?"

The *Community Guide* was developed and is continually updated by the nonfederal Task Force on Community Preventive Services. The Task Force, which is comprised of public health experts who are appointed by the director of the CDC, is charged with reviewing and assessing the quality of available evidence and developing appropriate recommendations.

Finally, when preparing a rationale to gain the support of decision makers, planners should not overlook the most important resource of any community—the people who make up the community. Promoting, maintaining, and in some cases restoring human health should be at the core of any health promotion program. Whatever the setting, better health of those in the priority population provides for a better quality of life. For those planners who end up practicing in a worksite setting, the importance of protecting the health of employees (i.e., protecting human resources) should be noted in developing a rationale. "Labor costs typically represent 60% to 70% of total annual operating costs for most organizations" (Chapman, 2006, p. 10); thus people are a company's single biggest asset. "Fit and healthy people are more productive, are better able to meet extraordinary demands and deal with stress, are absent less, reflect better on the company or community as exemplars, and so forth" (Chapman, 2006, p. 29).

Step 2: Title the Rationale

Once planners have identified and are familiar with the sources of information and data that can be used to sell program development, they are ready to begin the process of putting a rationale together. Thus, the next step is giving a title to the rationale. This can be quite simple in nature, such as "A Rationale for (Title of Program): A Program to Enhance the Health of (Name of Priority Population)." Immediately following the title should be a listing of who contributed to the authorship of the rationale.

Step 3: Writing the Content of the Rationale

The first paragraph or two of the rationale should identify the health problem from a "global perspective." By global perspective we mean presenting the problem using information and data at the most macro level (whether it be international, national, regional, state,

Examples of Sources of Evidence

The Campbell Collaboration

Type of evidence: Produces systematic reviews on the effects of social interventions in crime and justice, education, international development, and social welfare.

Website: http://www.campbellcollaboration.org/

Centre for Reviews and Dissemination; The University of York

Type of evidence: Synthesized research evidence on various topics including health technology assessment, public health, and child health.

Website: http://www.york.ac.uk/crd/

Cochrane

Type of evidence: Synthesized research evidence on health and health care. Can be searched using various terms including health education and health promotion.

Website: http://www.cochrane.org/

Canadian Task Force on Preventive Health Care

Type of evidence: Practice guidelines that support primary care providers in delivering preventive health care. Also, has information for general public.

Website: http://www.canadiantaskforce.ca

Health Evidence, McMaster University, Canada

Type of evidence: Effectiveness of public health interventions in Canada.

Website: http://healthevidence.org

National Cancer Institute

Document: *Research-tested Intervention Programs*

Type of evidence: A searchable database of cancer control interventions and program materials that are designed to provide program planners and public health practitioners easy and immediate access to research-tested materials.

Website: http://rtips.cancer.gov/rtips/index.do

Substance Abuse and Mental Health Services

Document: *National Registry of Evidence-based Programs and Practices*

Type of Evidence: Searchable online registry of substance abuse and mental health interventions.

Website: http://nrepp.samhsa.gov

Task Force on Community Preventive Services

Document: *Guide to Community Preventive Services*

Type of evidence: Programs and policies to improve health and prevent disease in communities.

Website: http://www.thecommunityguide.org

U.S. Preventive Services Task Force

Document: *The Guide to Clinical Preventive Services*

Type of evidence: Recommendations on the use of screening, counseling, and other preventive services that are typically delivered in primary care settings.

Website: http://www.ahrq.gov/professionals/clinicians-providers/guidelines-recommendations/uspstf/index.html

World Health Organization

Document: *Health Evidence Network (HEN)*

Type of evidence: Summarized evidence for public health, health care, and health systems policymakers.

Website: http://www.euro.who.int/en/data-and-evidence/evidence-informed-policy-making/health-evidence-network-hen or local) possible. In other words, begin the rationale by presenting the problem at the most macro level for which supporting data are available. So, if there is international information and data on the problem, say for example HIV/AIDS, begin describing the problem at that level. If data are not available to present the problem at the international level, say for example people without health insurance, move down to next level where the presentation can be supported with data. If available, also include the economic costs of such a problem; it will strengthen the rationale. "Much of the decision-making that occurs, for change to take place in an organization is based on financial considerations, and any change within an organization typically must be supported by a positive return on investment. Lacking sound financial support or a firm understanding of the financial implications, a good idea may not be realized in practice" (Gambatese, 2008, p. 153). Most health problems are also present at other levels. Presenting the problem at these higher levels shows decision makers that dealing with the health problem is consistent with the concerns of others.

Showing the relationship of the health problem to the "bigger problem" at the international, national, and/or state levels is the next logical step in presenting the rationale. Thus, the next portion of the rationale is to identify the health problem that is the focus of the rationale. This declaration of the health problem is referred to as the *problem statement* or *statement of the problem*. The problem statement should begin with a concise explanation of the issue that needs to be addressed (WKKF, 2004). The statement should also include *why* it is a problem and *why* it should be dealt with (see **Box 2.5**). If available, the statement should also include supporting data for the problem. Such data may come from a needs assessment if it has already been completed or from related literature.

BOX

2.5

Focus On

Examples of Problem Statements

For a local-level program

The number of children entering kindergarten who have not received two doses of the measles-mumps-rubella (MMR) vaccine in Mitchell County continues to increase. In the 2011–12 school year, 95% of the children who entered kindergarten had received two doses, while only 91% were immunized properly in 2015–16. Because the number of cases of MMR does not seem too high to parents/guardians, many do not feel it is necessary to subject their children to immunizations. Infectious diseases remain a major cause of illness, disability, and mortality. "Vaccines are among the most cost-effective clinical preventive services and are a core component of any preventive services package. Childhood immunization programs provide a very high return on investment" (USDHHS, 2015c, para. 6).

For a state-level program

Overweight and obesity are critical health threats facing the state of ABC. Between 2012 and 2015, the percentage of overweight adults in ABC increased from 34% to 35%, while the percentage of obese adults increased from 30% to 32%. Overweight and obesity are caused by an imbalance in the calories consumed vs. calories burned ratio. Both overweight and obesity increase the risks for heart disease, stroke, diabetes, and cancer. The annual costs (direct and indirect) of these diseases to the state have been estimated at $25 billion. There is good evidence that shows both the physical and financial costs of overweight and obesity are preventable.

In presenting the problem statement you may find it useful to use the technique of social math. **Social math** has been defined as "the practice of translating statistics and other data so they become interesting to the journalist, and meaningful to the audience" (Dorfman, Woodruff, Herbert, & Ervice, 2004, p. 112). In other words, data, especially large numbers, are presented in such a way that makes them easier to grasp by putting them in a context that gives instant meaning. "It is critical to select a social math fact that is 100 percent accurate, visual if possible, dramatic, and appropriate for the target audience" (NCIPC, 2008, 17). For example, $2.9 trillion was spent on health in 2013 in the United States (CMS, 2015b); 2.9 trillion is a large number and hard "to put our heads around." But equating that number with spending $9,255 for every person in the United States (CMS, 2015b) that year makes the number more comprehensible. Or, we could present the $2.9 trillion in social math terms by saying if every dollar equaled one second, then $2.9 trillion would equal 92,211 years! (See **Box 2.6** for other examples.)

BOX

2.6

Focus On

Examples of Social Math

● *Break the numbers down by time.*

If you know the amount over a year, what does that look like per hour? Per minute? For example, the average annual salary of a childcare worker nationally is $15,430, roughly $7.42 per hour. While many people understand that an annual salary of $15,430 is low, breaking the figure down by the hour reinforces that point—and makes the need for some kind of intervention even more clear.

● *Break down the numbers by place.*

Comparing a statistic with a well-known place can give people a sense of the statistic's magnitude. For instance, approximately 250,000 children are on waiting lists for childcare subsidies in California. That's enough children to fill almost every seat in every Major League ballpark in California. Such a comparison helps us visualize the scope of the problem and makes a solution all the more imperative.

● *Provide comparisons with familiar things.*

Providing a comparison to something that is familiar can have great impact. For example, "While Head Start is a successful, celebrated educational program, it is so underfunded that it serves only about three-fifths of eligible children. Applying that proportion to social security would mean that almost a million currently eligible seniors wouldn't receive benefits."

● *Provide ironic comparisons.*

For example, the average annual cost of full-time, licensed, center-based care for a child under age 2 in California is twice the tuition at the University of California at Berkeley. What's ironic here is how out of balance our public conversation is. Parents and the public focus so much on the cost of college when earlier education is dramatically more expensive.

● *Localize the numbers.*

Make comparisons that will resonate with community members. For example, saying, "Center-based childcare for an infant costs $11,450 per year in Seattle, Washington," is one thing. Saying, "In Seattle, Washington, a father making minimum wage would have to spend 79 percent of his income per year to place his baby in a licensed care center," is much more powerful because it illustrates why it is nearly impossible.

Source: National Center for Injury Prevention and Control (2008; revised 2010). *Adding Power to Our Voices: A Framing Guide for Communicating About Injury.* Atlanta, GA: Author. Retrieved May 14, 2015, from http://www.cdc.gov/injury/pdfs/cdcframingguide-a.pdf

At this point in the rationale, propose a solution to the problem. The solution should include the name and purpose of the proposed health promotion program, and a general overview of what the program may include. Since the writing of a program rationale often precedes much of the formal planning process, the general overview of the program is often based upon the "best guess" of those creating the rationale. For example, if the purpose of a program is to improve the immunization rate of children in the community, a "best guess" of the eventual program might include interventions to increase awareness and knowledge about immunizations, and the reduction of the barriers that limit access to receiving immunizations. Following such an overview, include statements indicating what can be gained from the program. Do your best to align the potential values and benefits of the program with what is important to the decision makers.

Next, state why this program will be successful. This is the place to use the results of *evidence-based practice* to support the rationale. It can also be helpful to point out the similarity of the priority population to others with which similar programs have been successful. And finally, using the argument that the "timing is right" for the program can also be useful. By this we mean that there is no better time than now to work to solve the problem facing the priority population.

Step 4: Listing the References Used to Create the Rationale

The final step in creating a rationale is to include a list of the references used in preparing the rationale. Having a reference list shows decision makers that you studied the available information before presenting your idea. (See **Box 2.7** for an example of a program rationale.)

BOX

2.7

Application

Example Program Rationale

A Rationale for a Comprehensive Tobacco Control Program in Philadelphia County, Pennsylvania

The World Health Organization (WHO) has noted that tobacco "is one of the biggest public health threats the world has ever faced, killing nearly six million people a year. More than five million of those deaths are the result of direct tobacco use while more than 600,000 are the result of non-smokers being exposed to second-hand smoke. Approximately one person dies every six seconds due to tobacco, accounting for one in 10 adult deaths" (WHO, 2014, para. 4). In addition, it has been estimated that up to 50% of current users will die of a tobacco-related disease (WHO, 2014). To further quantify the burden of tobacco on the people of the world is to note that six million deaths is the equivalent of losing the entire population of the state of Maryland each year.

The impact of tobacco use and secondhand smoke exposure has also been a problem in the United States. In 2013, the percentage of adult (> 18 years of age) smokers in United States was 17.8%, which is the lowest it has ever been, but it still totals 42.1 million people. Tobacco is the single most preventable cause of disease, disability, and death in the United States (CDC, 2014), and accounts for approximately 480,000 deaths per year. It has been estimated that 41,000 of those deaths are of non-smokers exposed to secondhand smoke (CDC, 2015b). In total, tobacco use and secondhand smoke exposure are responsible for 20% of all deaths in the United States each year. In addition, more than 16 million Americans are living with a disease caused by smoking (CDC, 2015b). That means for every person who dies because of smoking, at least *continued*

BOX

2.7

30 people live with a serious smoking-related illness. Smoking causes cancer, heart disease, stroke, lung diseases, diabetes, and chronic obstructive pulmonary disease (COPD), which includes emphysema and chronic bronchitis, and it also increases risk for tuberculosis, certain eye diseases, and problems of the immune system, including rheumatoid arthritis (CDC, 2015d).

In addition to the costly physical burden of tobacco use and secondhand smoke exposure in the United States, there is also a significant economic cost. The total financial burden of tobacco to the United States is more than $300 billion per year. This includes $170 billion in direct medical costs and more than $156 billion in lost productivity due to premature death and exposure to secondhand smoke (CDC, 2015c).

Tobacco use and secondhand smoke exposure are also concerns for the residents of Pennsylvania. While the current national percentage of adult cigarette smokers is 17.8%, the current percentage of smokers in Pennsylvania is 21.0% (CI 19.9-22.0%) (CDC, 2015a). In addition, just over 4% of those residing in Pennsylvania use chewing tobacco, snuff, or snus (CDC, 2015a). Locally, the burden of tobacco use is even greater. Philadelphia County Pennsylvania, which is conterminous with the City of Philadelphia, is home to more than 1.5 million people. The current percentage of adult smokers in Philadelphia County is 23% (CI 22-25%) (University of Wisconsin [UW], 2015), which is clearly above both the state and national averages. In fact, Philadelphia has the highest rate of adult smoking among the 10 largest U.S. cities (CDC, 2013). Further, Philadelphia County is ranked last out of the 67 counties in Pennsylvania in both health outcomes and health factors (UW, 2015). The three leading causes of death in Philadelphia County are heart diseases, cancer, and stroke. All three of these causes have a common risk factor—smoking. Philadelphia County has implemented several interventions to reduce smoking including a public education program to encourage adults to quit, a clean indoor air ordinance, an ordinance to eliminate smoking at the city-owned outdoor recreational facilities, and compliance checks to ensure retailers are properly checking for identification before selling tobacco products (CDC, 2013). Although each of these efforts can contribute to the reduction in smoking, more needs to be done.

To reduce the prevalence of smoking in a community the CDC has recommended a comprehensive approach, which it has outlined in a document titled *Best Practices for Comprehensive Tobacco Control Programs–2014* (CDC, 2014). The program includes five components: 1) state and community interventions, 2) mass-reach health communication interventions, 3) cessation interventions, 4) surveillance and evaluation, and 5) infrastructure administration and management.

The goals of such a program are to:

- "Prevent initiation among youth and young adults.
- Promote quitting among adults and youth.
- Eliminate exposure to secondhand smoke.
- Identify and eliminate tobacco-related disparities among population groups" (CDC, 2014, p. 9).

This approach is not without its merits, it is recommended based on solid evidence. "The Community Preventive Services Task Force recommends comprehensive tobacco control programs based on strong evidence of effectiveness in reducing tobacco use and secondhand smoke exposure. Evidence indicates these programs reduce the prevalence of tobacco use among adults and young people, reduce tobacco product consumption, increase quitting, and contribute to reductions in tobacco-related diseases

BOX

2.7

continued

and deaths. Economic evidence indicates that comprehensive tobacco control programs are cost-effective, and savings from averted healthcare costs exceed intervention costs" (CPSTF, 2014, para. 1).

After reviewing the data, it is clear that there is a significant smoking problem in Philadelphia County Pennsylvania. In order to deal with this problem, it is recommended that the Coalition for a Smokefree Philadelphia County build a comprehensive tobacco control program based on *Best Practices for Comprehensive Tobacco Control Programs– 2014* but adapt it to fit the population of Philadelphia County. The National Association of County and City Health Officials has created the "Guidelines for Comprehensive Local Tobacco Control Programs" (CDC, 2014) to show how the best practice guidelines can be adapted to a local level. It is also recommended that the Coalition begin its work by reviewing the existing tobacco prevention programs in the county. Those current activities that are in line with best practices should be keep, and those that are not should either be modified to be in line with the best practices or be dropped.

A comprehensive tobacco program has great potential for success in Philadelphia County for several reasons. First, it would be an evidence-based program with solid science to back it up. Second, similar programs in other large cities in the United States have been successful (CDC, 2014). And third, the program will be well planned and tailored to the residents of Philadelphia County. There is no better time than now to invest in the health of the people of Philadelphia County Pennsylvania!

References

Centers for Disease Control and Prevention. (2015a). *Behavioral risk factor surveillance system: Prevalence and trends data, Pennsylvania – 2013*. Retrieved May 16, 2015 from http://apps.nccd .cdc.gov/brfss/page.asp?cat=TU&yr=2013&state=PA#TU

Centers for Disease Control and Prevention. (2014). *Best practices for comprehensive tobacco control programs–2014*. Atlanta, GA: U.S. Department of Health, CDC, National Center for Chronic Disease Prevention and Health Promotion, Office of Smoking and Health. Retrieved May 16, 2015 from http://www.cdc.gov/tobacco/stateandcommunity/best_practices/pdfs/2014/comprehensive.pdf

Centers for Disease Control and Prevention. (2013). *Community profile: Philadelphia, Penn-sylvania*. Retrieved May 16, 2015 from http://www.cdc.gov/nccdphp/dch/programs /CommunitiesPuttingPreventiontoWork/communities/profiles/both-pa_philadelphia.htm

Centers for Disease Control and Prevention. (2015b). *Current cigarette smoking among adults in the United States*. Retrieved May 16, 2015 from http://www.cdc.gov/tobacco/data_statistics /fact_sheets/adult_data/cig_smoking/

Centers for Disease Control and Prevention. (2015c). *Economic facts about U.S. tobacco production and use. tobacco use:* Retrieved May 16, 2015 from http://www.cdc.gov/tobacco/data_statistics /fact_sheets/economics/econ_facts/index.htm#costs

Centers for Disease Control and Prevention. (2015d). *Smoking and tobacco use: Fast facts*. Retrieved May 16, 2015 from http://www.cdc.gov/tobacco/data_statistics/fact_sheets/fast_facts/index.htm

Community Preventive Services Task Force (CPSTF). (2014). *Reducing tobacco use and secondhand smoke exposure: Comprehensive tobacco control programs*. Retrieved May 16, 2015 from http: //www.thecommunityguide.org/tobacco/comprehensive.html

University of Wisconsin Population Health Institute (2015). *County health rankings & roadmaps*. Retrieved May 16, 2015 from http://www.countyhealthrankings.org/

World Health Organization. (2014). *Tobacco*. Retrieved May 16, 2015 from http://www.who.int /mediacentre/factsheets/fs339/en/

World Health Organization. (2015). *WHO global report on trends in prevalence of tobacco smoking 2015*. Retrieved May 16, 2015 from http://apps.who.int/iris/bitstream/10665/156262/1/9789241564922 _eng.pdf?ua=1

▷ Planning Committee

The number of people involved in the planning process is determined by the resources and circumstances of a particular situation. "One very helpful method to develop a clearer and more comprehensive planning approach is to establish a committee" (Gilmore, 2012, p. 35). Identifying individuals who would be willing to serve as members of the **planning committee** (sometimes referred to as a **steering committee** or **advisory board** or **planning team**) becomes one of the planner's first tasks. Because an effective planning committee is usually composed of interested and well-respected individuals, it is important to establish it carefully (Chapman, 2009).

When composing a planning committee it is also a good time to consider the concept of *partnering* to meet the eventual goals of the program that will be planned. **Partnering** can be defined as the association of two more entities (i.e., individuals, groups, agencies, organizations) working together on a project of common interest. Such associations usually means sharing of resources and tasks to be completed. There are a number of reasons to partner and include things such as: 1) meeting the needs of a priority population which could not be met by the capacities of an individual partner, 2) sharing of financial and other resources, 3) solving a problem or achieving a goal that is a priority to several partners, 4) bringing more stakeholders to the "table," 5) bringing more credibility to the program, 6) working with others that have the same values (Picarella, 2015), 7) seeing and solving a problem from multiple perspectives and thus creating different effects (Schiavo 2014), and 8) creating a greater response to a need because there is strength in numbers.

In looking for partners (sometimes referred to as collaborators) planners should consider these questions: 1) Who is also interested in meeting the needs of the priority population? 2) Who also sees the unmet need of a priority population as a problem? 3) Who has unused resources that could help solve a problem? and 4) Who would benefit from being your partner? The Prevention Institute has created an interactive framework and tool for analyzing collaborative efforts. The framework/tool, called the *Collaborator Multiplier*, is "based on the understanding that sectors often have different understandings of issues and divergent reasons for engaging in the same effort" (Prevention Institute, 2011, para. 2) (see the link for the Website in the Weblinks section at the end of the chapter). Here are some examples of groups who could become partners: two non-governmental health agencies who are both interested in seeing the reduction in smoking rates, a local service organization (i.e., Lions Club, Kiwanis) and a school-based clinic to improve student health, an employer and a health insurance carrier to improve the quality of life for employees, and a local health department and pro-environmental group working to improve the air quality in a community.

After consideration is given to forming partnerships, thought needs to be given to the size of the planning committee. The number of individuals on a planning committee can differ depending on the setting for the program and the size of the priority population. For example, the size of a planning committee for an obesity program in a community of 50,000 people would probably be larger than that of a committee planning a similar program for a business with 50 employees. There is no ideal size for a planning committee, but the following 10 guidelines, which have been presented earlier (McKenzie, 1988) and are given here in a modified form with updates, should be helpful in setting up a committee.

1. The committee should be composed of individuals who represent a variety of subgroups within the priority population. To the extent possible, the committee should have representation from all segments of the priority population (e.g., administrators/students/teachers, age groups, health behavior participants/ nonparticipants, labor/management, race/ethnic groups, different genders, socioeconomic groups, union/nonunion members). The greater the number of individuals who are represented by committee members, the greater the chance of the priority population developing a feeling of **program ownership**. With program ownership there will be better planned programs, greater support for the programs, and people who will be willing to help sell the program to others because they feel it is theirs (Strycker et al., 1997).

2. If the program that is being planned deals with a specific health risk or problem, then it would be important that someone with that health risk (e.g., smoker) or problem (e.g., diabetes) be included on the planning committee (Bartholomew, Parcel, Kok, Gottlieb & Fernández, 2011).

3. The committee should include willing individuals who are interested in seeing the program succeed. Select a combination of **doers** and **influencers**. Doers are people who will be willing to "roll up their sleeves" and do the physical work needed to see that the program is planned and implemented properly. Influencers are those who with a single phone call, email, or signature on a form will enlist other people to participate or will help provide the resources to facilitate the program. Both doers and influencers are important to the planning process.

4. The committee should include an individual who has a key role within the organization sponsoring the program—someone whose support would be most important to ensure a successful program and institutionalization.

5. The committee should include representatives of other stakeholders (any person or organization with a vested interest in a program) not represented in the priority population. For example, if health care providers are needed to implement a health promotion program they need to be represented on the planning committee.

6. The committee membership should be reevaluated regularly to ensure that the composition lends itself to fulfilling program goals and objectives.

7. If the planning committee will be in place for a long period of time, new individuals should be added periodically to generate new ideas and enthusiasm. It may be helpful to set a *term limits* for committee members. If terms of office are used, it is advisable to stagger the length of terms so that there is always a combination of new and experienced members on the committee.

8. Be aware of the "politics" that are always present in an organization or priority population. There are always some people who bring their own agendas to committee work.

9. Make sure the committee is large enough to accomplish the work, but small enough to be able to make decisions and reach consensus. If necessary, subcommittees can be formed to handle specific tasks.

10. In some situations there might be a need for multiple layers of planning committees. If the priority population is highly dispersed geographically and/or broken into decentralized subgroups (e.g., various offices of the same corporation, or several

different local groups within the same state, or different buildings within a school corporation), these various subgroups may need their own local planning committee that operates with some latitude but maintains and complements the core planning committee as the base of the program (Chapman, 2009).

The actual means by which the committee members are chosen varies according to the setting. Five commonly used techniques are:

1. Asking for volunteers by word of mouth, a newsletter, a needs assessment, or some other widely distributed publication

2. Holding an election, either throughout the community or by subdivisions of the community

3. Inviting/recruiting people to serve

4. Having members formally appointed by a governing group or individual

5. Having an application process then selecting those with the most desirable characteristics

Once the planning committee has been formed, someone must be designated to lead it. This is an important step (Strycker et al., 1997). The leader (chairperson) should be interested and knowledgeable about health promotion programs, and be organized, enthusiastic, and creative (McKenzie, 1988). One might think that most planners, especially health education specialists, would be perfect for the committee chairperson's job. However, sometimes it is preferable to have someone other than the program planners serve in the leadership capacity. For one thing, it helps to spread out the workload of the committee. Planners who are not good at delegating responsibility may end up with a lot of extra work when they serve as the leaders. Second, having someone else serve as the leader allows the planners to remain objective about the program. And third, the planning committee can serve in an advisory capacity to the planners, if this is considered desirable. **Figure 2.2** illustrates the composition of a balanced planning committee.

Once the planning committee has been organized and a leader is selected, the committee needs to be well organized and well run to be effective. The committee should meet regularly, have a formal agenda for each meeting, and keep minutes of the meetings (Hunnicutt, 2007). Further, the committee meetings should be efficient, not long and boring (Johnson & Breckon, 2007). In other words, meetings should be productive and represent a good use of the committee members' time. In addition, it is important for the committee to communicate frequently both with the decision makers and those in the priority population so that all can be kept informed. By communicating regularly, the committee has the unique opportunity to educate and inform others about health and the specific priorities of the program (Hunnicutt, 2007).

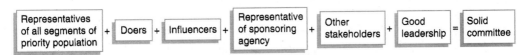

▲ **Figure 2.2** Makeup of a Solid Planning/Steering Committee

▷ Parameters for Planning

Once the support of the decision makers has been gained and a planning committee formed, the committee members must identify the **planning parameters** within which they will work. There are several questions to which committee members should have answers before they become too deeply involved in the planning process. In an earlier work (McKenzie, 1988), several such questions were presented, using the example of school-site health promotion programs. The questions are modified for presentation here. It should be noted, however, that not all of the questions would be appropriate for every program because of the different circumstances of each setting and the answers to some of the questions may have already been obtained during pre-planning.

1. What is the decision makers' philosophical perspective on health promotion programs? What are the values and benefits of the programs to the decision makers (Chapman, 1997)? Do they see the programs as something important or as "extras"?

2. What type of commitment are decision makers willing to make to the program? Are they interested in the program becoming **institutionalized**? That is, are they interested in seeing that the "program becomes imbedded within the host organization, so that the program becomes sustained and durable" (Goodman et al., 1993, p. 163)? Or are they more interested in providing a one-time or pilot program? (Note: Goodman and colleagues [1993] have developed a scale for measuring institutionalization.)

3. What type of financial support are decision makers willing to provide? Does it include personnel for leadership and clerical duties? Released/assigned time for managing the program and participation? Space? Equipment? Materials?

4. Are decision makers willing to consider changing the **organizational culture** so that there is a culture of health (Terry, 2012)? That is, are decision makers interested in establishing a health supporting culture (Golaszewski, Allen, & Edington, 2008) that is based on health-related values, beliefs, and practices? Among other things, such a culture might include health-supporting policies, services, and facilities. For example, are they interested in "well" days instead of sick days? Are they as interested in *presenteeism*—that is, showing up for work even if one is too ill, stressed, or distracted to be productive—as much as they are interested in absenteeism? Would they like to create employee nonsmoking and safety belt policies? Change vending machine selections to more nutritious foods? Set aside an employee room for meditation? Develop a health promotion page on the organization's Website?

5. Will all individuals in the priority population have an opportunity to take advantage of the program, or will it be available to only certain subgroups?

6. What type of committee will the planning committee be? Will it be a *permanent* or a *temporary (ad hoc)* committee (Hitt, Black, & Porter, 2012)? A permanent committee would indicate that decision makers want the planning committee to be a part of the ongoing structure of the organization.

7. What is the authority of the planning committee? Will it be an advisory group or a programmatic decision-making group? What will the chain of command be for program approval?

After the planning parameters have been defined, the planning committee should understand how the decision makers view the program, and should know what type and number of resources and amount of support to expect. Identifying the parameters early will save the planning committee a great deal of effort and energy throughout the planning process.

Summary

Creating a program rationale to gain the support of decision makers is an important initial step in program planning. Planners should take great care in developing a rationale for "selling" the program idea to these important people. The rationale should show how the benefits of the program align with the values of the decision makers, address the potential return on investment, and be backed by the best evidence available. A program rationale can be written using the following four steps: (1) Identify appropriate background information, (2) title the rationale, (3) write the content of the rationale, and (4) list the references used to create the rationale. A planning committee can be most useful in helping with some of the planning activities and in helping to sell the program to the priority population. When the planning committee is being formed consider potential collaborating partners. Planning committee members should include program stakeholders including interested individuals, doers and influencers, and others who are representative of the priority population. If the planning committee is to be effective, it will need to work efficiently and to know the planning parameters set for the program by the decision makers.

Review Questions

1. What is the reason for creating a program rationale?
2. Why is the support of decision makers important in planning a program?
3. What kinds of reasons should be included in a rationale for planning and implementing a health promotion program?
4. How important is selling the idea of a program to decision makers?
5. What items should be addressed when creating a program rationale?
6. What is a problem statement? What does it include?
7. What is social math? Give an example of how it could be used in a program rationale.
8. Who would make good planning partners?
9. Who should be selected as the members of a planning committee?
10. What are *planning parameters?* Give a few examples.
11. Why is it important to know the planning parameters at the beginning of the planning process?

Activities

1. Write a two-page rationale that sells a program you are planning to decision makers, using the guidelines presented in this chapter.

2. Write a two-page rationale for beginning an exercise program for a company with 200 employees. A needs assessment of this priority population indicates that the number one cause of lost work time in this cohort is back problems and the number one cause of premature death is heart disease.

3. Select a disease (e.g., diabetes, cancer, heart disease) or a health behavior (e.g., physical inactivity, smoking) and write a paragraph describing the health problem using social math.

4. Visit the Websites of the Community Preventive Services Task Force (CPSTF) and U.S. Preventive Services Task Force (USPSTF)—see Box 2.4 for URLs of the Websites. At the two sites, find out what the recommendations are for clinical skin cancer screenings and educational programs for skin cancer. Summarize your findings in one to two paragraphs. Based on the recommendations, write another one to two paragraphs describing what advice you would give with regard to future health promotion programming to a community coalition that is trying to reduce the number of cases of skin cancer in its community.

5. For a program you are planning, write a two-page description of the individuals (by position/job title, not name) who will be asked to serve on the planning committee, and provide a rationale for asking each to serve. Also, list any other agencies/organization who you believe would make good partners.

6. Provide a list (by position/job title, not name) and a rationale for each of the 10 individuals you would ask to serve on a community-wide safety belt program. Use the town or city in which your college/university is located as the community.

7. Read the example rationale presented in Box 2.7 and then critique it using the guidelines presented in this chapter. Critique by describing the following: (a) the strengths of the rationale, (b) the weaknesses, and (c) how you would change the rationale to make it stronger. Be critical! Closely examine the content, reasoning, and references.

Weblinks

1. http://www.thecommunityguide.org

   Guide to Community Preventative Services

   This Webpage includes evidence-based recommendations for programs and policies to promote population-based health from the Community Preventive Services Task Force (CPSTF).

2. https://new.wellsteps.com/

   WellSteps

   This is the home page for WellSteps, a company that helps other companies create worksite wellness programs. At the site you will find a number of different resources and tools that can assist you as you begin the planning process. One tool found at this site is the return on investment (ROI) calculator for health care costs [https://www.wellsteps .com/roi/resources_tools_roi_cal_health.php] that can help you determine if a health promotion for a company would make good economic sense.

3. http://www.countyhealthrankings.org

   County Health Rankings

   At this Website you will find a set of reports that rank the overall health of every county in the United States. If you are planning county-wide programs you will find this to be a valuable resource when creating rationales. The *County Health Rankings* are a part of the a collaboration between the Robert Wood Johnson Foundation and the University of Wisconsin Population Health Institute.

4. **http://www.astho.org**

   Association of State and Territorial Health Officials (ASTHO)

   ASTHO is the national nonprofit organization representing the state and territorial public health agencies of the United States, the U.S. Territories, and the District of Columbia. This Website has links to all the state and territorial health departments. If you are planning a program for the community setting, this site contains a lot of information that could help you develop a rationale for your program.

5. **http://www.preventioninstitute.org/index.php**

   Prevention Institute

   This Website is the home page of the Prevention Institute, a California-based organization that works from the approach of what can be done before people become ill or injured.

6. **http://www.cdc.gov/chronicdisease/calculator/index.html**

   Chronic Disease Cost Calculator, Version 2

   This Webpage presents background information and download links to the user guide and Chronic Disease Cost Calculator, Version 2.

Program Planning Models in Health Promotion

A key role, if not the central role, of the health education specialist is planning, implementing, and evaluating programs. **Box 3.1** identifies the responsibilities and competencies for health education specialists that pertain to the material presented in this chapter. Good health promotion programs are not created by chance; they are the product of coordinated effort and are usually based on a systematic planning model or approach. Planning models, which are visual representations and descriptions of steps or phases in the planning process are the means by which structure and organization are given to the successful development and delivery of health promotion programs. Models provide planners with direction and a framework from which to build interventions that can improve the health of individuals and communities.

Through the years, various planning models have been developed and presented for health promotion with varying degrees of acceptance and use. Although these models share common elements, they often label and describe these elements differently, giving the impression that something unique and meaningful has been offered. However, when new models emerge and appear novel, they are usually quite similar to the existing models. For this reason, we use what we call the *Generalized Model* to teach basic principles of planning and evaluation emphasized in most planning models. With this as a backdrop, it is

BOX 3.1

Responsibilities and Competencies for Health Education Specialists

This chapter covers planning models as well as other considerations and criteria necessary to develop a planning sequence from start to finish. Responsibilities and competencies related to the credentialing of health education specialists in this chapter include the following:

Area II: Plan Health Education/Promotion

    Competency 2.1: Involve priority populations, partners, and other stakeholders in the planning process

    Competency 2.4: Develop a plan for the delivery of health education/promotion

Source: *A Competency-Based Framework for Health Education Specialists—2015.* Whitehall, PA: National Commission for Health Education Credentialing, Inc. (NCHEC) and the Society for Public Health Education (SOPHE). Reprinted by permission of the National Commission for Health Education Credentialing, Inc. (NCHEC) and the Society for Public Health Education (SOPHE).

important to note that the Generalized Model is not a new or unique model either but rather a simple composite of what is represented in most, if not all other models. It is presented here as both a teaching model and framework for professional practice.

As illustrated in **Figure 3.1**, the Generalized Model consists of five basic phases or steps: (1) assessing needs; (2) setting goals and objectives; (3) developing interventions; (4) implementing interventions; and (5) evaluating results. In addition, pre-planning is a quasi-phase in the model but is not included formally since it involves actions that occur before planning technically begins. The first phase in the Generalized Model, assessing needs, is the process of collecting and analyzing data to determine the health needs of a population and usually includes priority setting and the identification of a priority population. Setting goals and objectives identifies *what* will be accomplished while interventions or programs are the means by which the goals and objectives will be achieved (i.e., the how). Implementation is the process of putting interventions into action and evaluation focuses on both improving

▲ **Figure 3.1** The Generalized Model

the quality of interventions (formative evaluation) as well as determining their effectiveness (summative evaluation). Collectively, these phases define planning and evaluation at its core. To illustrate how planning models in general are aligned with the phases outlined in the Generalized Model, we briefly describe seven prominent models used in health promotion settings. As you read the following descriptions, also note the many similarities these models have in common.

▷ Evidence-Based Planning Framework for Public Health

The ultimate goal of any planning effort is to improve health outcomes. To help ensure that health outcomes are improved, it is important to use evidence-based (i.e. effective or proven) approaches in all phases of planning. Ross Brownson, one of the premier authorities in evidence-based public health, and by association, health promotion, has written extensively on evidence-based outcomes (Brownson, Baker, Leet, Gillespie, & True, 2011; Brownson, Fielding, & Maylahn, 2009). Brownson and associates at the Prevention Research Center (PRC) at Washington University in St. Louis have developed a set of seven skills that collectively serve as an **evidence-based planning framework for public health** (Washington University Prevention Research Center, 2015). This framework, while not developed as a planning model per se, is in fact, very similar to most planning models, including the Generalized Model. **Box 3.2** displays the seven skills or phases of this framework.

Phases 1–2, *community assessment* and *quantifying the issue*, essentially represent a needs assessment common to most planning models. In this framework, community assessment requires planners to understand the **community context**, or the characteristics and circumstances that define the community, and also understand the health concerns of community members and how to implement programs most effectively to them. Most often, this requires collecting new data, including a process defined in the framework as community audits (i.e. documenting observations about the community). The community assessment also involves organizing and examining existing data (e.g. mortality, morbidity, risk factor data, etc.). Quantifying the issue (Phase 2), closely related to Phase 1, is the process of using descriptive epidemiology (i.e., occurrence and distribution of disease by person, place, and time) derived from surveillance systems and other secondary data sets (i.e., existing data) to

---

BOX	**Evidence-Based Planning Framework for Public Health**

3.2

Focus On

PHASE 1 Community Assessment
PHASE 2 Quantifying the Issue
PHASE 3 Developing a Concise Statement of the Issue
PHASE 4 Determining What is Known using Scientific Literature
PHASE 5 Developing and Prioritizing Program and Policy Options
PHASE 6 Developing an Action Plan and Implementing Interventions
PHASE 7 Evaluating the Program or Policy

Source: Washington University Prevention Research Center (2015). Evidence based public healthcourse. Retrieved from http://prcstl.wustl.edu/training/Pages/EBPH-Course-Information.aspx

analyze and display disease frequencies. In this step, data are also presented in tables and figures as prevalence or incidence rates, or as percentages, to help stakeholders make decisions about health concerns in the community. Combined with data from community members, the most significant health problems in the community begin to emerge (Washington University Prevention Research Center, 2015).

Phase 3, *developing a concise statement of the issue,* summarizes an analysis of root causes of the most significant health problems in the community. For example, root causes may include lack of interventions that address primary risk factors related to a health problem or inadequate policies to protect the community from a known threat. Root causes may also take the form of social determinants (i.e. inadequate education, low employment, high crime, etc., related to health disparities). This analysis leads to a concise written statement of root causes, or statement of the issue (Washington University Prevention Research Center, 2015).

Phase 4, *determining what is known using scientific literature,* directs planners to identify evidence-based solutions related to the root causes and related problems identified in the statement of the issue (Phase 3). Planners search resources such as the *Guide to Community Preventive Services* (CDC, 2015), or scientific journals, books, government reports, etc., and categorize potential solutions as recommended with strong evidence, recommended with sufficient evidence, insufficient evidence, and not recommended (no evidence). This process leads planners to various interventions that may effectively address the root causes of the health problems identified (Washington University Prevention Research Center, 2015).

Once potential interventions are examined, Phase 5, *developing and prioritizing program and policy options,* directs planners to prioritize specific interventions or actions steps using methods such as the Delphi technique, Nominal Group technique, Basic Priority Rating model, multi-level voting, or any other process that is systematic, objective, and allows for standardized comparisons (see Chapter 4 for descriptions of these methods). Planners are encouraged to identify priorities related to actions that lead to improved health outcomes (Washington University Prevention Center, 2015).

Phase 6, *developing an action plan and implementing interventions,* is what most planners would call *implementation.* In this step, goals and objectives are developed and action strategies (i.e. interventions) are planned. Logic models are developed to visually display the relationship between inputs (resources) and outputs (what will be accomplished). Management of action strategies, personnel, and communication with partners and community members are also addressed in this step (Washington University Prevention Center, 2015).

Finally, in Phase 7, *evaluating the program or policy,* planners take measures to improve the existing program or policy (i.e. formative evaluation) as well as measure effectiveness (i.e. summative, or impact and outcome evaluation). Basic decisions are made such as whether to conduct quantitative or qualitative evaluation and whether to use descriptive or inferential statistics (see Chapter 15 for descriptions). Planners decide on appropriate outcomes to measure, then decide how to collect, record, analyze and disseminate data (Washington University Prevention Center, 2015). A close examination of the planning approach used by Brownson and associates, who are clearly well respected in the field of evidence-based strategies, not only validates steps used in the Generalized Model, but also supports the argument that most planning models are composed of the same basic elements.

▷ Mobilizing for Action Through Planning and Partnerships (MAPP)

In 1997, the CDC and the National Association of County and City Health Officials (NACCHO) collaborated on the development of a new model and released the **MAPP** model—Mobilizing for Action through Planning and Partnerships in 2000 (NACCHO, 2001). While the MAPP model was presented as a foundational approach to planning and evaluation in public health settings, particularly among local (i.e. city or county) health departments, it has broad relevance to all health promotion settings. In fact, the MAPP model is considered a very robust model in practice today. Hershey (2011) provides an in-depth case study of how MAPP can be used successfully at the local level.

Use of the MAPP model is intended to improve health and quality of life through mobilized partnerships and taking strategic action (NACCHO, 2001). **Figure 3.2** displays the six phases of MAPP as well as the four MAPP assessments.

In the first phase of MAPP, *organizing for success and partnership development*, planners assess whether the MAPP process is timely, appropriate, or even possible. This involves assessing resources (including budgets), the expertise of available personnel, support of key decision makers and other stakeholders, and the general interest of community members. If resources are not available, the process is not undertaken. If the decision is made to proceed with a MAPP process, the following work groups are created: (1) a core support team, which prepares most, if not all of the material needed for the planning process; (2) the MAPP committee, composed of key sponsors (usually influential people or organizations

▲ **Figure 3.2** Display of the Six Phases of MAPP and the Four MAPP Assessments

Source: *Achieving Healthier Communities through MAPP: A User's Handbook.* Copyright © 2009 by the National Association of County and City Health Officials. Reprinted with permission.

from the private sector who lend support and other resources) and stakeholders who guide and oversee the process; and (3) the community itself, which provides input, representation, and decision making. This phase answers basic questions about the general feasibility, resources, and appropriateness of the MAPP process (NACCHO, 2001).

Phase 2 of the MAPP process, *visioning*, guides the community through a process that results in a shared vision (what the ideal future looks like) and common values (principles and beliefs that will guide the remainder of the planning process) (NACCHO, 2001). Generally, a facilitator conducts the visioning process and involves anywhere from 50 to 100 participants including the advisory committee, the MAPP committee, and key community leaders (NACCHO, 2001). This process is typical of what should occur in pre-planning (see the Generalized Model).

Phase 3, the *four MAPP assessments*, represents the defining characteristic of the MAPP model. The four assessments include (1) the community themes and strengths assessment (community or consumer opinion), (2) the local public health assessment (general capacity of the local health department and the local health system), (3) the community health status assessment (measurement of the health of the community by use of mortality, morbidity, risk factor and other related data, etc.), and (4) the forces of change assessment (forces such as legislation, technology, and other environmental or social phenomena that do or will impact the community). Collectively, the MAPP assessments provide insight on the gaps that exist between current status in the community and what was learned in the visioning phase as well as strategic direction for goals and strategies (NACCHO, 2001). The MAPP assessments provide an excellent framework for the types of data collection that should be part of any comprehensive needs assessment (see Chapter 4).

In Phase 4 of MAPP, *identify strategic issues*, planners develop a prioritized list of the most important issues facing the health of the community. Only issues that jeopardize the vision and values of the community are considered. Important tasks in this phase include consideration of what would happen if certain issues were not addressed, understanding why an issue is strategic, consolidating overlapping issues, and identifying a prioritized list. In Phase 5, *formulate goals and strategies*, planners create goals related to the vision and prioritize strategic issues then select strategies to accomplish the goals. Finally, Phase 6, the *action cycle*, is similar to implementation and evaluation phases in other planning models. In this phase, implementation details are considered, evaluation plans (i.e. gathering credible evidence) are developed, and plans for disseminating results are made (NACCHO, 2001).

▷ MAP-IT

More recently, in December 2010, *Healthy People 2020*, a national planning framework, was released to help guide public health and health promotion planning efforts for the next decade (USDHHS, 2015c). **MAP-IT** (Mobilize, Assess, Plan, Implement and Track) was introduced as a planning model to assist communities in implementing their own adaptations of *Healthy People 2020*. A few case studies have demonstrated how this can transpire (Offiong, Oji, Bunyan, Lewis, Moore, Olusanya, 2011; Devito-Staub, 2014). The phases in MAP-IT are displayed in **Box 3.3**.

Phases of MAP-IT

PHASE 1 Mobilize

PHASE 2 Assess

PHASE 3 Plan

PHASE 4 Implement

PHASE 5 Track

MAP-IT starts by mobilizing key individuals and organizations into a coalition that can work together to improve the health of the community (USDHHS, 2011c). Once partners are identified and the coalition is organized, roles are established for each partner and responsibilities are assigned. These responsibilities may include facilitating community input through meetings and other events, developing and presenting educational and/or training programs, leading fundraising or policy initiatives, and providing technical assistance in planning or evaluation (USDHHS, 2011c). In essence, the *mobilize* phase of MAP-IT is the same thing as pre-planning in the Generalized Model.

The second phase of MAP-IT, *assess,* is the equivalent of a needs assessment. This phase directs planners to ask and answer questions such as: (1) Who is affected by key health problems in our community? (2) What resources do we have to address the problems that we identify? And (3) What resources are required to have a meaningful impact? This phase of the model examines both the problems as well as the assets within a community to help planners focus on what the community can do versus what it would like to do (USDHHS, 2011c).

In the assess phase, both state and local data are collected and analyzed to help coalition members set priorities. In addition, the MAP-IT model directs planners to examine the social determinants, or root causes of the problems associated with the data collected. This might include an investigation of how the physical or social environments affect the health of the community, how a lack of access to health services contributes to death and illness, and how individual behavior as well as biology and genetics affect the health issues identified as priorities (USDHHS, 2011c).

The third phase of MAP-IT, *plan,* involves developing goals and objectives, measures, baselines, and targets. This means that as part of the objectives that are developed, planners determine what will be measured (e.g., a decrease in smoking among adults), the baseline (e.g., percent of adults in the community who smoke), and the targeted decrease (e.g., a decrease of three percent in five years). In this phase, planners also identify the specific interventions that will be used to accomplish the identified goals and objectives. This means addressing the following questions: (1) What do we need to do to reach our goals? And (2) How will we know when we have reached our goals? This phase is the equivalent of developing goals and objectives as well as interventions.

The fourth phase in MAP-IT, *implement,* involves organizing the coalition so it can put the plan into action. Here, a detailed work plan, including all of the information developed in Phase 3, is assembled to identify clear action steps, describe who is responsible for completing the action steps, and display a timeline with related deadlines. A communication plan is also produced in this phase to outline how program partners will reach and recruit participants and communicate the benefits of engaging in the program.

The final phase of MAP-IT, *track*, is the equivalent of evaluation. Here, coalition partners ask and answer specific questions such as: (1) Are we evaluating our work appropriately (i.e., formative evaluation)? (2) Did we follow the plan (i.e., process evaluation)? (3) What did we change (i.e., impact evaluation)? And, (4) Did we reach our goal (i.e., outcome evaluation) (USDHHS, 2011c)? MAP-IT encourages regular evaluations to measure and track progress over time and draws special attention to the quality of data being collected, the limitations of self-reported data, and the validity and reliability of data collected (USDHHS, 2011c). Progress on the impact of related interventions is shared often with stakeholders (USDHHS, 2011c).

▷ PRECEDE-PROCEED

"PRECEDE is an acronym for *p*redisposing, *r*einforcing, and *e*nabling *c*onstructs in *e*ducational/*e*cological *d*iagnosis and *e*valuation" (Green & Kreuter, 2005, p. 9). "PROCEED stands for *p*olicy, *r*egulatory, and *o*rganizational *c*onstructs in *e*ducational and *e*nvironmental *d*evelopment" (Green & Kreuter, 2005, p. 9). The model is very robust with hundreds of published papers citing evidence of its usefulness in improving health outcomes. It is perhaps one of the oldest and most enduring planning models used in health promotion. In the last few years it has been cited as integral in better understanding women's decisions to seek clinical breast exams (Hayes-Constant, Winkler, Bishop, & Taboada-Palomino, 2014), designing an oral health strategy (Binkley & Johnson, 2013), developing an intuitive eating approach to weight management (Cole & Horacek, 2009) and improving the quality of life in elders (Mazloomymahmoodabad, Masoudy, Fallahzadeh, & Jalili, 2014).

The first half of the model, PRECEDE, "consists of a series of planned assessments that generate information that will be used to guide subsequent decisions" (Green & Kreuter, 2005, p. 8). The second half of the model, PROCEED, "is marked by the strategic implementation of multiple actions based on what was learned from the assessments in the initial phase" (Green & Kreuter, 2005, p. 9).

The Eight Phases of PRECEDE-PROCEED

As displayed in **Figure 3.3**, **PRECEDE-PROCEED** is composed of eight phases. The underlying approach of this model is to begin by identifying the desired outcome, to determine what causes it, and finally to design an intervention aimed at reaching the desired outcome. In other words, PRECEDE-PROCEED begins with the final consequences and works backward to the causes. Once the causes are known, an intervention can be designed.

Phase 1 in the model is called *social assessment and situational analysis* and seeks to subjectively define the quality of life (problems and priorities) of those in the priority population while involving individuals in the priority population in an assessment of their own needs and aspirations. Social indicators of quality of life include achievement, alienation, comfort, crime, discrimination, happiness, self-esteem, unemployment, and welfare (Green & Kreuter, 2005).

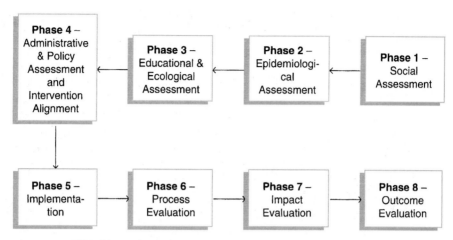

▲ **Figure 3.3** PRECEDE-PROCEED Model for Health Promotion Planning and Evaluation

In Phase 2, *epidemiological assessment*, planners use data to identify and rank the health goals or problems that may contribute to or interact with problems identified in Phase 1. These data include traditional indicators analyzed in needs assessments (e.g., mortality, morbidity, and disability data) as well as genetic, behavioral, and environmental factors (Green & Kreuter, 2005). It is important to note that ranking the health problems in this phase is critical, because there are rarely, if ever, enough resources to deal with all or even multiple problems. Also, this phase of the model is used to plan health programs. Note that in Figure 3.3, arrows work backward to connect the genetics, behavior, and environment boxes of Phase 2 with the health box and with the quality of life box of Phase 1.

Once identified, the risk factors or conditions related to broader health problems need to be prioritized. This can be accomplished by first ranking these factors by importance and changeability and then using a 2 × 2 matrix with "more important" and "less important" on the horizontal axis and "more changeable" and "less changeable" along the vertical axis (Green & Kreuter, 2005). The risk factors that fall into the "more important" and "more changeable" quadrant in the matrix will be the highest priorities.

Phase 3, *educational and ecological assessment*, identifies and classifies the various factors that have the potential to influence a given behavior into three categories: predisposing, reinforcing, and enabling. **Predisposing factors** include knowledge and many affective traits such as a person's attitude, values, beliefs, and perceptions. These factors can facilitate or hinder a person's motivation to change and can be altered through direct communication. Barriers or facilitators created mainly by societal forces or systems make up **enabling factors**, which include access to health care facilities or other health-related services, availability of resources, referrals to appropriate providers, transportation, negotiation and problem-solving skills, among others. **Reinforcing factors** involve the different types of feedback and rewards that those in the priority population receive after behavior change, which may either encourage or discourage the continuation of the behavior. Reinforcing behaviors can be delivered by, but not limited to, family, friends, peers, teachers, self, and others who control rewards (Green & Kreuter, 2005).

Phase 4 is composed of two parts: (1) *intervention alignment*; and (2) *administrative and policy assessment*. The intent of intervention alignment is to match appropriate strategies and interventions with projected changes and outcomes identified in earlier phases (Green & Kreuter, 2005). In administration and policy assessment, planners determine if the capabilities and resources of existing personnel and participating organizations are available to develop and implement the program. It is between Phases 4 and 5 that PRECEDE (the assessment portion of the model) ends and PROCEED (implementation and evaluation) begins. However, there is no distinct break between the two phases; they actually run together, and planners can move back and forth between phases.

The four final phases of the model—Phases 5, 6, 7, and 8—make up the PROCEED portion. In Phase 5—*implementation*—with appropriate resources secured, planners select interventions and strategies and implementation begins. Phases 6, 7, and 8 address *process, impact,* and *outcome evaluation* (see Chapter 13 for definitions), respectively, and are based on the earlier phases of the model, when objectives were outlined in the assessment process. Whether all three of these final phases are used depends on the evaluation requirements of the program. Usually, the resources needed to conduct evaluations of impact (Phase 7) and outcome (Phase 8) are much greater than those needed to conduct process evaluation (Phase 6) (Green & Kreuter, 2005).

▷ Intervention Mapping

Intervention mapping was designed to fill a gap in health promotion practice by translating data collected in the PRECEDE phases of PRECEDE-PROCEED (i.e., social, epidemiological, educational, ecological, administrative, organizational, and policy assessments) into theoretically based and otherwise appropriate interventions (Green & Kreuter, 2005). Once planners identify program objectives, they are guided by diagrams and matrices that incorporate outputs of the assessment process with relevant theory (Green & Kreuter, 2005). Intervention Mapping as a planning model has been refined and described more comprehensively by Bartholomew, Parcel, Kok, Gottlieb, and Fernandez (2011). The model has been used to develop a breast and cervical cancer screening program for Hispanic farmworkers (Fernandez, Gonzales, Tortolero-Luna, Partida, & Bartholomew, 2005), to develop a worksite physical activity intervention (McEachan, Lawton, Jackson, Conner, & Lunt, 2008), to explore the development of existing sex education programs for people with intellectual disabilities (Schaafsma, Joke, Kok, & Curfs, 2012), and in reducing heavy drinking among college students (Voogt, Poelen, Kleinjan, Lemmers, & Engels, 2014).

Box 3.4 outlines the six phases of Intervention Mapping. The first phase, *conduct a needs assessment*, is conducted by using the PRECEDE phases of the PRECEDE-PROCEED model and includes establishing a participatory planning group, assessing community capacity, and linking the needs assessment to health outcomes and quality of life goals (Bartholomew et al., 2011). Phase 2, *create matrices of change objectives*, specifies who and what will change as a result of the intervention (Bartholomew et al., 2011). Although the identification of goals and objectives is common to all planning models, intervention mapping makes a significant contribution in this regard and is considered the basic tool of the model. In this phase,

Phases of Intervention Mapping

PHASE 1   Conduct a Needs Assessment

PHASE 2   Create Matrices of Change Objectives

PHASE 3   Select Theory-Based Intervention Methods and Practical Applications

PHASE 4   Organize Methods and Applications into an Intervention Program

PHASE 5   Plan for Adoption, Implementation, and Sustainability of the Program

PHASE 6   Generate and Evaluation Plan

Source: Bartholomew, L.K., Parcel, G.S., Kok, G., Gottlieb, N.H., & Fernandez, M.E. (2011). *Planning Health Promotion Programs: An Intervention Mapping Approach* (3rd ed.). San Francisco, CA: Jossey-Bass.

planners create a matrix of change objectives which "state what needs to be achieved in order to accomplish performance objectives that will enable changes in behavior or environmental conditions that will in turn improve the health and quality of life program goals identified in Step 1" (Bartholomew et al., 2011, p. 239). This is perhaps the defining strength and unique contribution of the model.

Phase 3, *theory-based intervention methods and practical applications*, guides the planner through a process of selected theory-based interventions and strategies that hold the greatest promise to change the health behavior(s) of individuals in the priority population. Phase 4, *organize methods and applications into an intervention program*, describes the scope and sequence of the intervention, the completed program materials, and program protocols (Bartholomew et al., 2011). In addition, program materials are pretested with the priority population prior to implementation.

Phase 5 of intervention mapping is *plan for adoption, implementation, and sustainability of the program*. This phase requires the same development of matrices as in Phase 2, except in these matrices, the focus is on adoption and implementation of performance objectives (Bartholomew et al., 2011). In other words, instead of focusing on who and what will change within the priority population, the focus is on what will be done by whom among planners or program partners. Finally, Phase 6 is *generate an evaluation plan*. In this phase, planners decide if determinants were well specified, if strategies were appropriately matched to methods, what proportion of the priority population was reached, and whether or not implementation was complete and executed as planned (Bartholomew et al., 2011).

▷ Healthy Communities

Healthy Communities (or Healthy Cities) is a movement that began in the 1980s in Canada and, with the assistance of the World Health Organization, spread to various locations throughout Europe. As a result, organizations like California Healthy Cities and Indiana Healthy Cities were created in the United States. The movement is characterized by community ownership and empowerment and driven by the values, needs, and participation of community members with consultation from health professionals. Another characteristic of Healthy Communities is diverse partnership. It is not uncommon to see partners from business or labor, transportation, recreation, public safety, or even politicians partici-pate in the Healthy Communities process.

In the past few decades, the Centers for Disease Control and Prevention (CDC) has worked intensively with hundreds of communities to cultivate Healthy Communities and has reported that the following factors predict success: (1) local investment in com-munities; (2) providing a venue for local communities to learn about effective strategies; (3) mobilizing networks for change; and (4) providing tools to communities to achieve health equity and prevent chronic disease (Giles, Holmes-Chavez, & Collins, 2009). One of the lessons learned from Healthy Communities is the idea that the pursuit of shared values in the context of ownership and empowerment is a viable approach to improving health in the community. The Healthy Communities Program at the CDC has created the **CHANGE (Community Health Assessment aNd Group Evaluation) tool** to enable stakeholders and community team members to gather data on community strengths and assets as well as provide opportunities to create policy, systems, and environmental change through a community action plan (CDC, 2010a). This tool or model represents a viable planning framework for organizations and communities engaging in the Healthy Communities approach.

Box 3.5 displays the eight phases (described as action steps by CDC) of the CHANGE tool. Phase 1, *assemble the community team*, organizes 10-12 individuals, including key decision makers, representing diverse sectors from the community who are willing to collect and analyze data, translate data to an action plan, and oversee implementation of related interventions (CDC, 2010a). Phase 2, *develop a team strategy*, directs the community team to make decisions about how to operate most efficiently and effectively. This might include reorganizing the larger team into smaller work groups with specific tasks. It also includes creating decision-making procedures, including how to reach consensus (CDC, 2010a). Phase 3, *review all five CHANGE sectors*, divides the work of data collection and analysis into five sectors: (1) the community at large sector; (2) the community institu-tion/organization sector (i.e. institutions or organizations in the community that provide human services and access to facilities); (3) the health care sector; (4) the school sector; and

---

BOX

3.5

Highlights

Phases of the CHANGE Tool

PHASE 1	Assemble the Community Team
PHASE 2	Develop a Team Strategy
PHASE 3	Review All Five CHANGE Sectors
PHASE 4	Gather Data
PHASE 5	Review Data Gathered
PHASE 6	Enter Data
PHASE 7	Review Consolidated Data
PHASE 8	Build the Community Action Plan

Source: Centers for Disease Control and Prevention (2010a). Community Health Assessment aNd Group Evaluation Action Guide: Building a Foundation of Knowledge to Prioritize Community Needs. Atlanta: U.S. U.S. Department of Health and Human Services.

(5) the worksite sector. Each sector contains specific questions with related data elements associated with policy, systems, or environmental change that need to be addressed (CDC, 2010a). Phase 4, *gather data*, begins the assessment phase. Here, "sites" or locations that have data related to the questions associated with each sector are identified and specific data collection strategies such as observations, interviews, focus groups and surveys are used to gather new or existing data (CDC, 2010a). In Phase 5, *review data gathered*, team members discuss what was discovered and "rate" (or rank) each item (specific questions related to each sector) using a five-point scale. This involves making judgments about whether the condition of each item (e.g. condition and safety of sidewalks that increase or decrease the likelihood of physical activity, or structured physical activity classes in grades 9-12, etc.) is improving, getting worse, or staying the same (CDC, 2010a). Phase 6, *enter data*, incorporates CHANGE Sector Excel files, which organizes data for analysis. Phase 7, *review consolidated data*, transfers data into "CHANGE summary statements for quick reference of all sites with related ratings across all five sectors (CDC, 2010a). In essence, this step summarizes data to accommodate prioritization and decision making. Finally, Phase 8, *building the community action plan*, involves translating prioritized data from the summary statements to measurable objectives and action steps with assignments, and creates strategies for evaluation and reassessment (CDC, 2010a). The CHANGE action guide (CDC, 2010a) provides adequate instructions on how to complete the eight phases of this process. But in general, it includes pre-planning and visioning, needs assessment, priority setting, selecting appropriate policy, systems, or environmental interventions, and evaluating the quality and effectiveness of interventions.

▷ SMART

Although most planning models try to involve members of the priority population in the planning process at some level and some go so far as to incorporate consumer data (see MAPP for a good example), planning models such as **SMART** (Social Marketing Assessment and Response Tool [Neiger & Thackeray, 1998]), with a social marketing focus, generally do a better job of orienting program interventions to the preferences of consumers throughout the entire planning process (see Chapter 11 for more information on marketing/social marketing). Consumer data are collected continually, first to understand the wants and needs of consumers and then to test all aspects of intervention and communication strategies. There is some evidence to suggest that this planning approach may be more effective than traditional approaches used in health promotion (Neiger & Thackeray, 2002). SMART is one of the more robust social marketing models currently in practice; the other being the Community Based Prevention Marketing Model (Bryant, Forthofer, McCormack-Brown, Landis, & McDermott, 2000). Within the last few years, the SMART Model has been used in service-learning to teach community health (Buckner, Ndjakani, Banks, & Blumenthal, 2010), in the development of an educational intervention to treat schizophrenia (Bradshaw, Lovell, Bee, & Campbell, 2010), and in developing a support program for patients with diabetic kidney disease (Pagels, Hylander, & Alvarsson, 2015).

The SMART model, influenced primarily by Walsh and colleagues (1993), is also a composite of several social marketing planning frameworks but differs from most planning models used in health promotion settings due to its multistep focus on the consumer. Unlike some social marketing planning models, SMART has been used from start to finish in successful social marketing interventions (Neiger & Thackeray, 2002).

As displayed in **Box 3.6**, SMART is composed of seven phases. Like other social marketing planning models, the central focus of SMART is consumers. The heart of this model, composed of Phases 2 through 4, directs planners to acquire a broad understanding of the consumers who will be the recipients of a program and its interventions. These three phases seek to understand consumers before interventions are developed or implemented. Though these phases (2–4) are displayed in linear fashion, and for clarity will be described in sequence, they are typically performed simultaneously with members of the priority population.

BOX

3.6

Highlights

The SMART Model

Phase 1: Preliminary Planning

- Identify a health problem and name it in terms of behavior
- Develop general goals
- Outline preliminary plans for evaluation
- Project program costs

Phase 2: Consumer Analysis

- Segment and identify the priority population
- Identify formative research methods
- Identify consumer wants, needs, and preferences
- Develop preliminary ideas for preferred interventions

Phase 3: Market Analysis

- Establish and define the market mix (4Ps)
- Assess the market to identify competitors (behaviors, messages, programs, etc.), allies (support systems, resources, etc.), and partners

Phase 4: Channel Analysis

- Identify appropriate communication messages, strategies, and channels
- Assess options for program distribution
- Identify communication roles for program partners
- Determine how channels should be used

Phase 5: Develop Interventions, Materials, and Pretest

- Develop program interventions and materials using information collected in consumer, market, and channel analyses
- Interpret the marketing mix into a strategy that represents exchange and societal good
- Pretest and refine the program

Phase 6: Implementation

- Communicate with partners and clarify involvement
- Activate communication and distribution strategies
- Document procedures and compare progress to timelines
- Refine the program

Phase 7: Evaluation

- Assess the degree to which the priority population is receiving the program
- Assess the immediate impact on the priority population and refine the program as necessary
- Ensure that program delivery is consistent with established protocol
- Analyze changes in the priority population

Source: Adapted from Walsh et al. (1993) by Neiger & Thackeray (1998).

The Phases of SMART

Phase 1, *preliminary planning,* is critical for any type of health promotion program and in this model includes the planning elements of pre-planning and needs assessment as described earlier. Preliminary planning allows program planners to objectively assess all health problems and determine which one is most appropriate to address. This is most often accomplished through analysis of epidemiologic data, including various mortality and morbidity rates and associated risk factor data. It also includes objective priority setting with predetermined criteria. Sometimes planners do not undergo a process to select a priority health problem because the decision has already been made or the organization is dedicated to a specific health problem (e.g., the American Heart Association focuses on heart disease). Once a single health problem is determined, it is defined in terms of behaviors. Risk factors, or contributing factors, then become the focus of the social marketing process. This is similar to most health promotion programs.

Some social marketing practitioners and those who engage in community-based participatory research would argue that the priority population itself should determine the focus of an intervention or program. Good arguments can be made for this approach, including the idea that priority populations are capable of identifying their own problems and solutions and that they will be more vested in long-term involvement if they have ownership in the process. The SMART model suggests that planners, as trained health professionals, have both the expertise and responsibility to use various data sets to oversee and determine priority health problems within a community in partnership with members of the priority population. Once a priority or priorities are identified, the remainder of the process becomes almost exclusively consumer-driven.

While health professionals may determine initial program direction, the SMART model directs that consumers drive the development and implementation of interventions. This is not unlike most ventures in commercial marketing where a product or service is developed internally then tested with consumers and modified prior to distribution. For example, a company such as Coca-Cola develops its own identity and mission and creates the basic essence of its products. But it engages in complex marketing campaigns to better understand how to modify, improve, position, and deliver these products to its consumers in a way that offers benefits at reasonable costs.

Although goals are outlined in Phase 1, objectives are not. This makes sense from a social marketing perspective, since consumer research has not yet been performed. The goals are general statements of intent or direction, but they do not specify program components or direct the planner into specific courses of action.

Another task in Phase 1 is to develop preliminary plans for evaluation. Theoretically, it will make sense to most planners to consider evaluation early in the planning process. In reality, evaluation is too often an afterthought. Preliminary decisions regarding evaluation outcomes must be made early in the planning process in order to account for personnel, time, and budget requirements. Therefore, it is also important to determine how baseline and post-program (posttest) data will be collected and to identify valid survey or data collection instruments. Planners can also control for various kinds of bias or error in data collection if these basic evaluation concepts are considered before the program is implemented.

Finally, program costs need to be projected before the social marketing project begins. Social marketing can be an expensive proposition in terms of staff costs and direct expenses.

When performed correctly, a social marketing project can take several months or up to a year before implementation even begins. Program planners and organizations must decide if they are ready to make these kinds of time and financial commitments.

At the end of Phase 1, the social marketing planners have (1) identified the focus of interest in terms of modifiable behaviors, (2) developed goals that provide general direction, (3) outlined preliminary plans for evaluation, and (4) estimated total project costs. Based on this information, the planners and organizations can make an informed decision about the potential costs and benefits of the project as well as the application of social marketing.

Phase 2 of SMART is *consumer analysis*. In social marketing language, the process of performing consumer analysis is called **formative research**, defined as a process that identifies differences among subgroups within a population, identifies a subgroup, determines the wants and needs of the subgroup, and identifies factors that influence its behavior, including benefits, barriers, and readiness to change (Bryant, 1998).

It is important to remember that no single type of data collection technique is necessarily best in performing formative research. To the contrary, it is helpful to use multiple methods to gain a better perspective of the priority population. It is a mistake for those who engage in social marketing to perform one or two focus groups in the name of formative research and claim they understand their consumers. Ordinarily, however, formative research will involve the use of focus groups, in-depth interviews, and surveys, and so on, to understand consumer preferences.

At the conclusion of Phase 2, a priority population is also identified. Adequate formative research has been performed yielding data about major themes, directions, and consumer preferences related to the health problem and related interventions. Although Phases 2 through 4 are often performed simultaneously, information collected in Phase 2 can provide context for the other two phases. For example, knowing about consumer preferences related to some type of behavior change allows planners to more effectively understand consumer preferences related to the market mix and communication strategies.

Phase 3, *market analysis*, examines the fit between the focus of interest (desired behavior change) and important market variables within the priority population. *Marketing mix* is a term that is often used in both commercial and social marketing. It is composed of four components, also known as the 4Ps: product, price, place, and promotion (see Chapter 11 for more on the 4Ps).

At the conclusion of this phase, consumer analysis is enriched by a better understanding of important market variables that influence consumers. Combined with consumer analysis and channel analysis, market analysis provides a powerful combination of useful information about consumers, the environment they live in, and strengths and weakness associated with potential social marketing interventions.

The fourth phase of SMART is *channel analysis*. Although communication may not be the focal point of a social marketing campaign, it will play a secondary role in communicating important messages about the product. In addition to messages and related strategies, formative research includes specific questions about the type of communication channels consumers believe are most appropriate for the behavior change being addressed.

At the conclusion of Phase 4, communication channels are identified that are consistent with preliminary messages, and product distribution points and potential communication and intervention partners are identified.

Phase 5 of SMART is *develop interventions, materials and pretesting.* Once formative research is performed, it is critical that the data are transferred or infused adequately into the design of programs, interventions, and communication strategies. To do this, data must be analyzed and categorized appropriately to assure that planners understand what they have seen, heard, and observed. As planners meet to design programs and materials, they should keep formative research data in front of them and refer to them often. Discussion and decisions should reflect all data and represent a consensus among all planners. In other words, materials and methods should represent what was learned in formative research.

Once a program prototype is developed, it is imperative to return to the priority population and test the concepts before implementing a widespread campaign. In fact, social marketing represents a process of continually returning to the consumers until the program and all its support mechanisms are consistent with their views and preferences. Several mechanisms are available to perform pretesting. One example is a pilot test where the program can be implemented with the priority population on a smaller, less expensive scale. Phase 6 of SMART is *implementation.* This phase is concerned with clarifying everyone's role, including external partners. This means that procedures are communicated and documented, and that timelines are developed and followed. In this phase, the communication and distribution plans are activated and the actual program and its interventions are offered. In addition, the program is refined continually, based on consumer feedback.

The seventh and final phase of SMART is *evaluation.* The preliminary evaluation strategies that were identified in Phase 1 now take effect. Evaluation always has at least two major objectives: improve the quality of the program and determine the effectiveness of the program. With respect to quality, program planners assess the degree to which the priority population is actually receiving the program or interventions. Planners also assess the immediate impact the program is having and whether the interventions and related support strategies are acceptable and engaging to the priority population. In addition, planners ensure that program delivery is consistent with program protocol or at least consistent with developed timelines.

Ultimately, social marketing, and all its related work, is of little value unless behavior change occurs and health is improved. Evaluation also concerns itself with measuring these outcomes. Effective planners and evaluators also make sure that evaluation results are folded back into the program so that it can be improved before it is too late. This requires communicating evaluation results effectively to stakeholders.

▷ Other Planning Models

The Evidence-Based Planning Framework for Public Health, MAPP, MAP-IT, PRECEDE-PROCEED, Intervention Mapping, Healthy Communities (CHANGE tool), and SMART are all theoretically good models and can each be used to successfully plan, implement, and evaluate programs. While these specific models may be used more commonly in health promotion settings, still other models have been useful in various settings including Community-Based Prevention Marketing (Bryant, Forthofer, McCormack-Brown, Landis, & McDermott, 2000), PATCH (Lancaster & Kreuter, 2002), the Health Communication Model (National Cancer Institute, n.d.), Healthy Plan-It (Centers for Disease Control and Prevention, 2000), and SWOT (Strengths, Weaknesses, Opportunities, and Threats) (Panagiotou, 2003), which is more of a decision-making strategy than a traditional planning model. Technically, its use should be limited to the preliminary stages of decision making in preparation for more comprehensive strategic planning (Bartol & Martin, 1991; Johnson, Scholes, & Sexty, 1989).

▷ An Application of the Generalized Model

In practice, planners will often encounter situations where it is not feasible to use a model in its entirety or where it is necessary to combine parts of different models to meet specific needs. For this reason, the Generalized Model is used in this book to help you adapt and respond to complex planning challenges you will experience in professional practice. With planning expertise associated with your working knowledge of the Generalized Model, you will be able to more quickly assimilate and interpret varying or competing stakeholder preferences for planning into a guiding paradigm that will generally keep you on track. Although there is nothing unique about the Generalized Model itself, its principles are the building blocks for all other planning models. This likely became apparent to you as you reviewed the preceding planning models and noticed their many similarities. Each of these models in one form or another includes: pre-planning, assessing needs, setting goals and objectives, developing interventions, implementing interventions and evaluating results.

Another benefit of understanding the Generalized Model is an increased ability to apply an important process closely related to program planning—grant writing. Requirements listed in *requests for applications* (RFAs) or *requests for proposals* (RFPs) related to grant announcements will be developed by the funding agency/organization and include their preferences for language and terminology. But the steps or requirements related to requests for health funding often relate back to the steps displayed in the Generalized Model.

For example, funding requests from the CDC and other federal or national organizations generally require applicants to organize proposals with the following types of sections: background and statement of need; work plan; management plan; evaluation; and budget. These sections parallel closely with the Generalized Model: the background and statement of need relate to the needs assessment; the work plan includes goals and objectives as well as a description of interventions; and the management plan generally includes requirements for program implementation. The Community Tool Box (see Weblinks at the end of this chapter), a Website designed to assist health professionals with various tasks, outlines the standard components of a grant proposal. Sections include the statement of the problem/ needs assessment; project description (goals and objectives and methods/activities); the evaluation plan; and the budget request and justification (University of Kansas, 2015b).

To help you better understand how the Generalized Model might work in practice, we will use a hypothetical example to walk you through its five steps. Of course, in practice, stakeholders may choose a different approach than what is presented here. But at least you can see how the steps in the model build upon each other. While this example is hypothetical in nature, it is drawn from the 96 years of combined experience we as authors have with planning and evaluation in health promotion settings. In other words, it represents a realistic accumulation of our experience.

Let's assume Jane Doe, CHES, a recent health promotion graduate, has just been hired by a medium-sized county health department in California. She has been asked to lead a planning process to identify a health problem that will become the health department's key priority for the next three years.

The first thing Jane decides to do is some pre-planning. She sets out to identify key stakeholders who can help guide the process as well as partners who will help her carry out the work. She organizes a few meetings with stakeholders to discuss the collective vision for the process including purpose, scope, and deliverables as well as the leadership structure (i.e., authority, roles, and responsibilities). She ensures that a few partners are community residents who have volunteered previously with the health department and can help represent the community in general. Jane begins discussions with her partners to identify and secure resources to be able to implement a program once a priority health problem and priority population have been identified. Although Jane realizes she does not need to spend months or even weeks pre-planning, she understands the value of getting all stakeholders on the same page with respect to vision, leadership, and resources. This will help ensure a more positive and successful planning approach.

The actual planning and evaluation process begins with a *needs assessment*. Stakeholders determine together that they will collect data in three main categories: chronic diseases, infectious diseases, and injuries. Three teams are assembled to address each of the categories and each team is charged with identifying 8–10 leading health problems or diseases within the three categories. Teams agree to use a recent data report produced by the California Department of Health Services (organized by county) that describes leading causes of mortality, morbidity, and hospitalizations to select the 8–10 health problems for each of the categories. Stakeholders further determine that they will collect the following types of data for each of the 8–10 health problems: county-specific mortality and morbidity data; hospital discharge data; economic data; years of potential life lost; disability data; data on disparities; social determinants and risk factors for each health problem; and evidence of successful interventions that relate to the preventable nature of each health problem. The planning team decides on a presentation template for each health problem that includes graphs as well as brief descriptions for each of the predetermined criteria. The three planning teams decide to allow two months to collect and organize all the data.

After two months have passed, all three teams come together to compile their work in a single report and to make an oral presentation of their findings. Afterward, Jane and the community residents are given the assignment to use the basic priority rating (BPR) model 2.0 (Neiger, Thackeray, & Fagen, 2011) to narrow the list of health problems within each category to five (see Chapter 4 for BPR). Jane serves as the moderator of priority setting to make sure everyone understands the process. Within a week, five chronic diseases (heart disease, breast cancer, lung cancer, diabetes, and arthritis), five infectious diseases (HIV/AIDS, pneumonia, chlamydia, E.coli, and meningitis), as well as five unintentional injuries (falls, drownings, motor vehicle injuries, bicycle crashes, and auto-pedestrian injuries) surface as leading health problems in the county.

After preliminary priority setting, the group of stakeholders decides it would like to supplement its needs assessment with a series of focus groups throughout the county to determine what community residents feel are the most significant health problems among the initial priorities. Stakeholders decide to hire an evaluation firm to conduct 20 focus groups across the county and prepare a report. The final bid for services is $8,500, which the community outreach office of a local hospital agrees to pay.

As the evaluation firm begins to organize and conduct focus groups, stakeholders use the BPR model to further prioritize the remaining 15 health problems. Jane leads all discussions but is assisted by a program coordinator from the local chapter of the American Cancer Society who has years of experience in health promotion and some experience with the BPR model. It takes the group two additional meetings to develop a list of their top five priorities: (1) motor vehicle injuries; (2) heart disease; (3) breast cancer; (4) chlamydia; and (5) diabetes.

Within a month, the contracted evaluation team returns with its findings from the focus groups. Data indicate that the community believes effective prevention should start with children and adolescents and that the county should focus on childhood obesity as a risk factor for heart disease as well as the prevention of sexually transmitted diseases (i.e., chlamydia) among adolescents.

With these findings, Jane and her stakeholders are faced with a difficult decision. The BPR model and process produced a convincing case that motor vehicle injuries should be the county's top priority. But community residents are not in agreement. After thoughtful deliberation, stakeholders decide to develop a safe driving program among high school students throughout the county as well as a childhood obesity prevention program among elementary and junior high students. They further decide to create two planning teams for each of the priorities, with each team taking responsibility for grant writing and funding in general. The teams are also tasked to identify appropriate partners with specific expertise and resources in each of the two priority areas.

With health problems and priority populations identified, each newly formed team develops *goals and objectives* for each of the two priorities. Using *Healthy People* 2020 as a starting point, the teams develop general goals for each of the priorities as well as process, impact, and outcome objectives. The teams carefully develop their baseline measurements (i.e., starting points) for each objective based on the data collected in the needs assessment. Again, using the targets in *Healthy People 2020*, each team develops its own targets for each objective, ensuring that each one is specific, measurable, achievable, realistic, and time-phased.

With goals and objectives developed, the planning teams turn to *developing the interventions*, the third step in the Generalized Model. Here, planners need to determine if they will use existing programs and tailor them to their priority population or develop their own programs. Jane remembers from her undergraduate coursework that interventions need to be evidence-based. She works with both teams to ensure that the interventions selected will offer a high probability of success. In the end, the childhood obesity team decides to adapt a program from Utah titled *Gold Medal Schools*. This program is selected for its successful track record and its multifaceted approach combining educational components with policies leading to healthy school environments. The safe driving team selects a program called *Driving School Home*, a successful defensive driving course involving high school students from Illinois. Both teams then begin the process of fully understanding their programs and drafting budgets, including an analysis of how many staff members and volunteers would be required to implement each program, how much funding would be required to purchase program materials or capital equipment, and how much money might be required for consultants. Program protocols are available for each program and in a matter of weeks, both teams feel they understand the basic sequence of tasks and activities required to implement each program.

The fourth phase of the Generalized Model, *implementing interventions*, is focused on delivering interventions to the community. Before implementation occurs however, both teams begin to lay the necessary groundwork with school personnel to establish partnerships and to receive approval to proceed as planned. This becomes more complicated than Jane had anticipated. However, protocols and policies previously developed by the various school districts need to be observed. For example, one thing all school districts require is that each program be implemented on a pilot basis first to determine whether the likelihood of success is high enough to justify full implementation of the programs on a broader basis. In total, this process takes three months. But afterward, strong partnerships are established and implementation is approved for each program.

Implementation is equivalent to program management. In this phase, program partners ensure that programs are implemented as per predetermined protocol. Regular meetings are held to ensure that everyone is doing his/her job as planned. Managers follow up with their staff and make sure that timelines are carefully followed and that monies from approved budgets are accessible for program support. Implementation also focuses on marketing and communication. It is important that an adequate number of members from the priority population is reached and that enough people actually participate in the programs. Jane and her teams conduct in-depth interviews with school administrators to understand how to best communicate the purpose of the programs to potential participants (e.g., schools, students, and parents).

Jane helps to coordinate all the work of implementation and discovers that it takes a great deal of assertiveness and diplomacy to keep people moving forward on schedule. She also learns that certain aspects of both programs need to be modified in the process of implementation in order to increase the likelihood of their success. Toward the end of year one of implementation, Jane realizes that while neither program was implemented perfectly, both programs are running smoothly with continued enthusiasm and support.

During program implementation, Jane, along with two colleagues from the county health department conduct formative evaluation to ensure that the quality of program components and implementation are being presented as planned and that modifications are made continually to improve the likelihood of success. This also proves to be a challenge for Jane. During the course of implementing the *Driving School Home* program, she has to replace an ineffective teacher. As the *Gold Medal Schools* program is evaluated, Jane discovers that the kick-off assembly is too long and that both teachers and students are losing attention. When the assembly is shortened by 20 minutes and more incentives and small prizes are distributed, everyone feels more energized. These come to represent just a few of the many program improvements that are made during year one.

In addition, both teams had decided prior to implementation that outcome evaluation, which would measure both changes in behavior as well as decreases in the actual health problems, would be conducted by faculty and graduate students from a nearby university. University personnel were willing to conduct the research at no cost, providing they could use all data for publications in scientific journals. While the researchers required certain things of Jane and her partners, it became a win-win situation in the end. The researchers collected data immediately after the programs concluded and then again at three months after the conclusion of the programs. Data indicated that the *Gold Medal Schools* program was moderately effective and that the *Driving School Home* program was moderately to highly effective. Jane communicated to stakeholders that the programs were more likely to experience higher levels of success in future implementations based on continual improvements as part of formative and process evaluation. After data had been collected and analyzed, Jane made several presentations to stakeholders reporting on what went well and what went poorly. These presentations helped ensure continued funding for both programs.

To reiterate, the preceding example could have played out in many different ways based on the vision and competency of those leading the planning efforts. The purpose of the example was to describe how the phases in the Generalized Model might unfold. In practice, selecting a specific planning model to apply will be based on many factors: (1) the preferences of stakeholders (e.g., decision makers, program partners, consumers); (2) how much time and funding are available for planning purposes; (3) how many resources are available for data collection and analysis; (4) the degree to which clients are actually involved as partners in the planning process or the degree to which your planning efforts will be consumer oriented (i.e., planning is largely based on the wants and needs of consumers or the planning process is owned by the community itself); and (5) preferences of a funding agency (in the case of a grant or contract award). Planners must have the capacity to not only lead a planning process, but also negotiate these important issues among a diverse set of stakeholders.

▷ Final Thoughts on Choosing a Planning Model

Three important criteria, or the **three Fs of program planning**: *fluidity*, *flexibility*, and *functionality*, should also help guide the selection of your model and govern the application of its use. *Fluidity* suggests that steps in the planning process are sequential, or that they build on one another. It is usually a problem if certain steps in the planning process are performed out of sequence as diagrammed in the Generalized Model. For example, a planner cannot develop goals and objectives until a needs assessment has been performed and a priority health problem has been identified.

Flexibility means that planning is adapted to the needs of stakeholders. Due to various circumstances, planning is usually modified as the process unfolds. For example, some health problems, such as an outbreak of influenza, require a rapid assessment and scan of the environment. Strict adherence to a model in light of unique and pressing circumstances will generally lead to frustration among partners and a less-than-desirable outcome. *Functionality* means that the outcome of planning is improved health conditions, not the production of a program plan itself. A plan is only a tool to help planners accomplish their real work—to improve health and decrease disease and disability.

In addition to the *three Fs,* when deciding on a planning model, it is also important to ensure that the model is conducive to planning a **population-based approach** and that it uses an **ecological framework**. Whereas systematic and strategic planning efforts can address smaller populations such as those found in a small community or worksite, many planning processes pertain to large population segments of even larger populations—thus the term *population-based approach*.

Planners must also understand the interaction between a priority population and the communities in which they live. The ecological framework helps planners better appreciate that families, schools, employers, social networks, organizations, communities, and societies exert an influence on individuals and priority populations as they attempt to change health behaviors and improve their health (Bartholomew et al., 2011). Thus, planners must work with priority populations within the context of broad environments.

In addition, during pre-planning, planners need to determine the extent to which members of the priority population will be involved in the planning process and in decision making. This varies widely in practice and may range from no community involvement on one end of a continuum to an approach like community-based participatory research where the community itself owns the program and is the unit of identity, solution, and practice involved in all aspects of program development and delivery (Trickett, 2011). Ideally, planning efforts in health promotion should use a partnership-based approach in the context of community empowerment and mobilization where professionals work in unison with community members in taking actions to improve health and reduce disease.

 ## Summary

A model can provide the framework for planning a health promotion program. Several different planning models have been developed and revised over the years. The planning models for health promotion presented in this chapter have included:

1. The Generalized Model
2. Evidence-Based Planning Framework for Public Health
3. MAPP (Mobilizing for Action through Planning and Partnership)
4. MAP-IT (Mobilize, Assess, Plan, Implement, Track)
5. PRECEDE-PROCEED
6. Intervention Mapping
7. Healthy Communities (CHANGE tool)
8. SMART (Social Marketing Assessment and Response Tool)

The Generalized Model is recommended as the template for learning the basic principles of planning and evaluation: (1) assessing needs; (2) setting goals and objectives; (3) developing interventions; (4) implementing interventions; and (5) evaluating results. Several other models used in health promotion also continue to make valuable contributions typically using these same elements.

 ## Review Questions

1. How does an understanding of the Generalized Model help you understand other planning models?
2. What are the elements or steps in the Generalized Model that are common in most, if not all, other planning models?
3. Why is it important to use a model when planning?

4. How does pre-planning relate to most of the models presented in this chapter?

5. Explain the degree to which you believe consumers or members of the community should be involved in the planning process. Do you believe they should own or control the process?

Activities

1. After reviewing the models presented in this chapter, create your own model by identifying what you think are the common components of the models. Provide a rationale for including each component. Then draw a diagram of your model so that you can share it with the class. Be prepared to explain your model.

2. In a one-page paper, defend what you believe is the best planning model presented in this chapter.

3. Using a hypothetical health problem for a specific priority population, write a paper explaining the steps/phases for one of the models presented in this chapter.

4. Identify a health promotion program reported as successful in a scientific journal. What elements of the Generalized Model are described in the paper? Could you engage in an effective planning process based on the amount of information provided in the article? Summarize your comments in a one-page paper.

Weblinks

1. http://www.healthypeople.gov/2020/default.aspx

   Healthy People

   At this Website, *Healthy People 2020* is outlined with several helpful links including: (1) About Healthy People (background and general information); (2) *Healthy People* 2020 topics and objectives; (3) Data Search; (4) Leading Health Indicators (measurement and progress); (5) Healthy People in Action (the Healthy People 2020 consortium and stories from the field); and (6) Tools and Resources. This is a site with which planners in health promotion should be familiar.

2. http://prcstl.wustl.edu/training/Pages/EBPH-Course-Information.aspx

   Evidence-Based Planning for Public Health

   This Website displays the evidence-based planning framework for public health described in this chapter. PowerPoint presentations are provided for each skill and phase associated with this framework.

3. http://www.naccho.org/topics/infrastructure/mapp/index.cfm

   National Association of County and City Health Officials

   At this Website, the MAPP model is comprehensively diagrammed and explained. The four MAPP assessments are described, including how they are implemented, how to use subcommittees for each assessment, and how to make linkages between assessments.

4. http://www.healthypeople.gov/2020/tools-and-resources/Program-Planning

   MAP-IT: A Guide to Using *Healthy People 2020* in Your Community

This Website provides a valuable resource to assist health promotion professionals in implementing *Healthy People 2020*. The site includes field notes for each of the phases in MAP-IT with examples or case studies from various health organizations, as well as other resources and tool kits for each planning phase.

5. **http://www.cdc.gov/nccdphp/dch/programs/healthycommunitiesprogram/tools/change.htm**

   CHANGE Model (Community Health Assessment aNd Group Evaluation)

   This Website provides a detailed description of CDC's CHANGE model associated with the implementation of the Healthy Communities Approach.

6. **http://ctb.ku.edu/**

   Community Tool Box

   This Website is an indispensable tool for all planners in health promotion. According to the site, "The Tool Box offers more than 300 educational modules and other tools, many of which pertain to planning steps and phases discussed in this chapter.

7. **http://www.communityhlth.org/communityhlth/resources/hlthycommunities.html**

   Association for Community Health Improvement

   This Website provides additional information on the Healthy Communities Initiative including current projects and links.

8. **http://www.cdc.gov/healthcommunication/**

   Gateway to Health Communication and Social Marketing Practice, Centers for Disease Control and Prevention

   This Website provides an overview of health communication and social marketing practice including how to develop programs, segmenting an audience, and selecting appropriate channels and tools for program delivery.

Chapter

4

Assessing Needs

<table>
<tr><td>

Chapter Objectives

After reading this chapter and answering the questions at the end, you should be able to:

- Define *need* and *needs assessment*.
- Define *capacity, community capacity,* and *capacity building*.
- Explain why a needs assessment is an important part of the planning process.
- Explain what should be expected from a needs assessment.
- Differentiate between primary and secondary data sources.
- List the various methods for collecting primary data.
- Locate secondary data sources that are in print and on the World Wide Web.
- Explain how a needs assessment can be completed.
- Explain what is meant by health impact assessment.
- Conduct a needs assessment within a given population.

</td><td>

Key Terms

action research
basic priority rating
  (BPR)
bias
BPR model 2.0
capacity
capacity building
categorical funds
community capacity
community forum
Delphi technique
focus group
health assessments
  (HAs)
health impact
  assessment (HIA)
HIPAA
key informants
mapping
need
needs assessment
networking

nominal group
  process
observation
obtrusive observation
opinion leaders
participatory data
  collection
participatory research
photovoice
primary data
proxy measure
random-digit dialing
  (RDD)
secondary data
self-assessments
self-report
significant others
single-step survey
unobtrusive
  observation
walk-through
windshield tour

</td></tr>
</table>

Once the planning committee is in place and a planning model has been selected, the next step in the planning process is to identify the needs of those in the priority population. Gilmore (2012) has defined **need** as "the difference between the present situation and a more desirable one" (p. 8). These needs can be expressed in many different ways. For example, there may be a need for better health, or a need for more knowledge, or a need to possess a certain skill, to name a few. Whether a need of the priority population is actual (*true* need) or perceived (*reported* need) does not matter (Gilmore, 2012). What matters is being able to identify all needs, actual and perceived, so that they can be addressed through appropriate program planning.

From an epidemiologic viewpoint, a *needs assessment* has been defined as "[a] systematic procedure for determining the nature and extent of problems experienced by a specific population that affect their health either directly or indirectly" (Porta, 2014, p. 195). From a program planning viewpoint, a **needs assessment** is defined as the process of identifying, analyzing, and prioritizing the needs of a priority population. Other terms that have been used to describe the process of determining needs include *community analysis, community diagnosis,* and *community assessment.* Conducting a needs assessment may be the most critical step in the planning process because it "provides objective data to define important health problems, sets priorities for program implementation, and establishes a baseline for evaluating program impact" (Grunbaum et al., 1995, p. 54).

There are many reasons why a needs assessment should be completed before the other steps of the planning process begin. First, it is a logical place to start (Gilmore, 2012). Before a need can be met, it first must be identified and measured. Second, a needs assessment can help ensure that scarce resources are allocated where they can give maximum health benefit (Rowe, McClelland, & Billingham (2001). Without determining and prioritizing needs, resources can be wasted on unsubstantiated programming. Third, a needs assessment allows planners to "apply the principles of equity and social justice in practice" (Rowe et al., 2001) by focusing on those in greatest need. Fourth, failure to perform a needs assessment may lead to a program focus that prevents or delays adequate attention directed to a more important health problem. For example, a health problem that tends to create a high emotional response, particularly among parents, is the trauma associated with bicycle injuries in children. Of course, it is a tragedy when a preventable death occurs. In 2013, 7% of the 743 bicyclists killed in the United States were children age 15 and under (NHTSA, 2015). But an even more significant determinant of childhood injury and death in the United States is the inadequate use of safety belts or car seats involved with motor vehicle crashes. In fact, motor vehicle crashes are the leading cause of death among children in the United States (Sauber-Schatz, West, & Bergen, 2014). A needs assessment that examined both bicycle and motor vehicle crashes would lead planners to determine in most locations, in most instances, that restraining children in motor vehicles with safety belts or approved car seats is a more important issue.

Fifth, a needs assessment can determine the capacity of a community to address specific needs. **Capacity** refers to the individual, organizational, and community resources, such as leadership, relationships, operations, structures, infrastructure, politics, and systems, to name a few, that can enable a community to take action (Brennan Ramirez, Baker, & Metzler, 2008; Gilmore, 2012). In other words, when related to health promotion, **community capacity** is the "characteristics of communities that affect their ability to identify, mobilize, and address social and public health problems" (Goodman et al., 1998, p. 259) (see Chapter 9 for mapping community capacity). "Assessing community capacity helps you think about existing community strengths that can be mobilized to address social, economic, and environmental conditions affecting health inequities. In general, you should look at the places (e.g., parks, libraries) and organizations (e.g., education, health care, faith-based groups, social services, volunteer groups, businesses, local government, law enforcement) in various sectors of the community" (Brennan Ramirez et al., 2008, p. 54). "It is also important to identify the nature of the relationships across these sectors (e.g., norms, values), with the community (e.g., civic participation), and among various subgroups within the community (e.g., distribution of power and authority, trust, identity)" (Sampson & Raudenbush, 1999, and Trachim, 1989, as cited in Brennan Ramirez et al., 2008, p. 54).

Sixth, a needs assessment can provide a focus for developing an intervention to meet the needs of the priority population. And finally, knowing the needs of a priority population provides a reference point to which future assessments can be compared.

Having just stated several reasons why a needs assessment should be completed, it may seem odd that there are a few planning scenarios in which a needs assessment would not be used. The first would be if another needs assessment had been conducted recently, possibly for another related program, and the funding or other resources to conduct a second needs assessment in such a short period of time were not available. A second scenario in which a needs assessment may not be used is one where the program planners are employed by an agency that deals only with a specific need that is already known (e.g., cancer and the American Cancer Society), or the agency for which they work has received **categorical funds** that are earmarked or dedicated to a specific disease (e.g., HIV/AIDS), health determinant (e.g., risk factor), or program (e.g., immunization).

Although a needs assessment has long been an important step in health promotion process, two recent events have made the public more aware of the importance of a needs assessment. In 2003, the Institute of Medicine (2003) recommended examination of health department accreditation as a means of improving public health agency performance. After such an examination, the Public Health Accreditation Board (PHAB) was created in 2007 to create an accreditation process for governmental public health departments operated by tribes, states, local jurisdictions, and territories (PHAB, 2013b). In July 2011, PHAB released the *Accreditation Standards and Measures*. In order for a health department to become accredited, it must show its work meets the standards and measures that are spread over 12 domains. The first domain, which is a needs assessment, is stated as "Conduct and Disseminate Assessments Focused on Population Health Status and Public Health Issues facing the Community" (PHAB, 2013a, p. 13).

The second event that has made needs assessments more visible to the public was the passing of the Patient Protection and Affordable Care Act (PPACA also known as the ACA) that added section 501(r) to the Internal Revenue Code. Under section 501(r) of the code, 501(c)(3) organizations that operate one or more hospitals (i.e., non-profit hospitals) must meet four general requirements in order for the organization to maintain its 501(c)(3) tax-exempt status. One of the four general requirements is to conduct a community health needs assessment (CHNA) and adopt an implementation strategy for addressing the needs at least once every three years (CDC, n.d.b). Further, the IRS guidelines require that these organizations partner with a public health agency in conducting the CHNA. Each of these events that require community needs assessments will add to improving the community's health.

The remaining portions of this chapter will present discussions on what to expect from a needs assessment, the types and sources of data used to conduct a needs assessment, and a suggested process for conducting a needs assessment. **Box 4.1** identifies the responsibilities and competencies for health education specialists that pertain to the material presented in this chapter.

BOX

4.1

Focus On

Responsibilities and Competencies for Health Education Specialists

The content of this chapter is associated with a single area of responsibility. That responsibility and related competencies include:

RESPONSIBILITY I: Assess Needs, Resources, and Capacity for Health Education/Promotion

Competency 1.1: Plan assessment process for health education/promotion

Competency 1.2: Access existing information and data related to health

Competency 1.3: Collect primary data to determine needs

Competency 1.4: Analyze relationships among behavioral, environmental, and other factors that influence health

Competency 1.5: Examine factors that influence the process by which people learn

Competency 1.6: Examine factors that enhance or impede the process of health education/promotion

Competency 1.7: Determine needs for health education/promotion based on assessment findings

Source: *A Competency-Based Framework for Health Education Specialists—2015*. Whitehall, PA: National Commission for Health Education Credentialing, Inc. (NCHEC) and the Society for Public Health Education (SOPHE). Reprinted by permission of the National Commission for Health Education Credentialing, Inc. (NCHEC) and the Society for Public Health Education (SOPHE).

▷ What to Expect from a Needs Assessment

Several authors have provided lists of questions that should be answered after completing a needs assessment. They include:

1. Who makes up the priority population? (Petersen & Alexander, 2011)

2. What are the needs of the priority population? (Petersen & Alexander, 2011)

3. Why do these needs exist? (NACCHO, n.d.)

4. What factors create or determine the need? (NACCHO, n.d.)

5. Which subgroups within the priority population have the greatest need? (Petersen & Alexander, 2011)

6. Where are these subgroups located geographically? (Petersen & Alexander, 2011)

7. What resources are available to address the needs? (NACCHO, n.d.)

8. What is currently being done to resolve identified needs? (Petersen & Alexander, 2011)

9. How well have the identified needs been addressed in the past? (Petersen & Alexander, 2011)

Indirectly, getting answers to the latter three questions, numbers 7, 8, and 9, provides some information about the community capacity and whether part of the identified needs may include the need to build capacity. **Capacity building** refers to activities that enhance the resources of individuals, organizations, and communities to improve their effectiveness to take action.

No matter how needs assessment is defined, the concept embedded in the definitions is the same: identifying the needs of the priority population and determining the degree to which the needs are being met. If needs are not being met, there may also be a need to enhance capacity of the community.

▷ Acquiring Needs Assessment Data

Two types of data are generally associated with a needs assessment: primary data and secondary data. **Primary data** are those data you collect yourself (via a survey, a focus group, in-depth interviews, etc.) that answer unique questions related to your specific needs assessment. Most methods of collecting primary data are ones in which those collecting the data interact with (e.g., interviewing) or minimally interact with (e.g., windshield tour) those from whom the data are being collected. Such methods have been labeled as *interactive contact methods* or *minimal contact observational methods* (Marti-Costa & Serrano-Garcia as cited in Hancock & Minkler, 2012). **Secondary data** are those data already collected by somebody else and available for your use. Thus, the methods to collect these data have been labeled as *no contact methods* (Marti-Costa & Serrano-Garcia as cited in Hancock & Minkler, 2012). The advantages of using secondary data are that (1) they already exist, and thus collection time is minimal, and (2) they are usually fairly inexpensive to access compared to primary data. Both of these advantages are important to planners because programs are often planned when both time and money are limited. However, a drawback of using secondary data is that the information might not identify the true needs of the priority population—perhaps because of how the data were collected, when they were collected, what variables were considered, or from whom the data were collected. A good rule is to move cautiously and make sure the secondary data are applicable to the immediate situation before using them.

Primary data have the advantage of directly answering the questions planners want answered by those in the priority population. However, collecting primary data can be expensive and when done correctly, take a great deal of time.

An overview of the means of acquiring primary and secondary data are presented in the following pages.

Sources of Primary Data

Primary data can be collected using a variety of methods. Those most commonly used in planning health promotion programs are presented in **Box 4.2**.

SINGLE-STEP OR CROSS-SECTIONAL SURVEYS

Single-step surveys, or as they are often called *cross-sectional* (point-in-time) *surveys,* are a means of gathering primary data from individuals or groups with a single contact—thus, the term *single-step*. Such surveys often take the form of written questionnaires and interviews. When individuals or groups (also sometimes called *respondents* or *participants*) are answering questions about themselves, the information that is provided is referred to as **self-report** data. Thus, respondents are asked to recall (e.g., "When was your last visit to your dentist?") and report accurate information (e.g., "On average, how many minutes do you exercise each day?"). Self-report measures are essential for many needs assessments and evaluations because of the need to obtain subjective assessments of experiences (e.g., feelings about available programs, self-assessments of health status, and health behavior, such as eating patterns) (Bowling, 2005). "For some behaviors, such as safer sex behaviors, this is the only way one can measure behavior" (Sharma & Petosa, 2014, p. 100). Even marketing data (e.g., the best location for a program, the best time to offer a program, and willingness to pay for a

BOX

4.2

Focus On

Sources of Primary Data

Single-Step or Cross-Sectional Surveys	Community Forum (Town Hall Meeting)
From priority population—self-report	Meetings
written questionnaires	Focus Group
telephone interviews	Nominal Group Process
face-to-face interviews	Observation
electronic interviews	Direct observation
group interviews	Indirect observation (proxy measures)
Proxy measures	"Windshield" or walk-through (walking tours)
From significant others	
From opinion leaders	Photovoice and videovoice
From key informants	Self-Assessments
Multistep Survey: Delphi Technique	

program) and capacity data (e.g., "What resources are needed to make this change?) can be collected through these assessments. In addition, self-report measures have a broad appeal to those who need to collect data, because "they are often quick to administer and involve little interpretation by the investigator" (Bowling, 2005, p. 15). However, planners should be aware that self-report data do have limitations. One such limitation is **bias** (Windsor, 2015)—those data that have been distorted because of the way they have been collected. (See the section in Chapter 5 on bias free data.) To overcome some of these limitations and to maximize the usefulness of self-report, Baranowski (1985) has developed eight steps to increase the accuracy of this method of data collection:

1. Select measures that clearly reflect program outcomes.
2. Select measures that have been designed to anticipate the response problems and that have been validated.
3. Conduct a pilot study with the priority population. (See Chapter 5 for pilot studies.)
4. Anticipate and correct any major sources of unreliability.
5. Employ quality-control procedures to detect other sources of error.
6. Employ multiple methods.
7. Use multiple measures.
8. Use experimental and control groups with random assignment to control for biases in self-report.

By following these steps, planners can enhance the accuracy of self-report, making this a more effective method of data collection.

For a variety of reasons, there are times when those in the priority population cannot respond for themselves or do not want to respond. For example, children who have not learned how to read yet or people with dementia (Streiner, Norman, & Cairrney, 2015). In such situations, planners will have to collect data indirectly by asking another (i.e., *proxy reporter*) (Streiner et al., 2015) or looking for indications of a behavior. Such a method is referred to as a proxy (or indirect) measure. A **proxy measure** is an outcome measure that provides evidence that a behavior has occurred. Or as Dignan (1995) stated, "indirect measures are unmistakable signs that a specific behavior has occurred" (p. 103). Examples of proxy measures include (1) lower blood pressure for the behavior of medication taking, (2) body weight for the behaviors of exercise and dieting, (3) cotinine in the blood for tobacco use, (4) empty alcoholic beverages in the trash for consumption of alcohol, or (5) another person reporting on the compliance of his/her partner (Cottrell & McKenzie, 2011). Proxy measurements of skills or behavior usually require more resources and cooperation to obtain than self-report or direct observation (Dignan, 1995). The greatest concern associated with proxy measures is making sure that the measure is both valid and reliable (Cottrell & McKenzie, 2011).

In addition to surveying the priority population, there are other groups of individuals who are commonly asked to respond to single-step surveys for the purpose of collecting primary needs assessment data. They include significant others of the priority population, community opinion leaders, and key informants. **Significant others** may include family members and friends. Collecting data from the significant others of a group of heart disease patients is a good example. Program planners might find it difficult to persuade heart disease patients themselves to share information about their outlook on life and living with heart disease. A survey of spouses or other family members might help elicit this information so that the program planners could best meet the needs of the heart disease patients.

Opinion leaders are individuals who are well respected in a community and who can accurately represent the views of the priority population. These leaders are:

1. Discriminating users of the media

2. Demographically similar to the priority group

3. Knowledgeable about community issues and concerns

4. Early adopters of innovative behavior (see Chapter 11 for an explanation of these terms)

5. Active in persuading others to become involved in innovative behavior

Opinion leaders include political figures, chief executive officers (CEOs) of companies, union leaders, administrators of local school districts, and other highly visible and respected individuals. (See **Figure 4.1** for a form for tallying opinion leader survey data.)

Key informants are individuals with unique knowledge about a particular topic. For example, it may be a person who has had a specific problem like losing weight being able to talk about the barriers of such an experience, or a person who has tried to get health insurance through an exchange only to be denied coverage. Because their information may only represent a single experience and thus be biased, planners need to be careful not to base an entire needs assessment on the data generated from a key informant survey.

Single-step surveys of those in the priority population, significant others, opinion leaders, and key informants can be administered, as noted earlier, several different ways. The primary means of collecting data from these individuals include written questionnaires, telephone interviews, face-to-face interviews, electronic interviews, and group interviews. A discussion of each follows.

WRITTEN QUESTIONNAIRES

One of the most often used methods of collecting self-reported data is the written questionnaire. It has several advantages, notably the ability to reach a large number of

Data collection method			Number of interviewers
Total number of people interviewed			From: _____ To: ____
			Date Collected _____

Rank	Health Problem	**Number of Persons Identifying Problem**	**Percentage of Persons Identifying Problem**
1.			
2.			
3.			
4.			
5.			
6.			
7.			
8.			
9.			
10.			

▲ **Figure 4.1** Form to Tally Opinion Leader Survey Data
Source: U.S. Department of Health and Human Services, Centers for Disease Control and Prevention (no date), p. A3–12.

respondents in a short period of time, even if there is a large geographic area to be covered. This method offers low cost with minimum staff time needed. However, it often has the lowest response rate.

With a written questionnaire, each individual receives the same questions and instructions in the same format, so that the possibility of response bias is lessened. The corresponding disadvantage, however, is the inability to clarify any questions or confusion on the part of the respondent. As mentioned, the response rate for mailed questionnaires tends to be low especially if respondents cannot remain anonymous, but there are several ways to overcome this problem. One way is to include with the questionnaire a postcard that identifies the person in some way (such as by name or identification number). The individual is asked to return the questionnaire in the envelope provided and to send the postcard back separately. Anonymity is thus maintained, but the planner/evaluator knows who has returned a questionnaire. The planner/evaluator can then send a follow-up mailing (including a letter indicating the importance of a response and another copy of the questionnaire with a return envelope) to the individuals who did not return a postcard from the first mailing. The use of incentives also can increase the response rate. For example, some hospitals offer free health risk appraisals to those who return a completed needs assessment instrument.

The appearance of the questionnaire is also extremely important when collecting data. It should be attractive, easy to read, and offer ample space for the respondents' answers. It should also be easy to understand and complete, because written questionnaires provide no opportunity to clarify a point while the respondent is completing the questionnaire. In addition, all mailed questionnaires should be accompanied by a cover letter, to help clarify directions for completion (see Chapter 5 for more information on questionnaire design).

Short questionnaires that do not take a long time to complete and questionnaires that clearly explain the need for the information are more likely to be returned. Planners/evaluators should give thought to designing a questionnaire that is as easy to complete and return as possible. For other strategies to increase response rates to written questions delivered via the postal service see the systematic review conducted by Edwards et al. (2009).

FACE-TO-FACE INTERVIEWS

At times, it is advantageous to administer the instrument to the respondents in a face-to-face interview setting. This method is time consuming because it may require not only time for the actual interview but also travel time to the interview site and/or waiting time between interviews. The interviewer must be carefully trained to conduct the interview in an unbiased manner. It is important to explain the need for the information in order to conduct the needs assessment/evaluation and to accurately record the responses. Methods of probing, or eliciting additional information about an individual's responses, are used in the face-to-face interview, and the interviewer must be skilled at this technique.

This method of self-report allows the interviewer to develop rapport with the respondent. The flexibility of this method, along with the availability of visual cues, has the advantage of gaining more complete data from respondents. Smaller numbers of respondents are included in this method, but the rate of participation is generally high. It is important to establish and follow procedures for selecting the respondents. There are also several disadvantages to the face-to-face interview. It is more expensive, requiring more staff time and training of interviewers. Variations in the interviews, as well as differences between interviewers, can influence the results.

TELEPHONE INTERVIEWS

Compared to mailed surveys or face-to-face interviews, the telephone interview offers a relatively easy method of collecting self-reported data at a moderate cost. But it is not as easy and inexpensive as it once was "due in part to the increasing use of cell phones" (SHADAC, 2009, p. 1). The number of households in the United States that do not have landline telephone service, known as *wireless-only households*, continues to grow. It has been estimated that more than two out of five American homes (44.0%) have only wireless telephones and another 2.6% do not have any phone service (Blumberg & Luke, 2014). The prevalence of such 'wireless-only' households now markedly exceeds the prevalence of households with only landline telephones (8.5%), and this difference is expected to grow (Blumberg & Luke, 2014). Those most likely to live in wireless-only households are younger, living with other nonrelated adults, renting their residence, and being non-white (Blumberg & Luke, 2014). Therefore, depending on whom planners/evaluators are trying to interview and how they plan to select the participants for interviews, some individuals may not have a chance of being selected and/or contacted.

Prior to so many people living in wireless-only households, participants who were to be interviewed by telephone were selected using some type of random process. One method was to randomly select people from a "list." For example, a program participants' list, a local telephone book, student directory, church directory, or employee directory. However, selecting people randomly from a list misses people with unlisted telephone numbers and/or cell phones. One way to overcome this problem is a method known as **random-digit dialing (RDD)**, in which telephone number combinations are chosen at random. This method would include businesses as well as residences and nonworking as well as valid numbers, making it more time consuming. The numbers may be obtained from a table of random numbers or generated by a computer. The advantage of random-digit dialing is that it includes the entire survey population with a telephone in the area, including people with unlisted numbers and cell phones. However, there are several drawbacks to using RDD. The first is that those with cell phones may not have a telephone number with an area code in which they live. This is a problem because in order to use the RDD technique both the area codes and the exchanges (i.e., the first three digits of the seven-digit telephone number) must be known. Another drawback is some peoples' resistance to answering questions over the telephone or resentment about being interrupted with an unwanted call. And finally, those conducting the interviews may also have a difficult time reaching individuals because of unanswered phones or answering machines.

Like face-to-face interviews, telephone interviewing requires trained interviewers; without proper training and use of a standard questionnaire, the interviewer may not be consistent during the interview. Explaining a question or offering additional information can cause a respondent to change an initial response, thus creating a chance for interviewer bias. The interviewer does have the opportunity to clarify questions, which is an advantage over the written questionnaire, but does not have the advantage of visual cues that the face-to-face interview offers.

ELECTRONIC INTERVIEWS

With more and more individuals having access to the Internet and email [87% of U.S. adults use the Internet, and 72% of Internet users say they looked online for health information during the past year (Pew Research Center, 2014)], it was only a matter of time until planners/evaluators used them to conduct interviews. Advantages to using this type of interviewing compared to using a written questionnaire include the reduced response time, cost of materials, ease of data collection, flexibility in the design and format of the questionnaire, control over the administration such as distribution to the recipients all at the same time on the same day, and recipient familiarity with the format and technology (Neutens & Rubinson, 2014). In addition, responses received can be formatted to enter directly into a spreadsheet/statistical package eliminating manual data entry or scanning (Cottrell & McKenzie, 2011). However, there are several drawbacks to using the Internet for interviewing: not everyone has access to the Internet, obtaining email addresses of the possible respondents can be difficult, and some people's lack of comfort in using a computer. To date, studies in the literature on the response rate to electronic interviews has been mixed, with some studies reporting good results and others reporting lower rates similar to written questionnaires sent via the U.S. mail (Cottrell & McKenzie, 2011).

With the expanded use of the Internet has come an increase in the number of commercial companies (e.g., FluidSurveys, Qualtrics, QuestionPro, SurveyMonkey, surveygizmo, Zoomerang) that offer services to assist those in using this method of interviewing. This is how they work. Customers sign up and pay a fee. For the most part, the fee is based on the amount of service provided and the length of time the service is used. Typical services offered include design and preparation of the questionnaire, translation of the questionnaire into another language, customizing the questionnaire with organization logo/branding, personalized email cover letter introducing the questionnaire, personalized email thank-you letters for those who complete the instrument, data tallying and analysis, various trainings, and customer support. The costs of the services vary depending on the type of customer, but most companies provide a discount for not-for-profit and educational organizations. Some companies provide free options for limited use. One drawback of such commercial services is that they may not meet the security policies of some potential users (e.g., medical centers).

GROUP INTERVIEWS

Interviewing individuals in groups provides for economy of scale. That is, data can be collected from several people in a short period of time. But there are some drawbacks of such data collection that primarily revolve around one or more group members' influencing the response of others. A specific form of group interview discussed later in this chapter is focus groups. Focus groups are useful in collecting information for a needs assessment, but can also be used to determine if programs are being implemented effectively or determine program outcomes.

MULTISTEP SURVEY

As its title suggests, a multistep survey is one in which those collecting the data contact those who will provide the data on more than one occasion. The technique that uses this process is called the **Delphi technique**. It is a process that generates consensus through a series of questionnaires, which are usually administered via mail or electronic mail. The process begins with those collecting the data asking the priority population to respond to one or two broad questions. The responses are analyzed, and a second questionnaire with more specific questions based on responses to the first questionnaire, is developed and sent to the priority population. The answers to these more specific questions are analyzed again, and another new questionnaire is created and sent out, requesting additional information. If consensus is reached, the process may end here; if not, it may continue for another round or two (Gilmore, 2012). Most often, this process continues for five or fewer rounds.

COMMUNITY FORUM

The **community forum**, also sometimes referred to as a *town hall meeting,* approach brings together people from the priority population to discuss what they see as their group's problems/ needs. It is not uncommon for a community forum to be organized by a group representing the priority population, in conjunction with the program planners. Such groups include labor, civic, religious, or service organizations, or groups such as the Parent Teacher Association (PTA). Once people have arrived, a moderator explains the purpose of the meeting and then asks those from the priority population to share their concerns. One or several individuals from the organizing group, called *recorders,* are usually given the responsibility for taking notes or recording the session to ensure that the responses are documented accurately. However, when moderating a community forum, it is important to be aware that the silent majority may not speak out and/or a vocal minority may speak too loudly. For example, an individual parent's view may be wrongly interpreted to be the view of all parents.

At a community forum, participants may also be asked to respond in writing (1) by answering specific questions or (2) by completing some type of instrument. **Figure 4.2** is an example of an instrument that could be used to collect data from participants in a community forum.

MEETINGS

Meetings are a good source of information for a preliminary needs assessment or various aspects of evaluation. For example, if a health department is planning to conduct a needs

Directions: Please rank the need for each program in the community by placing a number in the space to the left of the programs. Use 1 to rank the program of greatest need, 2 for the next greatest need, and so forth, until you have ranked all seven programs. The program with the highest number next to it should be the one that, in your opinion, is least needed. If you feel that a program should not be considered for implementation in our community, please place an X in the space to the left of the program instead of a number. Please note that the number you place next to each program represents its need in the community, not necessarily your desire to participate in it. After ranking the program, place an X to the right of the program in the column(s) that represent the age group(s) to which you feel the program should be targeted.

Program	All ages	Children 5–12	Teens 13–19	Adults 20–64	Older adults 65+
_____ Alcohol education:	_____	_____	_____	_____	_____
_____ Exercise/fitness:	_____	_____	_____	_____	_____
_____ Nutrition education:	_____	_____	_____	_____	_____
_____ Safety belt use:	_____	_____	_____	_____	_____
_____ Smoking cessation:	_____	_____	_____	_____	_____
_____ Smoking education:	_____	_____	_____	_____	_____
_____ Weight loss:	_____	_____	_____	_____	_____

▲ **Figure 4.2** Instrument for Ranking Program Need

Source: *Instrument for Ranking Program Need.* Amy L. Bernard. Copyright © 2011 by Amy L. Bernard. Reprinted with permission.

assessment and would like some direction on what health topics to key in on, planners may meet with a small group from the priority population to find out what they see as health issues in the community.

The meeting structure can be flexible to avoid limiting the scope of the information gained. The cost of this form of data collection is minimal. Possible biases may occur when meetings are used as the sole source of data collection. Those involved may give "socially acceptable" responses to questions rather than discussing actual concerns. There also may be limited input if relatively few participants are included, or if one or two participants dominate the discussion.

FOCUS GROUP

The **focus group** is a form of qualitative research that grew out of group therapy. Focus groups are used to obtain information about the feelings, opinions, perceptions, insights, beliefs, misconceptions, attitudes, and receptivity of a group of people concerning an idea or issue. Focus groups are rather small, compared to community forums, and usually include only 8 to 12 people. If possible, it is best to have a group of people who do not know each other so that their responses are not inhibited by acquaintance. Participation in the group is by invitation. People are invited about one to three weeks in advance of the session. At the time of the invitation, they receive general information about the session but are not given any specifics. This precaution helps ensure that responses will be spontaneous yet accurate. Once assembled, the group is led by a skilled moderator who has the task of obtaining candid responses from the group to a set of predetermined questions. In addition to eliciting responses to the questions, the moderator may ask the group to prioritize the different responses. As in a community forum, the answers to the questions are recorded through either written notes and/or audio or video recordings, so that at a later date the interested parties can review and interpret the results.

Focus groups are not easy to conduct. Special care must be given to developing the questions that will be asked. Poorly written questions will yield information that is less than useful. In addition, the moderator should be one who is skilled in leading a group. As might be surmised, the level of skill needed to conduct a focus group increases as the topic of discussion becomes more controversial.

Although focus groups have been shown to be an effective way of gathering data, they do have one major limitation. Participants in the groups are usually not selected through a random-sampling process. They are generally selected because they possess certain attributes (e.g., individuals of low income, city dwellers, parents of disabled children, or chief executive officers of major corporations). Participants may not be representative of the priority population. Therefore, the results of the focus group are not generalizable (CDC, 2008a). For more detail and information about preparing for and conducting focus groups, see Gilmore (2012), National Cancer Institute (n.d.), and Teufel-Shone & Williams (2010).

NOMINAL GROUP PROCESS

The **nominal group process** is a highly structured process in which a few knowledgeable representatives of the priority population (5 to 7 people) are asked to qualify and quantify specific needs. Those invited to participate are asked to record their responses to a question without discussing it among themselves. Once all have recorded a response, participants share their responses in a round-robin fashion. While this is occurring, the facilitator is recording the responses on a computer screen, chalkboard or flipchart for all to see. The responses are clarified through a discussion. After the discussion, the participants are asked to rank-order the responses by importance to the priority population. This ranking may be considered either a preliminary or a final vote. If it is preliminary, it is followed with more discussion and a final vote.

OBSERVATION

Observation, defined as "notice taken of an indicator" (Green & Lewis, 1986, p. 363), can also be an effective means of collecting data. Not only can people be observed, but the environment (i.e., those things around the priority population) can be observed as well. Because those doing the observation can "see" but do not interact with those in the priority, observation has been labeled a *minimal-contact method of data collection.*

Observation can be direct or indirect. *Direct observation* means actually seeing a situation or behavior. For example, direct observation may include watching the eating patterns of children in a school lunchroom, observing workers on an assembly line to see if they are wearing their protective glasses, checking the smoking behavior of employees on break, and observing drivers for safety belt use. This method is somewhat time consuming, but it seldom encounters the problem of people refusing to participate in the data collection, resulting in a high response rate.

Observation is generally more accurate than self-report, but the presence of the observer may alter the behavior of the people being observed. For example, having someone observe smoking behavior may cause smokers to smoke less out of self-consciousness due to their being under observation. When people know they are being observed it is referred to as **obtrusive observation**. **Unobtrusive observation** means just the opposite; the persons being studied are not aware they are being measured, assessed, or tested. Typically, unobtrusive observation provides less biased data, but some question whether unobtrusive observation is ethical.

Differences among observers may also bias the results, because different observers may not observe and report behaviors in the same manner. Some behaviors, such as safety belt use, are very easy to observe accurately. Others, such as a person's degree of tension, are more difficult to observe. This method of data collection requires a clear definition of the exact behavior to observe and how to record it (i.e., having an observation checklist), in order to avoid subjective observations. Observer bias can be reduced by providing training and by determining rater reliability. If the observers are skilled, observation can provide accurate needs assessment or evaluation data at a moderate cost.

As noted earlier in this chapter, *indirect observation* (or proxy measure) can also be used to determine whether a behavior has occurred. This can be completed by either "observing" the outcomes of a behavior (e.g., pills left in a bottle) or by asking others (e.g., spouse) to report on such outcomes (see the earlier discussion on proxy measures). In addition, these measures can be used to verify self-reports when observations of the actual changes in behavior cannot be observed.

Some specific methods of observation that have been useful in collecting data for health promotion programs are *windshield tours* or *walk-throughs* and *photovoice*. When using a **windshield tour** or **walk-through**, the person(s) doing the observation "walks or drives slowly through a neighborhood, ideally on different days of the week and at different times of the day, 'on the lookout' for a whole variety of potentially useful indicators of community health and well-being" (Hancock & Minkler, 2012, p. 164). Potentially useful indicators may include: "(A) Housing types and conditions, (B) Recreational and commercial facilities, (C) Private and public sector services, (D) Social and civic activities, (E) Identifiable neighborhoods or residential clusters, (F) Conditions of roads and distances most travel, (G) Maintenance of buildings, grounds and yards" (Eng & Blanchard, 1990–1991, p. 96–97).

Photovoice (formerly called photo novella) is the creation of Wang and Burris (1994, 1997). It is a form of **participatory data collection** (i.e., those in the priority population participate in the data collection) in which those in the priority population are provided with cameras and skills training (on photography, ethics, data collection, critical discussion, and policy), then use the cameras to convey their own images of the community problems and strengths (Kramer et al., 2010; Minkler & Wallerstein, 2012). "Photovoice has 3 main goals: (1) to enable people to record and reflect their community's strengths and concerns; (2) to promote critical dialogue and enhance knowledge about issues through group discussions of the photographs; and (3) to inform policy makers" (FYVPC, 2006, para. 2).

Photovoice has been used a lot with "marginalized groups of various ages that want their perspective seen and heard by those in power" (WCPH, 2009, p. 1). More recently it has been receiving increased attention because of its application to health promotion. There are a number of reports of its use in the literature that have resulted in successful policy and environmental changes (e.g., Goodhard et al., 2006; Kramer et al., 2010; Wang, Morrel-Samuels, Hutchinson, Bell, & Pestronk, 2004). It has also been used with a variety of community and public health problems.

The process for using photovoice involves the following steps: (1) defining the goals and objectives of the project; (2) identifying the community participants; (3) providing participants with the purpose and philosophy behind photovoice; (4) providing participants with training to carry out the project; (5) providing a theme for taking the pictures (e.g., "show what is unhealthy about our community"); (6) letting the participants take the pictures; (7) selecting the photographs that reflect the concerns of the project; (8) in groups, engaging in meaningful dialogue about the significance of each photograph; (9) contextualizing the photographs by writing captions based on the mnemonic SHOWeD created by Wallerstein (1987) (i.e., What do you See here? What's really Happening here? How does this relate to Our lives? Why does this problem or this strength exist? What can we Do about this?); (10) codifying the results by identifying the issues, themes, or theories that emerge; (11) identifying the stakeholders and venues to present the results; (12) making the presentation(s) to the community stakeholders (e.g., policy makers, decision makers) and the public; and (13) taking action based on results of the photovoice process (Downey, Ireson, Scutchfield, 2009; Kramer et al., 2010; STEPS Centre, 2015; University of Kansas, 2014; Wang & Burris, 1997; Wang, Morrel-Samuels, et al., 2004; Wang, Yi, Tao, & Carovano, 1998; WCPH, 2009).

For those interested in learning more about photovoice please see reviews by Catalani and Minkler (2010) and Hergenrather, Rhodes, and Bardhoshi (2009).

SELF-ASSESSMENTS

Data can also be collected by those in the priority population through **self-assessments**. "A majority of these approaches address primary prevention issues, such as the assessment of risk factors and protective factors in one's lifestyle pattern, and the secondary prevention process of the early detection of disease symptoms" (Gilmore, 2012, p. 179). Examples of such assessments include breast self-examination (BSE), testicular self-examination (TSE), self-monitoring for skin cancer, and **health assessments (HAs)**. "Health assessments include instruments known as health risk appraisals or health risk assessments (HRAs), health status assessments (HSAs), various lifestyle-specific (e.g., nutrition, stress, and physical activity) assessment instruments, wellness and behavioral/habit inventories" (SPMBoD, 1999, p. xxiii), and disease/condition status assessments (e.g., chances of getting heart disease or diabetes). HAs, specifically HRAs, have been used more in worksite health promotion programs than in other settings.

Of the different self-assessments, it is the HAs that have been most useful in the needs assessment process, because from such assessments planners can obtain "group data which summarize major health problems and risk factors" (Alexander, 1999, p. 5). And of the HAs, it is the HRAs that are most often included in the needs assessment process. HRAs are instruments that estimate "the odds that a person with certain characteristics will die from selected causes within a given time span" (Alexander, 1999, p. 5). Even though HRAs are used as part of needs assessments, this was not their original intent. The original purpose of HRAs was to engage family physicians and their patients in conversation about risks of premature death and preventive health behaviors (Robbins & Hall, 1970).

To use an HRA as part of a needs assessment, planners would have those in the priority population complete a questionnaire. The instruments include questions about health behavior (e.g., smoking, exercise), personal or family health history of diseases (e.g., cancer, heart disease), demographics (e.g., age, sex), and usually some physiological data (e.g., height, weight, blood pressure, cholesterol). The resulting risk appraisals, in most cases, are calculated by computers, but some HRAs are hand-scored by the participant or health professional (Alexander, 1999). Most HRAs generate both individual and group reports. Thus planners can use the individual reports as part of an educational program for the priority population and use the group reports as another source of primary needs assessment data.

There are many HA instruments on the market. Before using one, you need to review information about the instruments that are available. Hunnicutt (2008a) created 10 critical questions that need to be asked when a health risk appraisal is purchased from a vendor: (1) How long has the vendor been in business? (2) How many other clients have used the instrument? (3) Who was behind the development of the HRA? (4) What is the best price? (5) Is the vendor willing to share the names of other clients who have used the HRA? (6) Is there any litigation pending against the vendor? (7) Is the vendor Health Insurance Portability and Accountability Act (HIPAA) compliant? (8) Will the vendor store the HRA data at a site outside the United States? (9) Is customer service/technical assistance included with the purchase of the HRA? (10) Who is the key contact within the company of the vendor and what is his/her emergency number?

Although this discussion has revolved around the use of HRAs as means of providing information for a needs assessment, they have also been used to help motivate people to: act on their health, measure health status, increase productivity, increase awareness, serve as cues to action, and to contribute to program design and evaluation (Simpson, Hyner, & Anderson, 2013) (see Hunnicutt, 2008b, for benefits of using personal health assessments in a worksite). However, it should be noted that the Community Preventive Services Task Force (CPSTF) has conducted two separate reviews on the use of HRAs among employees. In the first review, it was found that there was insufficient evidence to recommend the use of HRAs with appropriate feedback to achieve improvements in health behavior. In the second review, it was found that there was sufficient evidence to recommend the use of HRAs with appropriate feedback when combined with health education programs, and with or without additional interventions for improving health behaviors of employees (CPSTF, 2006 & 2007).

Table 4.1 summarizes the advantages and disadvantages of the various methods of collecting primary data.

Sources of Secondary Data

Several sources of secondary needs assessment data are available to planners. The main sources include data collected by government agencies at multiple levels (federal, state, or local), data available from nongovernment agencies and organizations, data from existing records (e.g., medical records), and data or other evidence that are presented in the literature (see **Table 4.2**).

DATA COLLECTED BY GOVERNMENT AGENCIES

Certain government agencies collect data on a regular basis. Some of the data collection is mandated by law (e.g., census, births, deaths, notifiable diseases), whereas other data are collected voluntarily (e.g., usage rates for safety belts). Because the data are collected by the government, program planners can gain free access to them by contacting the agency that collects the data, or by finding them on the Internet, or in a library that serves as a United States government depository. Many college and university libraries and large public libraries serve as such depositories.

TABLE 4.1 **Methods of Collecting Primary Data**

Method	Advantages	Disadvantages
Self-Report		
Written questionnaire via mail	Large outreach	Possible low response rate
	No interviewer bias	Possible problem of representation
	Convenient	No clarification of questions
	Low cost	Need homogenous group if response is low
	Minimum staff time required	
	Easy to administer	No assurance addressee was respondent
	Quick	Wait time for returns**
	Standardized	
Telephone interview	Moderate cost	Respondent can hang up**
	Relatively easy to administer	Telemarketers have made it harder**
	Permits unlimited callbacks	Possible problem of representation
	Can cover wide geographic areas	Possible interviewer bias
	Faster than mail or interview techniques**	Requires trained interviewers
		Wireless-only households
		Unlisted number households
Face-to-face interview	High response rate	Expensive
	Flexibility	Requires trained interviewers
	Gain in-depth data	Possible interviewer bias
	Develop rapport	Limits sample size
	Can observe nonverbal behavior**	Time-consuming
	No help from others in answering**	
Electronic interview	Low cost	Must have Internet access
	Ease and convenience	Self-selection
	Almost instantaneous	May lack anonymity
	Commercial companies' services	Respondent can easily delete request to participate**
	Wide geographic coverage**	Email addresses hard to get sometimes
Group interview	High response rate	May intimidate and suppress individual differences
	Efficient and economical	
	Can stimulate productivity of others	Fosters conformity
		Group pressure may influence responses
Delphi technique*	Pooled responses	High cost and time commitment
	Spans time and distance	Reduced clarification opportunities
	High motivation and commitment	Reduced immediate reinforcement
	Reduced influence of others	
	Enhanced response quality and quantity	
	Equal representation	
	Consistent participant contact	

(continued)

TABLE 4.1 *Continued*

Method	Advantages	Disadvantages
Community forum (town hall meeting)*	Relatively straightforward to conduct	Often difficult to achieve good attendance
	Relatively inexpensive	Participants in the community forum may tend to represent special interests
	Access to a broad cross-section of the community	Forum could degenerate into gripe session
	People participate on own terms	Data analysis can be time consuming
	Can identify most interested	
Meetings	Good for formative evaluation	Possible result bias
	Low cost	Limited input from participants
	Flexible	
Focus groups*	Low cost	Qualitative information
	Convenience	Limited representativeness
	Creative atmosphere	Dependence on moderator skill
	Ease of clarification	Preliminary insights
	Flexibility	Participant involvement
Nominal group process*	Direct involvement of priority groups	Time commitment
	Planned interactivity	Competing issues
	Diverse opinions	Participant bias
	Full participation	Segmented planning involvement
	Creative atmosphere	
	Recognition of common ground	
Observation	Accurate behavioral data	Requires trained observers
	Can be obtrusive	May bias behavior
	Moderate cost	Possible observer bias
		May be time-consuming
Self-assessments	Convenient	Possible low response rate
	No interviewer bias	Possible problem of representativeness
	Moderate cost	Self-selection
	Minimum staff time required	
	Easy to administer	
	Flexibility	

*From Gilmore (2012);   **From Neutens & Rubibson (2014)

DATA AVAILABLE FROM NONGOVERNMENT AGENCIES AND ORGANIZATIONS

In addition to the data available from government agencies, planners should also consult with nongovernment agencies and groups for data. Included among these are health care systems, voluntary health agencies, business, civic, and commerce groups. For example, most of the national voluntary health agencies produce yearly "facts and figures" booklets that include a variety of epidemiological data. In addition, local agencies (e.g., local health department), health care facilities (e.g., non-profit hospitals) and organizations (e.g., United Way) often have data they have collected for their own use.

TABLE 4.2 **Sample Sources of Secondary Data Available from Governmental and Nongovernmental Agencies and Organizations**

Type of Agency/Organization	Type of Data	URL (Web Address)
Government Agencies		
U.S. Bureau of Census	Demographic	http://www.census.gov
	U.S. Census *Statistical Abstract of the United States*	http://www.census.gov/prod/www/ statistical_abstract.html
Centers for Disease Control and Prevention (CDC)	Health and Vital Statistics	
	National Center for Health Statistics (NCHS)	http://www.cdc.gov/nchs/
	Morbidity Mortality Weekly Report (MMWR)	http://www.cdc.gov/mmwr/
	CDC WONDER	http://wonder.cdc.gov
	Behavioral Risk Factors	
	Behavioral Risk Factor Surveillance System (BRFSS)	http://www.cdc.gov/brfss/
	Youth Risk Behavior Surveillance System (YRBSS)	http://www.cdc.gov/healthyyouth /data/yrbs/index.htm
Food & Drug Administration (FDA)	Food, Drugs and Medical Device Data	http://www.fda.gov
Environmental Protection Agency (EPA)	Environmental Data and Statistics	http://www.epa.gov
Substance Abuse & Mental Health Services Administration (SAMHSA)	Substance & Mental Health Statistical Information	http://www.samhsa.gov
National Cancer Institute	Cancer Statistics	http://www.cancer.gov
Nongovernmental Agencies and Organizations		
American Cancer Society	Cancer Information and Statistics	http://www.cancer.org
American Heart Association	Heart Disease and Stroke Information and Statistics	http://www.heart.org/HEARTORG/
County Health Rankings	Health Data by U.S. Counties	http://www.countyhealthrankings.org
Henry J. Kaiser Family Foundation	Health Data by States	http://kff.org/statedata/

DATA FROM EXISTING RECORDS

These are health data that are often collected as a part of normal operations of an organization. These data can also serve as useful secondary needs assessment data. Using such data may be an efficient way to obtain the necessary information for a needs assessment (or an evaluation) without the need for additional data collection. The advantages include low cost, minimum staff needed, and ease in randomization. The disadvantages include difficulty in gaining access to the necessary records and the possible lack of availability of all the information needed for a needs assessment or program evaluation.

Examples of the use of existing records include checking medical records to monitor blood pressure and cholesterol levels of participants in an exercise program, reviewing insurance usage of employees enrolled in an employee health promotion program, and comparing the academic records of students engaging in an after-school weight loss program with those who are not. In these situations, as with all needs assessments using existing records, the cooperation of the agencies that hold the records is essential. At times, agencies may be willing to collect additional information to aid in the needs assessment for (or an evaluation of) a health promotion program. Keepers of records are concerned about confidentiality and the release of private information. The importance of privacy for those planners working in health care settings was further emphasized in 2003 with the enactment of the *Standards for Privacy of Individually Identifiable Health Information* section (The Privacy Rule) of the Health Insurance Portability and Accountability Act of 1996 (officially known as Public Law 104-191 and referred to as **HIPAA**, pronounced "hip-a"). The rule sets national standards that health plans, health care clearinghouses, and health care providers who conduct certain health care transactions electronically must implement to protect and guard against the misuse of individually identifiable health information. Failure to implement the standards can lead to civil and criminal penalties (USDHHS, OCR, n.d.). Planners can deal with these privacy issues by getting permission from all participants to use their records or by using only anonymous or *de-identified* (i.e., information removed so individuals cannot be identified) data.

DATA FROM THE LITERATURE

Planners might also be able to identify the needs of a priority population by reviewing any available current literature about that priority population. An example would be a planner who is developing a health promotion program for individuals infected by the human immunodeficiency virus (HIV). Because of the seriousness of this disease and the number of people who have studied and written about it, there is a good chance that present literature could reflect the need of a certain priority population.

The best means of accessing data from the literature is by using the available literature databases. Most literature databases today are available in several different forms, including electronic databases and the Internet. Depending on the database used, planners can expect to find comprehensive listings of citations for journal articles, book chapters, and books, and, in some databases, abstracts of the literature. Within the listings, most databases cite sources by both author and subject/title. **Figure 4.3** provides an example of what planners might find when searching a database.

Many literature databases are available to planners. Next is a short discussion of those databases that have proved helpful to health promotion planners.

PSYCINFO

PsycINFO®, which is produced by the American Psychological Association (APA), is an abstracting (not full-text) "and indexing database with more than 3 million records devoted to peer-reviewed literature in the behavioral sciences and mental health (APA, 2015, para. 1)

MEDLINE

Medline, the primary component of and accessed through PubMed®, is the U.S. National Library of Medicine's® (NLM) premier bibliographic database that contains over 22 million

Author Citation

Authors   Article title
↓   ↓

Neiger, B. L., Thackeray, R., & Fagan, M. C. Basic priority rating model 2.0: current
applications for priority setting in health promotion practice. *Health Promotion Practice*.
2011; 12(2), 166–171.

↑   ↑   ↑
Journal Volume Pages   Journal
(number)

Subject/Title Citation

Article title
↓

Basic priority rating model 2.0: current applications for priority setting in health
promotion practice. Neiger, B. L., Thackeray, R., & Fagan, M. C., *Health Promotion Practice*.
2011; 12(2), 166–171.

▲ **Figure 4.3** Sample Citations

references from more than 5,600 journals covering the life sciences with a concentration on
biomedicine. "A distinctive feature of Medline is that the records are indexed with NLM's
Medical Subject Headings (MeSH®)" (U.S. NLM, 2015, para. 1).

EDUCATION RESOURCE INFORMATION CENTER (ERIC)

ERIC is an online digital library of education literature sponsored by the Institute of
Education Sciences (IES) of the U.S. Department of Education. ERIC provides free access to
educational journal articles and other education-related materials.

CUMULATIVE INDEX TO NURSING & ALLIED HEALTH LITERATURE (CINAHL)

The CINAHL, which is updated monthly, provides indexing of journals from the fields of
nursing and other allied health disciplines. It also provides indexing for healthcare books,
dissertations from the field of nursing, selected conference proceedings, and standards of
practice. Subject headings follow the NLM's MeSH® structure.

PUBMED

PubMed includes "more that 24 million citations from biomedical literature from MEDLINE,
life science journals, and online books" U.S. NLM (n.d.). Some of the citations provide links
to full-text content.

Steps for Conducting a Literature Search

GENERAL SEARCH PROCEDURES

The process of searching a database is not difficult, and with the exception of a few individual differences, most indexes are arranged in a similar format. As Figure 4.3 indicated,
most indexes include both an author and a subject/title index. An item that is specific to
each index is its thesaurus, a listing of the key words the indexes used to index the subject/

titles. Planners can find the thesauri online or in a separate volume with or near a hard copy of the indexes.

Figure 4.4 provides planners with a literature search strategy in the form of a flowchart. The chart begins by identifying the need of the priority population or topic to be searched. At this point, planners can search either by subject/title or by author. If planners know of an author who has done work on their topic, they can search the database using the author's last name. If they do not have information on authors, they will need to match their topic with the key words presented in the thesaurus. Since there are times when a topic is not expressed in the same terms used in the thesaurus, planners will need to look for related terms. Once they have a list of key words, they need to search the database for possible matches. In conducting this search, they need to ensure that they are using the database that covers the years of literature in which they are interested. This search should identify possible sources and citations.

Once sources are identified, planners may review abstracts (or entire documents) online or locate a hard copy of the document. Then, planners must determine the quality and usefulness of the publication in the needs assessment process. One means by which planners can judge the quality of the literature is to examine the references at the end of the publications. First, this reference list may lead planners to other sources not identified in the original search. Second, if the sources found in the database include all those commonly cited in the literature, this can verify the exhaustiveness of the search.

SEARCHING VIA THE WORLD WIDE WEB

The continued development of the World Wide Web (WWW) has enhanced the opportunities for planners to obtain a variety of needs assessment data with the "touch of a button" from their home or office. Many of the government and nongovernment agencies and organizations, as well as the databases, discussed in this chapter have Websites that planners can access if they have the Web address, also known as the uniform resource locator (URL). If the Web address is unknown, planners can use a search engine to identify appropriate Websites.

Popular search engines include Yahoo, DuckDuckGo, Ask, AOL, Google, and bing. Planners can experiment with and select the sites that best fit their needs. If planners are using a term that has more than one word (i.e., *heart disease*), it is best to use quotation marks around the term when entering it on the search engine. "This will let the search engine know that the exact phrase, as contained in the quotation marks, is to be used when seeking sites that match. If the quotation marks are not used, the search engine will find sites that contain any of the words in the query" (Cottrell et al., 2015, p. 300) and thus many of the sites found may not be of use.

As with any data source, planners need to be aware that not all data found via the Web are valid and reliable. Thus planners need to scrutinize sources just as they would data found in hard copies. Librarians at Meriam Library at California State University, Chico created the Currency, Relevance, Authority, Accuracy, Purpose (CRAAP) Test that is most useful for evaluating information obtained via the Internet (see the link for the Website in the Weblinks section at the end of the chapter).

Using Technology to Map Needs Assessment Data

As has already been mentioned in this chapter, more and more needs assessment data are being obtained through the use of technology (i.e., electronic interviews, computerized searchers of the World Wide Web and databases).

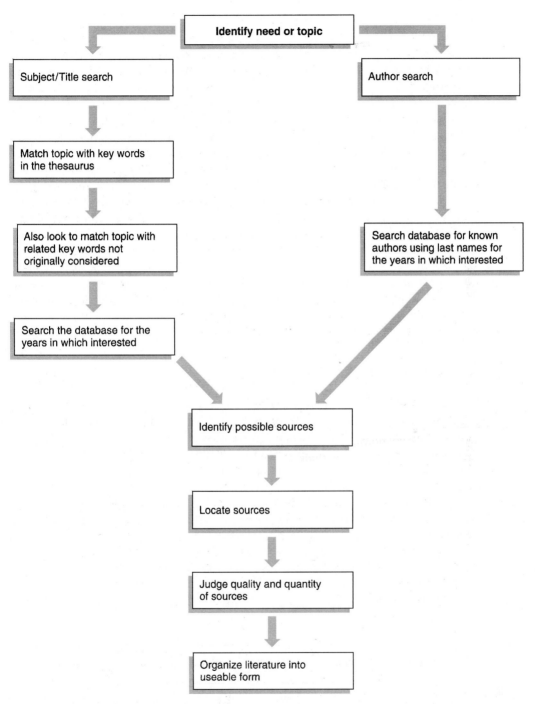

▲ **Figure 4.4** Literature Search Strategy Flowchart
Source: Adapted from Deeds (1992) and Marcarin (1995).

One other process that is being used more frequently is the use of geographic information systems (GIS) to help provide meaning to collected data. "GIS helps us analyze spatially referenced data and make well-informed decisions based on the association between data and the geography" (CDC, 2006). In other words, the data are mapped. **Mapping** "is the visual representation of data by geography or location, linking information to a place to support social and economic change on a community level. Mapping is a powerful tool for two reasons: (1) it makes patterns based on place much easier to identify and analyze, and (2) it provides a visual way of communicating those patterns to a broad audience, quickly and dramatically" (Kirschenbaum & Corburn, 2012, p. 444). The process of mapping involves (1) identifying the geographic area that the map will cover, (2) collecting the necessary data, (3) importing the data into GIS software so that the data can be placed on maps, and (4) analyzing what is found in the maps. Mapping has taken on more meaning recently because it has been noted that "when it comes to your health, your zip code is more important than your genetic code" (Iton, 2014, para. 8). Mapping has been used to address a number of different health problems. Some examples include blood pressure (Mendy, Perryman, Hawkins, & Dove, 2014), cancer (Beyer & Rushton, 2009; Richards et al., 2010), diabetes (Ruberto & Brissette, 2014), fruit and vegetable consumption (Lucan, Hillier, Schechtner, & Glanz, 2014), and lead screening (Graff, 2013). The use of GIS in the needs assessment process will continue to grow as the development of such software becomes more widely available and easier to use.

▷ Conducting a Needs Assessment

A number of different approaches can be used to determine the needs of the priority population. "Need assessments range from informal approaches, using educated and informed observations to formal, comprehensive research projects. However, the informal approaches are less reliable than a planned and scientifically developed research approach" (Timmreck, 2003, p. 89). Often, informal approaches are used because of limited resources, usually time, personnel, and money. However, as noted in the beginning of this chapter, needs assessment may be the most critical step in the planning process and should not be taken lightly. Resources used on need assessments usually pay dividends many times over. Therefore the authors present a six-step process that is more formal in nature: (1) determining purpose and defining the scope of the needs assessment, (2) gathering data, (3) analyzing the data, (4) identifying the risk factors linked to the health problem, (5) identifying the program focus, and (6) validating the need before continuing on with the planning process (see **Figure 4.5**).

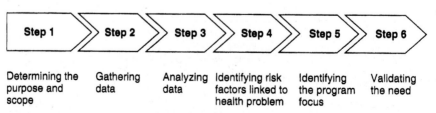

▲ **Figure 4.5** Steps in Conducting a Needs Assessment

Step 1: Determining the Purpose and Scope of the Needs Assessment

The initial step in the needs assessment process is to determine the purpose and the scope of the needs assessment. In other words, what is the goal of the needs assessment? What does the planning committee hope to gain from the needs assessment? How extensive will the needs assessment be? What kind of resources will be available to conduct the needs assessment? In reality, the first challenge associated with conducting a needs assessment is determining whether an assessment should even be performed, and if so, what type of needs assessment is appropriate. As noted earlier in the chapter a comprehensive needs assessment may not be warranted because a need may be obvious or an agency/organization has received categorical funding to address a specific health problem. However, a more focused needs assessment may be appropriate to gather more specific information about the need or health problem. For example, if the priority health problem is breast cancer, it is still necessary to collect current information on the degree to which women are either dying or suffering from the disease. It will be important to know how prevalent breast cancer is and where it is most prevalent in the population, as well as the high-risk subpopulations, economic costs, and general trends over time. The extent to which a needs assessment is necessary and appropriate should be determined by stakeholders, including key decision makers.

In other cases, a planner may be in a situation where a needs assessment has never been performed, not been performed for a long period of time, or where categorical funding does not dictate what health problem(s) should be addressed. This will require planners and their partners to collect a wide range of data, compare the importance of multiple health problems, and set priorities. In a general sense, this is the process that is often referred to as a *community health needs assessment* (CHNA). This implies that all significant health problems are examined to assess their relative significance. Stakeholders and planning groups will also usually determine how many health problems will be analyzed in the needs assessment. This will be influenced by how much time, and how many resources, can be directed to the needs assessment.

Another important decision that must be made is the extent to which those in the community where the needs assessment is being conducted will be involved in the needs assessment process. The term **participatory** or **action research** has gained popularity in recent years, though it is often misunderstood or used inappropriately. *Participatory research* has been "defined as systematic inquiry, with the collaboration of those affected by the issue being studied, for the purposes of education and of taking action or effecting change" (Mercer et al., 2008, p. 409).

Once the basic purpose and scope of the needs assessment is identified, planners may proceed to data collection. However, planners must not take this first step too lightly. Although a natural tendency is to move forward quickly, an understanding of why a needs assessment is being performed will give proper direction to all other steps that follow.

Step 2: Gathering Data

The second step in the needs assessment process is gathering data. As noted earlier in this chapter, there are many different sources of needs assessment data. A part of the art of conducting a needs assessment is to be able to identify the most relevant data possible. By *relevant data,* we mean those data that are most applicable to the planning situation and that will do the best job of helping planners to identify the actual needs of the priority population. Because of the cost and availability, it is recommended that planners begin the data-gathering process by trying to locate relevant secondary data. For example, if a national program is being planned, then national secondary data should be sought from appropriate national government and nongovernment agencies. If a local program is being planned, then appropriate local data should be sought. When planning a local program, it is not unusual to find that local data do not exist. If that is the case, planners may need to use state, regional, or national data (in that order) and apply them to the local area. For example, let's assume diabetes mellitus mortality data are needed for local planning and the only data available are national level data. Planners could use national data (e.g., 21.2 per 100,000 people died of diabetes in 2013) to estimate the number of deaths in a local community. If the population of a local city is 250,000, planners could infer that the number of deaths due to diabetes in the city during 2013 totaled 53 (i.e., 21.2 × 2.5). If the city's population were older, 53 deaths could be viewed as a low estimate because diabetes deaths are more prevalent in older populations. Conversely, if the population were younger, 53 deaths could be viewed as a high estimate. Obviously, as noted at the beginning of this chapter, there are disadvantages of using secondary data, but good planners use and interpret them in light of their limitations (McDermott & Sarvela, 1999).

Once relevant secondary data have been identified, planners need to turn their attention to gathering the appropriate primary data in order to fill in the "data gaps" to better understand the needs of the priority population. For example, if secondary data show that there is a need for cancer education programming, but does not specifically identify the type of cancer or segment the priority population by useful demographic characteristics (e.g., age or sex), then efforts should be made to collect such data. Or, it may be that all the secondary data are *quantitative data* such as how frequently a service is used, and thus it might be very useful to collect primary data that are *qualitative* in nature such as detailed explanations of why a service was not used. It should be noted that primary data collection could have a dual purpose. Not only do primary data collections provide valuable information about the specific planning situation that cannot be obtained from secondary data, they also provide an opportunity to get those in the priority population actively involved and contributing to the program planning process. Thus, planners need to decide what primary data are needed, from whom they should be collected (e.g., All? Some? Just certain demographic groups?), and what methods (e.g., Interviews? Questionnaires? Focus groups? Photovoice?) would be best for not only collecting the needed information but also in getting active participation from the priority population.

It should also be noted that the planning model used to develop a program might also drive the types of data collected for the needs assessment. For example, when the Social Marketing Assessment and Response Tool (SMART) model is used planners would be interested in collecting data that would assist with Consumer Analysis (Phase 2), Market Analysis (Phase 3), and Channel Analysis (Phase 4). When the Mobilizing for Action through Planning and Partnerships (MAPP) model is being used planners should be collecting data that would provide information for the Assessments (Phase 3) which yield a list of challenges and opportunities in a community (see Chapter 3 for more information about SMART and MAPP).

In addition to using a planning model to help guide the types of data to be collected, planners may also want to use theoretical constructs to help guide data collection. For example, it may be important for planners to know what stages of change (see Chapter 7 for information on the Transtheoretical Model) the priority population is in for a specific health behavior (i.e., exercise) in order to create a more focused intervention.

As planners conclude the second step in the needs assessment process, they must remember that each planning situation is different. It is desirable to have both primary and secondary needs assessment data in order to gain a clear picture of needs; however, depending on the resources and circumstances, planners may have access to only one or the other. In addition, there is usually a trade-off between quality and quantity of data. Planners must use the best data available under the challenges and constraints facing them.

Step 3: Analyzing the Data

At this point in the needs assessment process, planners must analyze all the data collected, with the goal of identifying and prioritizing the health problems. The goal of data analysis is easily stated, but this step may be the most difficult to complete. There are those rare occasions when the data analysis is not very complicated because the need is obvious. For example, the data may clearly show that breast cancer rates have continued to rise in a community, while the number of breast screenings has dropped, and those in the priority population recognize the problem. Or, in another setting the data analysis shows a very clear correlation between the health status of the priority population and the lack of primary health care received. However, not all analyses of data yield such obvious needs. More often than not, planners are faced with trying to compare data that are not easily compared. The data may be mixed (i.e., apples and oranges) or confusing. For example, they may have mortality data for one health problem, morbidity data for another, and perhaps behavioral risk factor data for yet another. Or, if planners are working with a multicultural priority population, data analysis may even be more confusing, because health concepts held by one culture may be very different than the health concepts held by the planners. When working with diverse communities, it is important to find "out more information about what is going on and why and how cultural issues may or may not influence a health problem or related risk behaviors" (Vaughn & Krenz, 2014, p. 178). A failure to understand and appreciate these differences in the priority population can have serious implications for success of any health promotion/disease prevention effort (Kline & Huff, 1999).

One systematic way to analyze the data is to use the first few phases of the PRECEDE-PROCEED model for guidance. Start by asking and answering the following questions:

1. What is the quality of life of those in the priority population?
2. What are social conditions and perceptions shared by those in the priority population?
3. What are the social indicators (e.g., absenteeism, crime, discrimination, performance, welfare, etc.) in the priority population that reflect the social conditions and perceptions?
4. Can the social conditions and perceptions be linked to health promotion? If so, how?
5. What are the health problems associated with the social problems?
6. Which health problem is most important to change?

The last question in this list is really asking the question: Which problem/need should get priority? The problems/needs must be prioritized not because the lowest-priority problems/ needs are not important, but because organizations have limited resources to deal with all identified problems/needs. Thus, "priority setting is critical in narrowing the scope of activity to reflect the availability of resources within the context of stakeholders' values and preferences. In addition, priority setting helps health promotion practitioners stay focused on problems that actually affect the health status of the population" (Neiger, Thackeray, & Fagen, 2011, p. 166). There are several benefits to effective priority setting. They include: (a) building consensus among the stakeholders for the allocation of resources in areas most likely to yield positive and sustainable outcomes; (b) clarifying expectations for the use of resources in a constrained environment, (c) helping to establish focus on issues based on objective criteria, and (d) helping establish a chain of accountability for the stakeholders (Barnett, 2012).

Priority setting is not easy and planners should be aware that there might be conflict among stakeholders. "Obstacles to the effective implementation of priority setting include, but are not limited to the following; (a) lack of quality data, (b) conflicting political dynamics and agendas, (c) stakeholder fatigue with assessment process, (d) poorly developed and/or understood criteria, and (e) lack of equity in stakeholder participation and processes" (Barnett, 2012, p. 46).

When setting priorities, the planners should seek answers to these questions:

1. What is the most pressing need? Why?
2. Are there resources adequate to deal with the problem?
3. Can the problem best be solved by a health promotion intervention, or could it be handled better through another means?
4. Are effective intervention strategies available to address the problem?
5. Can the problem be solved in a reasonable amount of time?

The actual process of setting priorities can take many different forms and can range from subjective approaches such as simple voting procedures, forced rankings, and the nominal group process with stakeholders to more objective but time-consuming processes such as the Delphi technique (Gilmore, 2012) and the **basic priority rating (BPR)** model. The BPR model, which was first known as the "priority rating process," was introduced more than 60 years ago (Hanlon, 1954) in an attempt to prioritize health problems in developing countries. During this span of time, the BPR has been most useful to program planners. Although the BPR model has provided basic direction in priority setting, it does not represent the broad array of data available to decision makers today (Neiger et al., 2011). In addition, "elements in the model give more weight to the impact of communicable diseases as compared to chronic diseases" (Neiger et al., 2011, p. 166). As such, Neiger and his colleagues have proposed changes to the BPR model and suggested a new name for the model; **BPR Model 2.0**. To provide both background and currency, both the BPR model (Pickett & Hanlon, 1990) and the BPR model 2.0 (Neiger et al., 2011) are presented here.

BPR MODEL

The BPR model requires planners to rate four different components of the identified needs and insert the ratings into a formula in order to determine a priority rating between 0 and 100. The components and their possible scores (in parenthesis) are:

A. size of the problem (0 to 10)

B. seriousness of the problem (0 to 20)

C. effectiveness of the possible interventions (0 to 10)

D. propriety, economics, acceptability, resources, and legality (PEARL) (0 or 1)

The formula in which the scores are placed is:

$$\text{Basic Priority Rating (BPR)} = \frac{(A + B)C}{3} \times D$$

Component *A*, size of the problem, can be scored by using epidemiological rates or determining the percentage of the priority population at risk. The higher the rate or percentage, the greater the score.

Component *B*, seriousness of the problem, is examined using four factors: economic loss to community, family, or individuals; involvement of other people who were not initially affected by the problem, as with the spread of an infectious disease; the severity of the problem measured in mortality, morbidity, or disability; and the urgency of solving the problem because of additional harm. Because the maximum score for this component is 20, raters can use a 0 to 5 score for each of the four factors.

Component *C*, effectiveness of the interventions, is often the most difficult of the four components to measure. The efficacy of some intervention strategies is known, such as immunizations (close to 100%) and smoking cessation classes (around 30%), but for many, it is not. Planners will need to estimate this score based upon the work of others or their own expert opinions. In scoring this component, planners should consider both the effectiveness of intervention strategies in terms of behavior change, as well as the degree to which the priority population will demonstrate interest in the intervention strategy.

Component *D*, PEARL, consists of several factors that determine whether a particular intervention strategy can be carried out at all. The score is 0 or 1; any need that receives a zero will automatically drop to the bottom of the priority list because a score of zero (a multiplier) for this component will yield a total score of zero in the formula. Examples of when a zero may result are if an intervention is economically impossible, unacceptable to the priority population or planners, or illegal. Ideally, some of these assessments will be made before a health problem is considered in the priority setting process.

Once the score for the four components is determined, an overall priority rating for each need can be calculated, and the prioritizing can take place.

BPR MODEL 2.0

Building on the BPR model, Neiger and his colleagues (2011) offered the following adaptations to the model and suggested calling the revised model the BPR model 2.0.

A. Size of the problem. "Depending on the availability of data and preferences of the stakeholders use one of the following:

  1. Use incidence *and* prevalence data and score each on a scale of 0 to 5 for a total of 10 points (it is recognized that incidence represents a proportion of prevalence).
  2. Use incidence *or* prevalence data and score each health problem on a scale of 0 to 10 points.
  3. Use age-adjusted cause-specific mortality rates *and* proportional mortality ratios for each health problem and score each on a scale of 0 to 5 for a total of 10 points.
  4. Use age-adjusted cause-specific mortality rates *or* proportional mortality ratios and score each health problem on a scale of 0 to 10 points" (p. 168).

B. Seriousness of the problem. Both the definitions for the components of "seriousness" and the scoring for the components be changed as follows:

  1. Urgency—defined "as the degree to which a health problem is increasing, stabilizing, or decreasing and that 5-year mortality trend data be used to score it" (p. 168). Scores should be assigned as follows: increasing trend data (5 or 4 points); stabilized trend data (3 or 2 points); and decreasing trend data (1 or 0 points).

2. Severity—expand the definition of the criterion to include: (a) the lethality of a health problem (as measured by five-year survival rate), (b) premature mortality (as measured by years of potential life lost or years of productive life lost), and (c) disability (as measured by disability-adjusted life years [DALYs]). Scores should be assigned as follows: 0- to 5-point scale (i.e., 5–4 is high, 3–2 is medium, and 1–0 is low).

3. Economic loss—defined as the accumulation of costs (direct and indirect) borne by society associated with the health problem. Scores should be assigned as follows: 0- to 5-point scale (i.e., 5–4 is high, 3–2 is medium, and 1–0 is low).

4. Impact on others—expand the definition of the criterion to include: "(a) as the communicable nature of the health problem (particularly when analyzing communicable diseases); (b) the behavioral effects related to the health problem on others (e.g., secondhand smoke, driving while under the influence of alcohol or other drugs, violence perpetrated on others, etc.); or (c) the emotional and physical impact the health problem (with attendant disabilities) has on others with respect to care giving" (p. 169). Scores should be assigned as follows: 0- to 5-point scale (i.e., 5–4 is high, 3–2 is medium, and 1–0 is low).

C. Effectiveness of the possible interventions. Limit the definition of "effectiveness" to evidence of a successful intervention and not rate the "reach" of the intervention. The scoring of effectiveness should be based on the typology of evidence developed by Brownson, Fielding, and Maylahn (2009). Scores should be assigned as follows: 0- to 10-point scale (i.e., 10–9 reflect evidence-based interventions, 8–7 reflect effective programs, 6–5 reflect promising interventions, 4–3 reflect emerging interventions, and 2–0 reflect unproven interventions).

D. PEARL. The calculation of PEARL should remain the same. However, if secondary data are available to calculate the PEARL it should be calculated prior to collecting primary data so that the needs assessment may be more focused.

For an example application of the BPR model 2.0 readers should refer to Neiger et al. (2011).

Finally, how will planners know when they have completed Step 3 (Analyzing the Data) of the needs assessment process? Planners should be able to list in rank order the problems/needs of the priority population.

Step 4: Identifying the Risk Factors Linked to the Health Problem

Step 4 of the needs assessment process is parallel to the second part of Phase 2 of the PRECEDE-PROCEED model: epidemiological assessment. In this step, planners need to identify the determinants of the health problem identified in the previous step. That is, what genetic, behavioral, and environmental risk factors are associated with the health problem? Because most genetic determinants either cannot be changed or interact with the behavior and/or environment, the task in this step is to identify and prioritize the behavioral and environmental factors that, if changed, could lessen the health problem in the priority population. Also, it should be noted that the term *environmental factors* applies to more than just the physical environment (e.g., clean air and water, proximity to facilities). Environment is multidimensional and can include economic environment (e.g., affordability, incentives, disincentives); service environment (e.g., access to health care, equity in health care, barriers to health care); social environment (e.g., social support, peer pressure); psychological environment (e.g., emotional learning environment); and the political environment (e.g., health policy). In essence then, modifying behavioral and/or environmental factors or determinants is the real work of health promotion. Thus, if the health problem is lung cancer, planners should analyze the health behaviors and environment of the priority population for known risk factors of lung cancer. For example, higher than expected smoking behavior may be present in the priority population, and the people may live in a community where smokefree public environments are not valued. Once these risk factors are identified, they too need to be prioritized (see Figure 3.4 for a means of prioritizing these risk factors).

Step 5: Identifying the Program Focus

The fifth step of the needs assessment process is similar to the third phase of the PRECEDE-PROCEED model: educational and ecological assessment. With behavioral, environmental, and genetic risk factors identified and prioritized, planners need to identify those predisposing, enabling, and reinforcing factors that seem to have a direct impact on the risk factors. In the lung cancer example, those in the priority population may not have (1) the skills necessary to stop smoking (predisposing factor), (2) access to a smoking cessation program (enabling factor), or (3) people around them who support efforts to stop smoking (reinforcing factor). "Study of the predisposing, enabling, and reinforcing factors automatically helps the planner decide exactly which of the factors making up the three classes deserve the highest priority as the focus of the intervention. The decision is based on their importance and any evidence that change in the factor is possible and cost-effective" (Green & Kreuter, 1999, p. 42).

In addition, when prioritizing needs, planners also need to consider any existing health promotion programs to avoid duplication of efforts. Therefore, program planners should seek to determine the status of existing health promotion programs by trying to answer as many questions as possible from the following list:

1. What health promotion programs are presently available to the priority population?
2. Are the programs being utilized? If not, why not?
3. How effective are the programs? Are they meeting their stated goals and objectives?
4. How were the needs for these programs determined?
5. Are the programs accessible to the priority population? Where are they located? When are they offered? Are there any qualifying criteria that people must meet to enroll? Can the priority population get to the program? Can the priority population afford the programs?
6. Are the needs of the priority population being met? If not, why not?

There are several ways to seek answers to these questions. Probably the most common way is through **networking** with other people working in health promotion and the health care system—that is, communicating with others who may know about existing programs. (See Chapter 9 for a more detailed discussion of networking.) These people may be located in the local or state health department, in voluntary health agencies, or in health care facilities, such as hospitals, clinics, nursing homes, extended care facilities, or managed care organizations.

Planners might also find information about existing programs by checking with someone in an organization that serves as a clearinghouse for health promotion programs or by using a community resource guide. The local or state health department, a local chamber of commerce, a coalition, the local medical/dental societies, a community task force, or a community health center may serve as a clearinghouse or produce such a guide. Another avenue is to talk with people in the priority population. Although they may not know about all existing programs, they may be able to share information on the effectiveness and accessibility of some of the programs. Finally, some of the information could be collected in Step 2 through separate community forums, focus groups, or surveys.

Step 6: Validating the Prioritized Needs

The final step in the needs assessment process is to validate the identified need(s). *Validate* means to confirm that the need that was identified is the need that should be addressed. Obviously, if great care were taken in the needs assessment process, validation should be a perfunctory step. However, there have been times when a need was not properly validated; much energy and many resources have thereby been wasted on unnecessary programs.

Validation amounts to "double checking," or making sure that an identified need is the actual need. Any means available can be used, such as (1) rechecking the steps followed in the needs assessment to eliminate any bias, (2) conducting a focus group with some individuals from the priority population to determine their reaction to the identified need (if a focus group was not used earlier to gather the data), and (3) getting a "second opinion" from other health professionals.

Application of the Six-Step Needs Assessment Process

In the previous sections, a six-step approach for conducting a needs assessment was presented. Now we would like to present an example of how this process may be applied. Let's assume that a committee has been appointed by the health administrator of a local health department to plan a cancer prevention program for the county, and that the composition of the committee closely represents the greater community. Let's also assume that the parameters for the authority of the planning committee have also been set. Here is how this needs assessment may be carried out.

Step 1: Determining the Purpose and Scope of the Needs Assessment—After an organizational meeting and a couple subsequent meetings, the planning committee decided that the purpose of the needs assessment was fourfold. To determine (1) what types of cancers were of greatest concern in the county, (2) which subpopulations within the county were at the greatest risk for the cancers identified, (3) what the most common risk factors were for the cancer(s) and subpopulation(s) identified, and (4) the focus of the proposed program. The committee members also decided that the scope of the needs assessment would be defined by the collection of both primary and secondary data, and that they wanted part of the primary data collection to be participatory in nature. That is, they wanted some of those in the priority population to participate in the data collection process.

Step 2: Gathering Data—The committee members decided to begin data collection by identifying available sources of secondary data. Initially they gathered secondary data for the past five years for both the state and the county in which they lived from the state health department for the incidence of invasive cancer; cancer mortality rates (i.e., crude and age-adjusted); mortality rates for various types of cancer broken down by sex, age, and race/ethnicity; and behavioral risk factors that were known to contribute to or cause the various types of cancer. In addition, committee members were able to get secondary data from the state environmental agency regarding the levels of air and water pollution in all 92 counties of the state.

The secondary data were good but they did not present a complete picture of the cancer issue in their county. What was not available in the secondary data were information and data related to cancer education programs, cancer screening programs, access to health care providers that specialized in cancer care, and the county residents' interest in taking part in activities that would reduce the incidence and prevalence in their community. Therefore, the committee created three different questionnaires to be administered via single-step surveys. The three questionnaires dealt with cancer prevention activities (i.e., education and screenings), cancer treatment, and attitudes toward and willingness to participate in cancer programs if offered in the community.

To make part of the primary data collection a participatory process the committee sought out two groups of volunteers from the county who were interested in cancer control. The first group was asked to assist in data collection by administering the surveys to various individuals in the county by visiting places where residents were likely to gather such as service group meetings, religious organizations (i.e., churches, mosques, and synagogues), services, worksites, and neighborhood meetings. The second group of volunteers was asked to collect data via a photovoice process with a theme of "identify those unhealthy areas of the county that contribute to cases of cancer."

Step 3: Analyzing the Data—The committee members decided to analyze the data comparing their county data versus the state data using the informal technique of "eye-balling" the data. To help make sense of some of the data they created a few cross-tabulation tables comparing county data to state data. The analysis of the secondary cancer data from the state health department, the County Health Rankings (University of Wisconsin Population Health Institute, 2015), and the Kaiser Family Foundation's state health facts (KFF, 2015) showed:

- higher county incidence rate for invasive cancers (501/100,000 vs. 426/100,000)
- both higher county cancer crude mortality rates (177/100,000 vs. 157/100,000) and age-adjusted mortality rates (170.0/100,000 vs. 161.2/100,000)
- higher county prevalence rates for colorectal, lung, and pancreas cancers
- lower county prevalence rates for breast, cervix, and prostate cancers

The analysis of the secondary behavior risk data from the state's Behavior Risk Factor Surveillance System data showed:

- higher percentage of county residents who had not had either a sigmoidoscopy or colonoscopy in the recommended time period
- higher percentage of county women who had either a clinical breast examination (77.1% vs. 74.5%) or mammogram (76.3% vs. 73.1%) in the recommended time period
- higher percentage of county women who had a Papanicolaou smear (82.6% vs. 77.4%) in the recommended time period
- higher percentage of county residents who were physically inactive (55.7% vs. 48.9%)
- higher prevalence of county residents who smoked (25.3% vs. 21.0%)

The analysis of the primary data from the three surveys conducted by the committee showed county residents:

- would participate in free and/or inexpensive cancer screenings if they were convenient
- were in favor of creating more smokefree public areas
- felt, and the data showed, that there were too few health care providers in the county who dealt with cancer.

The analysis of the photovoice process identified two major themes in the county:

- many of the county residents were physically inactive and appeared to be either overweight or obese, and
- there were few smokefree public places in the county

Based on all the available primary and secondary data the committee prioritized the list of cancers using the BPR model 2.0. Those calculations yielded the following BPR scores: breast (38.7), colorectal (56.8), lung (51.8), cervix (30.4), pancreas (24.0), and prostate (41.7). Therefore, the committee decided to work to reduce the incidence of colorectal and lung cancers in the county.

Step 4: Identifying the Risk Factors Linked to the Health Problem—The risk factors associated with colorectal cancer include age (> 50 years), personal history of colorectal polyps or cancer, personal history of inflammatory bowel disease (IBD), family history of colorectal cancer, diets high in red meats, physical inactivity, obesity, smoking, heavy alcohol use, and type 2 diabetes (ACS, 2015). The risk factors associated with lung cancer include smoking, exposure to radon, exposure to asbestos, high levels of arsenic in the drinking water, personal or family history of lung cancer, and air pollution (ACS, 2015).

Step 5: Identifying the Program Focus—Based on the analysis of the data and the risk factors associated with identified priority cancers the planning committee decided to focus the cancer prevention program on two areas: working to offer more cancer screening programs in the county, and working toward a nonsmoking ordinance in the county in order to create smoke-free public places.

Step 6: Validating the Prioritized Needs—Before moving forward with the planning for the cancer prevention programs to deal with colorectal and lung cancer, the committee had representatives from both the state department of health's cancer prevention program and the American Cancer Society review their needs assessment to validate their findings. Both groups agreed with the program focus.

▷ Special Types of Health Assessments

Before leaving the topic of needs assessment we need to introduce two specific types of health assessments that have gained special attention in the last few years. They are *health impact assessment* and *organizational health assessment*.

Health Impact Assessment

Health impact assessment (HIA) is an important topic because a HIA could impact the focus of a needs assessment and it is "a rapidly emerging practice" (CDC, 2015d, para. 6) in the United States (see NRC, 2011, for examples of its use). A HIA has been defined as "a systematic process that uses an array of data sources and analytic methods and considers input from stakeholders to determine the potential effects of a proposed policy, plan, program, or project on the health of a population and the distribution of those effects within the population. HIA provides recommendations on monitoring and managing those effects" (NRC, 2011, p. 5). In other words, a HIA is an "approach that can help to identify and consider the potential—or actual—health impacts of a proposal on a population. Its primary output is a set of evidence-based recommendations geared to informing the decision-making process. These recommendations aim to highlight practical ways to enhance the positive aspects of a proposal, and to remove or minimise [sic] any negative impacts on health, well-being and health inequalities that may arise or exist" (Taylor & Quigley, 2002, pp. 2–3).

The World Health Organization (2015) has noted that HIAs are based on four values. They include 1) democracy (i.e., all who are impacted by the proposed change get to participate in the assessment), 2) equity (i.e., all who will be impacted by the proposed change are treated fairly in the assessment), 3) sustainable development (i.e., both short- and long-term impacts of the proposed change are considered are part of the assessment), and 4) ethical use of evidence (i.e., evidence used in the assessment includes both qualitative and quantitative evidence and is collected using best practices).

There are a number of different frameworks (i.e., guides) that can be used to conduct a HIA (see Mindell, Boltong, & Forde, 2008 for a review of guides) and they "can range from simple, fairly easy-to-conduct analyses to more in-depth, complex analyses" (Brennan Ramirez et al., 2008, p. 46), but most of these guides include the following major steps:

1. Screening (identify plans, projects, or policies for which an HIA would be useful)
2. Scoping (identify which health effects to consider)
3. Assessing risks and benefits (identify which people may be affected and how they may be affected)
4. Developing recommendations (suggesting changes to proposals to promote positive health effects or minimize adverse health effects)
5. Reporting (present the results to decision makers), and
6. Monitoring and evaluating (determining the effect of the HIA on the decision) (CDC, 2015d, para. 3)

As planners prepare for a needs assessment they must also consider whether an HIA should be a part of the process.

Organizational Health Assessment

Earlier in this chapter mention was made of the impact that the Patient Protection and Affordable Care Act had on non-profit hospitals and the requirement that the hospitals had to conduct a CHNA once every three years. Another section (i.e., 1201) of the same law amended Section 2705 of the Public Health Service Act that encourages employers to implement comprehensive worksite health promotion programs for their employees. Under the new law, employers can offer incentives (up to 30% of the total cost of coverage) to encourage participation. The program must be reasonably designed to promote health or prevent disease. A program complies with the *reasonably designed* provision "if it 1) has a reasonable chance of improving the health of, or preventing disease in, participating individuals; (2) is not overly burdensome; (3) is not a subterfuge for discrimination based on a health factor; and (4) is not highly suspect in the method chosen to promote health or prevent disease" (CMS, 2015a, p. 2). "Critics of this provision have voiced concern about the broad definition of a 'reasonably designed' wellness program" (Goetzel et al., 2013, p. TAHP-2). To deal with this issue, in recent years several organizational health assessments have been created to determine if best-practices are in place in employer-sponsored worksite health promotion programs (Goetzel et al., 2013). These organization health assessments can be thought of as needs assessments for reasonably designed employee-sponsored worksite health promotion programs. Three of these organizational health assessments—the HERO Employee Health Management Best Practices Scorecard (Health Enhancement Research Organization, 2014), the Wellness Impact Scorecard (WISCORE®) (National Business Group on Health, 2015), Optimal Healing Environment (OHE) Assessment™ (Samueli Institute, 2015) —have been reviewed by Goetzel et al. 2013.

Summary

This chapter presented definitions of needs assessment and a discussion of primary and secondary data. The sources of these data along with their pros and cons were discussed at length. Also, presented in this chapter was a six-step approach that planners can follow in conducting a needs assessment on a given group of people. It is by no means the only way of conducting an assessment, but it is one viable option. No matter what procedure is used to conduct a needs assessment, the end result should be the same. Planners should finish with a clearly defined program focus. Finally, the terms health impact assessment and organization health assessment were introduced.

Review Questions

1. What is a need? What does *needs assessment* mean?
2. What is meant by the terms *capacity, community capacity*, and *capacity building*?
3. What should program planners expect from a needs assessment?
4. What is the difference between primary and secondary data?
5. Name several different sources of both primary and secondary data.
6. What advice might you give to someone who is interested in using previously collected data (secondary data) for a needs assessment?
7. What is the difference between a single-step (cross-sectional) and a multistep survey?
8. Explain the difference between a community forum and a focus group.
9. What are the steps in the photovoice process?
10. What is a health assessment (HA)?
11. Describe the steps used to conduct a literature search.
12. What are the six steps in the needs assessment process, as identified in this chapter? What is the most difficult step to complete?
13. What is the difference between the BPR model and the BPR model 2.0?
14. What is health impact assessment (HIA) and how could it affect a needs assessment?
15. What is an organizational health assessment? What relationship does it have to the Affordable Care Act?

Activities

1. Assume a local health department (LHD) that serves a rural population of about 100,000 people has hired you. After a few months on the job, your supervisor has given you the task of conducting a needs assessment. The last one completed by this LHD was 15 years ago. Based on the annual reports of the LHD over the past 5 years, it has been determined that the needs assessment should focus on the needs of the elderly. For the purpose of this needs assessment, the LHD has defined elderly as those 65 years of age and older. Working with the six-step approach to needs assessment presented in this chapter, complete the first two steps. Complete Step 1 by writing a purpose and scope for the needs assessment. Complete the first part of Step 2 by identifying at least four sources of relevant secondary data. Also, describe what you think would be the best way to go about collecting primary data and defend your choice. Then complete this activity by creating a list of things you would like to find out by gathering primary data.

2. Visit the Website of a commercial company (e.g., FluidSurveys, Qualtrics, QuestionPro, SurveyMonkey, surveygizmo, Zoomerang) that is in the business of helping others collect primary data via the Internet. Once at the site, find out as much as you can about using the service. What specific services does the company offer? How much do the services cost? What group of program planners do you think would most benefit from using the services? Summarize the results of your fact-finding experience in a one-page paper.

3. Using secondary data provided by your instructor or obtained from the World Wide Web (such as data from a Behavioral Risk Factor Surveillance System, state or local secondary data, or data from the National Center for Health Statistics), analyze the data and determine the health problems of the priority population.

4. Using data from the County Health Rankings Website (http://www.countyhealthrankings .org), examine the data presented for the county in which you grew up or currently live. After reviewing the data, prepare a written response that summarizes the general health status of the county.

5. Administer an HHA/HRA to a group of 25 to 30 people. Using the data generated, identify and prioritize a collective list of health problems of the group.

6. Plan and conduct a focus group on an identified health problem on your campus. Develop a set of questions to be used, identify and invite people to participate in the group, facilitate the process, and then write up a summary of the results based on your written notes and/or an audiotape of the session.

7. Using the data (paper-and-pencil instruments, clinical tests, and health histories) generated from a local health fair, identify and prioritize a collective list of health problems of those who participated.

Weblinks

1. **http://ctb.ku.edu/en**

   The Community Tool Box

   This site provides excellent resources on community assessment, conducting surveys, identifying problems, and assessing community needs and resources. Topic sections include step-by-step instruction, examples, checklists, and related resources.

2. **http://www.csuchico.edu/lins/handouts/eval_websites.pdf**

   CRAAP Test– Meriam Library, California State University, Chico

   This link takes you to a handout that presents the CRAAP Test for evaluating materials found on the World Wide Web.

3. **http://www.cdc.gov/nchs/surveys.htm**

   National Center for Health Statistics

   This Webpage of the National Center for Health Statistics (NCHS) provides an overview of all of the surveys and data collections systems of the NCHS. In addition, it provides the results of many of the surveys and examples of the questionnaires used to collect the data.

4. **http://www.kff.org/statedata/**

   Kaiser Family Foundation State Health Facts

   This site contains current state-level data on demographics and the economy, health costs and budgets, health coverage and uninsured, health insurance and managed care, health reform, health status, HIV/AIDS, Medicaid and CHIP, Medicare, minority health, providers and service use, and women's health. Planners can access information as tables, trend graphs, or color-coded maps.

5. **http://wonder.cdc.gov**

   CDC WONDER

   This is the home page for the Centers for Disease Control and Prevention's (CDC) Wide-ranging Online Data for Epidemiologic Research (WONDER). CDC WONDER is an easy-to-use, menu-driven system that provides access to a wide array of secondary public health information.

Measurement, Measures, Measurement Instruments, and Sampling

Chapter Objectives

After reading this chapter and answering the questions that follow, you should be able to:

- Define *measurement*.
- Explain the difference between quantitative and qualitative measures.
- Explain the reasons that measurement is such an important process as it relates to program planning and evaluation as well as research.
- Briefly describe the four levels of measurement.
- List the variables that are often measured by health education specialists.
- List the four desirable characteristics of data.
- Explain the various types of validity.
- Define *reliability* and explain why it is important.
- Define *bias* in data collection and discuss how it can be reduced.
- Briefly describe the steps to identify, obtain, and evaluate existing measurement instruments.
- Be able to develop questions and response options for a data collection instrument.
- Briefly describe the process for creating appropriate presentation for a data collection instrument.
- Describe how a sample can be obtained from a population.
- Differentiate between probability and nonprobability samples.
- Describe how a pilot test is used.

Key Terms

bias
census
cluster sampling
cognitive pretesting
concurrent validity
construct validity
content validity
convergent validity
criterion-related validity
discriminant validity
equivalence reliability
face validity
instrumentation
internal consistency
inter-rater reliability
interval level measures
intra-rater reliability
levels of measurement
measurement
measurement instrument
nominal level measures
nonprobability samples
nonproportional stratified random sample
ordinal level measures
parallel forms
pilot testing
population
predictive validity
preliminary review
pre-pilots
probability sample
proportional stratified random sample
psychometric qualities
public domain
qualitative measures
quantitative measures
random selection
rater reliability
ratio level measures
reliability
sample
sampling
sampling frame
sampling unit
sensitivity
simple random sample (SRS)
specificity
stability reliability
strata
stratified random sample
survey population
systematic sample
universe
validity

I n this chapter, we will examine critical concepts necessary to maximize the quality of data, whether for a needs assessment or a program evaluation. Specifically, we will examine the (1) term *measurement*, (2) types of data generated from measurement, (3) importance of measurement, (4) levels of measurement, (5) types of measures, (6) desirable characteristics of measures, (7) measurement instruments, (8) sampling, and (9) the importance of pilot testing in the data collection process.

Box 5.1 identifies the responsibilities and competencies for health education specialists that pertain to the material presented in this chapter.

▷ Measurement

Measurement can be defined as the process of applying numerical or narrative data from an instrument (e.g., a questionnaire) or other data-yielding tools to objects, events, or people (Windsor, 2015). For example, if researchers collect data on height and weight from a group of people then translate those data to body mass index (BMI) values (weight in kilograms divided by height in meters squared), they can classify participants as either underweight (usually a BMI of < 18.50), normal (18.50-24.99), overweight (25-29.99) or obese (> 30). In order to measure something then, planners and evaluators (hereafter referred to collectively as planners) need to identify what instrument or tool will be used to collect data, how data

---

BOX	**Responsibilities and Competencies for Health Education Specialists**
5.1	Because of the importance of measurement to program planning and evaluation, the content of this chapter cuts across two different areas of responsibility. Those responsibilities and related competencies include the following:

RESPONSIBILITY I: Assess Needs, Resources, and Capacity for Health Education/Promotion

Competency 1.2: Access existing information and data related to health

Competency 1.3: Collect primary data to determine needs

Competency 1.4: Analyze relationships among behavioral, environmental, and other factors that influence health

Competency 1.6: Examine factors that enhance or impede the process of health education/promotion

Competency 1.7: Determine needs for health education/promotion based on assessment findings

RESPONSIBILITY IV: Conduct Evaluation and Research Related to Health Education/Promotion

Competency 4.3: Select, adapt and/or create instruments to collect data

Competency 4.4: Collect and manage data

Competency 4.6: Interpret results

Competency 4.7: Apply findings

Source: *A Competency-Based Framework for Health Education Specialists—2015.* Whitehall, PA: National Commission for Health Education Credentialing, Inc. (NCHEC) and the Society for Public Health Education (SOPHE). Reprinted by permission of the National Commission for Health Education Credentialing, inc. (NCHEC) and the Society for Public Health Education (SOPHE).

will be categorized using numbers or words, and how these categories of data will be classified (e.g., for BMI: high risk, medium risk, low risk or excellent health, good health, poor health, etc.).

The data generated by measurements can be classified into two broad categories, depending on the method by which they are collected. **Quantitative measures** "are numerical data collected to understand individuals' knowledge, understanding, perceptions, and behavior" (Harris, 2010, p. 208). Examples of quantitative data could include the mortality rates for diabetes over the last five years, the aforementioned BMIs of participants in a weight loss program, the prevalence of cigarette smoking among adolescents, the ratings on a patient satisfaction survey, and the pretest and posttest scores on a HIV knowledge test. **Qualitative measures** are "data collected with the use of narrative and observational approaches to understand individuals' knowledge, perceptions, attitudes and behaviors" (Harris, 2010, p. 208). Qualitative data are usually represented as words that are organized into codes and themes. Examples of qualitative data could include notes generated from observational studies, transcripts from focus groups, and taped recordings of in-depth interviews with key informants. Quantitative and qualitative measures both have their individual strengths and weaknesses, yet their greatest utility may occur when both are used together in the measurement process. While quantitative data with adequate sample sizes can accurately represent entire populations, qualitative data can provide rich contextual understanding of those same populations. One way to think about the difference is that quantitative data is like looking at a picture that is just black and white; all you see are the numbers. Qualitative data adds color and texture, or richness to those numbers. **Table 5.1** provides a comparison of many of the qualities and characteristics of quantitative and qualitative measures.

The Importance of Measurement in Program Planning and Evaluation

As noted earlier in the chapter (see Box 5.1), health education specialists are expected to have the knowledge and skills to plan and carry out the processes associated with measurement; for example, (1) when reviewing literature in order to justify a program, health education specialists need to be able to understand the data generated by measurement in order to determine if they have adequate and appropriate evidence for a proposed program; (2) when conducting a needs assessment, health education specialists must understand

TABLE 5.1 **Comparison of Quantitative and Qualitative Measures**

Quantitative Measures	Qualitative Measures
Measures level of occurrence	Provides depth of understanding
Asks how often? and how many?	Asks why?
Studies actions	Studies motivations
Is objective	Is subjective
Provides proof	Enables discovery
Is definitive	Is exploratory
Measures levels of actions and trends, etc.	Allows insights into behavior and trends, etc.
Describes	Interprets

Source: Cottrell & McKenzie (2011, p. 228) from Debus (1988).

the basic principles of measurement in order to select and use appropriate data collection instruments; (3) when health education specialists are planning an evaluation to measure whether program objectives have been met, they need to be able to measure related program outcomes; (4) when a funding agency wants evidence that a program it funds is making a dif-ference in a community, health education specialists must apply appropriate measurement techniques to generate the needed evidence; or (5) when health education specialists are asked to interpret the results of a program evaluation to a group of stakeholders, they need to be competent in determining and communicating whether program components actually produced the identified results. Each of these examples demonstrates the need for a sound understanding of the processes associated with measurement. In other words, measurement is an integral part of program planning, implementation, and evaluation.

Levels of Measurement

A fundamental question of measurement is deciding *how* something should be measured (McDermott & Sarvela, 1999). For example, consider a scenario in which planners need data on the income levels of program participants. They could ask about the participants' income level in any of the following three ways:

1. Which of the following categories most closely corresponds with your overall household income: poor, lower middle class, upper middle class, or wealthy?

2. What income category best describes your annual household income? $0 to 10,000; $10,001 to 25,000; $25,001 to 40,000; $40,001 to 55,000; $55,001 to 70,000; $70,001+

3. What is your annual household income? $ _____ per year

Although these questions all pertain to household income, each question generates a different type and level of data. Seventy years ago, Stevens (1946) proposed that four **levels of measurement**—nominal, ordinal, interval, and ratio—were the basis for all scientific measurement. In fact, these four levels of measurement are widely accepted in social and behavioral research. The four levels of measurement are considered "hierarchical" in nature. In other words, they progress from more simple or basic to more complex.

1. **Nominal level measures** constitute the lowest level in the measurement hierarchy and use names or labels to categorize people, places, or things. While nominal data represent different categories, they do not represent any particular value or order (i.e., they are simply grouped by name). "The two requirements for nominal measures are that the categories have to be mutually exclusive so that each case fits into one of the categories, and the categories have to be exhaustive so that there is a place for every case" (Weiss, 1998, p. 116). For example, a question that would generate nominal data is, "What is your current student status?" The possible answers include the categories of "undergraduate student" and "graduate student." These answers are exhaustive (contain all possible answers) and mutually exclusive (the respondent has to be one or the other, but not both). We can then assign numbers to these categories according to a particular rule we create (e.g., 1 = undergraduate, 2 = graduate).

2. **Ordinal level measures**, like nominal level measures, allow planners to put data into categories that are mutually exclusive and exhaustive, but also permit them to rank-order the categories. The different categories represent relatively more or less of something. However, the distance between categories cannot be measured. For example, the question "How would you describe your level of satisfaction with your

health care? (select one) very satisfied—satisfied—not satisfied" creates categories (very satisfied—satisfied—not satisfied) that are mutually exclusive (the respondent cannot select two categories) and exhaustive (there is a category for all levels of satisfaction), and the categories represent more or less of something (amount of satisfaction), thus there is a rank order. We cannot, however, measure the distance (or difference) between the levels of satisfaction. Is the distance between very satisfied and satisfied the same distance between satisfied and not satisfied? Ordinal data categories are not necessarily an equal distance apart. Another example is when a patient is asked how much pain he or she is experiencing on a scale from 1 to 10. While 7 is more severe than 5, this difference may not be the same as the difference between 3 and 1.

3. **Interval level measures** enable planners to put data into categories that are mutually exclusive and exhaustive, and rank-orders the categories, and are continuous. Furthermore, the widths or differences between categories must all be the same (Hurlburt, 2003), which allows for the distance between the categories to be measured. There is, however, no absolute zero value. For example, a question that generates interval data is, "What was the high temperature today?" We know that a temperature of 70°F is different than a temperature of 80°F, that 80° is warmer than 70°, that there is 10°F difference between the two, and if the temperature drops to 0° F there is still some heat in the air (though not much) because 0°F is warmer than –10°F. Examples of health-related variables that are commonly measured on the interval level include weight, cholesterol, height, blood pressure, age and so forth.

4. **Ratio level measures**, the highest level in the measurement hierarchy, enable planners to do everything with data that can be done with the other three levels of measures; however, those tasks are accomplished using a scale with an absolute zero. Example questions that generate ratio data include the following: "During an average week, how many minutes do you exercise aerobically?" "How much money did you earn last month?" and "How many hours of sleep did you get last night?" An absolute zero "point means that the thing being measured actually vanishes when the scale reads zero" (Hurlburt, 2003, p. 17).

Table 5.1 shows the type of questions on a data collection instrument that result in different levels of measurement. **Figure 5.1** shows how different levels of data may be presented as charts after data analysis has been completed.

Because interval and ratio data are continuous and rank-ordered values with equal distance between them, and because most statistical procedures are the same for both types of data (Valente, 2002), some have combined them into a single level of measurement and refer to the resulting data as *numerical data*.

The type of data gathered dictates the type of statistical analyses that can be used. Generally speaking, nominal and ordinal measures are associated with nonparametric tests (less likely to assume a normal distribution of data, i.e., bell shaped curve) while interval and ratio data are more often associated with parametric tests (more likely to assume a normal distribution of data). Parametric statistics are often more powerful in detecting differences between groups and are therefore preferred by researchers and evaluators (Siegel & Castellan, 1988). Thus, when planners begin to think about measurement and data collection, they need to consider both the wording of their questions and the response options and how that wording will impact the data analysis (see Chapter 15).

As presented earlier, many different methods can be used to collect both primary and secondary data (see Chapter 4). Any method selected will require a measurement instrument

Nominal data

Ratio/Interval data

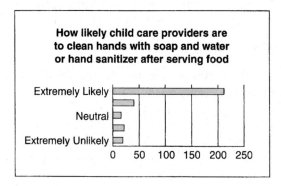

Ordinal data

▲ **Figure 5.1** How to Present Various Levels of Data

to collect the data. By **measurement instrument**, we mean the item used to measure the variables (e.g., demographic, psychosocial, behavioral) of interest. Measurement instruments are also sometimes referred to as tools or data collection instruments. The term **instrumentation** is "a collective term that describes all measurement instruments used" (Cottrell & McKenzie, 2011, p. 146).

Measurement instruments can take many different forms and sizes. They can range from the very simple, like a ruler or yardstick, to a questionnaire, to a very complicated piece of machinery that performs DNA sequencing. Although at times health education specialists may use machines or equipment as instruments (e.g., to check blood cholesterol), more commonly they employ a sequence of questions to measure variables of interest (Windsor, 2015). These sequences of questions most often take the form of *tests, questionnaires,* and *scales.* The term *test* is most often used in the context of educational measurement (DiIorio, 2005), such as an HIV/AIDS knowledge test. Questionnaires (sometimes called *survey instruments*) are instruments that gather information about a variety of factors (e.g., awareness, skills, behaviors, health status) related to one or more specific topics. For example, a questionnaire may be developed about sleep habits and include questions about the average number of hours slept per night, what time a person typically goes to sleep, use of sleep aids, and techniques used to fall a sleep. A questionnaire can include questions about several concepts or one or more scales. A scale is a set of questions that asks about one concept or construct, often related to a psychosocial variable like attitudes, beliefs, or opinions. For example, health education specialists may be interested in collecting data about attitudes related to water fluoridation in the priority population. The attitude scale would be a set of questions related to attitudes. In scales, often the response choice for every question is the same (e.g., always, sometimes, never). Sometimes the word *scale* is used in a general sense to refer to an entire questionnaire or instrument; however, it is not a technically correct use of the term.

Depending on the nature of the questions being asked, the instrument can vary in length. Some instruments can be as short as a single question, rating, or item to measure the variable, while others may be multipage instruments. There are advantages and disadvantages to various instrument lengths. Obvious advantages of a shorter instrument are the time for the participants to complete it and for the planners to organize and analyze the data. However, longer instruments may do a better job of measuring less stable (i.e., change over time) variables like attitudes (DiIorio, 2005), and longer instruments may be more suitable for statistical calculations (Bowling, 2005).

Types of Measures

Many different types of measures are used to conduct needs assessments or evaluate programs. Typically, health promotion programs focus on one or more of the following types of measures (also called variables) related to: demographics, awareness, knowledge, psychosocial characteristics, skills, behaviors, environmental attributes, health status, and quality of life indicators. **Table 5.2** illustrates some of these variables and the level of measurement.

▷ Desirable Characteristics of Data

The results of a needs assessment or program evaluation are only as good as the data that are collected and analyzed. If a questionnaire is filled with ambiguous questions and the respondents are not sure how to answer, it is highly unlikely that the data will reflect the true knowledge, attitudes, and so on, of those responding. Therefore, it is of vital importance that planners and evaluators make sure that the data they collect are reliable, valid, and unbiased. Collectively, these characteristics—reliability and validity—are referred to as an instrument's **psychometric qualities** (Cottrell & McKenzie, 2011).

TABLE 5.2 **Examples of Questions and Levels of Measurement**

Variable	Question Stem	Response Options	Level of Measurement
Demographic Height	About how tall are you without shoes?	__/__ ft/inches	Interval
Awareness			
Awareness of smoking cessation quitlines	A telephone quitline is a free telephone-based service that connects people who smoke cigarettes with someone who can help them quit. Are you aware of any telephone quitline services that are available to help people quit smoking?	Yes No	Nominal
Knowledge			
Knowledge of heart attack symptoms	Do you think pain or discomfort in the arms or shoulder are symptoms of a heart attack?	Yes No	Nominal
Psychosocial			
Social and emotional support	How often do you get the social and emotional support you need?	Always Usually Sometimes Rarely Never	Ordinal
Depression	During the past 30 days, for about how many days have you felt sad, blue, or depressed?	__ __ days	Ratio
Behaviors			
Visit to healthcare provider	About how many times in the past 12 months have you seen a doctor, nurse, or other health professional for your diabetes?	__ __ times	Ratio
Health status			
Arthritis diagnosis	Has a doctor, nurse, or other health professional EVER told you that you had some form of arthritis, rheumatoid arthritis, gout, lupus, or fibromyalgia?	Yes No	Nominal
Quality of life			
Overall measure of health	Would you say that in general your health is—	Excellent Very good Good Fair Poor	Ordinal

Source: Centers for Disease Prevention and Control, 2015a

Reliability

Reliability refers to consistency in the measurement process. That is, **reliability** "is an empirical estimate of the extent to which an instrument produces the same result (measure or score), applied once or two or more times" (Windsor, 2015, p. 196). However, no instrument will ever provide perfect accuracy in measurement because there will always be error. Reliability coefficients are highest if no error exists ($r = 1.0$) and lowest when there is only error or no association ($r = 0.0$) between two measures (Windsor, 2015). Error can come from many sources as will be discussed in the next section about reliability estimates. Planners need to strive to collect data under the best conditions that will produce reliable data. Several methods of estimating reliability are available.

Internal consistency is one of the most commonly used reliability estimates (Windsor et al., 2004). It refers to the intercorrelations among the individual items on a scale, that is, whether items on the scale are measuring the same domain. This can be done by examining the scale to ensure that the items reflect what is to be measured and that the level of difficulty of all items is consistent. Statistical methods can also be used to determine internal consistency by correlating the items on the test with the total score. A Cronbach's alpha reliability coefficient measures internal consistency and ranges from 0 to 1 with scores of greater than 0.70 typically classified as acceptable and scores of 0.80 classified as good (George & Mallery, 2003). While alpha coefficients of 0.90 or greater are generally considered to be excellent, scores this high can also indicate there is redundancy in the instrumentation (i.e., too many questions may be asking the same thing). If Cronbach's alpha is low that means there are errors due to item or content sampling, meaning all the questions on the scale are not interrelated. For example a researcher asked three questions related to people's perceptions about weight control ("The health and strength of my body are more important to me than how much I weigh;" "I honestly don't care how much I weigh as long as I am physically fit, healthy, and can do the things I want;" "I mostly exercise because of how it makes me feel physically"). The three items had a Cronbach alpha of 0.597. The item correlation matrix showed that last of the three items was not like the others and this contributed to the low reliability estimate. By removing the last item, the alpha increased to 0.633. This was still not at the .70 level, but it was improved.

Stability reliability estimates look for consistency over a period of time (Crocker & Algina, 1986). To establish this type of reliability, the same instrument is used to measure the same group of people under similar, or the same conditions, at two different points in time, and the two sets of data generated by the measurement are used to calculate a correlation coefficient (Cottrell & McKenzie, 2011). This is referred to as test-retest. An adequate amount of time should be allowed between the test and retest so that individuals are not responding on the basis of remembering responses they made the first time, but not be so long that other events could occur in the intervening time to influence their responses. To avoid the problems of retesting, parallel forms (equivalent forms) of the test can be administered to the participants and the results can be correlated. While a Cohen's kappa coefficient (Cohen, 1960) equal to or greater to than 0.70 is generally acceptable, a coefficient of 0.80 is ideal and should be documented (Harris, 2010; Windsor, 2015). There are many sources of error that can contribute to inconsistent scores over time including changes within the person (they did not get enough sleep the night before), or "errors due to administration, scoring, guessing, mismarking by examinees, and other temporary fluctuations in behavior" (Crocker & Algina, 1986, p. 133). Stability is important when implementing interventions over a long period of time and success is evaluated using pre and posttests. If there should be no change in the variables being measured among participants from pre- to posttest (i.e., the control group), then stability will be an important reliability estimate.

Rater reliability focuses on the consistency between individuals who are observing or rating the same item or when one individual is observing or rating a series of items. If two or more raters are involved, it is referred to as **inter-rater reliability**. If only one individual is observing or rating a series of events, it is referred to as **intra-rater reliability**. There are several different ways to calculate rater reliability. In a research study, most researchers would use Cohen's kappa to calculate rater reliability. However, a quicker and easier method is to calculate it as a percentage of agreement between/among raters or within an individual rater (DiIorio, 2005). An example of inter-rater reliability would be the percent of agreement between two observers who are observing passing drivers in cars for safety belt use. If raters observe 10 cars and the raters agree 8 out of 10 times on whether the drivers are wearing their safety belts, the inter-rater reliability would be 80%. Intra-rater reliability would be the degree to which one rater agrees with himself or herself on the characteristics of an observation over time. For example, when a rater is evaluating the CPR skills of participants in his or her program, the rater should be consistent while observing and evaluating participants.

Estimates of **equivalence reliability** focus on whether different forms of the same measurement instrument, when measuring the same subjects, will produce similar results (means, standard deviations, and inter-item correlations). The method used to establish equivalence is often referred to as **parallel forms**, equivalent forms, or alternate-forms reliability. One group is given both versions of an instrument and then the scores are correlated. The usefulness of having measurement instruments that possess parallel forms reliability is being able to test the same subjects on different occasions (e.g., using a pretest-posttest evaluation design) without concern that the subjects will score better on the second administration (posttest) because they remember questions from the first administration (pretest) of the instrument. Another time equivalent forms are used is when a researcher is trying to determine if a shorter form of a scale is just as reliable as a longer form. For example, the International Physical Activity Questionnaire (IPAQ) has both a short version (9 items) and a long version (31 items; Craig et al., 2003). If these instruments have equivalence it would not matter if a person filled out the short or long form, both instruments would give the same estimate of physical activity levels. If the forms are not equivalent, there is error due to item or content sampling.

Validity

When designing a data collection instrument, planners must ensure that it measures what it is intended to measure. This refers to **validity**. Using an instrument that produces valid results increases the chance that planners are measuring what they want to measure, thus ruling out other possible explanations for the results.

Face validity is the lowest level of validity. A measure is said to have face validity if, on the face, it appears to measure what it is supposed to measure (McDermott & Sarvela, 1999). Face validity differs from the other forms of validity in that it lacks some form of systematic logical analysis of the content (Hopkins, Stanley, & Hopkins, 1990). An example of face validity is when a planner/evaluator asks a group of colleagues to look over a series of questions to see whether they seem reasonable to include on a questionnaire about the risk for heart disease. Face validity is a good first step toward creating a valid measurement instrument, but is not a replacement for the other means of establishing validity (Cottrell & McKenzie, 2011).

Content validity refers to "the assessment of the correspondence between the items composing the instrument and the content domain from which the items were selected" (DiIorio, 2005, p. 213). This means that all essential elements of a domain or area are included in the instrument. For example, a person takes the certification exam to become a health education specialist (CHES) they want to be sure that the questions ask about everything a pesron should know and be able to do as a CHES certified health educator, and not just research and evaluation or another area of responsibility.

Content validity is usually established by using a group (jury or panel) of experts to review the instrument. After such a group is identified, they would be asked to review each element of the instrument for appropriateness. The collective opinion of the experts is then used to determine the content of the instrument. McKenzie and colleagues (1999) present a method of establishing content validity that includes both qualitative and quantitative steps.

With **criterion-related validity** we are interested in the usefulness of the score as an indicator of specific trait or behavior presently or in the future. To establish criterion validity for a scale, there must be a "gold standard" for the comparison with the scale. A gold standard is a measure that everyone agrees upon is the most accurate and valid measure of a trait, attribute, or behavior.

Concurrent validity means that the score on a measure (a scale) can predict the present standing or status of a trait, attribute or behavior, or even disease status. For example, a person fills out a survey about mental health and their score on that survey shows they have major depression. If the instrument has high concurrent validity that score is highly correlated with a counselor's diagnosis (the gold standard) of major depression. **Predictive validity** means that the score on a measure is able to predict future standing or status. For example, in prenatal screening a physician wants the amniocentesis test to accurately predict whether or not a baby will have (or not have) a birth defect when he or she is born. In physical activity measurement the gold standard is an accelerometer (think Fitbit or Fuel Band). When establishing validity for a new self-reported measure for how much physical activity a person got in the last 3 days, the score on the measure would be compared to the results from the accelerometer the person wore during the same time. If there is good concurrent validity then the scores from the self-report measure are highly correlated with the accelerometer results. Both measures are in agreement about a person's physically activity level.

Construct validity is concerned with whether the instrument is measuring the underlying construct. A construct is a label that we assign a set of attributes or behaviors; it is often abstract and sometimes theoretical. Examples of constructs in public health and the social sciences are: depression, body-image satisfaction, self-efficacy, worry, social support, perceived severity, religiosity, chronic disease self-management, anxiety, hopelessness, perceived stress, school satisfaction, job satisfaction, and so forth (see here for examples of more constructs http://cancercontrol.cancer.gov/brp/constructs/).

We cannot measure constructs with a simple question or an observation. That is we cannot ask a person "Are you depressed?" But if a person answers a set of questions (a scale) about their attitudes, behaviors, thoughts, and so forth, then the construct of depression can be measured. For example, a person answers the 21-item Beck Depression Inventory (BDI; Beck, Steer, & Carbin, 1988) and based on their score it can be determined whether or not they are depressed.

If we have construct validity then we can say that the scores from the scale represent the construct. We are confident that we are actually measuring what we said we are measuring. For example, we are confident the score on the BDI indicates a person has depression and is not a measure of a related (or unrelated) construct such as high social anxiety (i.e., the fear of negative evaluation by others).

Convergent validity is a type of construct validity evidence. It "is the extent to which two measures which purport to be measuring the same topic correlate (that is, converge)" (Bowling, 2005, p. 12). For example, researchers developing the Reynolds Adolescent Depression (RAD) scale (Krefetz, Steer, Gulab, & Beck, 2002) gave the RAD and the well-established BDI to a group on inpatient psychiatric adolescents. The scores revealed high correlation between the RAD and the BDI measures. This provided evidence that the RAD was in fact measuring depression. **Discriminant validity** "requires that the construct should not correlate with dissimilar (discriminant) variables" (Bowling, 2005, p. 12). The BDI is able to discriminate or distinguish between depression and anxiety (Beck, Steer, & Carbin, 1988). Again, this gives planners confidence that they are measuring what they intended to measure.

SENSITIVITY AND SPECIFICITY

When speaking about validity, planners should also be familiar with the terms *sensitivity* and *specificity*. These terms are used in health care settings as well as epidemiology to express the validity of screening and diagnostic tests (Cottrell & McKenzie, 2011). **Sensitivity** is defined as the ability of the test to identify correctly those who actually have the disease (Friis & Sellers, 2009). It is recorded as the proportion of true positive cases correctly identified as positive on the test (Timmreck, 1997). The better the sensitivity, the fewer the false positives. **Specificity** is defined as "the ability of the test to identify only non-diseased individuals who actually do not have the disease" (Friis & Sellers, 2009, p. 24). It is recorded as the proportion of true negative cases correctly identified as negative on the test (Timmreck, 1997). And the better the specificity, the fewer the number of false negatives. "An ideal screening test would demonstrate 100% sensitivity and 100% specificity. In practice this does not occur; sensitivity and specificity are usually inversely related" (Mausner & Kramer, 1985, p. 217).

Both validity and reliability are important. If an instrument does not measure what it is supposed to, then it does not matter if it is reliable (Windsor, 2015). If it is reliable planners may consistently get the same results, but the results will be of little value. **Box 5.2** summarizes the different types of reliability and validity.

BOX

5.2

Types of Reliability and Validity

Reliability—"an empirical estimate of the extent to which an instrument produces the same result (measure or score), applied once or two or more times" (Windsor, 2015, p. 196).

   Internal consistency—the intercorrelations among individual items on the instrument, that is, whether all items on the instrument are measuring part of the same domain.

   Stability—used to generate evidence of consistency over time" (Crocker & Algina, 1986).

   Rater (or observer)—associated with the consistent measurement (or rating) of an observed event by the same or different individuals (or judges or raters) (McDermott & Sarvela, 1999).

   Equivalence—focuses on whether different forms of the same instrument, or a shorter version of an instrument, when measuring the same participants will produce similar results. Also referred to as **parallel**, equivalent or alternate **forms reliability**.

Validity—whether an instrument correctly measures what it is intended to measure.

   Face—if, on the face, the measure appears to measure what it is supposed to measure (McDermott & Sarvela, 1999).

   Content—"the assessment of the correspondence between the items composing the instrument and the content domain from which the items were selected" (DiIorio, 2005, p. 213).

   Criterion-related—if the score is an indicator of specific trait or behavior presently (concurrent), in the future (predictive).

   Construct—scores on the instrument are measuring the underlying construct. There can be convergent and discriminant construct validity evidence.

Bias Free

Biased data are those data that do not accurately reflect the true level of a measure because of errors in the measurement process including how data were collected. In addition, **bias** can be introduced due to error in the selection of the study participants, in the study's design, or in the intervention phase which includes how participants were exposed to the treatment (Hartman, Forsen, Wallace, & Neely, 2002). In order to effectively plan and evaluate health promotion programs, planners must work to control bias. Windsor (2015) describes ways in which bias can occur in data collection—for example, when participants do not feel comfortable answering a sensitive question, when participants act differently because they know they are being watched, when certain characteristics of the interviewer influence a response, when participants answer questions in a particular way regardless of the questions being asked, or when a biased sample has been selected from the priority population (see information later in this chapter on sampling).

There are a number of steps planners can take to limit bias. For example, if data are being collected via observation, the observation should be as unobtrusive as possible. If sensitive questions are being asked of respondents, then those collecting such data need to ensure that the data are being collected in a confidential way (the identity of the respondent can be determined but not released), and consider collecting the data via an anonymous means (there is no way of identifying the respondent). No matter how data are collected, the use of techniques to reduce bias will increase the accuracy of the results.

▷ Measurement Instruments

Using an Existing Measurement Instrument

Before planners create their own measurement instrument, they should search for an existing instrument that will produce valid and reliable data and that meets their needs. As you will discover in the next section, it takes a great deal of time, effort, and resources to create a measurement instrument with good psychometric qualities. The main advantages of using an existing instrument include less planning time and thus lower costs. The major disadvantage—one that prevents the use of many existing instruments—is that the items on the existing instrument may not be relevant or appropriate for the program being planned or evaluated. Cottrell and McKenzie (2011) offer four steps for identifying, obtaining, and evaluating existing measurement instruments.

Step 1: Identifying measurement instruments. Start by searching the literature to see what others have used. You may not find an actual copy of the measurement instruments in the literature, but you may find a reference to the original source. As you are aware by now, the U.S. government has created many health-related data collection instruments. Conducting a search of applicable Websites (e.g., National Center for Health Statistics) can be useful. Remember, government publications are in the **public domain** (available for anyone to use) and thus free of charge and need no permission to use. Also, be aware that a number of commercial companies sell measurement instruments [e.g., Psychological Assessment Resources, Inc. (PAR)]. In addition, you may not find a measurement instrument that you can use in whole, but you may find specific questions or a scale that may work for you.

Step 2: Getting your hands on the instrument. Once you have identified potential measurement instruments, you then have to obtain a hard copy. Unless an instrument is copyrighted, or there are plans to do so in the future, most sources are willing to share their measurement instruments. A phone call, letter, or email requesting a copy of an instrument is usually all that it takes to get a copy. Once the source of the measurement instrument is known, be aware that you may have to pay for an instrument, and have to meet certain criteria (e.g., being a licensed psychologist, or agree to certain terms) to be able to obtain and use some measurement instruments.

Step 3: Is it the right instrument? Here are some questions to ask to determine whether an instrument is the right one for your purposes:

(1) Is there sufficient evidence of the psychometric qualities (validity and reliability) of the instrument? (2) Has it been used with participants similar to yours? (3) Are standard or normative scores available for various participants? (4) Is the instrument culturally appropriate for your participants? (5) Has the reading level of the instrument been determined? (6) Is there a cost to administer or have the instrument scored? Can you afford it? (Cottrell & McKenzie, 2011, p. 164)

Step 4: Final steps before proceeding. If you think you have found the right instrument, before proceeding make sure you have done everything necessary to be able to use it. Remember, for instruments that are not in the public domain, "you need the permission of the author for any use of the instrument, usually in writing, and particularly if you need to make any changes" (Dignan, 1995, p. 67). You also may need to fulfill other conditions placed on the use of the instrument by the owner of the copyright before you use it.

Creating a Measurement Instrument

Only when planners are unable to use or adapt another instrument for their use should they undertake the process of developing their own (Janz, Champion, & Strecher, 2002). The process for creating an instrument, particularly scales, with good psychometric qualities that will yield valid and reliable data is complex and beyond the scope of this text. For a detailed discussion of steps in this process, see Cottrell and McKenzie (2011) or Crocker and Algina (1986). However, often planners and evaluators will need to create questions for an instrument to conduct formative research or to measure program success. Next we will present a general discussion about the wording, sequencing, and presentation of questions on a measurement instrument.

WORDING QUESTIONS

The way in which questions are worded is extremely important in gaining the needed information. The result of a poorly worded question was evident to one health promotion planner who was planning a smoking cessation program for employees. When asked "Do you feel we need a smoking cessation program?" most employees said yes. The planner realized later that he should have also asked the question, "If offered, would you attend a smoking cessation program?" since very few employees participated. In general, always try to avoid questions that can be answered with a simple yes or no.

The following are guidelines to help you in wording structured questions, referred to as the question stem, with fixed response options.

First, avoid leading questions that guide the respondent's answer or suggest that you are looking for a specific type of response. For example, "Most people choose to get their health care at Intermountain Health Care. Where do you go when you need to get health care?"

Second, ask only about one thing at a time. Two-part questions, also called double-barreled, should also be avoided (e.g., "Do you brush and floss your teeth?"). The respondent may brush their teeth, but not floss.

Third, avoid jargon or use of words that people do not understand. (e.g., "What cardiovascular benefits do you feel are gained from aerobic exercise?"). If you need to use a technical term, like "cardiovascular" or "aerobic" define it before asking the question. For example, "The next questions will as about aerobic exercise. By aerobic we mean activities that are done for at least 30 minutes at a time, use large muscles, and cause you to breathe harder than normal."

Fourth, be specific. For example instead of asking, "How helpful was the diabetes education class," ask "How helpful were the classes in teaching you how to test your blood sugar." The first question is too broad and general. There may be many things about the class that was helpful. The second question asks about specific aspect of the class.

RESPONSE OPTIONS

In addition to the question stem, planners must determine the format for response options. Planners must give consideration to whether the type of question and the response options will generate the needed data. For example, assume planners were interested in identifying the ages of those in the priority population. A question like "How old are you?" could generate the best data (i.e., ratio level data), but some may not want to share their actual age and thus planners may not collect enough data to describe the priority population. In this case, a question that generates ordinal level data with response options such as: 15–24 years old; 25–44 years old; 45–64 years old; 65+ years old" may be a better choice.

For ease of data entry and analysis, close-ended or fixed response are the best. The drawbacks are that these types of questions do not allow individuals to elaborate on their answers. They may also force a person into a choice because of the limited number of responses to each question. One way to ensure that the most common responses to questions are included in the possible choices is to involve several individuals (especially those in the priority population) in the formation of the instrument and in pilot testing, discussed later in this chapter.

Common forced response options often include Likert scales. Likert scales allow respondents to select an answer choice along a continuum, generally ranging from a 5- to a 7-point scale. Likert scales can measure agreement, likelihood, frequency, importance, quality, and so forth. For example, responses to the question "How much do you agree with the following statement: I feel that it is important to limit my use of salt" might be rated on a 5-point scale ranging from "strongly disagree" (1) to "strongly agree" (5).

Always make sure that the question and the response options match. For example, if a question asks "How likely are you to attend another exercise class in the next month" the response options should *not* be "yes" and "no." Instead options should be on a Likert type scale from very unlikely (1) to very likely (5) as the question is asking about "how likely" they are to do a behavior.

Response options should be mutually exclusive and exhaustive. By mutually exclusive we mean that the options do not overlap and only one can be selected. For example, "Do you currently live in a: house, condo, or apartment?" Someone may live in a basement apartment of a house and thus select both house and apartment as response options. These options are not mutually exclusive. The list could be expanded to make it exhaustive. Exhaustive response options means that all the possible choices have been included. For example, if a question asked about race and only included Black and White, the list would not be exhaustive.

PRESENTATION

A survey instrument can have good questions, but if they are not presented in a way that is easy to read and understand there may be errors in the data or the response rate may be low. Therefore, presentation is just as important as wording of questions.

Every survey, whether administered in-person, by mail, or via the Internet should have the following six components.

1. A cover page. The cover page should include the title of the survey, indicate the survey sponsor, and contain an image that reflects the survey topic.

2. A survey title. The title should tell the reader what the survey is about. For example: "Live for Life Weight Loss Class Evaluation"

3. A purpose statement. This tells the respondent the reason for the survey. Do not be too specific so as to bias participant responses. For example, "The purpose of this survey is to learn about your experience with the Live for Life classes" is better than "The purpose of this survey is to find out about how often you eat fruit and vegetables and how often you exercise."

4. A statement about confidentiality of answers. This means that nobody will know what they put as answers and their responses will not be linked to them as a person.

5. Instructions for how they should fill out the survey. For example, "For each question, mark the one box that best reflects your opinion." These instructions may also appear throughout the survey before a set of questions. In that case, they are called "transition statements." For example, "The next group of questions asks about your opinion on the Live for Life curriculum. Mark whether you agree or disagree with each statement."

6. Instructions for what they are to do with the survey once they are completed. For example, "When you are finished with the survey, please place it in the box at the front of the room."

The visual appearance of the survey is very important. This allows respondents to easily answer the questions increasing accuracy and response rates. Here are six basic guidelines:

1. Allow for ample white space. There should be plenty of white space between response options and between the question stem and the response options.

2. Indent the response options from the question stem. This sets the responses apart from the question stem and makes them easy to identify.

3. Bold the question stem. This will make the question stem stand out from the response options.

4. Indicate skip patterns. Skip patterns are words that direct them to go to a specific question based on how they respond.

5. List all questions and response options vertically, from top to bottom. Our eyes naturally scan top to bottom, so it is easier and faster to read the options. Do not try to fit a lot of

questions on one page. Remember, white space is good. Layout can include two columns on a page, but make sure to separate the columns with a line.

6. Group related questions together. For example, when asking about foods a person eats, place all the food questions together. Also, group all questions that have similar response options together. For example, if there are several questions on a Likert scale of strongly agree to strongly disagree, place them together in the survey.

Lastly, ensure that the survey is designed and coded for easy data entry and analysis. If the survey is Internet-based many of these things will be done automatically. Specifically:

1. Use check boxes next to response options. It is better to have a box that they check rather than a "circle" your answer to reduce error due to mis-marking.

2. Code the response options. Coding means that there is a number associated with every response option. It is usually a number using 6-8 point font (or superscript or subscript number) to the left of the check box. Numbers are better than letters, because data entry can be done using the number key pad on a computer keyboard; it is much faster!

3. Never ask respondents to "check all that apply." Rather have them answer yes or no for each response option. This makes them evaluate each response option individually and again makes data entry and analysis much easier.

The first questions on an instrument should be ones that capture the respondent's attention, are easy to answer, and get them interested in answering the rest of the questions. For example, it is better to ask: "Which of the following did you like best about the Live for Life program?" than to ask, "How much do you currently weigh?" Questions that deal with sensitive topics should be posed at the end of the questionnaire or interview. Answers to questions about drug use, sexuality, or even demographic information, such as income level, are more readily answered when the respondents understand the need for the information, are assured of confidentiality or anonymity, and feel comfortable with the interviewer or the questionnaire. If the respondent ends the interview or does not complete the instrument when asked sensitive questions, the other information collected can still be used. To reduce the number of questions on an instrument, ask "is this a nice-to-know question or a need-to-know question?" Planners may be interested many questions but the answers to those questions do not fit the purpose for why the data are being collected. For example, it might be nice to know if people thought the chairs in the classrooms were comfortable but that answer does not help evaluate the success of the program.

Figure 5.2 includes sample survey questions and illustrates the key points for questions, response options, and presentation.

▷ Sampling

The need to select participants from whom data will be collected can occur at several times during the process of program planning or evaluation. Depending on the size of the priority population, planners may want to collect data from all participants, a **census**, or from only some of the participants, a **sample**. Each of the participants is referred to as a sampling unit. A **sampling unit** is the element or set of elements considered for selection as part of a sample (Babbie, 1992). A sampling unit "may be an individual, an organization, or a geographical area" (Bowling, 2005, p. 166).

1. Have you ever heard of the following viruses, bacteria, or parasites? (Choose yes or no for each one)

    a. Adenovirus   1☐Yes 2☐No
    b. Enterovirus   1☐Yes 2☐No   **Skip pattern noted**
    c. Giardia   1☐Yes 2☐No
    d. Cytomegalovirus 1☐Yes 2☐No– *Go to Question 3*

    Use "Yes" or "No" and not "check all that apply"

2. In your opinion, how likely is it that you will be exposed to the cytomegalovirus at your child care facility?

    1 ☐Extremely <u>unlikely</u>
    2 ☐Somewhat <u>unlikely</u>   **Use italics or underline for emphasis**
    3 ☐Unlikely
    4 ☐Likely
    5 ☐Somewhat likely
    6 ☐Extremely likely

3. As far as you know, when should the diaper changing surface be sanitized? (Choose one)

    1 ☐During the day, as needed
    2 ☐At the end of the day
    3 ☐Once a week
    4 ☐Once a month   **Coding number to the left of each box**
    5 ☐As needed
    6 ☐After every child

    Plenty of white space

    Line separates columns

4. On a typical day, for how many children does your child care facility provide care? (Include in your count children that are unrelated and related to you)

    1 ☐ 1–4
    2 ☐ 5–8   **Questions that go on to two lines are aligned flush left**
    3 ☐ 9–12
    4 ☐ 13–16

5. Not including yourself, do you employ another staff member (full-time or part-time) at your facility?

    1 ☐ Yes   **Indent response options**
    2 ☐ No

6. How many years have you been working as a child care provider?

    1 ☐ Less than 1 year
    2 ☐ 1–5 years   **Bold question stem**
    3 ☐ 6–10 years
    4 ☐ More than 10 years

7. What is your age?

    1 ☐ 18–19
    2 ☐ 20–29   **Age categories are mutually exclusive**
    3 ☐ 30–39
    4 ☐ 40–49
    5 ☐ 50–59
    6 ☐ 60 or older

8. What is the highest level of education that you have attained?

    1 ☐ High school diploma/GED, or less
    2 ☐ Some college
    3 ☐ Associate's degree
    4 ☐ Bachelor's degree or higher

▲**Figure 5.2** Example of Survey Questions, Response Options, and Presentation

Figure 5.3 illustrates the relationship between groups of individuals. All individuals, unspecified by time or place, constitute the **universe**—for example, all U.S. citizens, regardless of where they reside in the world. Within the universe is a **population** of individuals specified by time or place, such as all U.S. residents in the 50 states on January 1, 2016. Within this

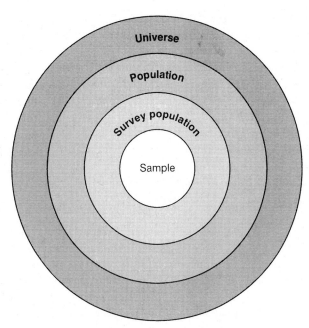

▲**Figure 5.3** Relationship of Study Populations

population is a **survey population**, composed of all individuals who are accessible to the researchers. The key term here is *accessible*. For example, all U.S. citizens who are accessible and can be reached by telephone would be a survey population. Obviously, this would not include those without telephones, such as those who choose not to own them, those institutionalized, and the homeless.

A survey population may still be too large to include in its entirety. For this reason, a sample is chosen from the survey population, a process called **sampling**. Those in the sample are the individuals who will be included in the data collection process. Using a sample rather than an entire survey population helps contain costs. For example, using a sample reduces the amount of staff time needed to conduct interviews, the cost of postage for written questionnaires, and the time and cost of travel to conduct observations.

How the sample is chosen is critical to the result of the needs assessment or evaluation: Does the information gained from the sample reflect the knowledge, attitudes, and behaviors of the survey population? According to Green and Lewis (1986), the sampling bias is the difference between the sampling estimate and the actual population value. Sampling bias can be reduced by controlling the sampling procedure—that is, how the sample is chosen. Furthermore, the ability to generalize the results to the survey population is greater when the sampling bias is reduced.

Probability Sample

Increasing the likelihood that the sample is representative of the survey population is achieved by **random selection**. Randomness minimizes the likelihood that a systematic source of selection bias will occur among the sample, thereby influencing the degree of representativeness of the population (Windsor, 2015). When random selection is used, each person in the survey population has an equal chance or probability of being selected, thus creating a **probability sample**.

There are a number of different methods for selecting a probability sample. The most basic of the probability sampling methods is selecting a **simple random sample (SRS)**. In order to select an SRS, or for that matter any probability sample, the planner must have a list or "quasi-list" (Babbie, 1992) of all sampling units in the survey population. This list is referred to as the **sampling frame**. Oftentimes, sampling frames have the names and contact information for everyone in the survey population such as with membership lists, patients of a clinic, and parents of children enrolled in a certain school or program. Other times the frame may simply be the title of an individual or organization, such as the director of environmental services in the 92 local health departments in Indiana, or a list of all the voluntary health agencies in the county (Cottrell & McKenzie, 2011).

Once the sampling frame has been identified, the planner can proceed with the process of selecting an SRS. It begins with assigning a number with an equal number of digits to each sampling unit in the frame. Suppose, for example, we have a frame of 200 individuals. The first person in the frame would be given the number 000. The rest of the individuals in the frame would be assigned consecutive numbers and the last person in the frame would be assigned the number 199. Once it is decided how large the sample should be, the sample can be selected. For the purpose of this example let's suppose a sample size of 20 is desired. To select these 20 individuals, a computer could be used to randomly select 20 numbers between 000 and 199, or it could be done manually by using a table of random numbers (Cottrell & McKenzie, 2011) (see **Table 5.3**).

In order to use a table of random numbers, the manner in which the table will be used needs to be set forth. Since these tables are generated randomly (by computer), it really does not matter which way one moves through the table as long as it is done in a consistent manner. For example, the process set forth could be to (1) use the first three digits in the columns of numbers (because all individuals in the example frame have a three-digit number, that is, 000 to 199); (2) proceed down the columns (as opposed to up or across the rows); (3) at the

TABLE 5.3 **Abbreviated Table of Random Numbers**

Row/Column	A	B	C	D	E
1	75 51	02 17	71 04	33 93	36 60
2	42 75	76 22	23 87	56 54	84 68
3	00 47	37 59	08 56	23 81	22 42
4	74 01	23 19	55 59	79 09	69 82
5	66 22	42 40	15 96	74 90	75 89
6	09 24	34 42	00 68	72 10	71 37
7	89 22	10 23	62 65	78 77	47 33
8	51 27	23 02	13 92	44 13	96 51
9	17 18	01 34	10 98	37 48	93 86
10	02 28	54 60	01 11	28 35	54 32

bottom of the column proceed to the top of the next column to the right; and (4) proceed in this same manner until the 20 individuals are selected. To ensure that this process is indeed random, the process must begin with a random start. That is, the planner cannot just pick the first number at the top of column one and proceed down through the column because every individual in the survey population would not have an equal chance of being selected. The planner can accomplish the random start by closing his or her eyes and pointing to a place on the table of random numbers then proceeding through the table in the way that was set forth above (Cottrell & McKenzie, 2011).

A **systematic sample** also uses a frame and takes every Nth person (determined by dividing the survey population size by the sample size, N/n), beginning with a randomly selected individual. For example, suppose that we want to choose a sample of 10 people from a survey population of 100. We start by randomly choosing a number between 001 and 100, such as 026, using a table of random numbers. We then choose every tenth ($N/n = 100/10 = 10$) person (036, 046, 056, 076, 086, 096, 006, 016) until we have the 10 subjects for the sample. In this way, everyone in the survey population has an equal chance of being selected. A simple random sample or systematic sample can also be used to select "naturally occurring groups or clusters, such as schools, clinics, worksites, or census tracks" (Gilmore, 2012, p. 74). When this occurs, it is called **cluster sampling**.

If it is important that certain groups be represented in a sample, a **stratified random sample** can be selected. Such a method would be used if the planners felt that a certain independent variable (e.g., size, income, or age, etc.) might have an influence on the data collected from the participants. A stratified random sample might also be used if it is believed that, due to small numbers of a certain group in the survey population, representatives from that group may not be selected using a simple random sample. That is, you may have a survey population of 100 participants and in that 100 there are only 8 of one group. If you were to select a sample of 10 from the 100, there is a good chance that none of the 8 from the small group might be selected (Cottrell & McKenzie, 2011).

Here is an example of the use of a stratified random sample. To begin, the planner first must divide the survey population into subgroups, or **strata**, then select a simple random sample from each stratum. Suppose we were interested in collecting data from companies within a particular state concerning the number of health education programs offered for employees. Based on past experience, we suspect the size of the business (i.e., number of employees) would affect the data we want to collect. That is, small companies might have fewer health education programs in general than large companies. Also, we know that relatively few companies in the state have a large number of employees. We could then divide the companies into strata by size, for example small (1–100 employees), medium (101–1,000), and large (1,001+). Once the planners decide how many to select from each stratum, they next decide whether to conduct a proportional stratified random sample or nonproportional stratified random sample. A **proportional stratified random sample** would be used if the planners wanted the sample to mirror, in proportion, the survey population. That is, draw out the companies in the same proportions that they are represented in the survey population. Say our example has 600 small companies, 350 medium companies, and 50 large companies, and the desired sample size is 100. Planners would then select simple random samples of 60 small, 35 medium, and 5 large companies (Cottrell & McKenzie, 2011).

A **nonproportional stratified random sample** may be used if the planners want equal representation from the different strata within the survey population. For example, suppose we want to collect information about the opinions of college students on a medium-size regional campus (the survey population) about a new alcohol use policy that was put in place by the administration and we want to hear equally from the different levels of students (freshmen [$n = 4,000$], sophomores [$n = 3,000$], juniors [$n = 2,000$], and seniors [$n = 1,000$]) because it is thought that the policy will affect each class differently. If a sample size of 200 is desired, we would randomly select (using a simple random sample method) 50 students from each of the classes (Cottrell & McKenzie, 2011). (See **Table 5.4** for a summary of probability sampling procedures.)

Nonprobability Sample

There are times when a probability sample cannot be obtained or is not needed. In such cases, planners can take **nonprobability samples** in which all individuals in the survey population do not have an equal chance or probability of being selected to participate in the needs assessment or evaluation. Participants can be included on the basis of convenience (because they have volunteered, are available, or can be easily contacted) or because they possess a certain characteristic.

Nonprobability samples have limitations in the extent to which the results can be generalized to the total survey population. Bias may also occur because those who are not included in the sample may differ in some way from those who are included. For example, including only the individuals who complete a health promotion program may bias the results; the findings might be different if all participants, including those who attended but did not complete the program, were surveyed.

Nonprobability samples can be used when planners are unable to identify or contact all those in the survey population. These samples can also be used when resources are limited and

TABLE 5.4 **Summary of Probability Sampling Procedures**

Sample	Primary Descriptive Elements
Simple Random	Each subject has an equal chance of being selected if table of random numbers and random start are used.
Systematic	Using a list (e.g., membership list or telephone book), subjects are selected at a constant interval (N/n) after a random start.
Nonproportional Stratified	The population is divided into subgroups based on key characteristics (strata), and subjects are selected from the subgroups at random to ensure representation of the characteristic.
Proportional Stratified	Like the nonproportional stratified random sample, but subjects are selected in proportion to the numerical strength of strata in the population.
Cluster or Area	Random sampling of groups (e.g., teachers' classes) or areas (e.g., city blocks) instead of individuals.

Source: Adapted from E. R. Babbie, *The Practice of Social Research*, 6th ed. (Belmont, CA: Wadsworth, 1992); P. C. Cozby, *Methods in Behavioral Research*, 3rd ed. (Palo Alto, CA: Mayfield, 1985); P. D. Leedy, *Practical Research: Planning and Design*, 5th ed. (New York: Prentice Hall); and R. J. McDermott and P. D. Sarvela, *Health Education Evaluation and Measurement: A Practitioner's Perspective*, 2nd ed. (New York: McGraw-Hill, 1999).

TABLE 5.5 **Summary of Nonprobability Sampling Procedures**

Sample	Primary Descriptive Elements
Convenience	Selecting people who are readily available and easy to reach; may be members of an intact group or people present at public location.
Homogeneous	People are selected who share similar characteristics or traits of interest.
Snowball	Method by which respondents are asked to identify others who fit study criteria; often used with difficult to find priority populations or to find information-rich respondents.
Quota	Choosing people based on whether they meet pre-established criteria; aiming to have certain number of respondents with specific characteristics.
Maximum variation	Ensuring diverse representation of the priority population by selecting a wide variety of people possessing characteristics or experiences.

a probability sample is too costly or time consuming. It is important that planners understand the limitations of this type of sample when reporting the results. (See **Table 5.5** for a summary of nonprobability sampling procedures.)

Sample Size

An often-asked question associated with sampling involves how many individuals are needed for planners to feel confident that sampling error is within an acceptable range so that reasonable conclusions can be drawn from the data collected. There is no easy answer to this question. Appropriate sample size is determined by both practical and statistical considerations. From a practical standpoint, often the resources (e.g., personnel, financial) available to collect data are the determining factor on how large the sample will be. Asked another way, is the desired sample size affordable?

When analyzing sample size from a statistical standpoint, three major theoretical considerations are used: central limit theorem (CLT), precision and reliability, and power analysis (Norwood, 2000). The CLT can provide the quickest answer to the sample size question. Mathematically, it has been shown that when a sample size approaches 30 in number, characteristics of that group approach the normal distribution of the group from which it was drawn. Thus, while a sample size of 30 may not properly estimate a research parameter or distinguish research results between groups, a general rule for comparison purposes is, no group should be smaller than 30.

Determining sample size using precision and reliability, or power analysis, is much more complicated (and is not within the scope of this book). **Table 5.6** is offered as an example of the application of these considerations. Detailed explanations of these concepts are presented in many statistics textbooks.

▷ Pilot Testing

Pilot testing (sometimes referred to as *piloting* or a *pilot study*) is a set of procedures used by planners to try out the program on a small group of participants prior to actual implementation. In other words, pilot testing can be thought of as a dress rehearsal for planners

TABLE 5.6 **Sample Sizes for Studies Describing Population Proportions When the Population Size Is Known**

Population Size	95% Confidence Interval Sample Size for Precision of		
	±1	±3	±5
500	*	*	222
1,000	*	*	286
5,000	*	909	370
10,000	5,000	1,000	385
100,000	9,091	1,099	398
S ∞	10,000	1,111	400

* = In these cases the assumption of normal approximation is poor, and the formula used to derive them does not apply.
Source: *Statistics: An Introductory Analysis*. Taro Yamane. Copyright © 1973 by Pearson Education. Adapted with permission.

(McDermott & Sarvela, 1999). The purpose of using pilot testing is to identify and, if necessary, correct any problems prior to implementation with the priority population. Thus, pilot testing permits a thorough check of all planned processes to help increase the chances of having a successful program. Throughout the program planning process, planners may use pilot testing to detect any problems with sampling, data collection instruments, data collection procedures, data analysis procedures, interventions, curricula, and program evaluation (McDermott & Sarvela, 1999). Because this chapter has focused on measurement and measures, the remaining portions of this discussion will focus on the pilot testing of data collection. Pilot testing will be discussed in later chapters, as it relates to the implementation of a program as well as its role in formative evaluation (see Chapter 12 and Chapter 14).

Once the data collection method has been determined and the instrument has been selected or created, a trial run of the instrument, data collection procedures, and analyses should be conducted. During the piloting process, it would not be uncommon for the planners to find problems, such as ambiguous questions, difficulty with coding sheets, and misunderstood directions. Further, the data collected during pilot testing should be statistically analyzed or compiled to make sure there is no difficulty with this step in the data collection process. Revising the data collection process using the information gained from the pilot testing helps ensure that the actual data collection will proceed smoothly.

Several authors have suggested processes for pilot testing (Borg & Gall, 1989; McDermott & Sarvela, 1999; Parkinson & Associates, 1982; Stacy, 1987). They have been combined here into a single process. Several of the preceding authors have presented hierarchies for pilot testing: preliminary review, pre-pilot, and pilot tests. The first and lowest level in the pilot testing hierarchy is a preliminary review. A **preliminary review** is conducted when those responsible for the data collection process ask colleagues, not people from the priority population, to review the data collection instrument. At a minimum, all data collection instruments should be subjected to this type of review. Specifically, in a preliminary review, colleagues would be asked to complete the instrument as if they were participants in hopes of identifying problems, and also respond to several other questions about the instrument, such as the appropriateness of (1) the instrument's title, (2) the introductory statement explaining the purpose of the data collection, (3) the directions, (4) the order or grouping of the questions, (5) the questions (e.g., unclear or too personal), (6) the length of the instrument, and (7) the method of returning the instrument, to name a few.

Next, pretesting is completed with members of the priority population. Respondents fill out the survey and then give feedback either orally or in writing about which questions and response options they found confusing. When you invite someone to come meet with you and fill out the survey this process is referred to as **cognitive pretesting** (Collins, 2003). In this process you ask the participant to talk out loud as they take the survey, tell you what they are thinking as they read the question and the responses. For example, if a question asked "How many residences have you lived in since you were born." The respondent might say, "I am thinking whether residences means houses or cities. I think it means cities, so I am going to write down five." You may actually be looking for number of houses, so you know you need to change the wording of that question. The same cognitive pretesting process can be used after a respondent fills out the survey instead of during the process. The planner holds a debriefing session after the respondent completes the instrument where inquiries are made about wording of questions, understanding, response options and so forth.

Pre-pilots (or mini-pilots) are used by planners with five or six members of the priority population to assess the quality of materials, instruments, and data collection techniques. The **pilot test** requires the actual implementation of the instrument. A representative sample of the priority population is used to determine the quality of the instrument. If enough subjects are used during the pilot study, it may be possible to check the validity and reliability of the instrument. If at all possible, the use of this sequence of pilot testing techniques is desirable, but planners are often limited by time and resources, and so not all the steps may be reasonable to complete.

▷ Ethical Issues Associated with Measurement

Whenever people are being measured as part of a needs assessment or an evaluation, planners need to be aware that many of their decisions made and actions taken throughout these processes could have ethical ramifications. Further, planners are obligated by law—via the Health Insurance Portability and Accountability Act of 1996—to guard against the misuse of individual identifiable health information.

Ethical issues associated with measurement begin with getting people to voluntarily participate in the process. Before people get involved they should be well informed about the nature of the process and what is expected when they do participate. Further, potential participants should not be coerced or deceived to participate. And, once participation has begun, planners should make it clear that participants have the right to discontinue participation at any time without penalty. A second issue is that of private and/or sensitive data. If planners need to ask questions that reveal private and sensitive data, they need to ensure anonymity or confidentiality. During data collection, planners may hear about illegal acts, such as drug use or other crimes, or they may be provided with access to confidential data. The planners must consider the ethical issues and the legal ramifications of such issues.

Once the data have been collected, several ethical issues could arise when the data are analyzed and reported. Inappropriate data analyses can lead to personal harm to participants, the continuation of inappropriate programs, policies or procedures, and the waste of time, effort, and resources (Cottrell & McKenzie, 2011). Regardless of the purposes for which the analyzed data are used, planners have an ethical obligation to ensure they do not mislead anyone who relies on them (Dane, 1990). Finally, when the results of a needs assessment or an evaluation are reported, planners must ensure not to reveal the identity of those who participated, or individual results of participants, without their permission.

Summary

This chapter focused on helping you understand the terms *measurement, measures, measurement instruments, sampling,* and *pilot testing.* A brief overview of measurement and measures was provided, along with the four levels of measurement: nominal, ordinal, interval, and ratio. Several different examples of questions used at each of the levels were also presented. Next, desirable characteristics of data were discussed, including reliability, validity, and the importance of being bias free. Background information was provided to assist you with processes to identify existing measurement instruments and create new ones. Information was also presented on writing measurement instrument questions. This was followed by a discussion of techniques used to draw the various probability and nonprobability samples, and when the various sampling techniques might be most useful. The chapter concluded with short presentations on the importance of using pilot testing and the ethical issues associated with measurement.

Review Questions

1. What is meant by *measurement,* and *qualitative* and *quantitative measures?*
2. What are the reasons that measurement is such an important process when it comes to program planning and evaluation?
3. Name and give an example of each of the four levels of measurement.
4. What are the most common types of measures (variables) used in needs assessments and evaluations? Give an example of each type of variable.
5. What are sources of validity evidence? What are the different types of reliability estimates? What are reasons that validity and reliability are important to measurement?
6. What is bias in data collection? Name three ways in which it can be controlled.
7. What are the steps one can follow when identifying, obtaining, and evaluating existing measurement instruments?
8. What are the advantages and disadvantages of using an existing measurement instrument?
9. What are the guidelines for wording questions and response options?
10. What are the guidelines for presentation when designing a data collection instrument?
11. Define *census, sample, sampling,* and *sampling frame.*
12. Using a table of random numbers, explain how a simple random sample is selected.
13. Describe three types of probability samples.

14. When, if ever, should nonprobability samples be used?

15. What is the purpose of a preliminary review, a pre-pilot (or mini-pilot), a pilot test, and cognitive pretesting? How is each conducted?

16. What ethical issues are associated with measurement?

Activities

1. Assume that your college or university has hired you to conduct a needs assessment on the student body for a new health promotion program. Because there are few secondary data on this group of people, other than national data on college students, you have decided to survey a random sample of students using a written instrument. Your task now is to develop the instrument. Create a draft of an instrument that includes questions that will collect data about the students' health behavior and demographic characteristics. Follow the guidelines in this chapter for wording questions as well as presentation.

2. Conduct a cognitive pretesting of your instrument developed in activity 1 on five or six of your friends, colleagues, or classmates. Make changes based on the feedback you receive. Next, pilot test the survey by asking 5–10 people to fill it out. Identify any flaws you see in the questionnaire or data collection process.

3. Assume that you are charged with the responsibility of collecting data from all the students on your campus who are interested in taking non-traditional physical activity classes such as yoga, spinning, or kickboxing. You do not have access to a list of students on campus that you can use as a sampling frame. Explain how you would obtain a representative sample from this population. Would probability or non-probability sampling be best? What are drawbacks and advantages of the method you selected?

4. Look in the peer reviewed literature or the Websites listed in this chapter to find a scale to measure a construct such as physical activity, social support, self-efficacy for stopping smoking, resilience, or something similar. Evaluate the quality of the scale by looking for evidence of validity and reliability in the scholarly literature (start with Google Scholar). Write a recommendation as to whether or not it would be an appropriate scale to use for a program evaluation or needs assessment.

Weblinks

1. http://ctb.ku.edu/tools/en/sub_main_1044.htm

Community Toolbox

This page from the Community Toolbox Website, created and maintained by the Work Group on Health Promotion and Community Development at the University of Kansas, defines and describes the process of developing baseline measures.

2. http://www.cdc.gov/nchs

National Center for Health Statistics (NCHS)

The NCHS Website is a rich source of data and measurement instruments used to collect the data about America's health.

3. http://www.surveysystem.com/resource.htm

   Creative Research Systems

   The Creative Research Systems Website includes a lot of information about survey instrument development data collection and includes a calculator for determining appropriate sample size.

4. http://www.socialresearchmethods.net/

   Web Center for Social Research Methods

   This Website is designed for people involved with social science research. Topics covered include measurement, statistics, study design, sampling, and more. There are several easy to understand examples provided.

5. http://www.qualtrics.com

   Qualtrics

   Qualtrics is one of the leading firms for conducting online surveys. You can set up an account and practice creating surveys.

6. http://www.eval.org/

   American Evaluation Association

   The American Evaluation Association is a professional association dedicated to improving the practice of evaluation in various sectors. There is an annual conference, an email list-serv, and several online resources. Student membership is relatively inexpensive.

7. http://cancercontrol.cancer.gov/brp/constructs/

   Health Behavior Constructs: Theory, Measurement and Research

   This Website provides definitions and measurement sources for major theoretical constructs related to behavioral research. This is a good place to start looking for measurement instruments.

Mission Statement, Goals, and Objectives

Chapter Objectives

After reading this chapter and answering the questions at the end, you should be able to:

- Explain what is meant by the terms *mission statement* and *vision statement*.

- Define *goals* and *objectives* and distinguish between the two.

- Identify the different levels of objectives as presented in the chapter.

- Describe a SMART objective.

- State the necessary elements of an objective as presented in the chapter.

- Specify an appropriate criterion for objectives.

- Write program goals and objectives.

- Describe the use for *Healthy People 2020*.

Key Terms

attitude objectives
awareness objectives
behavioral objectives
condition
criterion
environmental
   objectives
goal
impact objectives
knowledge objectives

learning objectives
mission statement
objectives
outcome
outcome objectives
process objectives
skill development
   objectives
SMART objectives
vision statement

To plan, implement, and evaluate effective health promotion programs, planners must have a solid foundation in place to guide them through their work. The mission statement, goals, and objectives of a program can provide such a foundation. If prepared properly, a mission statement, goals, and objectives should not only give the necessary direction to a program but also provide the groundwork for the eventual program evaluation (**Box 6.1**). There are two old sayings that help express the need for a mission statement, goals, and objectives. The first is: If you do not know where you are going, then any road will do—and you may end up someplace where you do not want to be, or you may eventually end up where you want to be, but after wasted time and effort. The second is: If you do not know where you are going, how will you know when you have arrived? Without a mission statement, goals, and objectives, a program may lack direction, and at best it will be difficult to evaluate. **Figure 6.1** shows the relationship between a mission statement, goals, and objectives. The size of the

Responsibilities and Competencies for Health Education Specialists

The content of this chapter focuses on the mission, goals, and objectives of a program. Because the mission, goals, and objectives provide the foundation on which programs are developed and the criteria used to evaluate the programs, the information presented in this chapter is applicable to three areas of responsibility:

RESPONSIBILITY II:	Plan Health Education/Promotion
	Competency 2.2: Develop goals and objectives
	Competency 2.3: Select or design strategies/interventions
RESPONSIBILITY III:	Implement Health Education/Promotion
	Competency 3.2: Train staff members and volunteers involved in implementation of health education/promotion
	Competency 3.4: Monitor implementation of health education/promotion
RESPONSIBILITY IV:	Conduct Evaluation and Research Related to Health Education/Promotion
	Competency 4.1: Develop evaluation plan for health education/promotion

Source: *A Competency-Based Framework for Health Education Specialists—2015.* Whitehall, PA: National Commission for Health Education Credentialing, Inc. (NCHEC) and the Society for Public Health Education (SOPHE). Reprinted by permission of the National Commission for Health Education Credentialing, Inc. (NCHEC) and the Society for Public Health Education (SOPHE).

▲ **Figure 6.1** Relationship of Mission Statement, Goals, and Objectives

rectangles presented in Figure 6.1 has special meaning. The rectangle that represents the mission statement is the largest, while the rectangle representing the objectives is the smallest, meaning that ideas presented go from broad to narrow in scope.

▷ Mission Statement

Sometimes referred to as a program overview or program aim, a **mission statement** is a short narrative that describes the purpose and focus of the program. The statement not only describes the current focus of a program but also may reflect the philosophy behind it. The mission statement also helps to guide planners in the development of program goals and objectives. **Table 6.1** presents examples of mission statements for programs offered in several different settings.

Some people mistake a vision statement for a mission statement. They are different. Whereas a mission statement provides a description of the current efforts of a program, a **vision statement** is a brief description of where the program will be in the future; typically, in three to five years. A vision statement answers the questions, "What do we want to be?" and "What will we look like in three to five years?" Vision statements are often part of a strategic planning process in which organizations define a strategy or direction for the

TABLE 6.1 **Examples of Mission Statements**

Setting	Mission Statement
Community Setting	The mission of the Walkup Health Promotion Program is to provide a wide variety of primary prevention activities for residents of the community.
Heath Care Setting	This program is aimed at helping patients and their families to understand and cope with physical and emotional changes associated with recovery following cancer surgery.
School Setting	School District #77 wants happy and healthy students. To that end, the district's personnel strive, through a Whole School, Whole Community, Whole Child model program, to provide students with experiences that are designed to motivate and enable them to improve or maintain their health.
Worksite Setting	The purpose of the employee health promotion program is to develop high employee morale. This is to be accomplished by providing employees with a working environment that is conducive to good health and by providing an opportunity for employees and their families to engage in behavior that will improve and maintain good health.

future. Items that are considered when creating a vision statement are future products (i.e., information, ideas, goods, services, events, and behavior), markets, customers, location, and staffing. Most programs do not include a vision statement. However, if a vision statement were added to Figure 6.1, it would be found in a larger rectangle to the left of the mission statement rectangle.

▷ Program Goals

Although some individuals use the terms *goals* and *objectives* interchangeably, they are not the same: There are important differences between them. **Goals** are broad statements that describe the expected outcomes of the program. They are less specific than objectives and are used to explain the general intent of a program to those not directly involved in the program (Cottrell & McKenzie, 2011; Neiger & Thackeray, 1998). "Goals set the fundamental, long-range direction" (NCCDPHP, n.d., p. 1). "Objectives break the goal down into smaller parts that provide specific, measurable actions by which the goal can be accomplished" (NCCDPHP, n.d., p. 1). In comparison to objectives, goals are expectations that: provide overall direction for the program, are more general in nature, do not have a specific deadline, usually take longer to complete, and are often not measured in exact terms.

Program goals are not difficult to write and need not be written as complete sentences. They should, however, be simple and concise, and should include two basic components: who will be affected, and what will change as a result of the program. Goals typically include verbs such as *evaluate, know, improve, increase, promote, protect, minimize, prevent, reduce,* and *understand* (Jacobsen, Eggen, & Kauchak, 1989). A program need not have a set number of stated goals. It is not uncommon for some programs to have a single goal while others have several. **Box 6.2** presents some examples of goals for health promotion programs.

BOX

6.2

Examples of Program Goals

- Reduce the incidence of cardiovascular disease in the employees of the Smith Company.
- Eliminate all cases of measles in the City of Kenzington.
- Prevent the spread of HIV in the youth of Indiana.
- Reduce the cases of lung cancer caused by exposure to secondhand smoke in Elizabethtown, PA.
- Reduce the incidence of influenza in the residents of the Delaware County Home.
- Increase the survival rate of breast cancer patients through the optimal use of community resources.

▷ Objectives

Objectives are precise statements of intended outcome (Gilbert, Sawyer, & McNeill, 2015). Objectives represent smaller steps than program goals—steps that, if completed, will lead to reaching the program goal(s) (Ross & Mico, 1980). Stated another way, objectives specify intermediate accomplishments or benchmarks that represent progress toward a goal (CDC, 2003). Objectives outline in measurable terms the specific changes that will occur in the priority population at a given point in time as a result of exposure to the program. "Objectives are crucial. They form a fulcrum, converting diagnostic data into program direction and resource allocation over time" (Green & Kreuter, 2005, p. 100). Objectives can be thought of as the bridge between needs assessment and a planned intervention. Knowing how to construct objectives for a program is a most important skill for planners.

Different Levels of Objectives

Several different levels of objectives are associated with program planning. The different levels are sequenced or placed in a hierarchical order to allow for more effective planning (Cleary & Neiger, 1998; Deeds, 1992; Parkinson & Associates, 1982). Objectives are created at each level in order to help attain the program goal. The "objectives should also be *coherent* across levels, with objectives becoming successively more refined and more explicit, and usually multiplied from one level to the next" (Green & Kreuter, 2005, p. 102). Achievement of the lower-level objectives will contribute to the achievement of the higher-level objectives and goals. **Table 6.2** presents the hierarchy of objectives and indicates their relationship to program outcomes and evaluation. Because the hierarchy of objectives was created from the work of several, the labels (names) given to the different levels of objectives have not been consistent. Thus, as we present the description of each type of objective, we identify various labels that have been used.

PROCESS OBJECTIVES

The **process objectives** are the daily tasks, activities, and work plans that lead to the accomplishment of all other levels of objectives (Deeds, 1992). They help shape or form the program and thus focus on all program inputs/resources (all that are needed to carry out a program), implementation activities (actual presentation of the program), and stakeholder reactions. More specifically, these objectives focus on such things as program resources

TABLE 6.2 **Hierarchy of Objectives and Their Relation to Evaluation**

Type of Objective	Program Outcomes	Possible Evaluation Measures	Type of Evaluation
Process objectives	Activities presented and tasks completed	Number of sessions held, exposure, attendance, participation, staff performance, appropriate materials, adequacy of resources, tasks on schedule	Process (form of formative)
Impact objectives			
Learning objectives	Change in awareness, knowledge, attitudes, or skills	Increase in awareness, knowledge, attitudes, or skill development/acquisition	Impact (form of summative)
Behavioral objectives	Change in behavior	Current behavior modified or discontinued, or new behavior adopted	Impact (form of summative)
Environmental objectives	Change in the environment	Measures associated with economic, service, physical, social psychological, or political environments, e.g., protection added to, or hazards or barriers removed from, the environment	Impact (form of summative)
Outcome objectives	Change in quality of life (QOL), health status, or risk, and social benefits	QOL measures, morbidity data, mortality data, measures of risk (e.g., HRA)	Outcome (form of summative)

Source: Adapted from Deeds (1992), Cleary & Neiger (1998), and Parkinson & Associates (1982).

(materials, funds, space); appropriateness of intervention activities; priority population exposure, attendance, participation, and feedback; feedback from other stakeholders such as the funding and sponsoring agencies; and data collection techniques, to name a few. They also form the groundwork for process evaluation (see the last column in Table 6.2).

IMPACT OBJECTIVES

The second level of objectives in the hierarchy is **impact objectives**. This level of objectives comprises three different types of objectives: learning objectives, behavioral objectives, and environmental objectives. They are called impact objectives because they describe the immediate observable effects of a program (e.g., changes in awareness, knowledge, attitudes, skills, behaviors, or the environment) and they form the groundwork for impact evaluation (see the last column in Table 6.2).

Learning Objectives. Learning objectives are the educational or learning tools needed in order to achieve the desired behavior change. They are based upon the analysis of educational and ecological assessment of the PRECEDE-PROCEED model.

Within this category of objectives, there is another hierarchy (Parkinson & Associates, 1982). This hierarchy includes four types of objectives, beginning with the least complex and moving toward the most complex. Complexity is defined in terms of the time, effort, and resources necessary to accomplish the objective. The learning objectives hierarchy begins with **awareness objectives** and moves through **knowledge, attitude**, and **skill development objectives**. This hierarchy indicates that if those in the priority population are going to adopt and maintain a health-enhancing behavior to alleviate a health concern or problem, they must first be aware of the health concern. Second, they must expand their knowledge and understanding of the concern. Third, they must attain and maintain an attitude that enables them to deal with the concern. And fourth, they need to possess the necessary skills to engage in the health-enhancing behavior.

Behavioral Objectives. **Behavioral objectives** describe the behaviors or actions in which the priority population will engage that will resolve the health problem and move you toward achieving the program goal (Deeds, 1992). Behavioral objectives are commonly written about adherence (e.g., regular exercise), compliance (e.g., taking medication as prescribed), consumption patterns (e.g., diet), coping (e.g., stress-reduction activities), preventive actions (e.g., brushing and flossing teeth), self-care (e.g., first aid), and utilization (e.g., appropriate use of the emergency room).

Environmental Objectives. **Environmental objectives** outline the nonbehavioral causes of a health problem that are present in the social, physical, psychological, economic, service, and/or political environments. Environmental objectives are written about such things as the state of the physical environment (e.g., clean air or water, proximity to facilities, removal of physical barriers), the social environment (e.g., social support, peer pressure), the psychological environment (e.g., the emotional learning climate), the economic environment (e.g., affordability, incentives, disincentives), the service environment (e.g., access to health care, equity in health care), and/or the political environment (e.g., health policy).

OUTCOME OBJECTIVES

Outcome objectives are the ultimate objectives of a program and are aimed at changes in health status, social benefits, risk factors, or quality of life. "They are outcome or future oriented" (Deeds, 1992, p. 36). If these objectives are achieved, then the program goal will be achieved. These objectives are commonly written in terms of health status such as the reduction of risk, physiologic indicators, signs and symptoms, morbidity, disability, mortality, or quality of life measures.

Consideration of the Time Needed to Reach the Outcome of an Objective

In addition to objectives being written at different levels within the hierarchy, they can also be written with consideration to the amount of time needed to reach the objective. Thus, the terms *short-term objective, intermediate objective*, and *long-term objective* have been used. Short-term objectives include a time frame in which an outcome is "expected immediately and can occur soon after the program or intervention is implemented, very often within a year" (NCCDPHP, n.d., p. 2). "Intermediate objectives result from and follow short-term outcomes" (NCCDPHP, n.d., p. 2), while "long-term objectives state the ultimate expected impact of the program or intervention" (NCCDPHP, n.d., p. 2). As an example, a short-term objective may be a process objective that focuses on capacity building indicating the number of health care providers would be increased. A corresponding intermediate objective may be written as an impact objective focusing on the number of people screened because of the increase in providers. And, the long-term objective, an outcome objective, could focus on risk reduction based on individuals being treated for a problem that was identified via the screening.

Developing Objectives

Does every program require objectives from each of the levels just described? The answer is no! However, too often, health promotion programs have too few objectives, all of which fall into one or two levels. Many planners have developed programs hoping solely to change the health behavior of a priority population. For example, a smoking cessation program may have an objective of getting 30% of the participants to stop smoking. Perhaps this program is offered, and only 10% of the participants quit smoking. Is the program a failure? If the program has a single objective of changing behavior, its sponsors would have a good case for saying that the program was not effective. However, it is quite possible that as a result of participating in the smoking cessation program, the participants increased their awareness of the dangers of smoking. They probably also increased their knowledge, maybe changed their attitudes, and developed skills for quitting or cutting back on the number of cigarettes they smoke each day. These are all very positive outcomes—and they could be overlooked when the program is evaluated, if the planner did not write objectives that cover a variety of levels.

Questions to be Answered When Developing Objectives

In addition to making sure that the objectives are written in an appropriate manner, planners also need to be consistent with other planning parameters. In this section we present six questions that planners should consider when writing objectives:

1. Can the objective be realized during the life of the program or within a reasonable time thereafter? It would be quite realistic to assume that a certain number of people will not be smoking one year after they have completed a smoking cessation program, but it would not be realistic to assume that a group of elementary school students could be followed for life to determine how many of them die prematurely due to inactivity.

2. Can the objective realistically be achieved? It is probably realistic to assume that 30% of any smoking cessation class will stop smoking within one year after the program has ended, but it is not realistic to assume that 100% of the employees of a company will participate in its fitness program.

3. Does the program have enough resources (personnel, money, and space) to obtain a specific objective? It would be ideal to be able to reach all individuals in the priority population, but generally there are not sufficient resources to do so.

4. Are the objectives consistent with the policies and procedures of the sponsoring agency? It may not be realistic to expect to incorporate a no-smoking policy in a tobacco company.

5. Do the objectives violate any of the rights of those who are involved (participants or planners)? Right-to-know laws make it illegal to withhold information that could cause harm to a priority population.

6. If a program is planned for a particular ethnic/cultural population, do the objectives reflect the relationship between the cultural characteristics of the priority group and the changes sought? It would not be realistic to have an objective that eliminates the use of tobacco in a priority population that is comprised of Native Americans because of the ceremonial pipe use in the Native American culture.

Elements of an Objective

For an objective to provide direction and be useful in the evaluation process, it must be written in such a way that it can be clearly understood, states what is to be accomplished, and is measurable. To ensure that an objective is indeed useful, it should include the following elements:

1. The *outcome* to be achieved, or what will change
2. The *conditions* under which the outcome will be observed, or when the change will occur
3. The *criterion* for deciding whether the outcome has been achieved, or how much change
4. The *priority population,* or who will change

The first element, the **outcome**, is defined as the action, behavior, or something else that will change as a result of the program. In an objective written as a sentence, the outcome is usually identified as the verb of the sentence. Thus words such as *apply, argue, build, compare, demonstrate, evaluate, exhibit, judge, perform, reduce, spend, state,* and *test* would be considered outcomes (see **Box 6.3** for a more comprehensive listing of

---

BOX
6.3

Focus On

Outcome Verbs for Objectives

abstract	copy	gather	offer	round
accept	count	(information)	order	score
adjust	create	generalize	organize	seek
adopt	criticize	generate	pair	select
advocate	deduce	group	participate	separate
analyze	defend	guess	partition	share
annotate	define	hypothesize	perform	show
apply	delay (response)	identify	persist	simplicity
approximate	demonstrate	illustrate	plan	simulate
argue	derive	imitate	practice	solve
(a position)	describe	improve	praise	sort
ask	design	infer	predict	spend
associate	determine	initiate	prepare	(money)
attempt	develop	inquire	preserve	state
balance	differentiate	integrate	produce	structure
build	discover	interpolate	propose	submit
calculate	discriminate	interpret	prove	subscribe
categorize	dispute	invent	qualify	substitute
cause	distinguish	investigate	query	suggest
challenge	effect	join	question	summarize
change	eliminate	judge	recall	supply
choose	enumerate	justify	recite	support
clarify	estimate	keep	recognize	symbolize
classify	evaluate	label	recommend	synthesize
collect	examine	list	record	tabulate
combine	exemplify	locate	reduce	tally
compare	exhibit	manipulate	regulate	test
complete	experiment	map	reject	theorize
compute	explain	match	relate	translate
conceptualize	express	measure	reorganize	try
connect	extend	name	repeat	unite
construct	extract	obey	replace	visit
consult	extrapolate	object	represent	volunteer
contrast	find	(to an idea)	reproduce	weigh
convert	form	observe	restructure	write

appropriate outcome words). It should be noted that not all verbs would be considered appropriate outcomes for an objective; the verb must refer to something measurable and observable. Words such as *appreciate, know, internalize,* and *understand* by themselves do not refer to something measurable and observable, and therefore are not good choices for outcomes. Some verbs work better than others for specific types of objectives. For example, the verb *list* is an appropriate verb for an awareness-level objective, but not for a knowledge-level objective. The verb *explain* would be much better suited for a knowledge-level objective.

The second element of an objective is the **condition** under which the outcome will be observed, or when it will be observed. "Typical" conditions found in objectives might be "upon completion of the exercise class," "as a result of participation," "by the year 2020," "after reading the pamphlets and brochures," "orally in class," "when asked to respond by the facilitator," "by year two of the program," "by May 15th," or "during the class session."

The third element of an objective is the **criterion** for determining when the outcome has been achieved, or how much change will occur. The purpose of this element is to provide a standard by which the planners/evaluators can determine if an outcome has been performed in an appropriate and/or successful manner. Examples might include "to no more than 105 per 1,000," "by 10% over the baseline," "300 pamphlets," "33% of the county residents," "75% of the motor vehicle occupants," "at least half of the participants," "according to CDC guidelines," or "all people who preregistered." One of the most difficult parts of creating appropriate objectives for a program is to determine what would be the appropriate criterion for an objective. Should program planners expect a 10% increase over baseline? Should they anticipate half of the employees to participate? What should be expected? There is no hard-and-fast rule for determining the criterion, but remember the criterion should be realistic and based on evidence whenever possible. Several different criterion-(target)-setting methods have been used in writing the objectives for the *Healthy People* initiative over the past three plus decades. **Box 6.4** provides a brief description of the target-setting methods used.

The last element that needs to be included in an objective is mention of the priority population, or who will change. Examples are "teachers of Smith Elementary," "employees of the company," "the people who participated in the program," and "those residing in the Muncie and Provo areas." **Figure 6.2** summarizes the key elements of a well-written objective. There is one exception to the priority population always being the *who* of an objective. That exception applies to process-level objectives. Because some of these objectives guide the work of the program planners and/or implementers. In those cases, the *who* is the staff or group entrusted with instituting the program instead of the priority population (Cottrell & McKenzie, 2011). (See **Box 6.5** for examples of objectives that would include the four primary elements.)

Objectives that include the elements described in this section are referred to as **SMART**. SMART stands for specific, measurable, achievable, realistic, and time-phased (CDC, 2003). Every objective planners write for their programs should be SMART! (See **Box 6.6** for a SMART Objectives Checklist.)

In summary, well-written objectives will always answer the question "WHO is going to do WHAT, WHEN, and TO WHAT EXTENT?" (NCCDPHP, n.d., p. 2). Although it is easy to describe the components of well-written objectives, it is not always easy to write them. **Box 6.7** provides a template to help program planners write objectives.

▲ **Figure 6.2** Elements of a Well-Written Objective

BOX

6.4

Focus On

Target Setting Methods for the Objectives of the *Healthy People* Initiative

- Better than best—When no baseline data were available, target was set based on a comparison to racial/ethnic group with best, or most favorable rate.
- Consistent with another program—Target was set based on the results of an already completed program.
- Consistent with national strategy—Target was set based on the national strategy to improve health.
- Consistent with regulations/policies/laws—Target was set based on data included in the regulations/policies/laws.
- Evidence-based approach—Target set based on results of completed research.
- Expert opinion—If no other data were available, the target was set based on the opinion of experts.
- Minimal statistical significance—Target was set using the smallest improvement that results in a statistically significant difference when tested against the baseline value.

- Modeling/projection of trend (or trend analysis)—Target was set using a model or based on trend data.
- No increase from baseline (maintain baseline)—Target was set based on the belief there would be no change from baseline.
- One state per year—Target was set based on getting one state (or the District of Columbia) to meet a criterion each year.
- Percent improvement—Target was based on a reasonable expected percent change in the priority population compared to previous improvement.
- Retain previous set of objectives target—Target was retained if the previous target was not reached and was still appropriate.
- Threshold analysis—Target was set after analyzing at what point change would begin to produce an effect.
- Total coverage or elimination—Target was set based on the belief that a criterion of 100% could be achieved.

Sources: Gurley (2007, April), USDHHS (2007), USDHHS (2015c).

▷ Goals and Objectives for the Nation

A chapter on goals and objectives would not be complete without at least a short discussion of the health goals and objectives of the nation. These goals and objectives have been most helpful to planners throughout the United States.

The goals and objectives of the nation, which have been referred to as the *health agenda* or the *blueprint of public health planning* for the United States, are the primary component of the U.S. *Healthy People* initiative. The *Healthy People* initiative was launched in 1978 and a year later released the publication of *Healthy People: The Surgeon General's Report on Health*

BOX

6.5

Focus On

Examples of Objectives to Support the Program Goal "To Reduce the Prevalence of Heart Disease in the Residents of Franklin County"

Process Objectives

A. By 2020, the program planners will increase the number of heart healthy educational sessions offered to the county residents from the baseline of 15 to 25 per year.

Outcome (what): Increase the number of heart healthy educational sessions

Priority Population (who): Program planners

Conditions (when): By 2020

Criterion (how much): From the baseline of 15 to 25 per year

B. By August 4, the volunteers will distribute the informational brochure to 33% of the county residents.

Outcome (what): Will distribute the informational brochure

Priority Population (who): Volunteers

Conditions (when): By August 4

Criterion (how much): 33% of the county residents

C. During the pilot testing, the program facilitators will receive a "good" rating from at least half of the participants.

Outcome (what): Will receive a "good" rating

Priority Population (who): Program facilitators

Conditions (when): During the pilot testing

Criterion (how much): At least half of the participants

D. Prior to the start of the program, the program staff will deliver the program notebooks to all people who preregistered for the program.

Outcome (what): Will deliver the program notebooks

Priority Population (who): Program staff

Conditions (when): Prior to the start of the program

Criterion (how much): All people who preregistered

Impact – Learning Objectives

A. Awareness level: After the American Heart Association's pamphlet on cardiovascular health risk factors has been placed in grocery bags, at least 20% of the shoppers will be able to identify two of their own risks.

Outcome (what): Identify their own risks

Priority population (who): Shoppers

Conditions (when): After distribution of the pamphlet

Criterion (how much): 20%

B. Knowledge level: When asked over the telephone, one out of three viewers of the heart special television show will be able to explain the four principles of cardiovascular conditioning.

Outcome (what): Able to explain the four principles of cardiovascular conditioning

Priority population (who): Television viewers

Conditions (when): When asked over the telephone

Criterion (how much): One out of three

BOX

6.5

continued

C. Attitude level: During one of the class sessions, 50% of the participants will defend their reason for regular exercise.

Outcome (what): Defend their reason for regular exercise

Priority population (who): Class participants

Conditions (when): During one of the class sessions

Criterion (how much): 50%

D. Skill development level: After viewing the video "How to Exercise," half of those participating will be able to locate their pulse and count it every time they are asked to do it.

Outcome (what): Locate their pulse and count it

Priority population (who): Those participating

Conditions (when): After viewing the video

Criterion (how much): Half of those participating

Impact—Behavioral Objectives

A. One year after the formal exercise classes have been completed, 40% of those who completed a majority of the classes will still be involved in a regular aerobic exercise program.

Outcome (what): Will still be involved

Priority population (who): Those who completed a majority of the classes

Conditions (when): One year after the classes

Criterion (how much): 40%

B. During the telephone interview follow-up, 50% of the residents will report having had their blood pressure taken during the previous six months.

Outcome (what): Will report having their blood pressure taken

Priority population (who): Residents

Conditions (when): During the telephone interview follow-up

Criterion (how much): 50%

Impact—Environmental Objectives

A. By the year 2020, 10% of the clinic patients will have been able to schedule an appointment either after 5 p.m. or on a Saturday.

Outcome (what): Will have been able to schedule

Priority Population (who): Clinic patients

Conditions (when): By the year 2020

Criterion (how much): 10%

B. By the end of the year, all senior citizens who want it will be provided transportation to the congregate meals.

Outcome (what): Provided transportation

Priority population (who): Senior citizens

Conditions (when): By end of year

Criterion (how much): All who want it

BOX

6.5

continued

Outcome Objectives

A. By the year 2020, heart disease deaths will be reduced to no more than 100 per 100,000 in the residents of Franklin County.

Outcome (what): Reduce heart disease deaths

Priority population (who): Residents of Franklin County

Conditions (when): By the year 2020

Criterion (how much): To no more than 100 per 100,000

B. By 2020, increase to at least 25% the proportion of men in Franklin County with hypertension whose blood pressure is under control.

Outcome (what): Blood pressure under control

Priority population (who): Men in Franklin County with hypertension

Conditions (when): By 2020

Criterion (how much): At least 25%

C. Half of all those in the county who complete a regular, aerobic, 12-month exercise program will reduce their "risk age" on their follow-up health risk assessment by a minimum of two years compared to their preprogram results.

Outcome (what): Will reduce their "risk age"

Priority population (who): Those who complete an exercise program

Conditions (when): After the 12-month exercise program

Criterion (how much): Half

D. Two-thirds of those who participate in a formal exercise program will use 10% fewer sick days during the life of the program than those who do not participate.

Outcome (what): Use 10% fewer sick days

Priority population (who): Those who participate

Conditions (when): During the life of the program

Criterion (how much): Two-thirds

BOX

6.6

Application

SMART Objective Checklist

Criteria to assess objectives

Yes No

1. Is the objective SMART?

- **Specific:** Who? (priority population and persons doing the activity) and What? (action/activity)
- **Measurable:** How much change is expected
- **Achievable:** Can be realistically accomplished given current resources and constraints
- **Realistic:** Addresses the scope of the health problem and proposes reasonable programmatic steps
- **Time-phased:** Provides a timeline indicating when the objective will be met

2. Does it relate to a single result?

3. Is it clearly written?

Source: CDC (2009b).

BOX

6.7

Application

Template for Writing Objectives for Health Promotion Programs

(Insert one *when* from list A here), (insert one *how much* from list B here) of the (insert one *who* from list C here), will (insert one *what* from list D here).

Column A—*When?*
- By December 2020
- After the program
- By year two of the program
- One year after the classes

Column B—*How much?*
- 10% improvement
- half
- a majority
- at least 25

Column C —*Who?*
- participants
- employees
- adolescents
- university students

Column D—*What?*
- be able to demonstrate how to prepare a low-fat meal
- be able to explain the difference between exercise and physical activity
- have stopped smoking
- list the risk factors for skin cancer

Promotion and Disease Prevention (USDHEW, 1979). Shortly thereafter, the first set of goals and objectives, *Promoting Health/Preventing Disease: Objectives for the Nation* (USDHHS, 1980) were published. The goals and objectives were written to cover the 10-year period from 1980 to 1990 and were divided into three main areas—preventive services, health protection, and health promotion—and included a total of 226 objectives. Since the creation of the first set of goals and objectives, three additional sets have been developed and published under the titles of *Healthy People 2000: National Health Promotion and Disease Prevention Objectives* (USDHHS, 1990), *Healthy People 2010* (USDHHS, 2000), and *Healthy People 2020* (USDHHS, 2015c). Formal reviews (i.e., measured progress) of these objectives are conducted both at midcourse half way through the 10-year period (i.e., "The Midcourse Review") and again at the end of 10 years. The midcourse review provides an opportunity to measure progress towards the 10-year targets and determine whether there are trends that need to be reversed. For example, in *Healthy People 2010*, a number of objectives were changed, updated, or deleted because of the events 9/11 and Hurricanes Katrina and Rita. Both the results of the midcourse and end reviews along with other available data are used to help create the next set of goals and objectives. Each set of goals and objectives has become more detailed than the previous. "The evolution from the first decade's objectives to each subsequent set of objectives reflected changing societal concerns, evidence-based technologies, theories, and discourses of those decades. Such accommodations changed the contours of the initiative over time in attempts to make it more relevant to specific partners and other stakeholders" (Green & Fielding, 2011, p. 451). At the time this text was being revised the "Healthy People 2020" midcourse review was just beginning.

Healthy People 2020, which was released at the end of 2010, will guide U.S. public health practice and health education specialists through 2020. *Healthy People 2020* includes a vision statement, a mission statement, four overarching goals, and almost 1,200 science-based objectives (see **Box 6.8**) spread over 42 different topic areas (see **Box 6.9**) (USDHHS, 2015c). On the Healthy People.gov Website each topic has its own Webpage. At a minimum each

BOX

6.8

Focus On

Example Goal and Objectives from *Healthy People 2020*

Educational and Community-Based Programs (ECBP)

Goal: Increase the quality, availability, and effectiveness of educational and community-based programs designed to prevent disease and injury, improve health, and enhance quality of life.

Objective: ECBP-10 Increase the number of community-based organizations (including local health departments, tribal health services, nongovernmental organizations, and state agencies) providing population-based primary prevention services in the following areas

ECBP 10.8 Nutrition

Target: 94.7%.

Baseline: 86.1% of community-based organizations (including local health departments, tribal health services, nongovernmental organizations, and state agencies) provided population-based primary prevention services in nutrition in 2008

Target setting method: 10% improvement.

Data source: National Profile of Local Health Departments (NPLHD), National Association of County and City Health Officials (NACCHO)

ECBP 10.9 Physical Activity

Target: 88.5%.

Baseline: 80.5% of community-based organizations (including local health departments, tribal health services, nongovernmental organizations, and state agencies) provided population-based primary prevention services in physical activity in 2008.

Target setting method: 10% improvement.

Data source: National Profile of Local Health Departments (NPLHD), National Association of County and City Health Officials (NACCHO)

Source: USDHHS (2015c).

page contains a concise goal statement, a brief overview of the topic that provides the background and context for the topic, a statement about the importance of the topic backed up by appropriate evidence, and references.

The importance of the *Healthy People* initiative serving as a blueprint for the nation's health agenda is evidenced by their widespread use. Since the publication of the first *Healthy People* goals and objectives in 1980, a number of other documents have been created that can help planners develop or adopt appropriate goals and objectives for their programs. A number of states and U.S. territories have taken the national objectives and created similar documents specific to their own residents. In addition, a number of agencies/organizations have taken similar steps to create documents that could be used by their members and clients in various planning efforts.

The national goals and objectives have been important components in the process of health promotion planning since 1980. It is highly recommended that planners review these objectives before developing goals and objectives for programs. The national objectives may also be helpful in providing a rationale for a program and in focusing program goals and objectives toward the areas of greatest need, as planners work toward the year 2020.

BOX

6.9

***Healthy People 2020* Topic Areas**

1. Access to Health Services
2. Adolescent Health
3. Arthritis, Osteoporosis, and Chronic Back Conditions
4. Blood Disorders and Blood Safety
5. Cancer
6. Chronic Kidney Disease
7. Dementias, Including Alzheimer's Disease
8. Diabetes
9. Disability and Health
10. Early and Middle Childhood
11. Educational and Community-Based Programs
12. Environmental Health
13. Family Planning
14. Food Safety
15. Genomics
16. Global Health
17. Health Communication and Health Information Technology
18. Health-Related Quality of Life and Well-Being
19. Healthcare-Associated Infections
20. Hearing and Other Sensory or Communication Disorders

21. Heart Disease and Stroke
22. HIV
23. Immunization and Infectious Diseases
24. Injury and Violence Prevention
25. Lesbian, Gay, Bisexual, and Transgender Health
26. Maternal, Infant, and Child Health
27. Medical Product Safety
28. Mental Health and Mental Disorders
29. Nutrition and Weight Status
30. Occupational Safety and Health
31. Older Adults
32. Oral Health
33. Physical Activity
34. Preparedness
35. Public Health Infrastructure
36. Respiratory Diseases
37. Sexually Transmitted Diseases
38. Sleep Health
39. Social Determinants of Health
40. Substance Abuse
41. Tobacco Use
42. Vision

Source: USDHHS (2015c).

Summary

The mission statement provides an overview of a program and is most useful in the development of goals and objectives. It should not be confused with a vision statement. The terms *goals* and *objectives* are sometimes used interchangeably, but they are quite different. Together, the two provide a foundation for program planning and evaluation. Goals are more general in nature and often are not measurable in exact terms, whereas objectives are more specific and consist of the steps used to reach the program goals. Objectives can and should be written for several different levels. For objectives to be useful, they should be written so as to be observable and measurable. At a minimum, an objective should include the following elements: a stated outcome (what), conditions under which the outcome will be observed (when), a criterion for considering that the outcome has been achieved (how much), and mention of the priority population (who). If an objective is written with the above stated elements it will conform to the SMART format. As planners develop their goals and objectives for their programs, they should find the *Healthy People 2020* document and other information at its Website very useful.

Review Questions

1. What is a mission statement? Why is it important? How is it different from a vision statement?

2. What is (are) the difference(s) between a goal and an objective?

3. What is the purpose of program goals and objectives?

4. What are the different levels of objectives?

5. What are the four different types of objectives found in "learning objectives hierarchy"?

6. What are the necessary elements of an objective?

7. What are the characteristics of a SMART objective?

8. Briefly explain the *Healthy People* initiative.

9. What are the goals and objectives for the nation? How can they be used by program planners?

10. How can planners use the *Healthy People 2020* goals and objectives in their program planning efforts?

Activities

1. Write a mission statement, a goal, and eight supporting objectives (one of each of the different types) for a program you are planning.

2. Which of the following statements include all four elements necessary for a complete objective? Revise those objectives that do not include all the elements.

   a. After the class on objective writing, the students will know the difference between a goal and an objective.

   b. The students will understand how a skinfold caliper works.

   c. After completing this chapter, the students will be able to write objectives for each of the levels based on the four elements outlined in the chapter.

   d. Given appropriate instruction, the employees will be able to accurately take blood pressure readings of fellow employees.

   e. Program participants will be able to list the reasons why people do not exercise.

3. Using data available from the County Health Rankings (http://www .countyhealthrankings.org) for the county in which you currently reside, write a goal aimed at improving a health behavior and write one process, three impact (i.e., one each for knowledge, behavior, and environment), and one outcome objective to help reach the goal.

4. Using data available from the Kaiser State Health Facts Website (http://kff.org /statedata) for the state in which you currently reside, write a goal aimed at improving a health status topic and write one process, three impact (i.e., one each for awareness, skill, and environment), and one outcome objective to help reach the goal.

5. Assume that you are a health education specialist working in a primary care clinic. Based on some data provided by personnel at the local hospital regarding birth outcomes for the clinic patients, your supervisor has asked that you create a new program to decrease the percentage of female patients of childbearing age who smoke. After completing a needs assessment you have found that the highest rate of smokers was among those patients who were 18–24 years of age, covered by a health insurance plan, and have more than one child. In addition, the average number of cigarettes smoked per day by the patients was 22. Write a mission statement, a goal, and at least six objectives to help reach the stated goal.

Weblinks

1. **http://www.cdc.gov/phcommunities/resourcekit/evaluate/index.html**

   Communities of Practice (CoP) for Public Health: Evaluate a CoP

   On this page of the Centers for Disease Control and Prevention Website, you will find more information about SMART objectives and some related resources that provide templates for writing SMART objectives.

2. **http://www.healthypeople.gov/2020/default**

   Healthy People 2020

   This is the home page for *Healthy People 2020*. At this site you can navigate to background information about *Healthy People 2020*, a listing of the 42 topic areas and the objectives, and suggestions for implementing *Healthy People 2020*.

3. **http://ctb.ku.edu/en**

   Community Tool Box

   On the home page of the Community Tool Box (CTB), you can use the "Search" function to locate information on creating mission statements, goals, and SMART objectives.

Theories and Models Commonly Used for Health Promotion Interventions

Chapter Objectives

After reading this chapter and answering the questions at the end, you should be able to:

- Define *theory, model, constructs, concepts,* and *variables.*

- Explain why health promotion interventions should be planned using theoretical frameworks.

- Describe how the concept of the ecological perspective applies to using theories.

- Explain the difference between a continuum theory and a stage theory.

- Briefly explain the theories and models presented in this chapter.

Key Terms

action stage

attitude toward the behavior

aversive stimulus

behavior change theories

behavioral capability

collective efficacy

community readiness

concepts

construct

contemplation stage

continuum theory

decisional balance

diffusion theory

direct reinforcement

early adopters

early majority

efficacy expectations

elaboration

emotional–coping response

expectancies

expectations

innovators

intention

laggards

lapse

late majority

likelihood of taking recommended preventive health action

locus of control

maintenance stage

model

negative punishment

negative reinforcement

outcome expectations

perceived barriers

perceived behavioral control

perceived benefits

perceived seriousness/ severity

perceived susceptibility

perceived threat

planning models

positive punishment

positive reinforcement

precontemplation stage

preparation stage

processes of change

punishment

recidivism

reciprocal determinism

reinforcement

relapse

relapse prevention (RP)

self-control

self-efficacy

self-regulation

self-reinforcement

social capital

social context

social network

socio-ecological approach (ecological perspective)

stage

stage theory

subjective norm

temptation

termination

theory

variable

vicarious reinforcement

Whenever there is a discussion about the theoretical bases for health education and health promotion, we often find the terms *theory* and *model* used. We begin this chapter with a brief explanation of these terms to establish a common understanding of their meaning.

One of the most frequently quoted definitions of **theory** is one in which Glanz, Lewis, and Viswanath (2008b) modified an earlier definition written by Kerlinger (1986). It states, "A *theory* is a set of interrelated concepts, definitions, and propositions that presents a *systematic* view of events or situations by specifying relations among variables in order to *explain* and *predict* the events of the situations" (p. 26). In other words, "a theory presents a systematic way of understanding events, behaviors and/or situations" (Glanz, n.d., p. 5). For health education specialists, theory helps "to develop an organized, systematic, and efficient approach to investigating health behaviors. Once these investigations produce satisfactory results and are replicated the findings can be used to inform the design of theory-based intervention programs" (Crosby, Salazar, & DiClemente, 2013, p. 32).

Nutbeam and Harris (1999) have stated that a fully developed theory would be characterized by three major elements: "It would explain:

- the major factors that influence the phenomena of interest, for example those factors which explain why some people are regularly active and others are not;
- the relationship between these factors, for example the relationship between knowledge, beliefs, social norms and behaviours [*sic*] such as physical activity; and
- the conditions under which these relationships do or do not occur: the how, when, and why of hypothesised [*sic*] relationships, for example, the time, place and circumstances which, predictably lead to a person being active or inactive" (p. 10).

In comparison, a **model** "is a composite, a mixture of ideas or concepts taken from any number of theories and used together" (Hayden, 2014, p. 2). Stated a bit differently: "Models draw on a number of theories to help understand a specific problem in a particular setting or content. They are not always as specific as theory" (Rimer & Glanz, 2005, p. 4). Unlike theories, models do "not attempt to explain the processes underlying learning, but only to represent them" (Chaplin & Krawiec, 1979, p. 68).

Though we just went to some effort to make a distinction between the words *theory* and *model*, when the terms *theory-based*, *theory-driven*, and *theory-informed* are used (such as in *theory-based/driven/informed planning*, *theory-based/driven/informed practice*, or *theory-based/driven/informed research*), it is commonly understood in our profession that the word *theory* is used in a general way to mean either theory or model. In fact, some of the best-known and often used theories in health education/health promotion use the word *model* in their title (e.g., Health Belief Model). Goodson (2010) provides an explanation for the discrepancy in the use of term *model* for things we refer to as "theory." She has indicated that when some of these models were created they were properly titled as models. They were created using theoretical constructs to explain specific phenomena. They had little empirical testing to prove their worth. Over time, these models have been tested and refined and thus have gained theory status. Goodson (2010) concludes by saying in our work "because we tend to borrow the theories we employ from other disciplines and fields and because our concern usually centers in applying these theories (or models) to practice or research, it seems to matter little to us whether we deal with theories or with models; it seems to matter even less what labels we attach to them" (p. 228). Thus, as we use the terms *theory* and *theory-based/driven/informed* throughout the remainder of this book, we use them to be inclusive of endeavors based on either a theory *or* a model.

Concepts are the primary elements or building blocks of a theory (Glanz et al., 2008b). When a concept has been developed, created, or adopted for use with a specific theory, it is referred to as a **construct** (Kerlinger, 1986). "The key concepts of a theory are its constructs" (Rimer & Glanz, 2005, p. 4). The operational (practical use) form of a construct is known as a **variable**. Variables "specify how a construct is to be measured in a specific situation" (Glanz et al., 2008b, p. 28). Thus, variables need to be matched "to constructs when identifying what needs to be assessed during evaluation of a theory-driven program" (Rimer & Glanz, 2005, p. 4).

> Consider how these terms are used in practical application. A personal belief is a *concept* related to various health behaviors. For example, people are more likely to behave in a healthy way—say exercise regularly—if they feel confident in their ability to actually engage in a healthy form of exercise. Such a concept is captured in a *construct* of the Social Cognitive Theory (SCT) called self-efficacy. (See the discussion of the SCT later in this chapter.) If health education specialists want to develop an intervention to assist people in exercising, the ability to measure the peoples' self-efficacy toward exercise will help create the intervention. The measurement may consist of a few questions that ask people to rate their confidence in their ability to exercise. This measurement, or operational form, of the self-efficacy construct is a *variable*. However, because of the complexity of getting a non-exerciser to become an exerciser, the health education specialist may need to use a *model*, composed of constructs from several theories, to plan the intervention (Cottrell et al., 2015, p. 98).

Based on these descriptions, it seems logical to think of theories as the backbone of the processes used to plan, implement, and evaluate health promotion interventions. They can help by (1) identifying why people behave as they do and why they are not behaving in healthy ways, (2) identifying information needed before developing an intervention, (3) providing a conceptual framework for selecting constructs to develop the intervention, (4) providing direction and justification for program activities, (5) providing insights into how best to deliver the intervention, (6) identifying what needs to be measured to evaluate the impact of the intervention, and (7) helping to guide research identifying the determinants of health behavior (Cowdery et al., 1995; Crosby, Kegler, & DiClemente, 2009; Glanz et al., 2008b; Simons-Morton, McLeroy, & Wendel, 2012). Theory also "provides a useful reference point to help keep research and implementation activities clearly focused" (Crosby et al., 2009, p. 11), and it infuses ethics and social justice into practice (Goodson, 2010). In addition, "[u]sing theory as a foundation for program planning and development is consistent with the current emphasis on using evidence-based interventions in public health, behavioral medicine, and medicine" (Rimer & Glanz, 2005, p. 5). Getting people to engage in health behavior change is a complicated process that is very difficult under the best of conditions. Without the direction that theories provide, planners can easily waste valuable resources in trying to achieve the desired behavior change. Therefore, program planners should ground their planning process in the theories that have been the foundation of other successful health promotion efforts.

There are many theories that health education specialists can use to guide their practice however, there is no best theory. "The 'best theory' is a function of how well it serves the objectives that must be met to achieve sustainable protective behaviors among a specified population. In essence, the range of behavioral and social science theories available for both health promotion practice and research affords the practitioner and researcher an opportunity to select the theories that are the most appropriate, feasible, and practical for a particular setting or population" (Crosby et al., 2009, p. 15). In addition, "No single theory or conceptual framework dominates research or practice in health promotion and education today" (Glanz et al., 2008b, p. 31). In a review of 10 leading health, medicine, and psychology journals, Painter, Borba, Hynes, Mays, and Glanz (2008) found that "dozens of theories and models" (Glanz, 2008b, p. 31) had been used in the reported literature. We have no intention of introducing all of them. However, approximately 10 theories and models are used regularly to plan programs. In the remaining sections of this chapter, and parts of several other chapters, we present an overview of the theories that are most often used in creating health promotion interventions. As you read about and study the various theories, you will find that some express the same general ideas, but employ "a unique vocabulary to articulate the specific factors considered to be important" (Glanz et al., 2008b, p. 28). Also, be aware that the presentation of theories that follows is by no means comprehensive in nature. For those readers who would like to examine these and other theories in more depth, we would recommend eight books: *Health Behavior and Health Education: Theory, Research and Practice* (Glanz, Rimer, & Viswanath, 2008a); *Emerging Theories in Health Promotion Practice and Research: Strategies for Improving Public Health* (DiClemente, Crosby, & Kegler, 2009); *Theory in Health Promotion Research and Practice* (Goodson, 2010); *Behavior Theory in Health Promotion Practice and Research* (Simons-Morton et al., 2012); *Theoretical Foundations of Health Education and Health Promotion* (Sharma & Romas, 2012); *Health Behavior Theory for Public Health* (DiClemente, Salazar, & Crosby, 2013); *Introduction to Health Behavior* (Hayden, 2014); and *Essentials of Health Behavior: Social and Behavioral Theory in Public Health* (Edberg, 2015). **Box 7.1** identifies the responsibilities and competencies for health education specialists that pertain to the material presented in this chapter.

▷ Types of Theories and Models

There are several ways of categorizing the theories and models associated with health education/promotion practice. One way of doing so is to divide them into two groups. The first group includes those theories and models used for planning, implementing, and evaluating health promotion programs. This group has been called **planning models**. The planning models were presented earlier (Chapter 3). The second group is referred to as **behavior change theories**. Behavior change theories help explain how change takes place.

▷ Behavior Change Theories

As noted earlier, there are many behavior change theories that health education specialists could use to plan programs. Because of the peculiarities of the theories and multitude of factors that could impact a specific planning situation, some theories work better in some situations than others. Before we present the theories focusing on behavior change, it is important to introduce the concept of the socio-ecological approach.

Responsibilities and Competencies for Health Education Specialists

The content of this chapter focuses on theories and models used in the practice of health promotion. Specifically, theories and models provide a "road map" for planners to use when creating interventions and evaluating the effectiveness of those interventions. The responsibilities and competencies related to these tasks include:

RESPONSIBILITY I: Assess Needs, Resources, and Capacity for Health Education/Promotion

Competency 1.1: Plan assessment process for health education/promotion

RESPONSIBILITY II: Plan Health Education/Promotion

Competency 2.3: Select or design strategies/interventions

Competency 2.4: Develop a plan for the delivery of health education/promotion

RESPONSIBILITY III: Implement Health Education/Promotion

Competency 3.3: Implement health education/promotion plan

RESPONSIBILITY IV: Conduct Evaluation and Research Related to Health Education/Promotion

Competency 4.1: Develop evaluation plan for health education/promotion

RESPONSIBILITY VII: Communicate, Promote, and Advocate for Health and Health Education/Promotion, and the Profession

Competency 7.1: Identify, develop, and deliver messages using a variety of communication strategies, methods, and techniques

Source: *A Competency-Based Framework for Health Education Specialists—2015*. Whitehall, PA: National Commission for Health Education Credentialing, Inc. (NCHEC) and the Society for Public Health Education (SOPHE). Reprinted by permission of the National Commission for Health Education Credentialing, Inc. (NCHEC) and the Society for Public Health Education (SOPHE).

The socio-ecological approach, which is grounded in the work of development psychologist Urie Bronfenbrenner (1979), gained traction in health promotion in the 1980s with the movement toward using a systems-approach for interventions. The underlying concept of the **socio-ecological approach** (sometimes referred to as the **ecological perspective**) is that human behavior shapes and is shaped by multiple levels of influences. "Individuals influence and are influenced by their families, social networks, the organizations in which they participate (workplaces, schools, religious organizations), the communities of which they are a part, and the society in which they live" (IOM, 2001, p. 26). In other words, the health behavior of individuals is shaped in part by the *social context* in which they live. **Social context** has been "defined as the sociocultural forces that shape people's day-to-day experiences and that directly and indirectly affect health and behavior (Burke, Joseph, Pasick, & Barker, 2009, p. 56S). Therefore, a central conclusion of the socio-ecological approach is that interventions must be aimed at multiple levels of influence in order to achieve substantial changes in health behavior (Sallis, Owen, & Fisher, 2008).

McLeroy, Bibeau, Steckler, and Glanz (1988) identified five levels of influence: (1) intrapersonal or individual factors, (2) interpersonal factors, (3) institutional or organizational factors, (4) community factors, and (5) public policy factors. More recently, Simons-Morton et al. (2012, p. 45) added two additional levels "(6) the physical environment and (7) culture." **Table 7.1** defines each of the seven levels, and **Box 7.2** provides an example of how the levels can impact health behavior.

TABLE 7.1 **An Ecological Perspective: Levels of Influence**

Concept	Definition
Intrapersonal Level	Individual characteristics that influence behavior, such as knowledge, attitudes, beliefs, and personality traits
Interpersonal Level	Interpersonal processes and primary groups, including family, friends, and peers that provide social identity, support, and role definition
Community Level	
Institutional Factors	Rules, regulations, policies, and informal structures that may constrain or promote recommended behaviors
Community Factors	Social networks and norms, or standards, that exist as formal or informal among individuals, groups, and organizations
Public Policy	Local, state, and federal policies and laws that regulate or support healthy actions and practices for disease prevention, early detection, control, and management
Physical Environment	Natural and built environment
Culture	Shared beliefs, values, behaviors and practices of a population

Sources: Rimer & Glanz (2005, p. 11); Simons-Morton et al., (2012, p. 45)

Because of the underlying concepts that are captured in the constructs of individual theories, certain theories are more useful in developing programs aimed at specific levels of influence. For example, some theories were developed to help explain behavior change in individuals, while others were developed to help explain change

BOX

7.2

Application

Application of the Socio-Ecological Approach

A good example of the use of the socio-ecological approach (ecological perspective) is the comprehensive method used to reduce cigarette smoking in the United States. At the *intrapersonal* (or *individual*) *level*, a large majority of smokers know that smoking is bad for them and a slightly smaller majority have indicated they would like to quit. Many have tried—some have tried on many occasions. At the *interpersonal level*, many smokers are encouraged by their physician and/or family and friends to quit. Some smokers may attempt to quit on their own or join a formal smoking cessation group to try to quit. At the *institutional* (or *organizational*) *level*, a number of institutions (e.g., churches and worksites) have developed policies that prohibit smoking in and/or on institution property (i.e., buildings and grounds). At the *community level*, a number of towns, cities, and counties have passed ordinances that prohibit smoking in public places. At the *public policy level*, a number of states have passed clean indoor air acts that limit smoking, and have passed laws increasing the tax on a package of cigarettes. Also at this level, the U.S. government has spent many dollars for public service announcements (PSAs) and other forms of media advertising the dangers of tobacco use. At the *physical environment level* new structures have been built to eliminate exposure to secondhand smoke with appropriate filtration systems and separate structures have been built to physically separate the smokers from the non-smokers. At the *culture level* a focus has been placed on establishing and reinforcing non-smoking as the cultural norm. Attacking the smoking problem from all levels has contributed to the decrease in the percentage of smokers in the United States.

at the community level. To assist program planners with matching theories appropriate to level of influence, we present our discussion of the theories using the simplified version of the socio-ecological model that condensed the multiple levels into three—intrapersonal, interpersonal, and community (Glanz & Rimer, 1995; Rimer & Glanz, 2005). "In practice, addressing the community level requires taking into consideration institutional and public policy factors, as well as social networks and norms" (Rimer & Glanz, 2005, p. 11). To this community level we add the sixth and seventh levels of influence-- physical environment and culture.

In addition to theories being placed into a level of influence at which they may be most useful, theories can also be categorized by the approach—continuum or stage theories—they use to explain behavior. **Continuum theories** are those behavior change theories that identify variables that influence actions (e.g., beliefs, attitudes) and combine them into a single equation that predicts the likelihood of action (Weinstein, Rothman, & Sutton, 1998; Weinstein, Sandman, & Blalock, 2008). "These theories acknowledge *quantitative* differences among people in their positions on different variables" (Weinstein et al., 2008, p. 124) and "thus, each person is placed along a continuum of action likelihood" (Weinstein et al., 1998, p. 291).

A **stage theory** is one that is comprised of an ordered set of categories into which people can be classified, and which identifies factors that could induce movement from one category to the next (Weinstein & Sandman, 2002a). More specifically, stage theories have four principal elements: (1) a category system to define the stages, (2) an ordering of stages, (3) common barriers to change facing people in the same stage, and (4) different barriers to change facing people in different stages (Weinstein et al., 1998; Weinstein & Sandman, 2002a). Advocates of stage theories "claim that there are *qualitative* differences among people and question whether changes in health behaviors can be described by a single prediction equation" (Weinstein et al., 2008, pp. 124–125). **Table 7.2** lists the theories presented in this book by level of influence and theory approach.

Intrapersonal Level Theories

The theories presented in this section of the chapter focus primarily on individual health behavior. The intrapersonal or "individual level is the most basic one in health promotion practice, so planners must be able to explain and influence the behavior of individuals" (Rimer & Glanz, 2005, p. 12). Intrapersonal theories focus on factors within the individual such as knowledge, attitudes, beliefs, self-concept, feelings, past experiences, motivation, skills, and behavior. Many health education specialists will use the theories we discuss in this section to assist individuals with behavior change, But be aware that some of these theories do not take into account social context and thus they may need to be combined with theories found in other levels of influence to reach their program goals.

STIMULUS RESPONSE (SR) THEORY

One of the theories used to explain and modify behavior is the stimulus response, or SR, theory (Thorndike, 1898; Watson, 1925; Hall, 1943). This theory reflects the combination of classical conditioning (Pavlov, 1927) and instrumental conditioning (Thorndike, 1898) theories. These early conditioning theories explain learning based on the associations among stimulus, response, and reinforcement (Parcel & Baranowski, 1981; Parcel, 1983). "In simplest terms, the SR theorists believe that learning results from events (termed 'reinforcements') which reduce physiological drives that activate behavior" (Rosenstock, Strecher, & Becker, 1988, p. 175). The behaviorist B. F. Skinner believed that the frequency of a behavior was determined by the reinforcements that followed that behavior.

TABLE 7.2 **Theories by Level of Influence and Category**

Level of Influence	Where Found in This Book
● Intrapersonal Level	
Continuum Theories	
Stimulus Response Theory	Chapter 7
Theory of Planned Behavior	Chapter 7
Health Belief Model	Chapter 7
Protection Motivation Theory	Chapter 7
Elaboration Likelihood Model of Persuasion	Chapter 7
Information-Motivation-Behavioral Skills Model	Chapter 7
Stage Theory	
Transtheoretical Model	Chapter 7
Precaution Adoption Process Model	Chapter 7
● Interpersonal Level	
Continuum Theories	
Social Cognitive Theory	Chapter 7
Social Network Theory	Chapter 7
Social Capital Theory	Chapter 7
● Community Level	
Continuum Theories	
Communication Theory	Chapters 8 & 11
Community Organizing	Chapter 9
Community Building	Chapter 9
Diffusion of Innovations	Chapter 7
Stage Theory	
Community Readiness Model	Chapter 7

In Skinner's view, the mere temporal association between a behavior and an immediately following reward is sufficient to increase the probability that the behavior will be repeated. Such behaviors are called *operants*; they operate on the environment to bring about changes resulting in reward or reinforcement (Rosenstock et al., 1988). Stated another way, operant behaviors are behaviors that act on the environment to produce consequences. These consequences, in turn, either reinforce or do not reinforce the behavior that preceded.

There are two broad categories of environmental consequences: *reinforcement* or *punishment* (McDade-Montez, Cvengros, & Christensen, 2005): Individuals can learn from both. **Reinforcement** has been defined by Skinner (1953) as any event that follows a behavior, which in turn increases the probability that the same behavior will be repeated in the future. Stated differently, reinforcement has "a *strengthening effect* that occurs when operant behaviors have certain consequences" (Nye, 1992, p. 16). Behavior has a greater probability of occurring in the future: (1) if reinforcement is frequent and (2) if reinforcement is provided soon after the desired behavior. This immediacy clarifies the relationship between the reinforcement and appropriate behavior (Skinner, 1953). Simons-Morton and colleagues (2012) have stated that when a behavior is sufficiently reinforced it tends to recur. If a behavior is complex in nature, smaller steps working toward the desired behavior with appropriate reinforcement will help to shape the desired behavior. This was found to be true in getting pigeons to play Ping-Pong, and it can be useful in trying to change a complex health behavior like smoking or exercise. Whereas reinforcement will increase the frequency of a behavior, punishment will decrease the frequency of a behavior. However, both reinforcement and punishment can be either positive or negative. The terms *positive* and *negative* in this context do not mean good and bad; rather, *positive* means adding something (effects of the stimulus) to a situation, whereas *negative* means taking something away (removal or reduction of the effects of the stimulus) from the situation.

If individuals act in a certain way to produce a consequence that makes them feel good or that is enjoyable, it is labeled **positive reinforcement** (or *reward*). Examples of this would be an individual who is involved in an exercise program and "feels good" at the end of the workout, or one who participates in a weight loss program and receives verbal encouragement from the facilitator, again making that person "feel good." Stimulus response theorists would note that in both of these situations, the pleasant experiences (internal feelings and verbal encouragement, respectively) should occur right after the behavior, which in turn increases the chances that the frequency of the behavior will increase.

While positive reinforcement helps individuals learn by shaping behavior, behavior that avoids punishment is also learned because it reduces the tension that precedes the punishment (Rosenstock et al., 1988). "When this happens, we are being conditioned by *negative reinforcement:* A response is strengthened by the *removal* of something from the situation. In such cases, the 'something' that is removed is referred to as a *negative reinforcer* or *aversive stimulus* (these two phrases are synonymous)" (Nye, 1979, p. 33). A good example of **negative reinforcement** is a weight loss program that requires weekly dues. When participants stop paying dues because they have met their goal weight, this removal of an obligation should increase the frequency of the desired behavior (weight maintenance). Or in the case of exercise, "negative reinforcements would include decreased poor self-image and decreased fatigue" (McDade-Montez et al., 2005, p. 64).

Some people think of negative reinforcement as a form of punishment, but it is not. While negative reinforcement increases the likelihood that a behavior will be repeated, **punishment** typically suppresses behavior. Skinner suggested "two ways in which a response can be punished: by *removing a positive reinforcer* or by *presenting a negative reinforcer* (aversive stimulus) as a consequence of the response" (Nye, 1979, p. 43). Punishment is usually linked to some uncomfortable (physical, mental, or otherwise) experience and decreases the frequency of a behavior. An aversive smoking cessation program that circulates cigarette smoke around those enrolled in the program as they smoke is an example of **positive punishment**. It decreases the frequency of smoking by presenting (adding) a negative reinforcer or **aversive stimulus** (smoke) as a consequence of the response. Examples of **negative punishment** (removing a positive reinforcer) would include not allowing employees to use the employees' lounge if they continue to smoke while using it, or reducing the health insurance benefits of employees who continue to participate in health-harming behavior such as not wearing a safety belt. Stimulus response theorists would note that taking away the privilege of using the employees' lounge or reducing health insurance benefits would decrease the frequency of smoking among the employees and increase the wearing of safety belts, respectively. **Figure 7.1** illustrates the relationship between reinforcement and punishment.

		Consequences	
		Positive (adding to)	Negative (taking away)
Behavior	Increase in frequency	Positive reinforcement (reward)	Negative reinforcement
	Decrease in frequency	Positive punishment	Negative punishment

▲ **Figure 7.1** 2 × 2 Table of the Stimulus Response Theory

Finally, if reinforcement is withheld—or, stating it another way, if the behavior is ignored—the behavior will become less frequent and eventually will not be repeated. Skinner (1953) refers to this as extinction. Teachers frequently use this technique with disruptive children in the classroom. If a child is acting up in class, the teacher may choose to ignore the behavior in hopes that the nonreinforced behavior will go away.

THEORY OF PLANNED BEHAVIOR (TPB)

The *theory of planned behavior* (TPB) is the first of several *value-expectancy theories* presented in this section. Value-expectancy theories were developed to explain how individuals' behaviors were influenced by beliefs and attitudes (Simons-Morton et al., 2012). Thus, the tendency to perform a particular act is a function of the expectancy that the act will be followed by certain consequences (e.g., 'How vulnerable am I to the danger?') and the value of those consequences (e.g., 'How severe is the danger?')" (Prentice-Dunn & Rogers, 1986, p. 157).

The theory of planned behavior has its foundation in the *theory of reasoned action* (TRA) (Fishbein, 1967). The TRA was developed to explain volitional behaviors, "that is, behaviors that can be performed at will" (Luszczynska & Sutton, 2005, p. 73). The TRA has proved to be useful when dealing with purely volitional behaviors, but complications are encountered when the theory is applied to behaviors that are not fully under volitional control. A good example of this is a smoker who intends to quit but fails to do so. Even though intent is high, nonmotivational factors—such as lack of requisite opportunities, skills, and resources—could prevent success (Ajzen, 1988).

The TPB (see **Figure 7.2**) is an extension of the TRA that addresses the problem of incomplete volitional control. Both the TRA and the TPB focus on determinants of behavioral intentions. In the TRA, Fishbein and Ajzen (1975) distinguished among *attitude, belief, intention,* and *behavior*. **Intention** "is an indication of a person's readiness to perform a given behavior, and it is considered to be an immediate antecedent of behavior" (Ajzen, 2006). According to this theory, individuals' intentions to perform given behaviors are functions of their *attitudes* toward the behavior and their *subjective norms* associated with the behaviors. **Attitude toward the behavior** "is the degree to which performance of the behavior is positively or negatively valued. According to the expectancy-value model, attitude toward a behavior is determined by the total set of accessible behavioral beliefs linking the behavior to various outcomes and other attributes" (Ajzen, 2006). Thus a person who has strong beliefs about positive attributes or outcomes from performing the behavior will have a positive attitude toward behavior (Montaño & Kasprzyk, 2008). For example, if a person feels strongly about exercise being able to help control weight, then that person will have a positive attitude toward exercise. The converse is true as well. Weak beliefs about the outcomes or attributes of exercise will produce a negative attitude toward it.

Subjective norm "is the perceived social pressure to engage or not engage in a behavior" (Ajzen, 2006). For many health behaviors, the social pressure comes from a person's peers, parents, partner, close friends, teachers, role models, boss, and co-workers, as well as experts or professionals like physicians or lawyers. Thus individuals who believe that certain people think they should perform a behavior and are motivated to meet the people's expectations will hold a positive subjective norm (Montaño & Kasprzyk, 2008). Similar to behavioral beliefs, the converse is also true. An example of a positive subjective norm are employees who see their co-workers as important people in their lives and believe that these people approve of them participating in a company exercise program.

The major difference between TPB and TRA is the addition of a third (the first being *attitude toward the behavior* and the second being *subjective norm*), conceptually independent determinant of intention—*perceived behavioral control*. Perceived behavioral control is similar to the Social Cognitive Theory's concept of self-efficacy. **Perceived behavioral control** "refers to people's perceptions of their ability to perform a given behavior" (Ajzen, 2006). Stated differently, perceived behavioral control refers to the perceived ease or difficulty of performing the behavior and is assumed to reflect past experience as well as anticipated impediments and obstacles. As a general rule, the more favorable the attitude and subjective norm with respect to a behavior, and the greater the perceived behavioral control, the stronger should be the individual's intentions to perform the behavior under consideration (Ajzen, 1988).

Figure 7.2 illustrates two important features of this theory. First, perceived behavioral control has motivational implications for intentions. That is, without perceived control, intentions could be minimal even if attitudes toward the behavior and subjective norm were

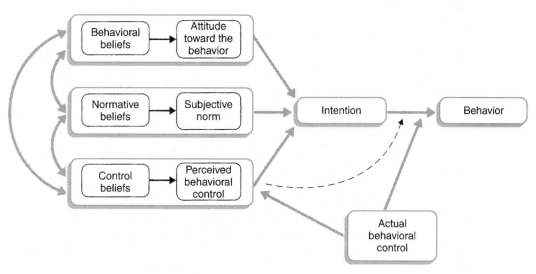

▲ **Figure 7.2** Theory of Planned Behavior Diagram

Source: *Theory of Planned Behavior Diagram.* Icek Ajzen. Copyright © 2006 by Icek Ajzen. Reprinted with permission.

strong. Second, there may be a direct link between perceived behavioral control and behavior. Behavior depends not only on motivation but also on actual control. *Actual behavioral control* "refers to the extent to which a person has the skills, resources, and other prerequisites needed to perform a given behavior. Successful performance of the behavior depends not only on a favorable intention but also on a sufficient level of behavioral control. To the extent that perceived behavioral control is accurate, it can serve as a proxy of actual control and can be used for the prediction of behavior" (Ajzen, 2006). To use the example of smoking once again as a behavior not fully under volitional control, TPB predicts that individuals will give up smoking if they:

- Have a positive attitude toward quitting
- Think others whom they value believe it would be good for them to quit
- Perceive that they have control over whether they quit

HEALTH BELIEF MODEL (HBM)

The *health belief model* (HBM) is also a value-expectancy theory. It was developed in the 1950s by a group of psychologists at the U.S. Public Health service to help explain why people would or would not use health services (Rosenstock, 1966). The HBM is based on Lewin's decision-making model (Lewin, 1935, 1936; Lewin et al., 1944). Since its creation, the HBM has been used to help explain a variety of health behaviors (Becker, 1974; Janz & Becker, 1984; Jones, Smith, & Llewellyn, 2014).

The HBM hypothesizes that health-related action depends on the simultaneous occurrence of three classes of factors:

1. The existence of sufficient motivation (or health concern) to make health issues salient or relevant.
2. The belief that one is susceptible (vulnerable) to a serious health problem or to the sequelae of that illness or condition. This is often termed **perceived threat**.
3. The belief that following a particular health recommendation would be beneficial in reducing the perceived threat, and at a subjectively acceptable cost. Cost refers to the **perceived barriers** that must be overcome in order to follow the health recommendation; it includes, but is not restricted to, financial outlays (Rosenstock et al., 1988, p. 177). In fact, the lack of self-efficacy is also seen as a perceived barrier to taking a recommended health action (Strecher & Rosenstock, 1997).

In recent years, self-efficacy has become a more meaningful concept in the perceived barriers construct of the HBM. When the HBM was first conceived, self-efficacy was not explicitly a part of it. "The original model was developed in the context of circumscribed preventive health actions (accepting a screening test or an immunization) that were not perceived to involve complex behaviors" (Champion & Skinner, 2008, p. 49). However, when program planners want to use the HBM to plan health promotion interventions for priority populations in need of lifestyle behaviors requiring long-term changes, self-efficacy must be included in the model. Therefore, "[f]or behavior change to succeed, people must (as the original HBM theorizes) feel threatened by their current behavioral patterns (perceived susceptibility and severity) and believe that change of a specific kind will result in a valued outcome at acceptable cost. They must also feel themselves competent (self-efficacious) to overcome perceived barriers to taking action" (Champion & Skinner, 2008, p. 50) (see **Figure 7.3**).

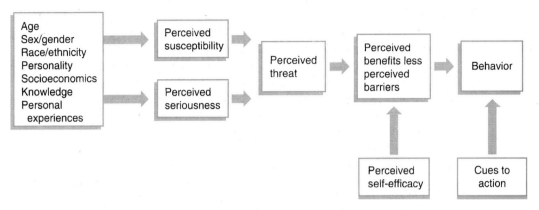

▲ **Figure 7.3** Health Belief Model

Here is an example of the HBM applied to exercise. Someone watching television sees an advertisement about exercise. This is a cue to action that starts her thinking about her own need to exercise. There may be some variables (demographic, sociopsychological, and structural) that cause her to think about it a bit more. She remembers her college health course that included information about heart disease and the importance of staying active. She knows she has a higher than normal risk for heart disease because of family history, poor diet, and slightly elevated blood pressure. Therefore, she comes to the conclusion that she is susceptible to heart disease (**perceived susceptibility**). She also knows that if she develops heart disease, it can be very serious (**perceived seriousness/severity**). Based on these factors, the individual thinks that there is reason to be concerned about heart disease (perceived threat). She knows that exercise can help delay the onset of heart disease and can increase the chances of surviving a heart attack if one should occur (**perceived benefits**). But exercise takes time from an already busy day, and it is not easy to exercise in the variety of settings in which she typically finds herself, especially during bad weather (perceived barriers). Her confidence in being able to overcome the barriers and exercise regularly will also be important (**self-efficacy**). She must now weigh the threat of the disease against the difference between benefits and barriers. This decision will then result in a likelihood of exercising or not exercising (**likelihood of taking recommended preventive health action**).

PROTECTION MOTIVATION THEORY (PMT)

The third value-expectancy theory presented in this section is the *protection motivation theory* (PMT). It was originally created by Rogers (1975) and "proposed to provide explanations of the effects of fear appeals on health attitudes and behavior" (Floyd, Prentice-Dunn, & Rogers, 2000, p. 409). The PMT was later revised and extended (Rogers, R., 1983) to a more general theory of persuasive communication that included reward and self-efficacy components. The PMT has some similarities to the HBM. Both contain a cost-benefit analysis in which the individual weighs the costs of taking a precautionary action against the expected benefits of taking action, and both share an emphasis on cognitive processes mediating attitudinal and behavioral change (Floyd et al., 2000; Prentice-Dunn & Rogers, 1986).

As explained by the PMT, inputs come from environmental sources of information such as verbal persuasion and observational learning, and from intrapersonal sources such as one's personality and feedback from personal experiences associated with the targeted mal-adaptive and adaptive responses (Floyd et al., 2000). Based on these inputs people make a cognitive assessment of whether there is a threat to their health. Information about a threat to one's health arouses two cognitive mediating processes: threat appraisal and coping appraisal (Floyd et al., 2000; McClendon & Prentice-Dunn, 2001).

The threat appraisal process is addressed first because a threat to one's health must be perceived or identified before there can be an assessment of the coping options (Floyd et al., 2000). Threat appraisal assesses maladaptive behaviors (e.g., physical inactivity, smoking, overeating, binge drinking). The assessment includes (1) a review of intrinsic (e.g., physical and psychological pleasure such as feeling "good") and extrinsic (e.g., peer approval such as receiving attention) rewards; and (2) a review of the perceived severity of and the perceived vulnerability to the threat. "Rewards increase the probability of selecting the maladaptive response (not to protect self or others), whereas threat will decrease the probability of selecting the maladaptive response" (Floyd et al., 2000, p. 410). "Thus the rewards minus the sum of severity and vulnerability indicate the amount of threat experienced by the individual" (McClendon & Prentice-Dunn, 2001, p. 322).

Coping appraisal assesses adaptive behaviors (e.g., health enhancing behaviors). This type of assessment includes (1) a review of response efficacy (e.g., belief that the coping action will avert the threat) and self-efficacy (i.e., belief that the person is capable of completing the coping action); and (2) a review of the response costs (e.g., "inconvenience, expense, unpleasantness, difficulty, complexity, side effects, disruption of daily life, and overcoming habit strength" [Rogers, 1984, p. 104]). "Response efficacy and self-efficacy will increase the probability of selecting the adaptive response, whereas response costs will decrease the probability of selecting the adaptive response" (Floyd et al., 2000, p. 411). In sum, the amount of coping appraisal experienced is indicated by the sum of response efficacy and self-efficacy minus the response costs" (McClendon & Prentice-Dunn, 2001, p. 322).

When the results of the threat appraisal and coping appraisal processes are combined it is the protective motivation that an individual possesses. Stated a bit differently, "The output of these appraisal-mediating processes is the decision (or intention) to initiate, continue, or inhibit the applicable adaptive responses (or coping modes)" (Floyd et al., 2000, p. 411). When using the PMT to design an intervention protection motivation has been measured using behavioral intentions (Floyd et al., 2000).

Prentice-Dunn and Rogers (1986, p. 156) offered the following summary of the PMT:

> PMT assumes that protection motivation is maximized when: (i) the threat to health is severe; (ii) the individual feels vulnerable; (iii) the adaptive response is believed to be an effective means for averting the threat; (iv) the person is confident in his or her abilities to complete successfully the adaptive response; (v) the rewards associated with the mal-adaptive behavior are small; and (vi) the costs associated with the adaptive response are small. Such factors produce protection motivation and, subsequently, the enactment of the adaptive, or coping, response.

Since its development, the PMT has been successfully used to create program interventions for a number of different health behaviors (Floyd et al., 2000). Some of the more recent applications of the theory have included: adolescent drug use intention (Wu et al., 2014), exercise among various groups (Bui, Mullan, & McCaffery, 2013; Gaston & Prapavessis, 2012), living wills (Allen, Phillips, Whitehead, Crowther, & Prentice-Dunn, 2009), pro-environmental behavior (Bockarova & Steg, 2014), social networks (Salleh et al.,

2012), sun protection behavior/skin cancer (Prentice-Dunn, McMath, & Cramer, 2009), and weight loss and bariatric surgery (Boeka, Prentice-Dunn, & Lokken, 2010).

ELABORATION LIKELIHOOD MODEL OF PERSUASION (ELM)

The *Elaboration Likelihood Model of Persuasion*, or the *Elaboration Likelihood Model* (ELM) for short, was initially developed to help explain inconsistencies in the results from research dealing with the study of attitudes (Petty, Barden, & Wheeler, 2009). Specifically, the model was designed to help explain how persuasion messages (communication) aimed at changing attitudes were received and processed by people. Though not created specifically for health communication, since its development the ELM has been used to help interpret and predict the impact of health messages (Petty & Briñol, 2012) (see **Figure 7.4**).

The utility of the ELM is that it does four essential things. First, the ELM proposes that modifying attitudes or other judgments can be formed as a result of a high degree of thought (i.e., central process route) or a low degree of thought (i.e., peripheral and processing route) (Petty et al., 2009). "That is, the elaboration continuum' ranges from low to high" (Petty & Briñol, 2012, p. 226). The distinction among the places on the continuum is the amount of elaboration. **Elaboration** refers to the amount of cognitive processing (i.e., thought) that a person puts into receiving messages.

Second, the ELM postulates that there are numerous specific processes of change that operate along the elaboration continuum (Petty & Briñol, 2011). The continuum stretches from one end anchored with processes requiring no thinking, like classical conditioning (see discussion on stimulus response theory earlier in the chapter), to processes requiring some effortful thinking such as inferences based on one's experiences, to processes requiring careful consideration (see value-expectancy theories presented earlier in the chapter) (Petty et al., 2009). The peripheral route processes involve minimal thought and rely on superficial cues or mental shortcuts (called *heuristics*) about issue-relevant information as primary means for attitude change (Petty et al., 2009). For example, people may form an attitude after hearing a persuasive message simply because the person delivering the message is someone that they admire. On the other hand, central route processes involve thoughtful consideration (or effortful cognitive elaboration) of issue-relevant information and one's own cognitive responses as the primary bases for attitude change (Petty et al., 2009). "Two conditions are necessary for effortful processing to occur—the recipient of the message must be both *motivated* and *able* to think carefully" (Petty et al., 2009, p. 188). An example of central route processing would be a motorcyclist's formation of an attitude about wearing a helmet based on thoughtful consideration of a message about the pros and cons of helmet use along with recalling knowledge gained in a motorcycle safety class and possibly the results of a motorcycle crash in which his or her cousin was involved.

It should be clear that the distinction between the peripheral and central routes is the amount of consideration given to the issue-relevant information and how the information is processed, not the type of information itself (Petty, Wheeler, & Bizer, 1999). "Of course, much of the time, persuasion is determined by a mixture of these processes" (Petty & Briñol, 2012, p. 226).

Third, when comparing the consequences of the two routes there are times when the result is similar. However, the two routes usually lead to attitudes with different consequences. "High effort central route processes are more likely to lead to attitudes that are persistent over time, resistant to counterattack, and influential in guiding thought and behavior than are peripheral process" (Petty et al., 2009, pp. 207–208).

▲ **Figure 7.4** The Elaboration Likelihood Model of Persuasion (ELM)

Source: "The Elaboration Likelihood Model of Persuasion" by R. E. Petty, J. Barden, and G. R. Alexander, from *Emerging Theories in Health Promotion Practice and Research: Strategies for Improving Public Health, 2e,* Ed. J. R. DiClemente, R. A. Crosby, and M. C. Kegler. Copyright © 2009 by Jossey-Bass. Reprinted with permission.

Fourth, and arguably the "most useful thing that the ELM does is to organize the many specific processes by which variables can affect attitudes into a finite set that operate at different points along the elaboration continuum" (Petty & Briñol, 2012, p. 226). The variables can have an influence on people's motivation to think or ability to think, as well as the valence of people's thought or the confidence in the thoughts generated (Petty et al., 2009). For example, variables that have an impact on how a message is processed are the source of the message (e.g., friend, expert), the message itself (e.g., funny, serious), the context (e.g., delivered person-to-person, on the Internet), and various characteristics of the recipient (e.g., intelligence, age, attentiveness).

The ELM has been used to develop a variety of interventions for health promotion programs. The one area where the ELM has been most useful in health promotion has been with message tailoring. *Tailored messages* are those that are "crafted for and delivered to each individual based on individual needs, interests, and circumstances" (NCI, n.d., p. 251). In other words, tailored messages are matched to the needs, interests, and circumstances of the intended recipient. It has been found that the more tailored the persuasive communication, the more relevant it is to the recipient, and the more likely the message will be processed through the central route. And, if a message is processed through the central route the more likely it will impact attitude and behavior change.

INFORMATION-MOTIVATION-BEHAVIORAL (IMB) SKILLS MODEL

The *information-motivation-behavioral* (IMB) *skills model* (see **Figure 7.5**) was initially created to address the critical need for a strong theoretical basis for HIV/AIDS prevention efforts (Fisher & Fisher, 1992). Since its development, there is evidence to support its usefulness with HIV/AIDS prevention (Fisher, Fisher, & Shuper, 2009) as well as other intervention strategies (Chang, Choi, Kim, & Song, 2014) including the management of diabetes (Osborn & Egede, 2010). According to the IMB model, the constructs of information, motivation, and behavioral skills are the fundamental determinants of preventive behavior. The information provided needs to be relevant, easily enacted based on the specific circumstances, and serve as a guide to personal preventive behavior. "In addition to facts that are easy to translate into behavior, the IMB model recognizes additional cognitive processes and content categories

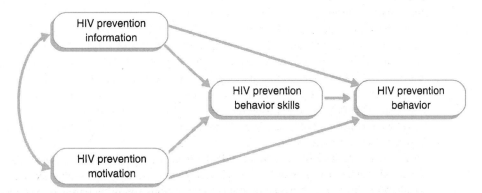

▲ **Figure 7.5** The Information-Motivation-Behavioral Skills Model of HIV Prevention

Source: "Changing AIDS-Risk Behavior." J. D. and W. A. Fisher from *Psychological Bulletin 111*(3). Copyright © 1992 by the American Psychological Association.

that significantly influence performance of preventive behavior" (Fisher et al., 2009, p. 27). Such as the simple decision rules a person may hold, like "if my best friend is willing to ride a motorcycle without a helmet, it must be okay."

Even though people are well informed about a particular health issue, they may not be motivated to act. According to the IMB model, prevention motivation includes both personal motivation to act (i.e., one's attitude toward a specific behavior) and social motivation to act (is there social support for the preventive behavior?) (Sharma, 2012). Both types of motivation are necessary for action to occur.

In addition to people being well informed and motivated to act, the IMB model also asserts that people must possess behavioral skills to engage in the preventive behavior. The behavioral skills component of the IMB model includes an individual's objective ability and his or her perceived self-efficacy to perform the preventive behavior.

In applying the IMB model, health education specialists cannot simply use their own judgment to determine what information to provide, how best to motivate, and what behavioral skills to teach to a given population. The process should begin by eliciting information from a subsample of the priority population to identify deficits in their health-relevant information, motivation, and behavior skills. Next health education specialists need to design and implement "*conceptually-based, empirically-targeted, population-specific*" (p. 29) interventions, constructed on the bases of the elicited findings (Fisher et al., 2009). Then, after the implementation of the intervention, health education specialists must evaluate the intervention to determine if it had significant and sustained effects on the information, motivation, and behavioral skill determinants of the preventive behavior and on the preventive behavior itself (Fisher et al., 2009).

THE TRANSTHEORETICAL MODEL (TTM)

The *transtheoretical model* (TTM), sometimes referred to as the Stages of Change Model, was developed to help explain how individuals and populations progressed toward adopting and maintaining health behavior change. The model uses stages of change to integrate processes and principles of change from across major theories, hence the name 'Transtheoretical'" (Prochaska, Johnson, & Lee, 1998). The model has its roots in psychotherapy and was developed by Prochaska (1979) after he completed a comparative analysis of therapy systems and a critical review of therapy outcome studies. From the analysis and review, Prochaska found that some common processes were involved in change.

As this model has evolved, researchers have applied it to many different types of health behavior change, including but not limited to alcohol and substance abuse, anxiety and panic disorders, delinquency, eating disorders and obesity, exercise, high-fat diets, handwashing, HIV/AIDS prevention, immunizations/vaccinations, mammography screening, medication adherence/compliance, unplanned pregnancy prevention, pregnancy and smoking, sedentary lifestyles, weight control, sun exposure, and physicians practicing preventive medicine (Angus et al., 2013; Prochaska, Redding, & Evers, 2008; Spencer, Adams, Malone, Roy, & Yost, 2006).

The core constructs of the TTM include the stages of change, the processes of change, decisional balance (i.e., the pros and cons of changing), self-efficacy, and temptation (see **Table 7.3**). In addition, this model is "based on critical assumptions about the nature of behavior change and interventions that can best facilitate change" (Prochaska et al., 1998, p. 60). A discussion of these constructs and assumptions follows.

TABLE 7.3 **Transtheoretical Model Constructs**

Constructs	Description
Stages of change	
Precontemplation	No intention to take action within the next 6 months
Contemplation	Intends to take action within the next 6 months
Preparation	Intends to take action within the next 30 days and has taken some behavioral steps in this direction
Action	Has changed overt behavior for less than 6 months
Maintenance	Has changed overt behavior for more than 6 months
Decisional balance	
Pros	The benefits of changing
Cons	The costs of changing
Self-efficacy	
Confidence	Confidence that one can engage in the healthy behavior across different challenging situations
Temptation	Temptation to engage in the unhealthy behavior across different challenging situations
Processes of change	
Consciousness raising	Finding and learning new facts, ideas, and tips that support the healthy behavior change
Dramatic relief	Experiencing the negative emotions (fear, anxiety, worry) that go with unhealthy behavioral risks
Self-reevaluation	Realizing that the behavior change is an important part of one's identity as a person
Environmental reevaluation	Realizing the negative impact of the unhealthy behavior, or the positive impact of the healthy behavior, on one's proximal social and/or physical environment
Self-liberation	Making a firm commitment to change
Helping relationships	Seeking and using social support for the healthy behavior change
Counterconditioning	Substitution of healthier alternative behaviors and/or cognitions for the unhealthy behavior
Reinforcement management	Increasing the rewards for the positive behavior change and/or decreasing the rewards of the unhealthy behavior
Stimulus control	Removing reminders or cues to engage in the unhealthy behavior and/or adding cues to reminders to engage in the healthy behavior
Social liberation	Realizing that social norms are changing in the direction of supporting the healthy behavior change

Source: *SPM Handbook for Health Assessment Tools.* Colleen A. Redding, Joseph S. Rossi, S. R. Rossi, W. F. Velicer, and J. O. Prochaska. Copyright © 1999 by the Society of Prospective Medicine. Reprinted with permission from the authors.

Behavioral change does not occur overnight. A person does not go to bed at night as a nonexerciser and wake up the next morning as an exerciser. Behavior change occurs over time. Thus, the **stage** construct, the core construct of the model, is comprised of categories of change (i.e., stages) along a continuum of motivational readiness to change a problem behavior (URI, 2015). On this continuum "people move from *precontemplation,* not intending to change, to *contemplation,* intending to change within 6 months, to *preparation,* actively planning change, to *action,* overtly making changes, and into *maintenance,* taking steps to sustain change and resist temptation to relapse" (Prochaska, Redding, Harlow, Rossi, & Velicer, 1994). The **precontemplation stage** is defined as a time in which "people do not intend to take action in the near term, usually measured as the next six months. The outcome interval may vary, depending on behavior. People may be in this stage because they are un-informed or under-informed about the consequences of their behavior. Or they may have tried to change a number of times and become demoralized about their abilities to change" (Prochaska et al., 2008, p. 100). People in this stage "tend to avoid reading, talking, or thinking about their high-risk behaviors" (Prochaska et al., 1998). The second stage, **contemplation** is the stage in which "people intend to change their behaviors in the next six months" (Prochaska et al., 2008, p. 100). It occurs when people are aware that a problem exists and are seriously thinking about a behavior change but have not yet made a commitment to take action. They are more open to feedback and information about the problem behavior than those in the precontemplation stage (Redding et al., 1999). For example, most smokers know that smoking is bad for them and consider quitting, but are not quite ready to do so. The third stage is called **preparation** and combines intention and behavioral criteria. In this stage, "people intend to take action soon, usually measured as the next month. Typically, they have already taken some significant step toward the behavior in the past year. They have a plan of action, such as joining a health education class, consulting a counselor, talking to their physician, buying a self-help book, or relying on a self-change approach" (Prochaska et al., 2008, p. 100). "These are the people we should recruit for such action-oriented programs as smoking cessation, weight loss, or exercise" (Prochaska et al., 1998, p. 61).

People are in the fourth stage, the **action stage**, when they have made overt changes in their behavior, experiences, or environment in order to overcome their problems within the past six months. This stage of change reflects a consistent behavior pattern, is usually the most visible, and receives the greatest external recognition (Prochaska, DiClemente, & Norcross, 1992). Since the behavior change is very new in this stage and the chance of relapse is high, considerable attention still must be given to relapse prevention (Redding et al., 1999). Also, "not all modifications of behavior count as action in this model. People must attain a criterion that scientists and professionals agree is sufficient to reduce risks of disease" (Prochaska et al., 2008, p. 102). For example, in smoking, reduction in the number of cigarettes smoked does not count, only total abstinence (Prochaska et al., 1998). If those making changes continue with their new pattern of behavior, they will move into the fifth stage, maintenance.

Working to prevent relapse is the focus of the **maintenance stage**. People in this stage have made specific, overt modifications in then lifestyles for at least six months and are increasingly more confident that they can continue their changes (Prochaska et al., 2008; Prochaska et al., 1998; Redding et al., 1999). The person's change has become more of a habit and the chance of relapse is lower, but it still requires some attention (Redding et al., 1999).

The final stage is **termination**. This stage is defined as the time when individuals who have changed have zero temptation to return to their old behavior and they have 100% self-efficacy—that is, a lifetime of maintenance. No matter what their mood, they will not return to their old behavior (Prochaska et al., 2008). This is a stage that few people reach with certain behaviors (e.g., drinking for alcoholics). Since this may not be a practical goal for the majority of people, it has been given less attention in the research (Prochaska et al., 2008). **Figure 7.6** provides a summary of the stages of change.

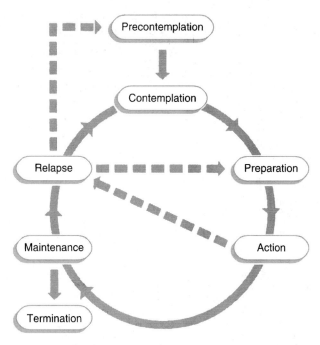

▲ **Figure 7.6** The Stages of Change

Source: *Models for Provider-Patient Interaction: Applications to Health Behavior Change.* M. G. Goldstein from The Handbook of Health Behavior Change by Shumaker, Sally Reproduced with permission of SPRINGER PUBLISHING COMPANY, INCORPORATED via Copyright Clearance Center.

The second major construct of the TTM is the **processes of change** (see Table 7.3 for an explanation of the 10 processes). "These are the covert and overt activities that people use to progress through the stages" (Prochaska et al., 2008, p. 101). Studies over the years have indicated that some of the processes are more useful at specific stages of change. The experimental set of processes (consciousness raising, dramatic relief, self-reevaluation, environmental reevaluation, and social liberation) are most often emphasized in earlier stages (precontemplation, contemplation, and preparation) to increase intention and motivation, whereas the behavioral set of processes (helping relationships, counterconditioning, reinforcement management, stimulus control, and self-liberation) are most often utilized in the later stages (preparation, action, maintenance) as observable behavior change efforts get underway and need to be maintained (Redding et al., 1999) (see **Table 7.4**).

The construct of **decisional balance** refers to the pros and cons of the behavioral change. That is, individuals' decisions to move from one stage to the next are based on the relative importance (pro), or the lack thereof (con), of the behavior change for the individuals. "Characteristically, the pros of healthy behavior are low in the early stages and increase across the stages of change, and the cons of the healthy behavior are high in the early stages and decrease across the stages of change" (Redding et al., 1999, p. 90).

The fourth construct of the TTM is **self-efficacy**. The developers of this model see self-efficacy as it was defined by Bandura (1977), as people's confidence in their ability to perform a certain behavior or task. The final construct of the TTM is temptation. **Temptation** "reflects the converse of self-efficacy—the intensity of urges to engage in a specific behavior when in

TABLE 7.4 **Progressing Through the Stages of the Transtheoretical Model**

		Stage Transitions			
		Precontemplation to Contemplation	Contemplation to Preparation	Preparation to Action	Action to Maintenance
Processes	Consciousness raising	X			
	Dramatic relief	X			
	Environmental reevaluation	X			
	Self-reevaluation		X		
	Self-liberation			X	
	Counterconditioning				X
	Helping relationships				X
	Reinforcement management				X
	Stimulus control				X

Source: Based on "The Transtheoretical Model and Stages of Change." J. O. Prochaska, C. A. Redding, K. E. Evers, in *Health Behavior and Health Education: Theory, Research, and Practice.* K. Glanz, B. K. Rimer, and K. Viswanath (eds.). Copyright © 2008 by Jossey-Bass.

difficult situations. Typically, three factors reflect the most common types of temptations: negative affect or emotional distress, positive social situations, and craving" (Prochaska et al., 2008, p. 102). As one might guess, temptation decreases as one moves through the stages; however, even in the maintenance stage temptation is still present.

As noted at the beginning of this discussion, the TTM not only includes the five core constructs but it is also based on five critical assumptions (Prochaska et al., 2008):

1. No single theory can account for all the complexities of behavior change. A more comprehensive model will most likely emerge from an integration across major theories.

2. Behavior change is a process that unfolds over time through a sequence of stages.

3. Stages are both stable and open to change just as chronic behavioral risk factors are stable and open to change.

4. The majority of at-risk populations are not prepared for action and will not be served by traditional action-oriented behavior change programs.

5. Specific processes and principles of change should be emphasized at specific stages to maximize efficacy (p. 103).

Since its development, the TTM has been useful in several different ways. The first is that it makes program planners aware that not everyone is ready for change "right now," even though there is a program that can help them modify their behavior. People proceed through behavior change at different paces. Second, if individuals are not ready for action right now, then other programs can be developed to help them become ready for action. **Box 7.3** provides an example how to "stage" a person with a series of TTM type questions. With such information, planners can match a person's stage to a specific intervention, which in turn can increase the chances that the intervention will have an effect.

BOX

7.3

Application

An Example of Using Questions Based on the Transtheoretical Model to "Stage" a Person

1. Do you eat at least five servings of fruits and vegetables each day?
   Yes—Move to question #2
   No—Skip to question #3
2. Have you been doing so for more than six months?
   Yes—Maintenance stage
   No—Action stage
3. Do you intend to in the next 30 days?
   Yes—Preparation stage
   No—Move to question #4
4. Do you intend to in the next six months?
   Yes—Contemplation stage
   No—Precontemplation stage

PRECAUTION ADOPTION PROCESS MODEL (PAPM)

The *precaution adoption process model* (PAPM) is more recent than the TTM (Weinstein, 1988; Weinstein & Sandman, 1992) and is based on decision theory (Simons-Morton et al., 2012). Its goal "is to explain how a person comes to the decision to take action, and how he or she translates that decision into action" (Weinstein et al., 2008, p. 126). Though the TTM and PAPM are both stage models and appear similar, "it is mainly the names that have been given to the stages that are similar. The number of stages is not the same in the two theories, and those with similar names are defined quite differently" (Weinstein & Sandman, 2002a, p. 125). The PAPM is most applicable for use with the adoption of a new precaution (e.g., getting an immunization), or the abandonment of a risky behavior (e.g., not using a safety belt or not wearing a motorcycle helmet) that requires a deliberate action. It can also be used to explain why and how people make deliberate changes in habitual patterns. It is not applicable for actions that require the gradual development of habitual patterns of behavior such as exercise and diet (Weinstein et al., 2008). It is also different from the TTM in that its stages are defined without reference to arbitrary time periods (Sutton, n.d.).

The PAPM includes seven stages along the full path from ignorance about a specific behavior to taking action to engaging in the behavior.

> At some initial point in time, people are unaware of the health issue (Stage 1) [Unaware]. When they first learn something about the issue, they are no longer unaware, but they are not yet engaged by it either (Stage 2) [Unengaged]. People who reach the decision-making stage (Stage 3) [Deciding about acting] have become engaged by the issue and are considering their response. This decision-making process can result in one of three outcomes: they may suspend judgment, remaining in Stage 3 for the moment; they may decide to take no action, moving to Stage 4 [Decide not to act] and halting the precaution adoption process, at least for the time being; or they may decide to adopt the precaution, moving to Stage 5 [Decide to act]. For those who decide to adopt the precaution, the next step is to initiate the behavior (Stage 6) [Acting]. A seventh stage, if relevant, indicates that the behavior has been maintained over time (Stage 7)

[Maintenance]. (Weinstein et al., 2008, p. 126; note: names of the stages were inserted by McKenzie, Neiger, & Thackeray.)

Figure 7.7 provides an example of the application of the PAPM to deciding whether or not to get the shingles vaccine. You will note in this example that Stage 7 is not applicable because only a single dose of the shingles vaccine is needed. However, if the flu vaccine was used as the example Stage 7 would read "Get the flu vaccine once a year, usually starting in September." As with the TTM, the usefulness of this model is its ability to identify various stages of the behavior change process (see **Box 7.4**). Once it is known what stage the program participants are in, then the program planners can develop a stage-specific intervention to move the participants toward action. **Table 7.5** presents the important issues that need to be addressed to move participants from one stage to the next.

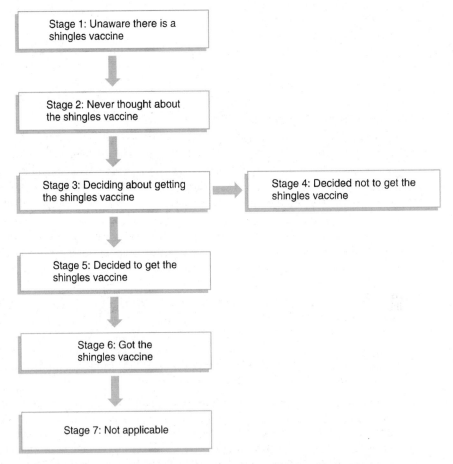

▲ **Figure 7.7** Application of the Precaution Adoption Process Model to shingles vaccine

An Example of Using a Question Based on the Precaution Adoption Process Model to "Stage" a Person

What are your intentions for receiving the new vaccine for shingles?

- I have already gotten it. (Stage 6)
- I have decided to get it. (Stage 5)
- I have thought about it and decided not to get it. (Stage 4)
- I am not sure. I am still trying to decide whether to get it or not. (Stage 3)
- I heard there was a vaccine, but I really haven't thought much about it. (Stage 2)
- I was not aware there was a vaccine for shingles. (Stage 1)

TABLE 7.5 **Progressing Through the Stages of the Precaution Adoption Process Model**

		Stage Transitions			
		Stage 1: (Unaware of issue) to Stage 2: (Unengaged by issue)	Stage 2: (Unengaged by issue) to Stage 3: (Deciding to act)	Stage 3: (Deciding to act) to Stage 4: (Decided not to act) or to Stage 5: (Decided to act)	Stage 5: (Decided to act) to Stage 6: (Acting)
Important Information for Stage-Specific Interventions	Information about hazard and precaution	X	X		
	Communication with significant other about hazard and precaution		X		
	Previous experience with hazard		X		
	Beliefs about hazard likelihood, severity and personal susceptibility			X	
	Perceived social norms and behaviors and recommendations of others			X	
	Personal fear and worry			X	
	Time, effort, and resources (including assistance) to act				X
	"How to" information and cues to action				X

Source: Based on *Health Behavior and Health Education: Theory, Research, and Practice*, by Karen Glanz, Barbara K. Rimer, and K. Viswanath. Copyright © 2008a by John Wiley & Sons, Inc.

Interpersonal Level Theories

Health behavior theories that focus on the interpersonal level assume individuals exist within, and are influenced by, a social environment (i.e., the people with whom they interact). That is to say, that an individual's attitudes and behaviors will be influenced by the actions, opinions, thoughts, attitudes, behavior, advice, and support of others. Further, an individual has a reciprocal effect on those people who make up their social environment (Rimer & Glanz, 2005). The individuals who have the greatest influence on others include spouse/partner, other family members, friends, peers (i.e., fellow students and coworkers), fellow members of social groups, health care providers, religious leaders, and others (Rimer & Glanz, 2005).

Although social relationships can have an impact on many different human behaviors, research has shown that they can be a powerful influence on health and health behaviors (Heaney & Israel, 2008). Therefore a number of theories have been created to explain concepts such as *social learning* (learning that occurs in a social context), *social power* (ability to influence others or resist activities of others), *social integration* (structure and quality of relationships), *social networks* ("web of social relationships and the structural characteristics of that web") (IOM, 2001, p. 7), *social support* ("aid and assistance exchanged through social relationships and interpersonal transactions" [Heaney & Israel, 2008, p. 191]), *social capital* ("relationships between community members including trust, reciprocity, and civic engagement" [Minkler, Wallerstein, & Wilson, 2008, p. 294]), and *interpersonal communication*. In the sections that follow, we present a detailed description of a well-established interpersonal theory—the social cognitive theory, and we present brief overviews of two newer theories—the social network theory and the social capital theory. These latter two theories may be theories in name only. Earlier in this chapter we made a distinction between theories and models. You may remember we said that there are some theories that have the term "model" in their title because that is the way they were initially identified and now that there is empirical evidence to call them theories the "model title" has remained because that is what we have gotten used to calling them. We believe that the social network and the social capital theories may have been prematurely called theories and are probably more in the model stage. But again as Goodson (2010) stated, "...it seems to matter little to us whether we deal with theories or with models; it seems to matter even less what labels we attach to them" (p. 228). Therefore, the important point of presenting the social network and social capital theories (or models) is to make you aware of the important concepts contained in each.

SOCIAL COGNITIVE THEORY (SCT)

The social learning theories (SLT) of Rotter (1954) and Bandura (1977)—or, as Bandura (1986) relabeled them, the *social cognitive theory (SCT)*—combine SR theory and cognitive theories. Stimulus response theorists emphasize the role of reinforcement in shaping behavior and believe that no "thinking" or "reasoning" is needed to explain behavior. However, Bandura (2001) stated, "If actions were performed only on behalf of anticipated external rewards and punishments, people would behave like weather vanes, constantly shifting directions to conform to whatever influence happened to impinge upon them at the moment" (p. 7). Cognitive theorists believe that reinforcement is an integral part of learning, but emphasize the role of subjective hypotheses or expectations held by the individual (Rosenstock et al., 1988). In other words, reinforcement contributes to learning, but reinforcement along with an individual's expectations of the consequences of behavior determine the behavior.

"Behavior, in this perspective, is a function of the subjective value of an outcome and the subjective probability (or 'expectation') that a particular action will achieve that outcome. Such formulations are generally termed 'value-expectancy' theories" (Rosenstock et al., 1988, p. 176). In brief, SCT explains human functioning in terms of triadic reciprocal causation (Bandura, 1986). "In this model of reciprocal causality, internal personal factors in the form of cognitive, affective, and biological events, behavioral patterns, and environmental influences all operate as interacting determinants that influence one another bidirectionally" (Bandura, 2001, pp. 14–15). The constructs of the SCT that have been most often used in designing health promotion interventions will be presented here.

As already noted, reinforcement is an important component of SCT. According to SCT, reinforcement can be accomplished in one of three ways: directly, vicariously, or through self-reinforcement (Baranowski, Perry, & Parcel, 2002). An example of **direct reinforcement** is a group facilitator who provides verbal feedback to participants for a job well done. **Vicarious reinforcement** is having the participants observe someone else being reinforced for behaving in an appropriate manner. This has been referred to as *observational learning* (Baranowski et al., 2002) or *social modeling*. In a system of reinforcement by **self-reinforcement**, the participants would keep records of their own behavior, and when the behavior was performed in an appropriate manner, they would reinforce or reward themselves.

If individuals are to perform specific behaviors, they must know first what the behaviors are and then how to perform them. This is referred to as **behavioral capability**. For example, if people are to engage in cardiovascular (i.e., "cardio") exercise, first they must know that cardiovascular exercise exists, and second they need to know how to do it properly. Many people begin exercise programs, only to quit within the first six months (Dishman, Sallis, & Orenstein, 1985), and some of those people quit because they do not know how to exercise properly. They know they should exercise, so they decide to run a few miles, have sore muscles the next day, and quit. Skill mastery is very important. The construct of **expectations** refers to the ability of human beings to think, and thus to anticipate certain things to happen in certain situations. For example, if people are enrolled in a weight loss program and follow the directions of the group facilitator, they will expect to lose weight. **Expectancies**, not to be confused with expectations, are the values that individuals place on an expected outcome. "Expectancies influence behavior according to the hedonic principle: if all other things are equal, a person will choose to perform an activity that maximizes a positive outcome or minimizes a negative outcome" (Baranowski et al., 2002, p. 173). Someone who enjoys the feeling of not smoking more than that of smoking is more likely to try to do the things necessary to stop. The construct of **self-regulation** or **self-control** states that individuals may gain control of their own behavior through monitoring and adjusting it (Clark et al., 1992). In writing about this construct, Bandura (1991) believed that self-regulation systems could have a big influence on behavior change. Later (Bandura, 1997) he expanded his thoughts about the construct and identified six methods for achieving self-regulation. They include (1) self-monitoring (i.e., self-observation) of one's behavior, (2) setting both incremental and long-term goals, (3) obtaining feedback on the quality of a behavior and how it can be improved, (4) rewarding self (or self-reinforcement) for meeting goals, (5) self-instructing both before and as the behavior is being performed, and (6) gaining social-support for the behavior. These six methods have been used extensively in health promotion programs. For example, when helping individuals to change their behavior (i.e., a goal of losing weight, quitting smoking, or exercising more), it is a common practice to have them monitor their behavior over a period of time, say through 24-hour diet or smoking records or exercise diaries, analyze their behavior based on data recorded, and then to have them reward (reinforce) themselves based on meeting their goals.

One construct of SCT that has received special attention in health promotion programs is self-efficacy (Strecher et al., 1986), which refers to the internal state that individuals experience as "competence" to perform certain desired tasks or behavior, "including confidence in overcoming the barriers to performing that behavior" (Baranowski et al., 2002, p. 173). "Unless people believe they can produce desired results and forestall detrimental ones by their actions, they have little incentive to act or to persevere in the face of difficulties" (Bandura, 2001, p. 10). Self-efficacy is situation specific; that is, individuals may be self-efficacious when it comes to regular exercise but not so when faced with reducing the amount of fat in their diet. People's competency feelings have been referred to as **efficacy expectations**. Thus, people who think they can exercise on a regular basis no matter what the circumstances have efficacy expectations. Even though people have efficacy expectations, they still may not want to engage in a behavior because they may not think the outcomes of that behavior would be beneficial to them. Stated another way, they may not feel that the reward (reinforcement) of performing the behavior is great enough for them. These beliefs are called **outcome expectations**. For example, in order for individuals to quit smoking for health reasons (behavior), they must believe both that they are capable of quitting (efficacy expectation) and that cessation will benefit their health (outcome expectation) (I. M. Rosenstock, personal communication, April 1986).

Individuals become self-efficacious in four main ways:

1. Through performance attainments (personal mastery of a task)
2. Through vicarious experience (observing the performance of others)
3. As a result of verbal persuasion (receiving suggestions from others)
4. Through emotional arousal (interpreting one's emotional state)

Not only can individuals be self-efficacious, so can groups of people. The term given to groups or organizations being efficacious is *collective efficacy*. **Collective efficacy** has been defined as the people's shared belief in their collective ability to act to produce specific changes. Like self-efficacy, collective efficacy is situation specific. It is a construct that has application when people seek to alter social systems (e.g., neighborhood watches and community organizing (see Chapter 9), but also has application in health promotion with regards to health policy (McAlister et al., 2008). Bandura (1982, p. 143) noted that "[p]erceived collective efficacy will influence what people choose to do as a group, how much effort they put into it, and their staying power when group efforts fail to produce results."

The construct of **emotional–coping response** states that for people to learn, they must be able to deal with the sources of anxiety that may surround a behavior. For example, fear is an emotion that can be involved in learning; according to this construct, participants would have to deal with the fear before they could learn the behavior.

The construct of **reciprocal determinism** states, unlike SR theory, that there is an interaction among the person, the behavior, and the environment, and that the person can shape the environment as well as the environment shape the person. All these relationships are dynamic. Glanz and Rimer (1995) provide a good example of this construct:

> A man with high cholesterol might have a hard time following his prescribed low-fat diet because his company cafeteria doesn't offer low-fat food choices that he likes. He can try to

change the environment by talking with the cafeteria manager or the company medical or health department staff, and asking that healthy food choices be added to the menu. Or, if employees start to dine elsewhere in order to eat low-fat lunches, the cafeteria may change its menu to maintain its lunch business (p. 15).

Finally, there is one other construct that grew out of the social learning theory of Rotter (1954) that needs to be mentioned because of its association with health behavior. "Rotter posited that a person's history of positive or negative reinforcement across a variety of situations shapes a belief as to whether or not a person's own actions lead to those reinforcements" (Wallston, 1994, p. 187). Rotter referred to this construct as **locus of control**. He felt that people with internal locus of control perceived that reinforcement was under their control, whereas those with external locus of control perceived reinforcement to be under the control of some external force. In the 1970s, Wallston and his colleagues at Vanderbilt University began testing the usefulness of this construct in predicting health behavior (Wallston, 1994). They explored the concept of whether individuals with internal locus of control were more likely to participate in health-enhancing behavior than those with external locus of control. They began their work by examining locus of control as a two-dimensional construct (internal versus external), then moved to a multidimensional construct (i.e., Multidimensional Health Locus of Control [MHLC]) when they split the external dimension into "powerful others" and "chance" (Wallston, Wallston, & DeVellis, 1978). Since developing the MHLC scale, a health/medical condition specific scale (Wallston, Stein, & Smith, 1994) and a religion and health scale (Wallston, 2007) for locus of control have been created. (Note: All scales are in the public domain and available from Wallston, 2007).

After a number of years of work by many different researchers, Wallston has come to the conclusion that locus of control accounts for only a small amount of the variability in health behavior (Wallston, 1992). The internal locus of control belief about one's own health status is a necessary but not sufficient determinate of health-enhancing behavior (Wallston, 1994). Since the rise of the construct of self-efficacy, Wallston (1994) feels that self-efficacy is a better predictor of health-promoting behavior than locus of control. This is not to say that locus of control is not a useful construct in developing health promotion programs. Knowing the locus of control orientation of those in the priority population can provide planners with valuable information when considering social support as part of a planned intervention. **Table 7.6** provides a summary of the constructs of the SCT and an example of how each construct might be operationalized.

SOCIAL NETWORK THEORY (SNT)

The term **social network** ("web of social relationships that surround people and the structural characteristics of that web" [IOM, 2001, p. 7]) arose in the 1950s from the work of a sociologist who studied Norwegian villages. Barnes (1954) created the term to describe social relationships and characteristics of the villagers that could not be described through traditional social units such as families (Edberg, 2015; Heaney & Israel, 2008). Since that time, the concept has continued to be used and studied by sociologists and professionals in various other disciplines including health education/health promotion. One primary reason for the growth in its use in recent years is that researchers have become dissatisfied with many of the other theories presented in this chapter. "For example, theories that show attitudes toward a behavior are associated with the behavior often do not help us to understand how to change those attitudes" (Valente, 2010, p. 7). To support the work of health education specialists

TABLE 7.6 **Often-Used Constructs of the Social Cognitive Theory and Examples of Their Application**

Construct	Definition	Example
Behavioral capability	Knowledge and skills necessary to perform a behavior.	If people are going to exercise aerobically, they need to know what it is and how to do it.
Expectations	Beliefs about the likely outcomes of certain behaviors.	If people enroll in a weight-loss program, they expect to lose weight.
Expectancies	Values people place on expected outcomes.	How important is it to people that they become physically fit?
Locus of control	Perception of the center of control over reinforcement.	Those who feel they have control over reinforcement are said to have internal locus of control. Those who perceive reinforcement under the control of an external force are said to have external locus of control.
Reciprocal determinism	"Environmental factors influence individuals and groups, but individuals and groups can also influence their environments and regulate their own behavior" (McAlister, Perry, & Parcel, 2008, p. 171).	Lack of use of vending machines could be a result of the choices within the machine. Notes about the selections from the nonusing consumers to the machine's owners could change the selections and change the behavior of the nonusing consumers to that of users.
Reinforcement (directly, vicariously, self-management)	Responses to behaviors that increase the chances of recurrence.	Giving verbal encouragement to those who have acted in a healthy manner.
Self-control, or self-regulation	Gaining control over one's own behavior through monitoring and adjusting it.	If clients want to change their eating habits, have them monitor their current habits for seven days.
Self-efficacy	People's confidence in their ability to perform a certain desired task or function	If people are going to engage in a regular exercise program, they must feel they can do it.
Collective efficacy	Beliefs about the ability of the group to perform concerted actions that bring desired outcomes (McAlister et al., 2008, p. 171).	If a group of people is going to work to change a community's culture toward healthy behavior, they must feel that they can do it.
Emotional-coping response	For people to learn, they must be able to deal with the sources of anxiety that surround a behavior.	Fear is an emotion that can be involved in learning, and people would have to deal with it before they could learn a behavior.

Source: *Principles and Foundations of Health Promotion and Education.* Randall R. Cottrell, James T. Girvan, James F. McKenzie, and Denise M. Seabert. Copyright © 2015 by Pearson Education. Reprinted with permission.

there is now evidence from social epidemiological observational studies that have clearly documented the beneficial effects of supportive networks on health status (Heaney & Israel, 2008; Valente, 2010). But is there enough evidence to suggest there is such a thing as a *social network theory* (SNT)? Heaney and Israel (2008) feel that the social network, and the closely related concept of social support, "do not connote theories per se. Rather, they are concepts that describe the structure, processes, and functions of social relationships" (p. 193). They feel that intervention studies are "needed to identify the most potent causal agents and critical time periods for social network enhancement" (p. 197). For example, it is not known how much social networking is enough to enhance health or how much is too much. It is also not known what are the characteristics of "good networks" that result in positive health behavior (e.g., regular exercise) versus "bad networks" that lead to negative health behavior (e.g., smoking). But what is known is that people who are part of social networks are as a whole healthier than those who are not involved in networks.

One person who has written about SNT is Edberg (2015). He has described different types of social networks (e.g., ego-centered networks and full relational networks) and indicated that the key components to SNT are the relationships between and among individuals and how the nature of those relationships influences beliefs and behaviors. He further states that those who use the SNT need to consider the items on the following list when assessing the role of a network on the health behavior of individuals who are part of the network (Edberg, 2015):

- Centrality versus marginality of individuals in the network—how much involvement does the person have in the network?
- Reciprocity of relationships—are relationships one-way or two-way?
- Complexity or intensity of relationships in the network—are the relationships between two people or are they multiplexed?
- Homogeneity or diversity of people in the network—do all members of the network have similar characteristics or are they different?
- Subgroups, cliques, and linkages—are there concentrations of interactions among some members and do they interact or are they isolated from others?
- Communication patterns in the network—how does information pass between the members in the network?

In summary, we know that social networks can impact health, but the specifics of who is most impacted and how best to set up and use social networks are unknown. Nevertheless, because of the impact of social networks, health education specialists planning interventions need to consider if social networks should be a part of the strategy they use to bring about change. And finally, with the power of the Internet and social networking, the impact of social networks in the work of health education specialists will to continue to grow.

SOCIAL CAPITAL THEORY

The often-quoted definition of **social capital** is "the relationships and structures within a community, such as civic participation, networks, norms of reciprocity, and trust, that promote cooperation of mutual benefit" (Putnam, 1995, p. 66). More recently, it has been defined as "the degree of social connectedness" (Simons-Morton et al., 2012, p. 410). "Social capital is a collective asset, a feature of communities rather than the property of individuals. As such, individuals both contribute to it and use it, but they cannot own it" (Warren, Thompson, & Saegert, 2001, p. 1). The term got its start in political science and has been used in the health education/promotion field since the mid-1990s. The influence of social capital is well documented (Crosby et al., 2009). There are epidemiological studies that show that greater social capital is linked to several different positive outcomes (i.e., reduced mortality, some access to health care). There are also correlational studies that show that lack of social capital is related to poorer health outcomes (e.g., Kawachi, Subramanian, & Kim, 2008). But as with social networks, a cause-effect relationship has not been established between social capital and better health. Social capital is an important descriptor of community wellness, but it is not a strategy and requires community organizing and capacity building in order to be strengthened (Minkler & Wallerstein, 2012).

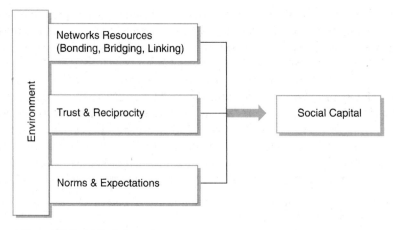

▲ **Figure 7.8** Social Capital
Source: Based on *Introduction to Health Behavior Theory*, by J. Hayden. Copyright © 2014 by Jones & Bartlett Learning.

Figure 7.8 provides a graphic representation of the social capital. This particular figure includes the key concepts of Putman's (1995) definition of social capital and three different types of network resources—bonding, bridging, and linking social capital. These three types are differentiated based on the strength of the relationships between/among those people in the social network (Hayden, 2014). Originally, *bonding social capital* (sometimes referred to as exclusive social capital) was defined as "the type that brings closer together people who already know each other" (Gittell & Vidal, 1998, p.15), but since then it has been expanded to encompass people who are similar or people who are members of the same group. Bonding social capital would come from those who are members in a service organization (e.g., Lions, Elks, American Legion) or religious community, for example. *Bridging social capital* (sometimes referred to as inclusive social capital), was originally defined as "the type that brings together people or groups who previously did not know each other" (Gittell & Vidal, 1998, p. 15), though now bridging social capital is seen more as the resources that people obtain from their interaction with people from outside their group, oftentimes from people with different demographic characteristics. An example would be people from different parts of a community working to create a community park.

The most recently recognized, and weakest, network resource is *linking social capital* (Hayden, 2014). In this type of network social capital comes from relationships between/among individuals with institutions and individuals who have relative power over them (Szreter & Woolcock, 2004). An example would be when a boss and an employee work together on a project.

Again, as with social networks it is important that health education specialists be aware of the concept of social capital when planning interventions. It is not an intervention in itself, but it is a concept that needs to be considered and monitored.

Community Level Theories

As noted earlier in this chapter, the community level theories include any theory that would apply to the last five levels of the ecological perspective—institutional, community, public policy, environmental, and culture. Community level theories "explore how social systems function and change and how to mobilize community members and organizations. They offer strategies that work in a variety of settings such as health care institutions, schools, worksites, community groups, and government agencies" (Rimer & Glanz, 2005, p. 22). Like the other levels already discussed in this chapter, a number of different community-level theories are available for health planners. Several community level theories involve community organizing and developing (see Chapter 9). The following section presents a discussion of two community level theories–- diffusion theory and the community readiness model.

DIFFUSSION THEORY

Diffusion theory (Rogers, 1962) provided an explanation for the spread of *innovations* (something new, such as a product, service, or program) in populations; stated another way, it provides an explanation for the pattern of adoption of the innovations. Like other processes discussed in this chapter, adoption is situation specific and it results from people going through a series of stages. Rogers (2003) outlined the following five stages: (1) knowledge (acquisition of about the innovation), (2) persuasion (i.e., attitude concerning the innovation); (3) decision (about adopting or not adopting); (4) implementation (beginning to use the innovation); and (5) confirmation (commitment to use, continue to use, or discontinue use of the innovation). If one thinks of a health promotion program as an innovation, the theory describes a pattern the priority population will follow in adopting the program.

The pattern of adoption can be represented by the normal bell-shaped curve (Rogers, 2003) (see **Table 7.7**). Those individuals who fall in the portion of the curve to the left of minus 2 standard deviations from the mean (this would be between 2% and 3% of the priority population) would probably become involved in the program just because they had heard about it and wanted to be first. These people are called **innovators**. They are venturesome, independent, and daring. They want to be the first to do things, although others in the social system may not respect them.

The second group of people to adopt something new includes those represented on the curve between minus 2 and minus 1 standard deviations. This group, which composes about 14% of the priority population, is called **early adopters**. These people are very interested in the innovation, but they are not the first to sign up. They wait until the innovators are already involved to make sure the innovation is useful. Early adopters are respected by others in the social system and looked upon as opinion leaders.

The next two groups are the **early majority** and the **late majority**. They fall between minus 1 standard deviation and the mean and between the mean and plus 1 standard

TABLE 7.7 **Diffusion of Innovations**

Group	% of Population	Place on a Bell-shaped Curve
Innovators	~2-3	Less than minus 2 standard deviations
Early Adopters	~14	Between minus 2 and minus 1 standard deviations
Early Majority	~34	Between minus 1 standard deviation and the mean
Late Majority	~34	Between the mean and plus 1 standard deviation
Laggards	~16	Greater than plus 1 standard deviation

deviation on the curve, respectively. Each of these groups comprises about 34% of the priority population. Those in the early majority may be interested in the health promotion program, but they will need external motivation to become involved. Those in the early majority will deliberate for some time before making a decision. It will take more work to get the late majority involved, because they are skeptical and will not adopt an innovation until most people in the social system have done so. Planners may be able to get them involved through a peer mentoring program, or through constant exposure about the innovation.

The last group, the **laggards** (16%), is represented by the part of the curve greater than plus 1 standard deviation. They are not very interested in innovation and would be the last to become involved in new health promotion programs, if at all. They are very traditional and are suspicious of innovations. Laggards tend to have limited communication networks, so they really do not know much about new things.

Because diffusion occurs over time, the cumulative prevalence of adopters at successive points can be represented by a S-shaped curve. At first, only a few people adopt (innovators). However, over time, the curve begins to climb as additional individuals decide to adopt the innovation (early adopters, early majority, and late majority). The curve then levels off as adoption of the innovation ceases, leaving a few who have not adopted (laggards) (Goldman, 1998; Rogers, 2003).

One of the more useful application of the diffusion theory is when marketing a health promotion program because "the distinguishing characteristics of the people who fall into each category of adopters from 'innovators' to 'early adopters' to middle majority categories to 'late adopters' [laggards] tend to be consistent across a wide range of innovations" (Green, 1989). Therefore, different marketing techniques can be used depending on the type of people the planners are trying to reach with a program. For example, program planners want rapid diffusion of innovations. They know that although innovators will adopt the program or product first, the key subgroups of the priority population are the early adopters and early majority. It is especially important to identify the early adopters (opinion leaders) as soon as possible in the implementation process since, according to diffusion theory, the sooner they adopt the innovation the sooner the rest of the population will follow. The challenge is how to identify and reach the early adopters.

The diffusion of innovations theory has been applied to many different types of health promotion programs. One of the more interesting uses of diffusion theory has been to "conceptualize the transference of health promotion programs from one locale to another" (Steckler, Goodman et al., 1992). Steckler, Goodman, and colleagues (1992) developed a series of six questionnaires to measure the extent to which health promotion programs are successfully disseminated. Planners should refer to this work if they are interested in using and measuring diffusion.

COMMUNITY READINESS MODEL (CRM)

Community readiness "is the degree to which a community is willing and prepared to take action on an issue" (Tri-Ethnic Center for Prevention Research at Colorado State University, 2014, p. 4). Like with individuals, communities are in different levels of readiness for change. The community readiness model (CRM) is a stage theory for communities. The concept of community readiness got its start back in the early 1990s, growing out of the need to understand the problems associated with developing and maintaining community programs. (See Edwards, Jumper-Thurman, Plested, Oetting, & Swanson, 2000, for a description of the origin of the CRM.) What was evident from the beginning is that few communities were alike. They may have had similar problems, but the dynamics in each community did not mean that the starting point for dealing with the problem could be the same. "Communities are fluid—always changing, adapting, growing" (Edwards et al., 2000, p. 291), and like individuals, communities are in various stages of readiness for change. Yet, the stages of change for communities are not the same as for individuals. "The stages of readiness in a community have to deal with group processes and group organization, characteristics that are not relevant to personal readiness" (Edwards et al., 2000, p. 296–297). Though the model was developed initially to deal with alcohol and drug abuse, it has been useful in helping with a variety of health and nutrition topics (e.g., AIDS awareness, elimination of heart disease, depression awareness, reduction of sexually transmitted diseases), environmentally centered programs (e.g., air quality and recycling), and social programs (e.g., intimate partner violence programs) (Edwards et al., 2000).

The CRM defines nine stages:

1. *No Awareness.* The problem is not generally recognized by the people in the community or the leaders of the community.

2. *Denial.* There is little or no recognition in the community that there is a problem; if so, the feeling is nothing can be done about it.

3. *Vague Awareness.* Feeling among some in the community that there is a problem and something should be done, but no motivation or leadership to do so.

4. *Preplanning.* The clear recognition by some that there is a problem and something should be done. There are leaders for action, but no focused or detailed planning.

5. *Preparation.* There is planning going on but it is not based on collected data. There is leadership, resources are being sought, and there is modest support for efforts.

6. *Initiation.* Information is available to justify and begin efforts. Staff is in, or has just completed, training. Leaders are enthusiastic and there is usually little resistance and involvement from the community members.

7. *Stabilization.* Program is running, staffed, and supported by community and decision makers. Program is perceived as stable with no need for change. May include routine tracking, but no in-depth evaluation.

8. *Confirmation/Expansion.* Standard efforts are in place and supported by the community and decision makers. Program has been evaluated and modified, and efforts are in place to seek resources for new efforts. Data are collected on an ongoing basis to link risk factors and problems.

9. *Professionalism.* Much is known about prevalence, risk factors, and cause of problems. Highly trained staff runs effective programs, aimed at general population and appropriate subgroups. Programs have been evaluated and modified. Community is supportive but should hold programs accountable (Edwards et al., 2000).

A community's readiness for addressing an issue can be assessed through a process in which interviews are conducted and scored with key informants. The interviews are based on five key dimensions of community readiness (i.e., community knowledge of efforts, leadership, community climate, community knowledge of the issue, and resources). Once the stage of readiness is known, like the other stage theories, there are suggested processes for moving

TABLE 7.8 **Community Readiness Stages and Goals**

Stage	Goal
1. *No awareness*	Raise awareness of the issue
2. *Denial*	Raise awareness that the problem or issue exists in the community
3. *Vague awareness*	Raise awareness that the community can do something
4. *Preplanning*	Raise awareness with the concrete ideas to combat condition
5. *Preparation*	Gather existing information to help plan strategies
6. *Initiation*	Provide community-specific information
7. *Stabilization*	Stabilize efforts/programs
8. *Confirmation/expansion*	Expand and enhance service
9. *Professionalism*	Maintain momentum and continue growth

Source: "Community readiness: Research to practice." Ruth W. Edwards, Pamela Jumper-Thurman, Barbara A. Plested, Eugene R. Oetting, Louis Swanson, in *Journal of Community Psychology 28*(3). Copyright © 2000 by John Wiley & Sons, Inc.

a community from one stage to the next. **Table 7.8** presents the nine stages and the goal for each stage. A handbook for using this model has been created and is available from the Tri-Ethnic Center for Prevention Research at Colorado State University (2014).

▷ Cognitive-Behavioral Model of the Relapse Process

For most people, relapse is a part of change. **Relapse** "refers to the breakdown or failure in a person's attempt to change or modify a particular habit pattern, such as stopping 'bad habits' or developing new, optimal health behaviors" (Marlatt & George, 1998, p. 33). Marlatt and George (1998) differentiate between relapse (an indication of total failure) and a **lapse** (a single slip or mistake). The first drink or cigarette following a period of abstinence would be considered a lapse. It has been said that getting people to change behavior is hard, but having them maintain the behavior is much harder. This is nicely illustrated by the old saying, "Giving up smoking is easy; I've done it a hundred times." At one time, it was enough for program planners just to get people to change their behavior; now they need to do more. Because of the difficulty of maintaining a new behavior, program planners need to give special attention to helping those in the priority population avoid slipping back to their previous behaviors.

Although much of the early research dealing with this concept of slipping back was conducted using addictive behaviors, such as substance abuse and gambling, the concept applies to all behavior change, including preventive health behaviors. Marlatt (1982) indicates that a high percentage of individuals who enter programs for health behavior change relapse to their former behaviors within one year. More specifically, researchers have warned program planners of **recidivism** problems with participants in exercise and diet (Gaesser, Angadi, & Sawyer, 2011), oral health care treatment (McCaul et al., 1990), weight loss (Grattan, & Connolly-Schoonen, 2012), and smoking cessation (Leventhal & Cleary, 1980) programs. Therefore, planners need to make sure that program interventions include the skills necessary for dealing with those difficult times during behavior change.

Marlatt (1982) refers to the process of trying to prevent slipping back as relapse prevention. Relapse prevention, which is based on the social cognitive theory, combines behavioral skill-training procedures, cognitive therapy, and lifestyle rebalancing (Marlatt & George, 1998). **Relapse prevention (RP)** is "a self-control program designed to help individuals to anticipate and cope with the problem of relapse in the habit-changing process" (Marlatt & George, 1998, p. 33). Relapse is triggered by *high-risk situations*. "A high-risk situation is defined broadly as any situation (including emotional reactions to the situation) that poses a threat to the individual's sense of control and increases the risk of potential relapse" (Marlatt & George, 1998, p. 38). Cummings, Gordon, and Marlatt (1980), in a study of clients with a variety of problem behaviors (e.g., drinking, smoking, heroin addiction, gambling, and overeating), found high-risk situations tend to fall into two major categories: intrapersonal and interpersonal determinants. They found that 56% of the relapse situations were caused by intrapersonal determinants, such as negative emotional states (35%), negative physical states (3%), positive emotional states (4%), testing personal control (5%), and urges and temptations (9%). The 44% of the situations represented by interpersonal determinants included interpersonal conflicts (16%), social pressure (20%), and positive emotional states (8%). These determinants can be referred to as the *covert antecedents* of relapse. That is to say, these high-risk situations do not just happen; instead, they are created by what Marlatt (1982) calls *lifestyle imbalances*.

People who have the coping skills to deal with a high-risk situation have a much greater chance of preventing relapse than those who do not. Marlatt has developed both global and specific self-control strategies for relapse intervention. Specific intervention procedures are designed to help participants anticipate and cope with the relapse episode itself, whereas the global intervention procedures are designed to modify the early antecedents of relapse, including restructuring of the participant's general style of life. A complete application of the relapse prevention model would include both specific and global interventions (Marlatt, 1982).

▷ Limitations of Theory

The major foci of this chapter have been to present an overview and the major constructs of the theories that are commonly used to design interventions for health promotion programs. Although all the theories presented have been found to be useful in certain situations and settings, no one theory has been shown to be useful in all situations and settings. In fact, each of the theories presented has its limitations. For example, the SR theory focuses on consequences (i.e., reinforcement or punishment) that result from behaviors acting on the environment. These consequences either increase or decrease the probability of the behavior being repeated but they do not take into consideration that thinking and reasoning also impact behavior. The value-expectancy theories presented in this chapter (i.e., TPB, HBM, PMT) focus on cognitive variables but fail to suggest that change takes place over time in stages. Yet the stage theories have been criticized because a number of psychologists feel that behavior is much more complex and that behavior change cannot be neatly placed within a stage. Several different author groups have reviewed the various theories and identified their weaknesses. Three sources (Angus et al., 2013; Boston University School of Public Health, 2013; Munro, Lewin, Swart, & Volmink, 2007) present limitations of many of the theories presented in this chapter. If you are interested in limitations of other theories not noted in these sources or are interested in other view points about limitations of a theory simply type the words "limitations of" and add the name of the theory into a Internet search engine and a number of sources will appear.

Summary

Many theories are available to program planners, and it is important to remember that no one theory is best. This chapter presented an overview of the theories that are most often used in health promotion programs. These theories are important for planners because they provide information about why people are, or are not, engaging in health-enhancing behaviors; what factors to consider when creating interventions; and what factors to look for when evaluating a program. Theories can be categorized in a number of ways. This chapter presents two categories. The first categorizes theories by the level of influence at which it is most effective; the second classifies theories as either the continuum or stage theories. Finally, a brief explanation is provided about the limitations of theory.

Review Questions

1. Define *theory*, using your own words.
2. How is a theory different from a model?
3. How do concepts, constructs, and variables relate to theories?
4. Why is it important to use theories when planning and evaluating health promotion programs?
5. How can the socio-ecological approach be used to select a theory for use?
6. What makes stage theories different from continuum theories?
7. What is the underlying concept for each of the following theories?
   a. Stimulus response theory
   b. Social cognitive theory
   c. Theory of planned behavior
   d. Health belief model
   e. Protection motivation theory
   f. Elaboration likelihood model of persuasion
   g. Information-motivation-behavioral skills model
   h. Transtheoretical model
   i. Precaution adoption process model
   j. Social network theory
   k. Social capital theory
   l. Diffusion of innovations
   m. Community readiness model
8. What is the major difference between the transtheoretical model and the precaution adoption process model?

9. How is the community readiness model different from the other stage models?

10. How can program planners help to prepare those in the priority population for relapse prevention?

Activities

1. Assume that you have identified a prioritized need for a given priority population. In a two-page paper:

   a. State who the priority population is and what the need is.

   b. Select a theory to use as a guide in developing an intervention to address the problem.

   c. Explain why you chose the theory that you did.

   d. Defend why you think this is the best theory to use.

   e. Show how the problem "fits into" the theory.

2. In a two-page paper, identify a theory that you plan to use in developing the intervention for the program you are planning. Explain why you chose the theory, and why you think it is a good fit for the problem you are addressing.

3. Write a paragraph on each of the following:

   a. Using the stimulus response theory, explain why a person might smoke.

   b. Using the social cognitive theory (SCT), explain how you could help people change their diets.

   c. Explain how the SCT construct of behavioral capability applies to managing stress.

   d. Explain the differences between, and the relationship of, the SCT constructs of expectations and expectancies.

   e. Explain what would have to take place for individuals to be self-efficacious with regard to taking their insulin.

   f. Use the information-motivation-behavioral skills model to explain how to encourage a person to eat a healthy diet.

   g. Use the theory of planned behavior to explain how a smoker stops smoking.

   h. Use protection motivation theory to explain how you could create a public service announcement to encourage people to exercise.

   i. Apply the health belief model to getting a person to get a flu shot.

   j. Apply the transtheoretical model to get a person to change any health behavior.

   k. Using the precaution adoption process model, explain how a person decides to get screened for blood cholesterol.

   l. Explain how a social network could be used to encourage people to adopt a healthy behavior.

   m. Explain how you might increase the social capital of a community.

   n. Explain who and when those in a priority population may join a new exercise program.

   o. Explain how the community readiness model could be used by planners who are interested in getting a citywide smoking ordinance passed.

4. Your supervisor at the local health department has asked you to create a new program to encourage people in your county to get the influenza vaccine. After conducting a needs assessment it was found that the priority population for the program would be senior

citizens who to seem lack enabling factors for getting vaccinated. Which theory/model do you feel would be the best to use as the foundation for the intervention you will create? Write a brief rationale defending your choice.

5. You have been asked to create a brief education program to prepare outpatients for a screening colonoscopy for the gastroenterology department at the hospital where you work. The request was made because feedback from a significant number of patients who received the screening last year indicated that they wished they would have known what to expect in advance. Which theory/model do you feel would be the best to use to plan the education program around? Write a brief rationale defending your choice.

6. After tallying the results of an employee satisfaction survey, the director of the human resources (HR) department in the company where you work wants to begin an incentive program to encourage more people to participate in the employee health promotion program. The HR director would like you to create the incentive-based intervention for the program. Which theory/model do you feel would be the best to use to create the incentive-based intervention? Write a brief rationale defending your choice.

 # Weblinks

1. **http://web.uri.edu/cprc/about-ttm/**

   Cancer Prevention Resource Center (CPRC), University of Rhode Island

   CPRC is the home of the Transtheoretical Model. At this Website, you can obtain information about the model, as well as measures that can be used to "stage" a person.

2. **http://www.cdc.gov/ViolencePrevention/overview/social-ecologicalmodel.html**

   National Center for Injury Prevention and Control, Division of Violence Prevention, Centers for Disease Control and Prevention

   This Website provides an application of the socio-ecological approach to violence prevention.

3. **http://sbccimplementationkits.org/demandrmnch/ikitresources**
   /theory-at-a-glance-a-guide-for-health-promotion-practice-second-edition/

   Health Communication Capacity Collaborative National Cancer Institute (NCI)

   At this Website you will be able to download a copy of the National Cancer Institute's publication *Theory at a Glance: A Guide for Health Promotion Practice.* This volume presents a single, concise summary of health behavior theories that is both easy to read and practical.

4. **http://people.umass.edu/aizen/tpb.html**

   Theory of Planned Behavior

   This is part of the Website of Dr. Icek Ajzen, creator of the theory of planned behavior. The site provides great detail about the theory, as well as sample questionnaires to show how data can be collected using this theory.

5. **http://cancercontrol.cancer.gov/brp/constructs/index.html**

   Cancer Control and Population Sciences, National Cancer Institute (NCI)

   This page at the NCI's Cancer Control and Population Sciences Website presents definitions, background information, references, published examples, and information about the best measures of a number of theoretical constructs used in health promotion practice and research.

Interventions

Chapter Objectives

After reading this chapter and answering the questions at the end, you should be able to:

- Define the word *intervention* and apply it to a health promotion setting.

- Provide a rationale for selecting an intervention strategy.

- Explain the advantages of using a combination of several intervention strategies rather than a single intervention strategy.

- List and explain the different categories of intervention strategies.

- Briefly explain motivational interviewing.

- Explain the terms *curriculum, scope, sequence, units of study, lessons, lesson plans, health advocacy, health literacy,* and *health numeracy*.

- Briefly explain the modified framework for instructional design.

- Explain how behavioral economics might shape incentives.

- Explain the difference between adopting and adapting an evidence-based intervention.

- Describe how to adapt an evidence-based intervention.

- Create a new intervention for a health promotion program.

Key Terms

behavioral economics	health communication
best experience	health literacy
best practices	health numeracy
best processes	incentive
built environment	intervention
communication	lessons
channel	lesson plan
community advocacy	literacy
community building	motivational
community	interviewing
organization	multiplicity
contest	numeracy
contingencies	penetration rate
contract	scope
cultural audit	segmenting
culturally sensitive	sequence
curriculum	social media
disincentives	strategy
dose	tailoring
GINA	unit plans
health advocacy	

Once the goals and objectives have been developed, planners need to decide on the most appropriate means of reaching or attaining those goals and objectives. The planners must adopt, adapt, or design an activity or set of activities that would permit the most *effective* (leads to desired outcome) and *efficient* (uses resources in a responsible manner) achievement of the outcomes stated in the goals and objectives. These planned activities make up the *intervention*, or what some refer to as *treatment*. When applied to the planning of health promotion programs, an **intervention** can be defined as the planned actions that are designed to prevent disease or injury or promote health in the priority population. For example, let's say that you want the employees of Company S to increase their use of safety belts while riding in company-owned vehicles. You can measure their safety belt use before doing anything else, by observing them driving out of the motor pool. This would be a pre-program measure. Then you can intervene in a variety of ways. For example, you could provide an incentive by stating that all employees seen wearing their safety belts would receive a $10 bonus in their next paycheck. Or you could put in each employee's pay envelope a pamphlet on the importance of wearing safety belts. You could institute a company policy requiring all employees to wear safety belts while driving company-owned vehicles. Each of these activities for getting employees to increase their use of safety belts would be considered part of an intervention. After the intervention, you would complete a post-program measurement of safety belt use to determine the success of the program. In the case of the example just given, health education specialists could use an incentive by itself and call it an intervention, or they could use an incentive, pamphlets, and a company policy all at the same time to increase safety belt use and refer to the combination as an intervention.

The above discussion about the number of activities that make up an intervention in part speaks to the *size* of an intervention. Two terms that relate to the size of an intervention are *multiplicity* and *dose*. **Multiplicity** refers to the number of components or activities that make up the intervention. We have known for a number of years (Erfurt et al., 1990; Kline & Huff, 1999; Shea & Basch, 1990) that interventions that include several activities are more likely to have an effect on the priority population than are those that consist of a single activity. What has become more apparent in recent years is that these intervention activities are more likely to be effective if they are aimed at multiple levels of influence that affect individuals' and populations' behaviors and health status (Glanz & Bishop, 2010). In other words, they have a greater chance of being successful if they use a socio-ecological approach. Some refer to this as a *systems approach*. Few people change their behavior based on a single exposure; instead, multiple exposures are generally needed to change most behaviors. It stands to reason that "hitting" the priority population at multiple levels or through multiple means should increase the chances of making an impact. Although research has shown that using several activities is better than one, it has not identified an exact number of activities or a specific combination of activities that will ensure the most effective results (Kline & Huff, 1999). The right combination of activities will depend on the needs of those in the priority population and the specific planning situation.

When speaking about the **dose** of an intervention, we are referring to the number of program units delivered. For example, say that it was decided that the intervention for a skin cancer program would consist of multiple activities (*multiplicity*) and those activities would include an educational class for the public, distribution of text messages to those at high risk, and radio and television public service announcements (PSAs). The dose questions related to these activities would be: How many times would the class be offered? How many text messages would be distributed? And, how many times would the PSAs run? Again, like multiplicity, we know that the greater the dose of an intervention, the greater the chance for change. (Chapter 14 includes additional information about multiplicity and dose as they relate to process evaluation.)

Box 8.1 identifies the responsibilities and competencies for health education specialists that pertain to the material presented in this chapter.

BOX

8.1

Responsibilities and Competencies for Health Education Specialists

The content of this chapter focuses on the creation or adaptation of the intervention that will be used in the program. The intervention is really the heart of a program. It is the component of the program that will cause the change in the priority population. The responsibilities and competencies related to the tasks of creating an intervention include:

RESPONSIBILITY I: Assess Needs, Resources, and Capacity for Health Education/Promotion

Competency 1.6: Examine factors that enhance or impede the process of health education/promotion

RESPONSIBILITY II: Plan Health Education/Promotion

Competency 2.3: Select or design strategies/interventions

Competency 2.4: Develop a plan for the delivery of health education/promotion

RESPONSIBILITY VI: Serve as a Health Education/Promotion Resource Person

Competency 6.2: Train others to use health education/promotion skills

RESPONSIBILITY VII: Communicate, Promote, and Advocate for Health, Health Education/Promotion, and the Profession

Competency 7.1: Identify, develop, and deliver messages using a variety of communication strategies, methods, and techniques.

Competency 7.2: Engage in advocacy for health education/promotion

Competency 7.3: Influence policy and/or systems change to promote health education

Source: *A Competency-Based Framework for Health Education Specialists—2015.* Whitehall, PA: National Commission for Health Education Credentialing, Inc. (NCHEC) and the Society for Public Health Education (SOPHE). Reprinted by permission of the National Commission for Health Education Credentialing, Inc. (NCHEC) and the Society for Public Health Education (SOPHE).

▷ Types of Intervention Strategies

As mentioned earlier, there are many different types of activities that planners can use as part of an intervention. Most activities can be placed in larger categories called strategies. By **strategy**, we mean "a general plan of action for affecting a health problem" (CDC, 2003, glossary). Here, we present several categories of intervention strategies based on a modification of the Centers for Disease Control and Prevention's (2003) terminology for intervention strategies. These categories cover the more common strategies used by planners, but in actuality the variety of strategies is limited only by the planners' imagination. Irrespective of the types of strategies used, health education specialists should seek to use strategies that are evidence-based. Note that the categories presented here are not always mutually exclusive—that is, some of the examples that we use to help explain the strategies could be used in more than one category. Even with this limitation, the strategies have been categorized into the following seven groups:

1. Health communication strategies
2. Health education strategies

3. Health policy/enforcement strategies

4. Environmental change strategies

5. Health-related community service strategies

6. Community mobilization strategies

7. Other strategies

Health Communication Strategies

Health communication has been defined as "the study and use of communication strategies to inform and influence individual and community decisions that affect health" (USDHHS, 2015a, para. 1). It can also be defined by the form it takes in health promotion programs (e.g., mass media, media advocacy, risk communication, public relations, entertainment education, print material, electronic communication). Of the various intervention strategies used in health promotion, we present health communication strategies first for several reasons. First, almost all health promotion interventions include some form of communication ranging from simple, such as speaking and listening, to the more complex communication campaigns delivered through various forms of media. Second, communication strategies are useful in reaching many of the goals and objectives of health promotion programs. They have been shown to create awareness of an issue, change attitudes toward a health behavior, encourage and motivate individuals to follow recommended health behaviors, reinforce attitude and behavior change, increase demand and support for services, and build social norms (Ammary-Risch, Zambon, & Brown, 2010; NCI, n.d.). Third, communication strategies probably have the highest **penetration rate** (number in the priority population exposed or reached) of any of the intervention strategies. And fourth, they are much more cost effective and less threatening than most other types of strategies. But be aware that health communication also has its limitations. For example, health communication alone is rarely sufficient to change behavior and reduce the risk of disease.

Although communication has always been an important strategy in health promotion programs, the means by which communication takes place has changed. In the traditional communication model, a sender relays a message through a channel to receivers (i.e., consumers)—a vertical or top-down process. In such a model, the sender is the gatekeeper of the information, while the consumers play a less active, almost passive, role in receiving the message (Thackeray & Neiger, 2009). An example is when a health department posts information on its Website for public consumption. However, with the enhanced capabilities of the Internet and the development of other emerging communication technologies, the means of delivering health communications have been greatly expanded and blurred the strict roles of the sender and receiver. With the new technology has come a new communication model: the multidirectional communication (MDC) model (Thackeray & Neiger, 2009) (see **Figure 8.1**). In the MDC model, communication occurs through a combination of: (1) sender top-down (vertical) messages, (2) consumer created bottom-up messages, (3) consumer shared horizontal (side-to-side) messages, and (4) consumers seeking information. Thus in the MDC model consumers not only receive information but also actively seek, develop, and share information (Thackeray & Neiger, 2009).

An underlying concept of the MDC model is that the sophistication with which health information is communicated has changed dramatically in recent years due in large part to

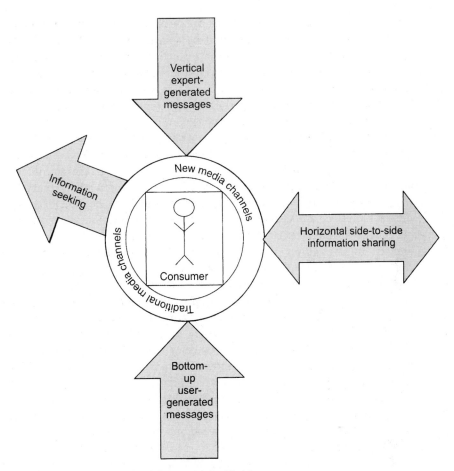

▲ **Figure 8.1** A Multidirectional Communication Model

Source: Thackeray, R., & Neiger, B. L. (2009). A multidirectional communication model: Implications for social marketing practice. *Health Promotion Practice,* 10(2), 171–175. © 2009 Sage Publications.

new technology. To compete for the attention and participation of consumers, those who plan health promotion programs must either develop a working knowledge of these communication technologies or have the foresight to access those who can provide the necessary expertise. A key characteristic of effective health communication campaigns is that they are people- (or audience-) centered (Schiavo, 2014). This requires that planners understand consumer tendencies, needs, and preferences before designing campaigns and messages.

There are literally hundreds of communication activities that could be used with a health communication strategy. Communication channels is one way to subdivide these activities. A **communication channel** is the route through which a message is disseminated to the priority population. "Understanding communication channels is imperative to conducting strategic, effective and user-centric health interventions, campaigns and outreach" (CDC, 2014b, para. 1). Selecting appropriate channels for a priority population is often related to, or in some cases limited by, the setting where the communication will be delivered (Kreps, Barnes, Neiger, & Thackeray, 2009). "For example, if the home is identified as the prime setting, appropriate channels could include one-on-one home visits, technology via the telephone, or mass media via television or radio" (Kreps et al., 2009, p. 91). The four traditional communication channels include intrapersonal (one-on-one communication), interpersonal (small group communication), organization and community, and mass media. These channels are hierarchical in nature with regards to the number of people they reach. The intrapersonal channel typically reaches the fewest number of people, while the mass media channel reaches the largest number of people.

Because of the Internet and the other emerging technologies we are adding *social media* as a fifth communication channel. **Social media**, or *interactive media*, is an overarching term for any type of media that uses the Internet and other technologies to enhance social interaction for sharing and discussing information. Unlike the other four communication channels, social media does not have a set place in the hierarchy because it "cuts across" several different levels. That is, depending on the type and purpose of social media, it can be used to generate social interaction at any of the levels of the traditional communication channel hierarchy. After we address each of the four traditional communication channels found in the hierarchy, we will present information on social media.

Over the years, the *intrapersonal channel* has most often been used, but by no means exclusively, in health care settings when the health care provider and patient interact. This is a familiar channel for most people and one they trust. It is typically an effective communication channel, but it is also typically the most time and resource intensive channel for the number of people reached. This is especially true when the health communication messages have some level of personal relevance. Means of creating personal relevance in a message include *personalizing* (i.e., placing the recipient's name on/in the communication), *targeting* (i.e., providing standardized information to a segmented group like Asian American adolescent girls), or *tailoring* it for the recipient. **Tailoring** has been defined as "any combination of information or change strategies intended to reach one specific person, based upon characteristics that are unique to that person, related to the outcome of interest, and have been derived from an individual assessment" (Kreuter & Skinner, 2000, p. 1). Tailoring takes more effort and resources than *personalizing* or *targeting* communication because it requires obtaining individual information on each member of the priority population (Kreuter, Farrell, Olevitch, & Brennan, 1999; Schmid, Rivers, Latimer, & Salovey, 2008; Suggs & McIntyre, 2009). Tailoring is best for helping to change complex behaviors, targeting is best when behavior is relatively simple (e.g., a one time behavior like getting a vaccination) (Schmid et al., 2008), while personalizing a message helps to get an individual's attention.

In more recent years, the tailoring of intrapersonal communication has been greatly enhanced by the use of technology. Tailoring of messages has been used with electronic mail messages (Kreuter et al., 1999) and with information delivered through Websites (Suggs & McIntyre, 2009). Another example involves the use of telephones. Although most people no longer think of the telephone, when it is used to talk with another person, as "technology," it too is used for health promotion interventions via the intrapersonal channel. Planners have used it for "gathering information, disseminating information, providing health education and counseling, promoting health education programs, offering cues to action and social support" (Soet & Basch, 1997, p. 760) on a variety of health topics ranging from asthma management (e.g., Raju, Soni, Aziz, Tiemstra, & Hasnain, 2012), to diabetes and hypertension (e.g., Goode et al., 2011), to weight management (e.g., Terry, Seaverson, Grossmeier, & Anderson, 2011). Health education delivered by telephone "can be classified into two broad categories: *individual initiated*, whereby the individual must actively seek contact and assistance from a health information hotline; and *outreach*, whereby the individual is called" (Soet & Basch, 1997, p. 760). Individual-initiated health information hotlines or help lines usually provide information, and sometimes education and counseling, whereas outreach activities range from brief, one-time preappointment reminders to long-term interactive professional health counseling (Soet & Basch, 1997) or coaching. Soet and Basch (1997) present a generic process for developing a telephone intervention activity that includes: (a) designing the intervention protocol, (b) selecting and training those delivering the intervention, and (c) developing the documentation and data collection protocol.

Within the intrapersonal channel, one health communication activity in particular that has received much attention is *health coaching*. Health coaching is the process by which a trained health coach, using the results from some type of personal health assessment (e.g., health risk appraisal), assists a client/consumer in identifying health-enhancing goals and uses behavioral psychology principles to help motivate the client to work toward the goals. This confidential communication relationship often takes place via a series of telephone conversations but can be conducted in face-to-face sessions. There are a number of commercial companies that offer health coaching services. Such services have been used as part of employee health promotion programs for a number of years (e.g., Chapman, Lesch, & Baun, 2007; Harris, Hannon, Beresford, Linnan, & McLellan, 2014) to help enhance employee health and reduce health care costs, and more recently in clinical settings to assist patients with health behavior change and management of chronic diseases (e.g., Willard-Grace et al., 2015).

A technique that is often used in health coaching is *motivational interviewing*. **Motivational interviewing** (MI) "is a collaborative, person-centered form of guiding to elicit and strengthen motivation for change (Miller & Rollnick, 2009, p. 137). Miller (1983) first used MI with individuals who had drinking problems. Since that time it has been used to help individuals with a wide variety of health problems in which a behavior change was needed (Rubak, Sandbaek, Lauritzen, & Christensen, 2005). At the heart of MI is helping a person explore and resolve the ambivalence associated with behavior change. "The operational assumption in MI is that ambivalent attitudes or lack of resolve is the primary obstacle to behavioral change, so that the examination and resolution of ambivalence becomes its key goal" (SAMHSA, 2015, para. 1). MI is not a process where a trained professional "gives advice" or "tells a person what to do," but rather is a process in which the trained professional helps guide an individual to identify internal motivation for change. **Box 8.2** presents the four principles of MI.

Examples of the *interpersonal channel* are support groups and small classes. This channel has many of the same characteristics of the intrapersonal channel, but reaches larger numbers of people with fewer resources.

Many people receive a lot of information through *organization* and *community channels*. Often health promotion programs have priority populations that are part of or entirely comprise already existing groups (e.g., workers of a particular company, social groups, or members of a religious organization), or who may participate in a community activity. As such, organizational and community channels provide excellent ways to reach priority populations. Thus church bulletins, company or agency newsletters, organizations or community bulletin boards, and community activities are often used as a part of communication activities.

Probably the most visible communication channel to most people is the *mass media channel*. Mass media interventions can seek to influence people either directly or indirectly. When done directly the intervention identifies a problem of concern and targets the people who can

BOX

8.2

Focus On

Principles of Motivational Interviewing

The four principles of MI are presented below. Each is followed by bulleted points that provide more detail about the principle and an example application of the principle. Note: The participant is the person who could benefit from a behavior change and the trained professional is the one providing the motivational interviewing.

Principle 1: Express Empathy – Expressing empathy towards a participant shows acceptance and increases the chance of the trained professional and the participant developing a rapport.

- Acceptance enhances self-esteem and facilitates change.
- Skillful reflective listening is fundamental.
- Ambivalence is normal.

—Example statement from the trained professional: "I understand that is has been difficult for you to quit smoking. Many people with whom I work find this to be difficult. It is still important for us to try to identify ways for you to work on this. What do you think you can do to stop smoking?"

Principle 2: Develop Discrepancy – Developing discrepancy enables a participant to see that his/her present situation does not necessarily fit into his/her values and what he/she would like in the future.

- The participant rather than the trained professional should present the arguments for change.
- Change is motivated by a perceived discrepancy between present behavior and important personal goals and values.

—Example statement from the trained professional: "You have told me that you would like to feel better. I think you know quitting will improve your health. Why do you think it has been hard for you to quit once and for all?"

Principle 3: Roll with Resistance – Rolling with resistance prevents a breakdown in communication between a participant and a trained professional and allows the participant to explore his/her views.

- Avoid arguing for change.
- Do not directly oppose resistance.
- New perspectives are offered but not imposed.
- The participant is a primary resource in finding answers and solutions.
- Resistance is a signal for the trained professional to respond differently.

—Example statement from the trained professional: I know you have tried to quit "cold turkey" in the past, would you like to know how some others have been successful at quitting?,

Principle 4: Support Self-Efficacy

- Self-efficacy is a crucial component to facilitating change. If a participant believes that he/she has the ability to change, the likelihood of change occurring is greatly increased.
- A participant's belief in the possibility of change is an important motivator.
- The participant, not the trained professional, is responsible for choosing and carrying out change.
- The trained professional's own belief in the participant's ability to change becomes a self-fulfilling prophecy.

—Example statement from the trained professional: "I know that it must seem like an impossible task to stop smoking, but now that we have discussed some options that have helped others stop, which ones do you think might work for you?

Source: Adapted from United States Department of Agriculture (n.d.).

change it while, when it is done indirectly, the interventions seek to influence people by creating beneficial changes in the places or environments (e.g., homes, schools, worksites, roads, grocery stores, cities) in which people live and work (Abroms & Maibach, 2008). For example, to increase the number of children who are immunized properly a direct mass media intervention would target the parents/guardians of the children. A mass media intervention to counter the advertising of unhealthy foods and drinks in a specific neighborhood would be an example of indirect mass media intervention. The mass media channel includes both print and electronic (e.g., distribution via the Internet) formats, such as billboards; direct mail; daily papers with national or local circulation; local weekly newspapers; local, public, and network television, including cable television; public and commercial radio stations; and magazines with either a broad readership or a narrow focus. There are many ways to convey a message using the mass media. These include news coverage, public affairs coverage, talk shows, public service roundtables, entertainment, public service announcements (PSAs), paid advertisements, editorials, letters to the editor, comic strips, and columnists' commentaries (Arkin, 1990).

With the growth of and the developments in technology, the *social media* channel has significantly changed the way people communicate both formally and informally. Social media, sometimes referred to as *interactive media* or *Web 2.0*, has several characteristics that set it apart from the other communication channels already discussed. The unique characteristics of social media include 1) it is user or consumer generated, organized, and distributed; (2) information can be revised or updated almost immediately; (3) it is typically low cost in terms of creation and maintenance; (4) it can reach broader, more diverse audiences, and (5) it is generally entertaining to use. There are many different forms of social media that allow for content management (collaborative writing, e.g., wikis), content sharing (e.g., podcasts, Webinars, widgets, eCards), social bookmarking (i.e., tagging, saving, searching, and rating Websites, e.g., Digg), social gaming, social journaling (e.g., blogs), social networking (e.g., Facebook, MySpace, LinkedIn, Twitter, text messaging), social news (i.e., tagging, voting for, and commenting on news articles, e.g., Newsvine), social video and photo sharing (e.g., YouTube, Flickr), and syndication (e.g., real simple syndication [RSS] feeds).

Though the use of social media in health promotion interventions may be limited only by planners' creativity, we feel that its greatest potential lies in three uses: (1) the Internet as a platform to deliver behavior change interventions (e.g., weight loss programs; see Bennett & Glasgow, 2009); (2) the Internet to promote health promotion programs (e.g., viral marketing; see Thackeray, Neiger, Hanson, & McKenzie, 2008); and (3) the Internet and mobile devices for community mobilization or advocacy (e.g., organizing youth to get involved in civic affairs; see Thackeray & Hunter, 2010). However, as with other channels of communication, when using social media planners need to think strategically about what they are trying to accomplish and then decide how to use technology to accomplish the program's goals. In other words, planners need to focus on the relationship between themselves and those in the priority population, and the ways people connect with each other, because social media is really all about developing relationships. Thackeray and Bennion (2009) have adapted the strategic thinking acronym POST, found in a book by Li and Bernoff (2008), to assist program planners in creating health promotion interventions that include social media (see **Table 8.1**).

The CDC has created two publications that provide information about and best practices for the use of social media. They include: CDC's *Guide to Writing Social Media* (CDC, 2012a) and *The Health Communicator's Social Media Toolkit* (CDC, 2011b). (Note: See the references for location of these publications.)

TABLE 8.1 **Using *POST* to Think Strategically About Social Media**

POST	Li & Bernoff (2008)	Thackeray & Bennion (2009)
People	What are they ready for?	What technology do they use? Why?
Objectives	Why do you want to pursue the groundswell?	What do you want to happen (i.e., a change in attitudes, knowledge, and/or behavior)?
Strategy	How do you want relationships to change (e.g., customers to carry your messages; customers to become engaged)?	How will you use the marketing mix (i.e., product, price, place, promotion)?
Technology	What technology to use?	What technology will you use, given what you are trying to accomplish?

Regardless of the communication channel used in creating a communication intervention, planners need to consider the literacy level of those in the priority population. **Literacy** "is the ability to use printed and written information to function in society, to achieve one's goals, and to develop one's knowledge and potential" (White & Dillow, 2005, p. 4). "Literacy can be thought of as currency in this society. Just as adults with little money have difficulty meeting their basic needs, those with limited literacy skills are likely to find it more challenging to pursue their goals—whether these involve job advancement, consumer decision making, citizenship, or other aspects of their lives" (Kirsch, Jungeblut, Jenkins, & Kolstad, 1993, p. xix). The last national assessment of adult literacy in the United States was conducted in 2003. That study, called the National Assessment of Adult Literacy (NAAL), assessed a representative sample of over 19,000 adults age 16 and older on *prose* (the knowledge and skills to perform prose tasks such as reading and comprehending a news story), *document* (the knowledge and skills to perform document tasks such as completing a job application), and *quantitative literacy*, sometimes referred to as **numeracy** (the knowledge and skills to perform quantitative tasks such as balancing a checkbook or calculating a tip) (USDE, n.d.). Results of the 2003 NAAL were reported using four literacy levels: *below basic* (indicates no more than the most simple and concrete literacy skills, e.g., searching a short, simple text to find out when to show up for an appointment), *basic* (skills necessary to perform simple and everyday literacy activities, e.g., finding specific information in a pamphlet), *intermediate* (skills necessary to perform moderately challenging literacy activities, e.g., consulting reference materials to determine which foods contain a particular vitamin), and *proficient* (skills necessary to perform more complex and challenging literacy activities, e.g., comparing viewpoints in two editorials). **Figure 8.2** provides a comparison of the percentage of adults in each literacy level for the two most recent national literacy assessments.

The 2003 NAAL included the first-ever national health literacy assessment of adults in the United States. The health literacy scale used in the assessment and the tasks that the adults were asked to perform were guided by the following definition of **health literacy**: "the capacity to obtain, process, and understand basic health information and services to make appropriate health decisions" (USDHHS, 2015b, para 1).

Like the general literacy assessment, health literacy results from the NAAL were reported using the same four literacy categories: below basic, basic, intermediate, and proficient. The results showed that 14% had below basic health literacy, 22% had basic health literacy, 53% had intermediate health literacy, and 12% had proficient health literacy (Kutner, Greenberg, Jin, & Paulsen, 2006). Stated a bit differently, this study showed that "nearly 9 out of 10 adults have

Literacy scale
and year

Prose	1992	14	28	42	15
Prose	2003	14	29	44	13
Document	1992	14	22	49	15
Document	2003	12*	22	58	13*
Quantitative	1992	26	32	30	13
Quantitative	2003	22	33	33	13

70 60 50 40 30 20 10 0 10 20 30 40 50 60 70 80 90 100

Percent below basic   Percent basic above

■ Below basic   ▨ Basic   ▨ Intermediate   ▨ Proficient

*Significantly different from 1992

Note: Detail may not sum to totals because of rounding. Adults are defined as people 16 years of age and older living in households or prisons. Adults who could not be interviewed due to language spoken or cognitive or mental disabilities (3 percent in 2003 and 4 percent in 1992) are excluded from this figure.

▲ **Figure 8.2** Percentage of Adults in Each Literacy Level: 1992 and 2003

Source: White & Dillow (2005). White, S., & Dillow, S. (2005). Key concepts and features of the 2003 National Assessment of Adult Literacy (NCES 2006-471). Washington, DC: National Center for Education Statistics, U.S. Department of Education.

difficulty using the everyday health information that is routinely available in our health care facilities, retail outlets, media, and communities" (USDHHS, 2010, p. 1). Though the problem of limited health literacy affects people of all ages, races, incomes, and education levels, it disproportionately affects lower socioeconomic and minority groups (Kutner et al., 2006).

Though the NAAL assessment of health literacy included a quantitative component, in recent years health numeracy has emerged as a separate and important issue (Golbeck, Ahlers-Schmidt, Paschal, & Dismuke, 2005). As with health literacy, health numeracy is not at the levels it should be and may have a significant impact on health status (Estrada, Martin-Hryniewicz, Peek, Collins, & Byrd, 2004). **Health numeracy** has been defined as "the degree to which individuals have the capacity to access, process, interpret, communicate, and act on numerical, quantitative, graphical, biostatistical, and probabilistic health information needed to make effective health decisions" (Golbeck et al., 2005, p. 375). This definition recognizes that there are degrees of health numeracy that fall along a continuum, and "that health numeracy is not simply about understanding (processing and interpreting), but also functioning (communicating and acting) on numeric concepts in terms of health" (Golbeck et al., 2005, p. 375). Further, Golbeck and her colleagues (2005) suggested that health numeracy consists of four skills: basic (e.g., counting the number of pills), computational (e.g., determining the number of calories consumed using a nutritional label), analytical (e.g., determining if test results are in the normal range), and statistical (e.g., determine risk with probability).

Because of the lack of health literacy and health numeracy in the United States, health education specialists need to work to ensure that the health communication interventions are appropriate for their priority population and consistent with the *National Action Plan to Improve Health Literacy* (USDHHS, 2010). The CDC has created a publication–*Simply Put:*

A guide for creating easy-to-understand materials (CDC, 2009a) (Note: See the references for location of this publication.)– that provides many useful ideas for creating health communication materials.

As noted in the *Simply Put* (CDC, 2009a) document, making sure written materials are presented at the appropriate reading level for the priority population is an important concept. Americans, on average, read at the 7th grade reading level (Mishoe, 2008). Therefore, when writing for the general public you should try to write at the 6th grade reading level. Reading levels can be checked using a readability test such as, the Fog-Gunning Index, Flesch-Kincaid Grade Level Readability Formula, the Fry Readability Formula, or the SMOG (stands for Simple Measure of Gobbledegook). Today many computer word-processing programs include a tool that can be used to check the reading level. In case yours does not, **Box 8.3** presents the steps in the process of testing readability using the SMOG.

BOX

8.3

Application

The SMOG Readability Formula

To calculate the SMOG reading grade level, begin with the entire written work that is being assessed, and follow these four steps:

1. Count off 10 consecutive sentences near the beginning, in the middle, and near the end of the text.
2. From this sample of 30 sentences, circle all of the words containing 3 or more syllables (polysyllabic), including repetitions of the same word, and total the number of words circled.
3. Estimate the square root of the total number of polysyllabic words counted. This is done by finding the nearest perfect square, and taking its square root.
4. Finally, add a constant of 3 to the square root. This number gives the SMOG grade, or the reading grade level that a person must have reached if he or she is to fully understand the text being assessed.

A few additional guidelines will help to clarify these directions:

- A sentence is defined as a string of words punctuated with a period (.), an exclamation point (!), or a question mark (?).
- Hyphenated words are considered as one word.
- Numbers that are written out should also be considered, and if in numeric form in the text, they should be pronounced to determine if they are polysyllabic.
- Proper nouns, if polysyllabic, should be counted, too.
- Abbreviations should be read as unabbreviated to determine if they are polysyllabic.

Not all pamphlets, fact sheets, or other printed materials contain 30 sentences. To test a text that has fewer than 30 sentences:

1. Count all of the polysyllabic words in the text.
2. Count the number of sentences.
3. Find the average number of polysyllabic words per sentence as follows:

$$\text{Average} = \frac{\text{Total \# polysyllabic words}}{\text{Total \# of sentences}}$$

4. Multiply that average by the number of sentences *short of* 30.

Source: The SMOG Readability Formula from "SMOG grading—a new reading formula" by H.G. McLaughlin, The Journal of Reading 12, 639-646. Copyright © 1969 by John Wiley & Sons. Reprinted with permission.

continued

BOX 8.3

5. Add that figure to the total number of polysyllabic words.
6. Find the square root and add the constant of 3.

Perhaps the quickest way to administer the SMOG grading test is by using the SMOG conversion table. Simply count the number of polysyllabic words in your chain of 30 sentences and look up the appropriate grade level on the chart.

SMOG Conversion Table*

Total Polysyllabic Word Counts	Approximate Grade Level (±1.5 Grades)
0–2	4
3–6	5
7–12	6
13–20	7
21–30	8
31–42	9
43–56	10
57–72	11
73–90	12
91–110	13
111–132	14
133–156	15
157–182	16
183–210	17
211–240	18

*Developed by Harold C. McGraw, Office of Educational Research, Baltimore County Schools, Towson, Maryland.

Health Education Strategies

Earlier (Chapter 1) *health education* was defined as "any planned combination of learning experiences designed to predispose, enable, and reinforce voluntary behavior decisions conducive to health in individuals, groups, or communities" (Green & Kreuter, 2005, p. G-4). You may be asking, "How is this definition different from the definition presented in the earlier section for health communication strategies?" There are some health communication strategies, because of the way they are designed, that could be classified as health education strategies. And, there are some health education strategies that could meet the definition of health communication strategies. There is no clear dividing line between these two categories of intervention strategies. That is, they are not mutually exclusive categories. In fact, it is for this reason that some authors have included health education strategies as part of the health communication strategies category or vice versa. Yet, we have decided to separate the two types of strategies. In general, we see health communication strategies as those that inform people (e.g., a brochure on skin cancer or a mass media campaign on preventing HIV), while health education strategies are those that are planned learning experiences that provide knowledge and skills to the learners in a more formal educational setting. We see health education strategies as those usually associated with settings such as classes, seminars, workshops, and courses, both face-to-face and online. Some examples include prenatal classes for expectant parents, a workshop for parents on how to better communicate with their teenager, or a first aid and CPR course for potential babysitters.

Prior to presenting information about creating health education interventions it is important to have some background in how people learn. Many theories/models have been put forth to help explain how people learn. While many of the theories/models include components that are unique to the theory/model, there is also much overlap in the content. Space does not allow for the review of those theories/models here. However, we are fortunate that other authors (Bryan, Kreuter, & Brownson, 2009; Minelli & Breckon, 2009) have reviewed those theories/models. Those reviewers have identified many of the common components and created lists of learning principles. Their lists can help guide planners as they create health education interventions. We present their lists here. Minelli and Breckon (2009) refer to their list as the 10 general principles of learning. For them, learning is facilitated: (1) if several of the senses (e.g., seeing, hearing, speaking) are used; (2) if the learner is actively involved in the process, rather than a passive participant; (3) if the learner is not distracted by discomfort or extraneous events; (4) if the learner is ready to learn; (5) if that which is to be learned is relevant to the learner and that relevance is perceived by the learner; (6) if repetition is used; (7) if the learning encountered is pleasant, if progress occurs that is recognizable by the learner, and if that learning is recognized and encouraged; (8) if the material to be learned starts with what is known and proceeds to the unknown, while concurrently moving from simple to complex concepts; (9) if application of concepts to several settings occurs, which generalizes the material; and (10) if it is paced appropriately for the learner.

The principles offered by Bryan and colleagues (2009) are specific to adult learners. The principles represent a synthesis of recurring themes that the authors found when reviewing existing theories/models related to adult education. Their adult learning principles include:

1. "Adults need to know why they are learning.
2. Adults are motivated to learn by the need to solve problems.
3. Adults' previous experience must be respected and built upon.
4. Adults need learning approaches that match their background and diversity.
5. Adults need to be actively involved in the learning process." (p. 559)

With this brief overview of learning principles, let's look at the makeup of a health education intervention. Though health communication strategies may be the most frequently used health promotion intervention strategy, health education strategies are the ones that provide the opportunity for the priority population to gain in-depth knowledge about a particular health topic. Well-designed health education strategies take an understanding of the educational process and take a great deal of effort to create. In order to better understand this process, several terms must be defined. The first is the word *curriculum*. **Curriculum** refers to "a planned set of lessons or courses designed to lead to competence in an area of study" (Gilbert, Sawyer, & McNeill, 2015, p. 437). Examples include the health education curriculum of a school district or the curriculum for a hospital's diabetes education program. To further define a curriculum it is important to understand the terms *scope* and *sequence*. **Scope** refers to the breadth and depth of the material covered in a curriculum, whereas **sequence** defines the order in which the material is presented. To

Title of Program: _____ Title of Lesson: _____ Page ___ of ___		
Unit: _____ Lesson No.: _____		
Priority Population: _____ Length of Lesson: _____		
Resources & References	Content	Teaching Method
	Introduction:	
	Body: 1. 2. 3.	
	Conclusion:	
Evaluation:		

▲ **Figure 8.3** Example Lesson Plan Format

further clarify these definitions, scope has been referred to as the horizontal organization of the substance of the curriculum (Goodlad & Su, 1992), while the sequence is the vertical relationship among the curricular areas (Ornstein & Hunkins, 1998). It is not unusual for the scope of a health education curriculum to be presented as *unit plans*. A **unit plan** is defined as "an orderly, self-contained collection of activities educationally designed to meet a set of objectives. Other terms for this are *curriculum plans, modules*, and *strands*" (Gilbert et al., 2015, p. 202). Thus, a school health curriculum may have units on exercise, nutrition, chronic diseases, communicable diseases, and so forth, while the diabetes education curriculum might include units on self-management, working with a health care professional, and avoiding emergencies. And finally, units of study are further subdivided into **lessons**—the amount of material that can be presented during a single educational encounter, say for example the amount of material that can be presented in a one-hour class. The written outline of a lesson is referred to as a **lesson plan** and typically includes three components—introduction, body, and conclusion. The introduction provides an overview of what will be covered, the body presents the health content, and the conclusion reviews what was presented. There is an old saying that summarizes these three parts that states *tell them what you are going to tell them* [introduction], *tell them it* [body], *and tell them what you told them* [conclusion]. (See **Figure 8.3** for an example lesson plan format.)

The heart of any lesson is the body or the content portion of the lesson. Gagne (1985) has created a framework, called the *Nine Events of Instruction*, for designing educational experiences that provides a nice outline for creating the body of a lesson. More recently, Kinzie (2005) modified Gagne's framework for application to health promotion applications. The modified framework includes five stages instead of the original nine created by Gagne: (1) *gain attention* (convey health threats and benefits); (2) *present stimulus material* (target or tailor the message to audience knowledge and values, demonstrate observable effectiveness, make behaviors easy to understand and do); (3) *provide guidance* (use trustworthy models to demonstrate); (4) *elicit performance and provide feedback* (to enhance *trailability*, and develop

TABLE 8.2 Application Instructional Design Framework for a Lesson on Breast Cancer

Stage	Content Covered	Method of Presentation
Gain attention	• Help participants identify personal risk to breast cancer • Share benefits of doing breast self-examinations (BSE), regular breast exams by physicians, and mammograms	• Use breast cancer risk appraisal or breast cancer pretest • Present a case study of women finding a lump in the breast early
Present stimulus material		
Target/tailor message to knowledge and values	• Using information from risk appraisal or pretest, target/tailor breast cancer information	• Lecture/discussion
Demonstrate observable effectiveness	• Explain importance of early diagnosis	• Use peer educators to role-play interaction with physician
Make desired behaviors easy to understand	• Present steps in BSE and making appointment with physician and for mammogram	• Use video showing correct steps for BSE or peer educators to demonstrate on models
Provide guidance	• Have others share experiences on how exams are conducted	• Use guest speakers who perform regular BSE and radiographers who do mammograms
Elicit performance and provide feedback	• Repeat steps in BSE and let participants practice BSE	• Use breast models for practice and provide critique
Enhance retention and transfer	• Encourage participants to share information learned with others and ways to remember to act	• Lecture/discussion • Brainstorm reminder ideas • Distribute BSE shower cards that explain importance of regular action for participants to place in their bathrooms

proficiency and self-efficacy); and (5) *enhance retention and transfer* (provide social support and deliver behavioral cues) (Kinzie, 2005). **Table 8.2** provides an example of how these five stages can be applied to a health topic.

There are many different ways of presenting health education such as lecture, discussion, group work, audiovisual materials, computerized instruction, laboratory exercises, and written materials (books and periodicals). **Box 8.4** provides a more complete listing of educational activities, and Gilbert et al. (2015) have provided a detailed discussion of these activities.

Health Policy/Enforcement Strategies

Health polices/enforcement strategies include executive orders, laws, ordinances, judicial decisions, policies, regulations, rules, and position statements. Though each of the different types of policy/enforcement strategies has its own definition, common to all of them is a decision made by an authoritative person, agency/organization, or body and that is presented in a statement or guidelines intended to direct or influence the actions or behaviors

BOX

8.4

Focus On

Commonly Used Educational Activities

A. Audiovisual materials and equipment
   1. Audiotapes, records, and CDs
   2. Bulletin, chalk, cloth, flannel, magnetic, and peg boards
   3. Charts, pictures, and posters
   4. Films and filmstrips
   5. Instructional television
   6. Opaque projector or Elmo
   7. Slides and slide projectors
   8. Transparencies, PowerPoint® slides, and overhead projector
   9. Video (DVDs and tapes)
B. Technology-assisted instruction
   1. World Wide Web
   2. Desktop publishing
   3. Photo and video voice
   4. Presentation programs
   5. Individualized learning programs
   6. Video conferencing (e.g., Skype)
   7. Social media
C. Printed educational materials
   1. Displays and bulletin boards
   2. Instructor-made handouts and worksheets
   3. Pamphlets
   4. Study guides (commercial and instructor-made)
   5. Text and reference books
   6. Workbooks
D. Teaching strategies and techniques for the classroom
   1. Brainstorming
   2. Case studies
   3. Cooperative learning
   4. Debates
   5. Demonstrations and experiments
   6. Discovery or guided discovery
   7. Discussion
   8. Group discussion
   9. Guest speakers
   10. Lecture
   11. Lecture/discussion
   12. Newspaper and magazine articles
   13. Panel discussions
   14. Peer group teaching/coaching
   15. Personal improvement projects
   16. Poems, songs, and stories
   17. Problem solving

BOX

8.4

continued

18. Puppets
19. Questioning
20. Role playing and plays
21. Simulation, games, and puzzles
22. Tutoring
23. Values clarification activities
24. Word games

E. Teaching strategies and techniques for outside of the classroom
1. Community resources
2. Field trips
3. Health fairs
4. Health museums
5. Health education centers

of others. Another way to think about them is as strategies that are mandated or regulated. Such strategies revolve around establishing some type of standard or requirement, sometimes associated with incentives or disincentives, to encourage or discourage actions by groups of individuals or society as a whole (Riegelman, 2014). This type of intervention strategy can regulate the behavior of individuals (e.g., use of safety belts and motorcycle helmets), organizations (e.g., paying taxes for certain activities), institutions (e.g., school board adopting a position statement that a district will only provide well-balanced meals in the cafeteria), or communities (e.g., housing codes for rental properties) (Brennan Ramirez et al., 2008). This type of intervention strategy can also be used to "affect the built environment, such as zoning related to new grocery stores or fast food restaurants, maintenance of sidewalks and streetscapes, or architectural design features such as neighborhood signage addressing the history and culture of the community" (Brennan Ramirez et al., 2008, p. 70).

Health policy/enforcement strategies may be controversial. Some have criticized this type of strategy because it mandates a particular response from those governed by it. It takes away individual freedoms and sometimes plays on a person's pride, "pocketbook," and psyche. Stated a bit differently, "it runs counter to a fundamental emphasis on property rights, economic individualism, and competition in American political culture. The exceptionalism of the United States lies in its antistatist beliefs: Americans are less concerned with what government will do to benefit individuals than what government might do to control them" (Oliver, 2006, p. 196). This type of strategy must be based on sound evidence and must be sold on the basis of "common good." That is, the justification for this type of societal action is to protect the public's health. Health policy/enforcement strategies exist for the protection of the community and of individual rights. For example, in order to establish herd immunity most in a population need to be immunized, thus the reasoning behind immunizing children prior to entering school.

Some would say that health policy/enforcement strategies do not allow for the "voluntary behavior conducive to health" suggested by Green and Kreuter (2005, p. G-4) in their definition of health education. But, at the same time, this kind of activity can get people to change their behavior when other strategies have failed. Brownson, Chriqui, and Stamatakis (2009) have pointed out that if we review the 10 great public health achievements of the 20th century (CDC, 1999b), we will find that each of them was influenced by policy. For example, before the passage of safety belt laws, a national study showed that about 11% of drivers and front-seat passengers of automobiles were observed using a safety belt (Goodwin et al., 2013). Now that safety belt laws are in effect, national safety belt use is 86%; in states where the law permits law enforcement officers to stop and cite a safety belt violator independent of any other traffic behavior (i.e., primary enforcement belt use law), usage rates average 90% (Goodwin et al., 2013).

Policymaking is complex and each setting in which policy is created has its own characteristics. For example, a state legislature where a law for smokefree public places is being debated would have many different characteristics from a boardroom of a private company where a no smoking policy is being created. Regardless of the setting, Block (2008) has identified six phases of policymaking—agenda setting, policy formulation, policy adoption, policy implementation, policy assessment, and policy modification—that we feel can be adapted and applied to the creation of any of the health policy/enforcement strategies for a health promotion program. The first phase, *agenda setting,* deals with determining what the health problem is, analyzing whether the cause of the problem can best be solved with a policy/ enforcement strategy, and identifying evidence to show that such a strategy will work. Phase 2, *policy formulation,* is the phase in which the policy or mandated action is actually developed. The actual wording of the policy is not easy work. It is difficult to move from a concept or idea to wording that effectively carries out the intent of the concept or idea and creates the most good for the most people. The simplest language possible should be the goal. If the policy being created is a legal document (e.g., law, ordinance), it is not unusual for various interest groups to try to influence those writing the document so that the resulting work best represents their interests. In other words, there are likely to be both pro and con feelings toward the policy and thus this phase can be very political. The third phase, *policy adoption* or approval, takes place when the authoritative individual or group "approves" the formulated policy. Again, depending on the policy being considered, politics can impact the outcome.

Once the policy has been approved it must be *implemented.* This is the fourth phase of the process. In this phase, the necessary human and financial resources must be assembled to make the policy work. As a part of this phase, it is important that those who are implementing the new policy use good judgment and show respect for others when doing so. Depending on the policy and its complexity there may be a need for education programs to ensure that the priority population understands the policy. Consideration may also need to be given to the enforcement of the policy. The fifth phase of the process, *policy assessment,* entails making sure that the policy is being carried out as written and that it is indeed working to solve the problem it was intended to solve. Based on the results of the policy assessment, the authoritative individual or group must consider the sixth and final phase—*policy modification.* In this phase some judgment and possible action must be made to determine whether the policy should be maintained, modified, or eliminated (Dunn, 1994). **Box 8.5** provides a list of questions that need to be considered when determining whether or not policy should be the *or* part of the health promotion intervention.

Questions to Consider When Creating Policy

- Is policy the best way to deal with the problem? Is it necessary?
- Is there evidence to show that the proposed policy has the potential to be effective?
- Is the proposed policy based on ethical principles that balance rights, interests, and values?
- Is the proposed policy stated clearly?
- Will the proposed policy include implementation and enforcement language?
- Is the policy culturally appropriate for the priority population?
- Has a representative group from the priority population been engaged and involved in the policy making process?
- Is there support for the proposed policy?
- Is there a need for the public to discuss/debate the proposed policy?
- What are the potential barriers to getting the policy enacted, implemented, sustained, and evaluated? Opposition? Resources? Political climate?
- Would it be useful to phase-in the policy overtime?

Environmental Change Strategies

Another group of strategies that has been used in meeting the goals and objectives of health promotion programs is environmental change strategies. Such strategies have been most useful in providing "opportunities, support, and cues to help people develop healthier behaviors" (Brownson, Haire-Joshu, & Luke, 2006, p. 342). As such, they help remove barriers in the environment. "Environmental barriers in a community can make modifying unhealthy behaviors challenging. Poor environmental quality; inadequate access to affordable, nutritious food; and safety issues often make healthy living impractical" (Flores, Davis, & Culross, 2007, para. 4). In other words, environmental change strategies are about creating health-enhancing environments (Hunnicutt & Leffelman, 2006). In the 1986 *Ottawa Charter for Health Promotion,* it was stated that the healthier choice should be the easier choice (WHO, 2009). Friedan (2010) stated it a bit differently when he said that the content of the environment should be changed to make healthy options the default choice so that individuals would have to expend significant effort not to benefit from them. Removing environmental barriers often helps to make the healthier choice the easier choice.

Environmental change strategies are characterized by changes "around" individuals and are not limited to the physical environment. Other environments include the economic environment (e.g., financial costs, affordability), service environment (e.g., accessibility to health care or patient education), social environment (e.g., social support, peer pressure), cultural environment (e.g., traditions of ethnic group), psychological environment (e.g., emotional learning environment), and political environment (e.g., support for healthy environments). Environmental change strategies have a close relationship to health policy/enforcement strategies because there are times when a policy change may be needed to make a change in the environment, for example a city or county ordinance that creates smokefree workplaces. Other examples of such strategies include equipping automobiles with safety belts, air bags, and child safety seats; placing speed bumps in parking lots by playgrounds to slow traffic where children are present; or installing fire and safety doors in apartment buildings to make them safer for the residents. Often environmental change strategies do not necessarily require action on the part of the priority population (CDC, 2003) as noted in the examples above. Yet, some of these strategies provide a "forced choice" situation, as when the selection of foods and beverages in vending machines or cafeterias are changed to include only healthful foods. If people want to eat foods from these places, they are forced to eat certain types of foods.

Other activities in this category may provide those in the priority population with health messages and environmental cues for certain types of behavior. Examples would be posting of no-smoking signs, eliminating ashtrays, providing lockers and showers, using role modeling by others, playing soft music in a work area, organizing a shuttle service or some other type of transportation system to get seniors to congregate for meals or to a health care provider, and providing point-of-purchase education, such as a sign on a vending machine or food labeling on the food options in the cafeteria.

One "environment" that has received increased attention in recent years is the built environment. The term **built environment** "generally refers to an interdisciplinary area of focus that describes the design, construction, management, and land use of human-made surroundings as an interrelated whole, as well as their relationship to human activities over time" (Coupland, Rikhy, Hill, & McNeil, 2011, p. 6). It includes, but is not limited to: transportation systems (e.g., mass transit); urban design features (e.g., bike paths, sidewalks, adequate lighting); parks and recreational facilities; land use (e.g., community gardens, location of schools, trail development); building with health enhancing features (e.g., green roofs, stairs); road systems; and housing free from environmental hazards (Coupland et al., 2011; Davidson, 2015; IOM, 2005). The built environment can be structured to give people more or fewer opportunities to behave in health enhancing ways. Earlier (see Chapter 4) we discussed the use of health impact assessments (HIAs) as a special type of needs assessment process "to determine the potential effects of a proposed policy, plan, program, or project on the health of a population and the distribution of those effects within the population" (NRC, 2011, p. 5). Although the major focus of an HIA is to make sure change is not made that could harm the health of a population, the results of a HIA could also lead to the modifications or additions to the built environment that provide more opportunities for enhancing health.

Finally, like so many of the other intervention strategies, environmental change strategies often are more effective when combined with intervention strategies from the other categories. An example of such multiplicity is combining the mandating of safety belts in automobiles, which is important alone, with strict enforcement of safety belt laws (a health policy/enforcement strategy), which makes for a much more effective intervention.

Health-Related Community Service Strategies

Health-related community service strategies include services, tests, treatments, or care to improve the health of those in the priority population (CDC, 2003). Examples of this type of intervention strategy include, but are not limited to, completing a health risk assessment (HRA) form (see Chapter 4 for a discussion of HRAs); offering low-cost flu shots or child immunizations; providing clinical screenings (sometimes called *biometric screenings*) for diabetes, blood pressure, or cholesterol; and providing professional health checkups and examinations. Because a health-related community service strategy requires action on the part of those in the priority population, an important component of this type of strategy is to reduce the barriers to obtaining the service. Thus planners must be mindful of the affordability and accessibility of such services. Also, planners must weigh the consequences of including this type of strategy in an intervention. For example, if abnormal readings are found during a screening, those conducting the screening have an ethical obligation to follow up and make sure appropriate referrals for care are made. Chapman (2003) has provided a nice review of many of the concerns associated with biometric screening.

Health-related community service strategies are often carried out by partnering organizations and are offered in a variety of settings including grocery stores, pharmacies, shopping malls, health fairs, worksites, personal residencies, mobile units (e.g., vans equipped with mammography units), and easily accessible health care facilities. Such strategies usually have high credibility with priority populations because of their link with health care providers.

Community Mobilization Strategies

"Community mobilization strategies involve helping communities identify and take action on shared concerns using participatory decision making, and include such methods as empowerment" (Barnes, Neiger, & Thackeray, 2003, p. 60). There is increasing evidence to support population-wide, community-level interventions to change health behaviors when community mobilizing strategies are combined with other strategies (Karwalajtys et al., 2013). In this book we present two subcategories of community mobilization strategies: (1) community organization and community building, and (2) community advocacy.

COMMUNITY ORGANIZATION AND COMMUNITY BUILDING

Other than defining the terms *community organization* and *community building*, little will be presented here about these terms because more information is presented elsewhere (Chapter 9). **Community organization** has been defined as "the process by which community groups are helped to identify common problems or change targets, mobilize resources, and develop and implement strategies to reach their collective goals" (Minkler & Wallerstein, 2012, p. 37). **Community building** is "an orientation to practice focused on community, rather than a strategic framework or approach, and on building capacities, not fixing problems" (Minkler, 2012, p. 10).

COMMUNITY ADVOCACY

Community advocacy is a process in which the people of the community become involved in the institutions and decisions that will have an impact on their lives. It has the potential for creating more support, keeping people informed, influencing decisions, activating nonparticipants, improving service, and making people, plans, and programs more responsive (Checkoway, 1989). Some individuals often confuse or use the words advocacy and lobbying interchangeably. There is a distinction. *Lobbying* is when individuals/organizations attempt to influence a specific piece of pending legislation by contacting elected officials or their representatives, while advocacy is trying to affect generalized change (e.g., healthier school lunches) by expressing opinions for or against causes or positions. Community advocacy can have a big impact on social change issues, including those dealing with health. The community advocacy that deals with health issues is called **health advocacy**. This type of advocacy has been defined as "the processes by which the actions of individuals or groups attempt to bring about social, environmental, and/or organizational change on behalf of a particular health goal, program, interest, or population" (Joint Committee on Health Education and Promotion Terminology, 2012, p. 17). Galer-Unti, Tappe, and Lachenmayr (2004) have

TABLE 8.3 **Advocacy Strategies: Good, Better, Best**

Strategy	Good	Better	Best
Voting behavior	Register and vote	Encourage others to register and vote	Register others to vote
Electioneering	Contribute to the campaign of a candidate friendly to public health and health education	Campaign for a candidate friendly to public health and health education	Run for office or seek a political appointment
Direct lobbying	Contact a policy maker	Meet with your policy makers	Develop ongoing relationships with your policy makers and their staff
Integrate grassroots lobbying into direct lobbying activities	Start a petition drive to advocate a specific policy in your local community	Get on the agenda for a meeting of a policy-making body and provide testimony	Organize a community coalition to enact changes that influence health
Use the Internet	Use the Internet to access information related to health issues	Build a Webpage that calls attention to a specific health issue, policy, or legislative proposal	Teach others to use the Internet for advocacy activities
Media advocacy: Newspaper letters to the editor and op-ed articles	Write a letter to the editor	Write an op-ed piece	Teach others to write letters and op-ed pieces for media advocacy
Media advocacy: Acting as a resource person	Respond to requests by members of the media for health-related information	Issue a news release	Develop and maintain ongoing relationships with the media personnel

Source: Galer-Unti, R. A., Tappe, M. K., Lachenmayr, S. (2004). Advocacy 101: Getting Started in Health Education Advocacy. *Health Promotion Practice* Vol 5(3) pp. 280-288. Copyright © 2004 by Society for Public Health Education. Reprinted by permission of SAGE Publications, Inc.

identified seven different ways of advocating for health and health education: (1) influencing voting behavior, (2) electioneering, (3) direct lobbying, (4) integrating grassroots lobbying into direct lobbying efforts, (5) using the Internet, (6) media advocacy—newspaper letters to the editor and opinion-editorial (op-ed) articles, and (7) media advocacy—acting as a resource person. They have further organized these seven advocacy strategies in a three-tiered approach to show the varying levels of involvement in the advocacy process. These levels and examples of each are presented in **Table 8.3**.

As noted in our earlier discussion of health communication strategies, the Internet and emerging technologies can be effective means to enhance advocacy efforts. Thackeray and Hunter (2010) have suggested that cell phones and social networking sites (SNS) on the Internet can be used for: (1) recruiting people to join the cause, (2) organizing collective action, (3) raising awareness and shaping attitudes, (4) raising funds to support the cause, and (5) communicating with decision makers. While both cell phones and SNS can be used for these advocacy-related purposes there are advantages and disadvantages to using one over the other in various situations. **Table 8.4** outlines the comparative qualities of each.

TABLE 8.4 **Comparative Qualities of Social Networking Sites and Cell Phones in Advocacy**

Technology	Advantages for Advocacy	Disadvantages for Advocacy
Social Networking Sites	Message sent on SNS can be stored indefinitely	Not all advocates may be able to attend in-person events because of geographic distances inherent in an online community
	Easy to invite friends and fans to join the advocacy cause	Older decision makers may not give as much credence to this form of communication
	Can organize events and post specifics about location, time, and purpose	Requires Internet access
	Reach a large number of people quickly	
	One central location for advocates to find information about the advocacy cause	
	Can post videos or photos	
	Unlimited space to post information	
	Can update posts from a Web-enabled cell phone or mobile device	
	Can check posts from a Web-enabled cell phone or mobile device	
Cell Phones	Reach a large number of people quickly in real-time	A text or video message may be quickly erased
	Text or video message will be received immediately	Decision makers may not be able to answer the phone when in a meeting
	Can use phones to take photos	Have to limit messages to 160 characters
	Decision maker can read a text message while in a meeting	Advocates' cell phone calling plans may be limited by the number of text messages they can send
	Can be used to send quick, brief reminders of events	Not all advocates may own a cell phone
	No need for Internet access	Cell phone numbers may be changed and contact with advocates is lost.
	Can talk to the other individual in person.	
	Can forward text or video messages to friends and other advocates	

Source: "Empowering Youth: Use of Technology in Advocacy to Affect Social Change." R. Thackeray and M. Hunter, from the *Journal of Computer–Mediated Communication*, *Volume 15*, pp. 575–591. Copyright © 2010 by John Wiley & Sons, Inc. Reprinted with permission.

For planners interested in improving their knowledge and skills related to community advocacy activities, the Society for Public Health Education (SOPHE) and the American Public Health Association (APHA) have created useful guides. SOPHE's document is titled *Guide to Effectively Educating State and Local Policymakers* (available at: http://www.sophe.org/CDP/Ed_Policymakers_Guide.cfm), while APHA's is titled *APHA Legislative Advocacy Handbook: A Guide for Effective Public Health Advocacy* (available at: http://www.iowapha.org/resources/Documents/APHA Legislative Advocacy Handbook1.pdf).

Other Strategies

The other strategies category includes a variety of intervention activities that do not fit neatly into one of the six categories discussed above.

BEHAVIOR MODIFICATION ACTIVITIES

Behavior modification activities, often used in intrapersonal-level interventions, include techniques intended to help those in the priority population experience a change in behavior. *Behavior modification* is usually thought of as a systematic procedure for changing a specific behavior. The process is based on the stimulus response and social cognitive theories. As applied to health behavior, emphasis is placed on a specific behavior that one might want either to increase (such as exercise or stress management techniques) or to decrease (such as smoking or consumption of fats). Particular attention is then given to changing the events that are antecedent or subsequent to the behavior that is to be modified.

In changing a health behavior, the behavior modification activity often begins by having those trying to make a change keep records (diaries, logs, or journals) for a specific period of time (24 to 48 hours, one week, or one month) concerning the behavior (such as eating, smoking, or exercise) they want to alter. Using the information recorded, one can plan an activity to modify that behavior. For example, facilitators of smoking cessation programs often will ask participants to keep a record of all the cigarettes they smoke from one class session to the next (see **Figure 8.4** for an example of such a record). After keeping the record, participants are asked to analyze it to see what kind of smoking habit they have. They may be asked questions such as: "What three cigarettes seem to be the most important of the day to you?" "In what three places or activities do you find yourself smoking the most?" "With whom do you find yourself smoking most often?" "Is there a primary reason or mood for your smoking?" "When during the day do you find yourself smoking the most and the least?" Once the participant has answered these questions, appropriate interventions can be designed to deal with the problem behavior. For example, if participants say they smoke only when they are by themselves, then activities would be planned so that they do not spend a lot of time alone. If other participants seem to do most of their smoking while drinking coffee, an activity would be developed to provide some type of substitute. If participants seem to smoke the most while sitting at the table after meals, activities could be planned to get them away from the table and doing something that would occupy their hands.

Another way of leading into a behavior modification activity is through a health status evaluation, or what is often referred to as a *health screening*. Such screenings could happen at home (e.g., BSE, TSE, hemocult), at a community health fair (e.g., blood pressure, cholesterol), or in the office of a health care professional (e.g., breast examination). Like record keeping via diaries, logs, or journals, health screenings can "grab the attention" (develop awareness) of those in the priority population to begin the behavior modification process.

Name _____

Date _____

Numbers of Cigarettes During the Day	Time of Day	Need Rating*	Place of Activity	With Whom	Mood or Reason
1.	_____	1 2 3	_____	_____	_____
2.	_____	1 2 3	_____	_____	_____
3.	_____	1 2 3	_____	_____	_____
4.	_____	1 2 3	_____	_____	_____
5.	_____	1 2 3	_____	_____	_____
6.	_____	1 2 3	_____	_____	_____
7.	_____	1 2 3	_____	_____	_____
8.	_____	1 2 3	_____	_____	_____
9.	_____	1 2 3	_____	_____	_____
10.	_____	1 2 3	_____	_____	_____
11.	_____	1 2 3	_____	_____	_____
12.	_____	1 2 3	_____	_____	_____
13.	_____	1 2 3	_____	_____	_____
14.	_____	1 2 3	_____	_____	_____
15.	_____	1 2 3	_____	_____	_____
16.	_____	1 2 3	_____	_____	_____
17.	_____	1 2 3	_____	_____	_____
18.	_____	1 2 3	_____	_____	_____
19.	_____	1 2 3	_____	_____	_____
20.	_____	1 2 3	_____	_____	_____
21.	_____	1 2 3	_____	_____	_____
22.	_____	1 2 3	_____	_____	_____
23.	_____	1 2 3	_____	_____	_____
24.	_____	1 2 3	_____	_____	_____
25.	_____	1 2 3	_____	_____	_____
26.	_____	1 2 3	_____	_____	_____
27.	_____	1 2 3	_____	_____	_____
28.	_____	1 2 3	_____	_____	_____
29.	_____	1 2 3	_____	_____	_____
30.	_____	1 2 3	_____	_____	_____

*Need rating: How important is the cigarette to you at this time?

    1 = Most important; I would miss it very much

    2 = Average

    3 = Least important; I would not miss it

▲ **Figure 8.4** Twenty-Four-Hour Cigarette Count

ORGANIZATIONAL CULTURE ACTIVITIES

Closely aligned with environmental change strategies are activities that affect organizational culture. Culture is usually associated with norms and traditions that are generated by and linked to a "community" of people and reflects the group's values, beliefs, and practices. Organizations, which are made up of people, also can have their own culture. The culture of an organization can be thought of as its personality. The culture expresses what is and what is not considered important to the organization. "Cultural norms are not statistical averages, but instead are related to social standards of appropriate behavior. Cultural norms are accepted and expected practice" (Golaszewski et al., 2008, p. 7). The nature of the culture depends on the type of organization—corporation, school, or nonprofit group and the importance that the organization's leadership places on it. Thus, the leadership of an organization could advance a culture that supports health, or stated a bit differently, could advance a culture that includes health-related values, beliefs, and practices (Terry, 2012). For example, if organizational decision makers believe exercise is important, they may provide employees with an extra 20 minutes at lunchtime for exercise. Similarly, it is surprising to see how many young executives will use a corporation's exercise facility because the chief executive officer does. Other examples of organizational culture activities that support health might include changing the types of foods found in vending machines, closing the "junk food" machines during lunch periods at school, offering discounts on the health foods found in the company cafeteria, and getting retailers to change the way they have done things in the past, such as moving their tobacco products from in front of a counter to behind a counter, so that an employee has to get them for the customer.

For organizational culture activities to be effective in supporting a culture of health there must be a consistency about the importance of health throughout the organization. It must be system-wide and delivered through multiple channels (Terry, 2014). For example, if a culture of health is to be achieved, if an organizational culture activity is associated with employee benefits (e.g., regular free health screenings), it would be counter productive to stock the organization's vending machines with unhealthy snack choices.

Like other health promotion strategies, the use of organizational culture activities should begin with an assessment. The term that has been given to assessments associated with organizational culture is a *culture* (or *cultural*) *audit*. A **cultural audit** is an evaluation of the assumptions, values, normative philosophies, and cultural characteristics of an organization in order to determine whether they support or hinder that organization's central mission (BusinessDictionary.com, 2015b). When applied to health, the audit would help determine whether the culture hinders or supports health. There are companies that will perform health culture audits for organizations (Note: search the Internet with key words "health culture audit" for sources). In addition, the Wellness Council of America (WELCOA) has created a free WELCOA Quick-Inventory (Hunnicutt, 2009) as a means to help assess the environment of a workplace.

Once the status of the organizational culture has been determined there are several steps that can be taken to work toward a health supporting culture. Golaszewski and his colleagues (2008) have identified the following influences on an organization's health supporting culture: (1) shaping cultural health values (e.g., raise the visibility of benefits of healthy lifestyles, raise the visibility of leadership promoting healthy lifestyles, encourage employee forums where they can discuss health, showcase the organization's involvement in health promotion); (2) shaping cultural health norms (e.g., identify key norms for health promotion in the organization, conduct interviews of those in the priority population to determine support or lack thereof for a healthy culture, evaluate idea versus actual norm levels); (3) use cultural touch points (e.g., mechanisms that support a healthy culture like committing resources to health, leaders' modeling healthy lifestyles, rewards and recognitions for health, include health promoting ideas in organizational recruitment, orientation, training, communication, relationships, and rites, symbols, and rituals); (4) encourage peer support (e.g., mobilize existing support systems, develop mutual support systems); and (5) building a supportive cultural climate for health (e.g., foster a sense of community, foster a shared vision, foster a positive outlook, and foster cultural climate with health promotion).

INCENTIVES AND DISINCENTIVES

The use of incentives (sometimes referred to as "carrots") and disincentives (sometimes referred to as "sticks") to influence health behaviors is a common type of activity, especially in worksite settings. However, it has also been applied to community and public health settings (Ashraf, 2013). An **incentive** is "an anticipated positive or desirable reward designed to influence the performance of an individual or group" (Chapman, 2005, p. 6). An incentive can increase the perceived value of an activity (Patton et al., 1986), motivate people to get involved, encourage health service use behavior (Chapman, 2005), encourage compliance with professional health advice (Chapman, 2005), remind program participants of their commitment to and goals for behavior change (Wilbur, 1983), promote short-term behavior change (French, Jeffery, & Oliphant, 1994; Robison, 1998), and maintain behavior change over time (Ashraf, 2013; Pescatello et al., 2001; Poole, Kumpfer, & Pett, 2001). Incentives can work because they make good health decisions easier and poor ones more difficult (Ashraf, 2013). The key to motivating people with incentives, either intrinsic or extrinsic, is knowing what will incite them to action. Thus for this type of activity to work, the planners need to match the incentives with the needs, wants, or desires of the priority population. However, this is not easy, for what is an incentive for one person may be a deterrent for another, and vice versa. If planners are not in touch with what program participants want, there is a chance of losing participant interest in the program (Hunnicutt, 2001). Therefore, incentives work best when they are tailored to the individual characteristics of the participants. For example, a financial incentive will typically generate less response from wealthy participants than lower income participants (Haveman, 2010).

Because incentives are used to assist individuals in making decisions about their health, it is important to better understand what influences decision making. We only need to look around us to see that individuals do not always make good health choices. Consider individuals who continue to smoke even though they know it is bad for their health. To help understand the reasoning behind such decisions, the concept of *behavioral economics* can help. Behavioral economics has been called "the hybrid offspring of economics and psychology" (Lambert, 2006, p. 53). *Neoclassical economics* or *traditional economics* assumes individuals make decisions based on rational thinking by weighting the gains (pros) and losses (cons) associated with the decision. **Behavioral economics** is a method of analysis that applies psychological insights into decision making. Thus, behavioral economists believe that decisions are not based solely on rational thinking but that they are highly dependent on the context in which the decision is made (Samson, 2014; Zimmerman, 2009). Here are some behavioral economic insights that help explain decision making. Individuals: (1) are more concerned about avoiding losses than acquiring gains, (2) are comfortable with status quo and do not want to change, (3) are aware of social norms and want to conform, (4) experience decision

> **BOX 8.6**
>
> *Highlights*
>
> ## Behavioral Economics
>
> To address some of the insights from behavioral economics program planners have used several different techniques to assist people to making good health decision. One of these techniques is message *framing*. Planners who frame their health promotion programs by emphasizing the "program benefits" versus "program obligations" have had better results in getting people to make good health decisions. For example, a smoking cessation program framed as "You are not alone in your battle to quit, come see what a smokefree life can mean for you," has a much better chance of resulting in a good health decision than one framed as "This smoking cessation program is science-based and has shown good results for those who stick with it." Another technique used to help people make good health decisions and sustain change overtime has been *commitment devices*. An example of a commitment device related to a weight loss program would have enrollees put up a bond, say $500, at the beginning of the program and would not be returned until their goal weight was reached. In addition, the bond could also be donated to a charity if the goal weight was not reached in a reasonable period of time. Such a program takes advantage of people's tendency to prefer avoiding losses to acquiring gains.

fatigue (i.e., choice overload) and put off difficult choices, (5) use heuristics (i.e., shortcuts or quick answers) because of decision fatigue, (6) have trouble evaluating probabilities associated with health decisions, and (7) overvalue the present outcomes of decision and discount the future outcomes (i.e., present bias) (Arhraf, 2013; Riedel & Calao, 2014). (See **Box 8.6** for an application of behavioral economics.)

For program planners, the task becomes one of matching the needs of the program participant or potential program participant with available incentives. A couple of different approaches can be used to accomplish this. The first is to include questions about incentives as part of any needs assessment conducted in program planning keeping in mind the insights from behavioral economics. For example, a needs survey or focus group might include a question on incentives, such as "What incentives would entice you to participate in the exercise program?" or "What would it take to get you to participate in this program?" or "What would it take to keep you involved in a health promotion program?" or "Would you continue to participate in an exercise program if you knew you were going to be given a nice T-shirt after logging 100 miles running or walking, or participating for 50 days in a yoga class or swimming program?" The responses to these questions should provide some indication of the type of incentives that would be most appropriate for this priority population.

A second approach would be to conduct an "experiment" with different incentives. This could be accomplished via a pilot study with a small group from the priority population using different incentives. In such a pilot study, half of the participants would receive one incentive, while the other half would receive another. The outcomes at which the incentives were aimed would then be compared to determine which incentive was more useful. A third approach would be use the most promising incentive based on previous experience or the experience reported by others (see discussion on best experiences later in the chapter). This third approach might be used when program resources are limited.

Based on the idea that incentives should meet the individual needs of those in the priority population, the possibility of different types of incentives is almost endless. Incentives are usually grouped into two major categories: material (i.e., financial) and nonmaterial.

Some examples of material incentives include providing any material item (e.g., food, clothing) of worth to those in the priority population, or actual money in the form of extra pay, bonuses, or rebates (Ashraf, 2013; Chapman 2005; Haveman, 2010; Pescatello et al., 2001; Poole, Kumpfer, & Pett, 2001); paying membership fees to health-related facilities (Chapman, 2005); giving gift certificates; or reducing health insurance premiums or deductibles. Examples of nonmaterial incentives include altruistic feeling like after giving blood (Ashraf, 2013; Serxner, 2013), giving special attention or recognition (e.g., name mentioned in a newsletter) (Chapman, 2005; Haveman, 2010), social support, or providing additional vacation days or "well" days (Chapman, 2005; Haveman, 2010).

Terry and Anderson (2011) noted that incentives should be safe, effective, participant-centered, timely, and equitable. In addition, Haveman (2010) has offered six principles that can assist program planners in creating effective incentives. His principles were intended for use with incentives associated with the delivery of health care, but we have adapted them to health promotion. Principle one is identifying the desired outcome or, stated a different way, what is the problem that needs to be addressed. This may seem obvious but is often overlooked. For example, if the desired outcome is to have program participants stop smoking, the incentives should be tied to quitting or the steps to quitting. The second principle is identifying the behavior change that will lead to the desired outcome. In the smoking cessation example, participants need to come up with a strategy to quit smoking, actually stop, and stay off cigarettes for a specified period of time. Principle three is determining the potential effectiveness of the incentive in achieving the behavior change. This is not easy because responsiveness to incentives varies greatly. "Understanding this response involves determining the extent to which the behavior targeted is amenable to change through the incentive" (Haveman, 2010, p. 2). The "size" of the incentive should be appropriate to the effort required. If the perceived benefit of the action is exceeded by its perceived cost, the incentive will be ineffective (Haveman, 2010). (See **Box 8.7** for a list of factors that determine the effectiveness incentives.) The fourth principle is to link the incentive directly to the desired outcome or behavior. In the smoking cessation example, any incentive should be linked to either the final outcome—no smoking for one year after the quit date—or to the actions leading up to it, for example, setting a quit date, deciding on a strategy to quit, actually quitting, not smoking for six months, and not smoking for one year. If the second option is used, an incentive could be attached to each step. Further if this second option is used the incentives could be graduated so that incentives are worth more than the one given at the previous step. Principle five is identifying any possible adverse effects of the incentive. In the smoking cessation example, nonsmokers may say that they have no chance to receive a smoking cessation incentive. So how could those creating the incentive deal with this situation? The sixth, and final, principle is to evaluate and report changes in the behavior or outcome in response to the incentive. If a case is going to be made for using incentives as part of health promotion programs in the future, planners will need to document their work and show that the incentives, at least in part, were responsible for the outcomes or desired behavior.

Just as incentives can be used to get people involved in behavior change, *disincentives* can be used to discourage a certain behavior. More formally, **disincentives** have been defined as "an anticipated negative or undesirable consequence designed to influence the performance of an individual or group" (Chapman, 2005, p. 6). For example, "[s]ustained increases in excise taxes, constraining advertising and marketing, constricting use in public places, and penalizing the sale and distribution to minors have all worked to help drive down the use of tobacco" (McGinnis et al., 2002, pp. 88–89).

BOX

8.7

Focus On

Factors That Determine the Effectiveness of Incentives

MAJOR FACTORS	MINOR FACTORS
● Dollar value of the reward(s)	● Importance to supervisor
● Convertibility into item of personal value	● Degree of fun experienced
● Amount of effort needed to qualify	● Language compatibility
● Clarity of messaging	● Convenience of record keeping
● Timing and repetition of messaging	● Amount of change in benefits
● Extent of distrust in employers' motives	● Availability of alternative standards
● Supporting messages from management	● Credibility of wellness staff
● Ease of enrollment	● Use of outside vendor
● Perceived complexity of requirements	● Adequacy of FAQs
● Fairness and defensibility of requirements	● Availability of FAQs
● Group or competitive nature	● Treatment of "gamers"
● Desirability of required behavior	● Utility of program documents
● Readiness composition of population	● Tax implications
● Combination of pay values	● Option to ask questions
● Spousal eligibility	● Time of the year
● Compatibility of incentives with culture	● Generational effects
● Past wellness incentive performance	● Reporting back to employees

Source: "The Changing role of incentives in health promotion and wellness." L. S. Chapman, D. Whitehead, and M. C. Connors, from *The Art of Health Promotion*. Copyright © 2008 by *American Journal of Health Promotion*. Reprinted with permission.

One final note that we need to mention before leaving this topic is the impact that federal legislation has had on incentives and disincentives. As we noted at the beginning of this section, though incentives and disincentives have been used in health promotion programs in a variety of settings, they have been used with great favor in worksite settings. Up until 1996, there were few limitations on how incentive and disincentives were structured (Chapman, 2005) and because of this some employers were creatively tying incentives and disincentives associated with health to individual and group health insurance plans. However, Congress was concerned that employers were being unfair to some employees in order to reduce their health care costs. Accordingly, Congress has now enacted three pieces of legislation that have impacted the way incentives and disincentives can be used. They include the Health Insurance Portability & Accountability Act of 1996 (more commonly referred to as HIPAA), the Genetic Information Nondiscrimination Act of 2008 (officially known as Public Law 110-233 and referred to as *GINA*), and the Affordable Care Act (ACA) (ACA actually refers to two separate pieces of legislation—the Patient Protection and Affordable Care Act [P.L. 111-148] and the Health Care and Education Reconciliation Act of 2010 [P.L. 111-152].

HIPAA created provisions in it that make it illegal for employers to discriminate against their employees because of a "health status related factor" with the outcome of affecting coverage or cost to the employee under a group or individual health plan (Chapman, 2005). That is, those who offer and administer health insurance plans cannot deny health care claim expenses, charge some employees more for their health insurance premiums, or place a surcharge on their premiums because of health status related conditions like high blood pressure, high blood cholesterol, or poor vision. For example, an employer cannot require employees to pay higher premiums than their coworkers because they have high blood pressure. However, the law does not preclude offering incentives—in the form of premium discounts or rebates or modifying applicable co-payments or deductibles—to those who participate in health promotion programs. So an employer could reduce employees' co-payment on a visit to a doctor or on the cost of a prescription medication if the employees participated in the company's employee health promotion program.

GINA, which amends portions of HIPAA by treating genetic information as *protected health information* (PHI), prohibits discrimination in health coverage and employment based on genetic information. GINA went into effect for health care plans starting on or after December 7, 2009. Though the bulk of GINA is aimed at health care coverage provided by employers, it also impacts health promotion/wellness programs. The area of health promotion programming that it most affected is the use of health risk assessments (HRAs). HRAs cannot request genetic information prior to enrollment in a health care "plan, and no rewards or penalties may be offered in conjunction with an HRA that requests genetic information, even if the request is made after the enrollment" (Grudzien, 2009, para. 6). As a result of these regulations, planners "should review all wellness and disease management plans to determine how a HRA is used and what information is requested; remove any financial incentives or penalties if genetic information is collected in the HRA; and remove any genetic information from the HRA if financial incentives or penalties want to be offered" (Grudzien, 2009, para. 6).

The ACA further refined rules associated with how incentives could be used in programs that are a part of group health insurance plans. These new rules apply to health plans that began on or after January 1, 2014. The ACA continued to support employee wellness programs but also included rules to ensure the programs would not discriminate based on health status. It did so by making a distinction between *participatory wellness programs* and *health-contingent wellness programs*. A participatory wellness program is one that does not provide an incentive or does not tie an incentive to a health factor. Examples of participatory program incentives include: fitness center membership reimbursements; paying employees who complete a health risk assessment without requiring them to take further action, or waiving an out-of-pocket cost for attending a smoking cessation program that is not contingent on quitting.

A health-contingent wellness program is one that requires individuals to meet a specific health-related standard to obtain an incentive. Examples include programs that provide an incentive to those who do not use, or decrease their use of tobacco, or programs that provide an incentive to those who achieve a specified cholesterol or blood pressure level (USDOL, n.d.).

Because health-contingent wellness programs have the potential to discriminate based on health status, the ACA also includes the following:

1. Programs must give those covered by the health insurance plan an opportunity to qualify for the incentive at least once per year.

2. Programs must be designed to have a reasonable chance of improving health or preventing disease and not be overly burdensome for individuals.

3. Programs must be reasonably designed to be available to all similarly situated individuals (i.e., those with same problems or circumstances).

4. Programs must include a reasonable alternative standard or waiver to qualify for the incentive for individuals whose medical conditions make it unreasonably difficult, or

for whom it is medically inadvisable, to meet the specified health-related standard. In addition, individuals must be given notice of the opportunity to qualify for the same incentive through other means.

5. The incentives for wellness program participants may not exceed 30% of the cost of health insurance coverage.

SOCIAL ACTIVITIES

The importance of social support for behavior change and its relationship to health have been known for a number of years (e.g., IOM, 2001). Many people find it much easier to change a behavior if those around them provide support or are willing to be partners in the behavior change process. Social support can be provided in a variety of ways. "There are at least four types of social support: (1) emotional, (2) instrumental, (3) informational, and (4) appraisal" (Valente, 2010, pp. 36-37). *Emotional support* is assistance from people close to a person that focuses on the person's feelings. *Instrumental support* deals with providing material items and services to people. *Informational support* comes in the format of providing various forms of information such as advice, knowledge, and suggestions to people. Appraisal support includes analysis and feedback that allows people to evaluate their situation (Valente, 2010). A discussion of several different types of social support activities that can provide these different types of social support follows.

SUPPORT GROUPS AND BUDDY SYSTEM

The importance of support groups as part of comprehensive interventions has been well established. One need only look to the 12-step programs (e.g., Alcoholics Anonymous, Overeaters Anonymous, and Gamblers Anonymous) and commercial programs (e.g., Weight Watchers) to realize the importance of people coming together to share their experiences and support one another's efforts. A support group need not be large; it might be as small as just two people. A buddy system is an example of a two-person group. A buddy system can take one of two different forms. In the first, both individuals are trying to change a behavior. In such a relationship, the two individuals support each other, whether this means helping each other stay on a special diet or meeting each other at 6 A.M. for exercise. In the other form, only one of the two is trying to change a behavior. The one not changing the behavior may have already changed (e.g., has already quit smoking or is exercising regularly) and is acting as a mentor to the one trying to change, or may not be trying to change but provides support at regular intervals or as problems arise.

To enhance the motivation provided by support groups and buddy systems it is not uncommon for these activities to also use a *contest* (also referred to competitions or challenges) or a *contract*. A **contest** can be described as a challenge between two individuals/groups in which the object is to outperform the competitor. Examples of contests include the competition between two individuals to see who can lose the most weight, who can walk/run the most miles, or who can go the longest without a cigarette. Contests could also be based on teams within the priority population (such as two different companies, two schools, or departments within an organization), using similar criteria but now based on group total figures (pounds, miles, or cigarettes). Contests have been useful in introducing and promoting health promotion programs and achieving significant initial participation rates, but they have not been as useful as an ongoing recruitment tool (Wilson, 1990).

A **contract** is an agreement between two or more parties that outlines the future behavior of those parties. Contracts are a common part of everyday living. People enter into contracts when they sign a lease for an apartment or a residence hall agreement, take out an insurance policy, borrow money, or buy something over a period of time. The same concept can be applied to getting and keeping people motivated in health promotion programs. Program participants would enter into a contract with another person (the program facilitator, a significant other, or a fellow participant) and then work toward an objective or agreement specified in the contract. The contract would also specify **contingencies**—that is, what happens as a result of the contract's term either being met or not being met.

For an exercise program, this system might work as follows: The program participant and program facilitator would draw up a contract based on the participant's present status in the program (e.g., exercising for 30 minutes once a week) and on what would be a reasonable goal for the near future (e.g., eight weeks). Thus the contract might state that the participant will exercise for 30 minutes twice a week for the first week, 30 minutes three times a week for the second week, and so forth, building up gradually to the final goal of exercising for 30 minutes most days of the week at the end of eight weeks. The outcome should focus on a behavior that can be maintained at the end of the contract period. For a weight loss program, the goal might be written as eliminating snacking in the evening, increasing fruits and vegetables in the diet to five servings per day, and walking for 30 minutes three times a week. These are behaviors that can reasonably be maintained after the weight loss.

The parties to the contract then decide on what the contingencies will be. Thus the participant might offer to make a contribution to some local charity or state that she will continue in the program for another eight weeks if she does not meet the contract goal. The facilitator might promise the participant a program T-shirt if she fulfills the contract during the specified eight-week period. Other ideas for contingencies might include granting a kickback on fees for completing a certain percentage of the classes, or earning points toward products or services. No matter what the contingencies are, it seems to help if the contract is completed in writing.

SOCIAL GATHERINGS

Social gatherings can be an important type of social intervention. Bringing together people who may be confronting similar problems for the purpose of purely social interaction not related to the problem can indirectly help them deal with the problem. Examples of such activities might be single parents having a cookout or a group of senior citizens attending a play. Although these gatherings do not deal directly with these people's common problems, they do help fill voids in their lives and thus indirectly help with the problem.

SOCIAL NETWORKS

Social networks are another type of social intervention. A *social network* is the "web of social relationships and the structural characteristics of that web" (IOM, 2001, p. 7). The nature of the structural characteristics can be quite varied, consisting of almost anything that creates a special feeling: need, concern, loyalty, frustration, power, affection, or obligation, to name just a few. When people are "networking," they are said to be looking for relationships that would be useful in helping them with their concerns, such as problem solving, program development, resource identification, and others. As part of a health promotion intervention, social networking may take many different forms and can range from informal networking where participants create relations on their own to more formal networking where program participants are "assigned" others with whom to network. The actual networking itself may take place face-to-face, via the telephone, or through some type of social media. An example would be when program smoking cessation participants trade contact information (e.g., email address, telephone numbers, or "friend" another) for the purpose of connecting when trying to resist a cigarette or trying to locate a needed resource to solve a problem.

It should also be noted that although most social support and buddy systems take place between individuals, they can also be established at the institutional level. Like individuals, institutions can be paired up to help one another. For example, if two companies are interested in establishing health promotion programs, they could work together on their programs and share information and resources where appropriate. Or, if one company has a well-established program in place, then that company could mentor another company in setting up a program.

▷ Creating Health Promotion Interventions

Once program planners have completed a needs assessment, written program goals and objectives, and considered different types of intervention strategies, they are in a position to begin identifying an appropriate intervention. Identifying an intervention is not as straight-forward as taking a new medical procedure from one hospital to the next. Most health promotion problems result from the interaction of complicated social dynamics that must be accommodated (Runyan & Freire, 2007). There is no one best way of intervening to accomplish a specific program goal that can be generalized to all priority populations. Each priority population has unique needs and wants that must be addressed, and each setting has its own peculiarities. Nevertheless, well planned and successful health promotion programs have common characteristics such as: (1) addressing one or more risk factors of the priority population, (2) being theory-driven, (3) being based on the best possible evidence (see the discussion of scientific evidence later in the chapter), (4) adhering to professional ethical standards, (5) being culturally appropriate, (6) being consistent with professional criteria, guidelines, or codes of practice (e.g., America College of Sports Medicine's guidelines for exercise programs (ACSM, 2014)), (7) using resources efficiently, and (8) including an evaluation component. Such characteristics help standardize and ensure the quality of the program, give credibility to a program, help with program accountability, provide a legal defense if a liability situation might arise, and identify ethical concerns that need to be addressed as a part of planning, implementing, and evaluating programs.

Intervention Planning

When deciding on how best to intervene to reach the program goals and objectives, program planners have three possible avenues available to them. They could *adopt* an existing intervention that is supported by evidence showing that the intervention was effective when used elsewhere. They could *adapt* an existing intervention that is supported by evidence showing it was effective elsewhere but the circumstances or setting in which it was used were different that the proposed setting. Or, the planners could design a new intervention. Irrespective of the avenue used to identify an intervention, interventions should be based on a sound rationale backed by the best available evidence as opposed to chance; a strategy should not be selected just because the planners think it "sounds good" or because they have a "feeling" that it will work. Too often, intervention decisions are "based on perceived short-term opportunities, lacking systematic planning and review of the best evidence regarding effective approaches" (Brownson, Fielding, & Maylahn, 2009, p. 175). As mentioned earlier, planners should choose or create an intervention that will be both effective and efficient.

Adopting a Health Promotion Intervention

In order for program planners to adopt an intervention for use in their program there are several questions they must be able to respond to with a "Yes" answer. The questions include: (1) Is there sufficient evidence to show that the intervention has been successful in dealing with the problem in question? (2) Is there sufficient evidence to show that the intervention has been successful in dealing with the problem in question in a population with similar characteristics (e.g., age, sex, culture, racial/ethnic make-up, social circumstances) to the population in the new setting? (3) Is there evidence to show that the intervention was successful in more than one setting? (4) Are there similar resources available in the new setting to ensure the fidelity of the intervention? and (5) Is the new environment setting similar to the environmental setting identified in the evidence? If "No" is the answer to any of these questions then planners should consider either adapting the existing intervention or developing a new intervention. If the answers to the questions are not clearly "Yes" or "No" Runyan and Freire, (2007) have noted that planners might "benefit from discussion among several people knowledgeable about the problem, the setting, and program planning" (p. 423).

Adapting a Health Promotion Intervention

If the evidence supporting the successful use of an intervention is different (e.g., social context or other unique characteristics) than the one in which the planners are currently working, the question becomes "Can the intervention that was successful in another setting (i.e., evidence-based intervention [EBI]) be adapted to work in the new setting?" That is, can an intervention be adapted to the circumstance in which the priority population lives? To help answer this question, the CDC's Division of HIV/AIDS, along with some external partners, developed draft guidance to adapt EBIs (McKleroy et al., 2006). The approach of this framework emphasizes both the planners' experience working with the priority population and the resources available for adaption and implementation, while still maintaining fidelity to the core elements of the intervention, the theory on which it was based, and internal logic of the original intervention (McKleroy et al., 2006).

The adaptation framework is a five-step approach that is presented graphically in a linear format (see **Figure 8.5**). However, like other planning models presented in this book, the steps are interconnected and thus overlap in terms of their timing and ordering. McKleroy et al. (2006) have presented the following description of the five steps.

> The first action step, assess, involves assessing the target population, the EBIs being considered for implementation, and the agency's capacity to implement the intervention. The second, select, is determining whether to adopt the intervention without adaptation, implement the intervention with adaptation, or choose another intervention and repeating the assess action step before moving forward. The third action step, prepare, falls within the preparation phase and involves actually adapting the intervention materials, pre-testing the adapted materials with the target population, and increasing agency capacity and developing collaborative partnerships when necessary to implement the intervention. The fourth action step, pilot, is pilot testing the adapted intervention or its components if it is not feasible to pilot the entire

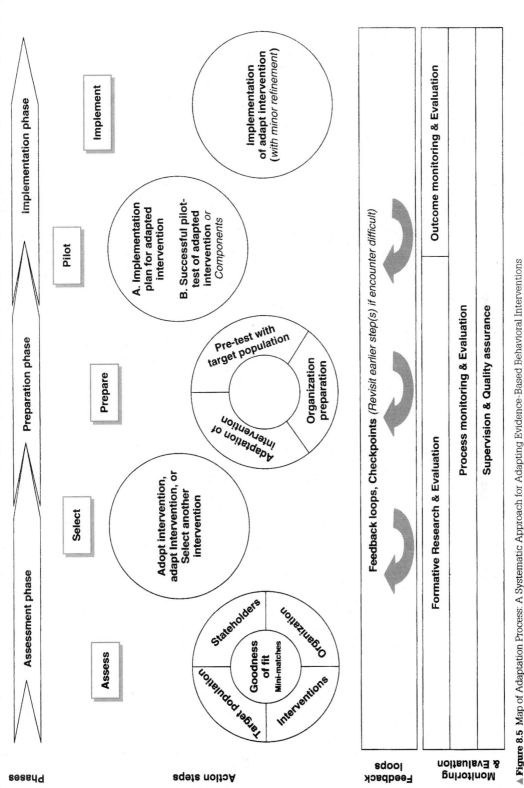

▲ **Figure 8.5** Map of Adaptation Process: A Systematic Approach for Adapting Evidence-Based Behavioral Interventions

Source: **McKleroy**, V. S., Galbraith, J. S., Cummings, B., Jones, P., Harshbarger, C., Collins, C., Gelaude, D., Carey, J. W., & ADAPT Team (2006). Adapting evidence-based behavioral interventions for new settings and target populations. *AIDS Education and Prevention, 19*(Suppl. A), 59–73.

227

intervention and developing an implementation plan. The fifth, implement, is conducting the entire adapted intervention with minor revision as needed. Additionally, the guidance includes feedback loops and checkpoints to ensure each action step is addressed adequately, and to provide an opportunity to revisit earlier action steps should difficulties occur. Process monitoring and evaluation, and routine supervision and quality assurance are also important considerations for the guidance. Credible evidence collected during the adaptation process should be evaluated to determine the success of the adaptation process as well as the effectiveness of the adapted intervention (p. 64).

If you are interested in adapting an EBI, we strongly recommend that you review McKleroy et al. (2006) for a more in-depth description and practical examples of the five-step framework.

Designing a New Health Promotion Intervention

If there is not sufficient evidence to support the adoption or adaptation of an intervention to a new setting then planners are faced with creating a new intervention. Although no prescription for an appropriate intervention has been developed, experience has indicated that the results of some interventions are more predictable than others. In this section, we present eight major questions that planners need to consider when creating new health promotion interventions. **Figure 8.6** summarizes these major considerations.

1. *What needs to change? And, where is the change needed?* Designing an appropriate intervention begins by going back to the early steps in the program planning process and examining the results of the needs assessment and reviewing the goals and

▲ **Figure 8.6** Items to Consider When Creating a Health Promotion Intervention

objectives of the proposed program. The needs assessment identified the behavioral, environmental, and genetic determinants or risk factors of the health problem. (Note: Remember that because genetic determinants either cannot be changed or often interact with behavior and environment, the planners' focus should be on behavioral and environmental factors.) For example, after identifying the determinants of a health problem, planners then determine the predisposing, enabling, and reinforcing factors that need to be addressed in their proposed program. These factors should be reflected in the program goals and objectives. If the single purpose of a program were to increase the awareness of the priority population, the intervention would be very different from what it would be if the purpose were to change behavior.

Knowing what must be changed is critical to creating an intervention, but just as critical is understanding the context in which the change will take place. Understanding the context has been referred to as the *settings approach* (Baric, 1993) to health promotion. More specifically, a settings approach means addressing the contexts (physical, organizational, and social) "within which people live, work, and play and making these the object of inquiry and intervention as well as the needs and capacities of the people found in the different settings" (Poland, Krupa, & McCall, 2009, p. 505). Therefore when creating an intervention, planners need to analyze the setting—"who is there; how they think or operate; implicit social norms, hierarchies of power; accountability mechanisms; local moral, political, and organizational culture; physical and psychosocial environment; broader sociopolitical and economic context, etc." (Poland et al., 2009, p. 506)—to make sure the intervention is a good "fit" for those in the priority population. For those interested in more of what to consider when analyzing the setting, we recommend the questions posed by Poland et al. (2009).

2. *At what level of prevention will the program be aimed?* Because of the needs and wants of those in the priority population, planners need to consider at which level or levels of prevention—primary, secondary, and tertiary—the program will be aimed. For example, a program aimed at increasing the level of exercise is likely to be received differently by asymptomatic nonexercisers (primary prevention) than by a patient recovering from a heart attack (tertiary prevention).

3. *At what level(s) of influence will the intervention be focused?* Program planners must recognize that those in the priority population "live in social, political, and economic systems that shape behaviors and access to the resources they need to maintain good health" (Pellmar et al., 2002, p. 210). As such, planners need to decide at what level or levels of influence they can best obtain the goals and objectives of the program. For example, if the goal of the program is to increase safety belt use, can that be best accomplished by trying to intervene at an intrapersonal level with an individual education program, at the institutional level with a company policy, at the public policy level with an enhanced state safety belt law, or at multiple levels? Though it is possible that an intervention can be aimed at a single level of influence, the evidence is mounting that there is a greater chance of changing and maintaining health behaviors if interventions are aimed at multiple levels of influence (Glanz & Bishop, 2010). Therefore, planners need to ask and answer the question, "What levels of influence should be addressed to provide the best chances of achieving the program goal and objectives?"

4. *What types of intervention strategies are known to be effective (i.e., have been successfully used in previous programs) in dealing with the program focus?* In other words, what does the evidence show about the effectiveness of various interventions to deal with the problem that the program is to address? (Refer back to Chapter 2 for the definition of and available sources

of evidence.) Using evidence does not mean finding a specific intervention to deal with the problem but rather going through a process of decision making that is based on the evaluation of reliable data and previous work (Baker, Brownson, Dreisinger, McIntosh, & Karamehic-Muratovic, 2009). To assist planners in identifying the best available evidence, Green and Kreuter (2005) and Brownson and colleagues (2009) have put forth typologies for classifying interventions based on the level of scientific evidence. Green and Kreuter (2005) have suggested three sources of guidance for selecting intervention strategies—best practices, best experiences, and best processes. **Best practices** refer to "recommendations for an intervention, based on critical review of multiple research and evaluation studies that substantiate the efficacy of the intervention in the populations and circumstances in which the studies were done, if not its effectiveness in other populations and situations where it might be implemented" (p. G-1).

When best practice recommendations are not available for use, planners need to look for information on *best experiences*. **Best experience** intervention strategies are those of prior or existing programs that have not gone through the critical research and evaluation studies and thus fall short of best practice criteria but nonetheless show promise in being effective. Best experiences can be found by networking with other professionals and by reviewing the literature.

If neither best practices nor best experiences are available to planners, then the third source of guidance for selecting an intervention strategy is using *best processes*. **Best processes** intervention strategies are original interventions that the planners create based upon their knowledge and skills of good planning processes including the involvement of those in the priority population and appropriate theories and models (see Chapter 7). (See **Table 8.5** for a matrix of aligning objectives, program outcomes, methods, theory, intervention strategies, and activities.)

Whereas the Green and Kreuter (2005) typology for classifying interventions has three levels, the typology put forth by Brownson and colleagues (2009) has four—*evidence-based, effective, promising,* and *emerging.* The first level, evidence-based, includes interventions that are peer reviewed via a systematic or narrative review (e.g., those contained in the *Guide to Community Preventive Services* [CDC, 2015c]). This first level is parallel to the best practices level of Green and Kreuter (2005). The interventions found in the second level, *effective*, have been peer reviewed but are not part of a systematic or narrative review (e.g., article that appears in the scientific literature). Those interventions that are deemed effective via a program evaluation but without formal peer review make up the third level, *promising* (e.g., state or federal government reports that have not gone through peer review). Levels two and three, effective and promising respectively, are parallel to the best experiences described by Green and Kreuter (2005). The fourth and final level is *emerging*. This level includes ongoing works, practice-based summaries, or evaluation works in progress (e.g., pilot studies).

5. *Is the intervention an appropriate fit for the priority population?* Intervention strategies need to be designed to "fit" the priority population. Each priority population has certain characteristics that impact how it will receive an intervention. Two processes that help to "fit" an intervention to the priority population are tailoring and segmenting. The rationale for tailoring an intervention activity is based on research that shows people pay more attention to information that is personally relevant to them (NCI, n.d.). Because we presented information on tailoring earlier in the chapter in our discussion of health communication section, we will use this space to present information on segmenting. **Segmenting** is the process of dividing a broader population into smaller groups with similar characteristics that are likely to exhibit similar behavior/ reaction to an intervention (see information in Chapter 11 about segmenting a priority

TABLE 8.5 Matrix of Type of Objectives, Program Outcomes, Methods, Theory, Intervention Strategy, and Activities

Type of Objective	Program Outcome	Method	Theory—Construct*	Intervention Strategy	Possible Activities
Learning	• Awareness of risk perception/services/resources	Information	HBM—perceived susceptibility PMT—perceived severity TTM—processes of change	Health communication	• Informational session • Completion of HRA
		Raising awareness	SCT—expectations	Health communication	• Brochure on risks
	• Knowledge	Active learning	SCT—behavioral capability HBM—perceived seriousness HBM—perceived benefits/barriers	Health education	• Classes, seminars, workshops • Printed materials
		Tailoring	PAPM—stages TTM—stages	Health communication and education	• Classes, seminars, workshops
	• Attitudes	Persuasive communication	SCT—expectancies	Health communication and education	• Classes, seminars, workshops • Panel discussions
		Processing information	TTM—decisional balance ELM—central route TPB—attitude toward the behavior SCT—reinforcement IMB—prevention motivation		• Guest speakers
	• Skills	Skills training and practice	SCT/HBM/TTM—self-efficacy TPB—perceived behavioral control	Health communication and education	• Classes, seminars, workshops • Simulations
			SCT—self-control	Behavior modification	

231

TABLE 8.5 *continued*

Type of Objective	Program Outcome	Method	Theory—Construct*	Intervention Strategy	Possible Activities
Behavioral	• Behavior	Modeling	SCT—reinforcement		• Scenarios, role playing
		Coping response	C-BMRP—self-control		
		Reinforcement	HBM—cues to action	Incentives	• Determine and provide incentives
			SRT—punishment/ reinforcement	Behavior modification	• 24-hour behavior records
		Counterconditioning	TTM—processes of change	Health communication and education	• Keeping journals
				Organizational culture	• Classes, seminars, workshops
		Modeling	SCT—reinforcement		• Peer education
Environmental	• Physical environment	Facilitation	SCT—reciprocal determinism	Health policy/ enforcement	• Regulations/ ordinances
		Barriers	HBM—perceived barriers	Environmental change	
			C-BMRP—high-risk situation		
		Organizational building	CRM—stages	Community mobilization	• Create a coalition
	• Social environment	Social support	TPB—subjective norm	Social activities	• Create networks/ buddies
			SNT—ego/alter	Social Networks	

Abbreviations for theories: C-BMRP = cognitive–behavior model of relapse prevention; CRM = community readiness model; ELM = elaboration likelihood model of persuasion; HBM = health belief model; IMB = information—motivation—behavioral skills model; PAPM = precaution adoption process model; PMT = protection motivation theory; SCT = social cognitive theory; SNT = social network theory; SRT = stimulus response theory; TPB = theory of planned behavior; TTM = transtheoretical model.

population). Segmentation allows planners to create an intervention to fit the needs and characteristics of a priority population (Pasick, D'Onofrio, & Otero-Sabogal, 1996). Following are a few examples of how priority population segmentation can be applied. If program planners are developing written materials as part of their intervention, they need to make sure that the materials are written at an acceptable reading level for the priority population. From a developmental stage perspective, it is not reasonable to expect kindergartners to sit still for a one-hour lesson. Interventions also need to "fit" culturally within the priority population (Pérez & Luquis, 2014) and be **culturally sensitive**. Culturally sensitive interventions are those "that are relevant and acceptable within the cultural framework of the population to be reached" (Frankish, Lovato, & Shannon, 1998). In attempts to be culturally sensitive, because culture is often context specific, planners need to be careful not to perpetuate harmful cultural stereotypes.

One final item to consider when thinking about the appropriateness of an intervention strategy for the priority population is to ask if there is any chance that the strategy could cause any unintended effects in the priority population. For example, could the strategy threaten the physical safety or raise undue anxiety in the priority population (CDC, 2003)?

6. *Are the necessary resources available to implement the intervention selected?* Obviously some intervention strategies require more money, time, personnel, or space to implement than others. For example, it may be prudent to provide each person in the priority population with a $100 incentive for participating in the health promotion program, but it may not be possible because of budget limitations.

7. *Would it be better to use an intervention that consists of a single strategy or one that is made up of multiple strategies?* Again, we refer to the principle of multiplicity. A single-strategy intervention would most likely be easier and less expensive to implement and easier to evaluate. There are, however, some real advantages to using several strategies at multiple levels of influence: (1) "hitting" the priority population with a message in a variety of ways from multiple levels of influence; (2) appealing to the variety of learning styles within any priority population; (3) keeping the health message constantly before the priority population; (4) hoping that at least one strategy appeals enough to the priority population to help bring about the expected outcome; (5) appealing to the various senses (such as sight, hearing, or touch) of each individual in the priority population; and (6) increasing the chances that the combined strategies would help reach the goals and objectives of the program (e.g., communication used to publicize a policy change) (CDC, 2003). When interventions include multiple strategies offered at multiple levels of influence to multiple groups, they often include several interacting components or "active ingredients." Such interventions are now being referred to as *complex interventions* (Hawe, 2015). Probably the biggest drawback to using complex interventions is the difficulty of separating the effects of one strategy from the effects of others in evaluating the impact of the total program and of individual components. However, Glasgow, Vogt, and Boles (1999) have developed an evaluation model titled RE-AIM (acronym for reach, efficacy, adoption, implementation, and maintenance) for use with multi-strategy interventions.

▷ Limtations of Interventions

Finally, before leaving this chapter on interventions we would be negligent if we did not mention that even well-planned interventions are not always successful in achieving the expected outcomes. That is, most interventions come with some limitations. In a keynote address on the impact of injuries as a public health problem, Sleet (2015) identified some of the limitations associated with the three major approaches to intervening to prevent injuries namely—innovations in engineering and technology, legislation and enforcement, and education for behavior change. Sleet (2015) noted in order for engineering and technology innovations to be successful in preventing injuries they must be: effective and reliable; acceptable to those for whom they were intended; easy to use; and used properly. Consider how these criteria apply to child-resistant cigarette lighters and medicine bottles, bicycle helmets, smoke and carbon monoxide detectors, and microwave-safe baby bottles.

In order for legislative and enforcement interventions to prevent injuries the laws must: be widely known to the people; be fair and acceptable to the people; insure that the probability of being caught for not obeying is high; and outline punishment that is swift and certain if the law is broken. Think about how these criteria might limit laws associated with child-safety restraints for motor vehicles, safety belts, motorcycle helmets, and speeding. In order for educational interventions to be effective in preventing injuries people must: be exposed to the information; understand and believe the information; have the resources to make the necessary changes; and be reinforced when they make the changes. Reflect on how these criteria may limit educational programs on smoke detector maintenance, drinking and driving, and texting while operating a motor vehicle. Although Sleet's (2015) examples were restricted to injury prevention and three major intervention strategies, the same or similar limitations could be applied to the other categories of intervention strategies presented in this chapter.

 ## Summary

Interventions are those actions that are designed to prevent disease or injury or promote health in the priority population. Interventions are also sometimes referred to as *treatments*. Although many times an intervention is made up of a single strategy, it is more common for planners to use a variety of strategies aimed at multiple levels of influence to make up an intervention for a program. In this chapter, intervention strategies were categorized into the following groups: (1) Health communication strategies; (2) Health education strategies; (3) Health policy/enforcement strategies; (4) Environmental change strategies; (5) Health-related community service strategies; (6) Community mobilization strategies, and (7) Other strategies. Additionally, this chapter presented three avenues for designing health promotion interventions including adopting, adapting, or creating a new intervention. And, finally, the chapter provided some limitations of interventions.

 ## Review Questions

1. What is an intervention?

2. What are the advantages of using a multistrategy intervention (i.e., principle of multiplicity) over one that includes a single strategy? Are there any disadvantages? If so, what are they?

3. What does *dose* mean in terms of an intervention?

4. What are the major categories of interventions? Explain each.

5. Define each of the following terms as they relate to health education strategies: *curriculum, scope, sequence, unit of study, lessons*, and *lesson plans*.

6. What is motivational interviewing? How can it best be used in a health promotion program?

7. State and briefly describe the five stages of Kinzie's (2005) modified framework for instructional design.

8. Define *health literacy* and *health numeracy* and explain how they impact health promotion programs.

9. What is health advocacy?

10. What special issues are there related to incentives with which planners working in the worksite setting need to be concerned? How can behavioral economics be used to shape incentives?

11. Why should program planners be concerned with program guidelines that have been developed by professional organizations and other groups?

12. What is the difference between adopting and adapting an evidence-based intervention?

13. Identify and briefly explain the five steps in the framework for adapting an evidence-based intervention for a new setting.

14. Briefly discuss the questions set forth in this chapter that should be considered before creating a new intervention.

15. What are some of the limitations associated with interventions?

Activities

1. Create a multi-strategy intervention for a program you are planning.

2. Create a multi-strategy intervention for a program that has as its goal "to get third-grade students to wear helmets while riding their bicycles."

3. Using evidence found at the *Guide to Community Preventive Services*, adapt a multi-strategy intervention for a setting of your choice.

4. Create a multi-strategy intervention for a program that has as its goal "the rehydration of young children in the small village of Y in the developing country of Q."

5. Design and present on an 8½" × 11" piece of paper a bulletin board that could be used as part of the multi-activity intervention you are planning. Divide the piece of paper that represents the bulletin board into six equal sections and indicate what you will include in each section.

6. Interview a classmate to find out information about his or her health risks. Then, assuming you are a patient educator in a health clinic, create a one-page *tailored* letter to the person, urging him or her to seek an appropriate screening for the health risk(s).

7. Develop a three-fold pamphlet that can be used as an informational piece for a program you are planning.

8. With other students in your class, write a PSA script for a program you are planning. Then rehearse the script and record it.

9. Write a two-page, double-spaced news release that describes a program you are planning.

10. Write a letter to your state or federal senators or representatives and request their support of a piece of health-related legislation that is currently being considered.

Weblinks

1. **http://www.cdc.gov/socialmedia/**

    Social Media at CDC

    This page on the CDC's Website deals with the use of social media. From here you can link to the various social media tools of CDC and to a page that provides guidelines that have been developed to provide critical information on lessons learned, best practices, clearance information, and security requirements.

2. **http://nccc.georgetown.edu**

    National Center for Cultural Competence (NCCC)

    At this site you will find a lot of resource material dealing with cultural competence including a listing of publications, self-assessments, and current projects and initiatives.

3. **http://www.cdc.gov/healthliteracy/**

    Health literacy

    This page on the CDC's Website focuses on health literacy. The site provides information, tools, and links on health literacy research, practice, and evaluation. It also provides links to the National Action Plan to Improve Health Literacy, CDC's Action Plan to Improve Health Literacy, and the federal Plain Writing Act.

4. **http://www2a.cdc.gov/phlp/**

    Public Health Law Program

    This page on the CDC's Website focuses on public health law and policy. From here you can link to public health law news and other materials and resources that examine the authority of the government at various jurisdictional levels to improve the health of the general population within societal limits and norms.

5. **http://www.thecommunityguide.org/index.html**

    Guide to Community Preventive Services

    This Webpage includes evidence-based recommendations for programs and policies to promote population-based health.

6. **http://www.cdc.gov/healthcommunication/index.html**

    Gateway to Health Communication & Social Marketing Practice

    This page on the CDC's Website provides resources to help build health communication or social marketing campaigns and programs. It includes tips for analyzing and segmenting an audience, choosing appropriate channels and tools, and evaluating the success of messages or campaigns.

Community Organizing and Community Building

Chapter Objectives

After reading this chapter and answering the questions at the end, you should be able to:

- Define *community, community organizing, community building, task forces,* and *coalitions.*

- Outline the processes for organizing and building a community.

- Explain the term *mapping community capacity.*

Key Terms

active participants
bottom-up
citizen-initiated
coalition
community
community building
community organizing
executive participants
gatekeepers
grassroots
mapping community capacity

occasional participants
ownership
potential building blocks
primary building blocks
secondary building blocks
supporting participants
task force

There are a number of different processes involved in planning health promotion programs and those processes vary based upon the circumstances of the planning situation. The processes selected and used to plan programs are in part predicated on the level of the influence (i.e., intrapersonal, interpersonal, and/or community), and the level of influence is often predicated on the size of the priority population. For example, certain processes are more useful when planning programs for relatively small groups or communities of people such as those found in worksites, clinics, and schools, whereas other processes must be considered when working with larger communities. By community, we do not mean only those groups of people within a certain geographic area, though that could define a community, but more specifically, a **community** is defined as "a collective body of individuals identified by common characteristics such as geography, interests, experiences, concerns, or values (Joint Committee on Health Education and Promotion Terminology, 2012, p. 15). Israel and colleagues (1994) have stated that communities are characterized by the following elements: (1) membership—a sense of identity and belonging; (2) common symbol systems—similar language, rituals, and ceremonies; (3) shared values and norms; (4) mutual influence—community members have influence and are influenced by each other; (5) shared needs and commitment to meeting them; and (6) shared emotional connection—members share common history, experiences, and mutual support. Thus communities can be defined by location, race, ethnicity, age, occupation, interest in particular problems (e.g., domestic violence), outcomes (e.g., breast cancer survivors), or other common bonds (e.g., people with a disability) (Turnock, 2012). Today, we can also talk about a cyber community (Minkler, Wallerstein, & Wilson, 2008).

Although many of the planning processes are applicable regardless of the size of the community, when working with large communities an additional process is needed in order to have a successful program. This additional process is organizing those in the community to come together to work as a group to deal with the needs of the community. This chapter addresses the fundamental elements of organizing communities for action. **Box 9.1** identifies the responsibilities and competencies for health education specialists that pertain to the material presented in this chapter.

▷ Community Organizing Background and Assumptions

In recent years, there has been a shift in the focus of the work of planners and others in the helping professions. Where once the work of planners focused almost solely on the individual, today the focus is on broadening to the community. *Community-based, community empowerment, community participation, community partnerships* and *systems change* are among the many terms that are being used more frequently by health agencies, outside funders, and policy makers (Minkler, 2012). There are good reasons for the use of these terms and most revolve around the need for communities to organize.

With the evidence to show that interventions aimed at the community level (also referred to as *population-based approaches*) can have a positive affect on the health of a community, it is important that health education specialists have community organizing skills. In the early history of the United States, a sense of community was inherent in everyday life (Green, 1989). It was natural for communities to pool their resources to deal with shared problems. More recently, the need to organize communities has seemed to increase. "Advances in electronics (e.g., handheld digital devices) and communications (multifunction cell phones and Internet), household upgrades (e.g., energy efficiency), and increased mobility (e.g., frequency of moving and ease of worldwide travel) have resulted in a loss of a sense of community. Individuals are much more independent than ever before. The days when people knew everyone on their block are past. Today, it is not uncommon for people to never meet their neighbors" (McKenzie & Pinger, 2015, p. 135). Because of these changes in community social structure and the resources necessary to meet the needs of communities, it now takes a concerted effort to organize a community to act for the collective good.

"The term *community organization* was coined by American social workers in the late 1880s to describe their efforts to coordinate services for newly arrived immigrants and the poor" (Minkler & Wallerstein, 2012, p. 38). More recently, *community organization* has been used by a variety of professionals, including health education specialists, and refers to various methods of intervention to deal with social problems. "Community organization is important in fields like health education and social work partially because it reflects one of their fundamental principles, that of 'starting where the people are' (Nyswander, 1956)" (Minkler & Wallerstein, 2012, p. 37-38). "The health education professional who begins with the community's felt needs, is more likely to be successful in the change process and in fostering true community ownership of programs and actions" (Minkler et al., 2008, p. 288).

BOX

9.1

Focus On

Responsibilities and Competencies for Health Education Specialists

This chapter focuses on the fundamental elements of organizing communities. As such, the content presented cuts across several different areas of responsibility for health education specialists. The responsibilities and competencies related to these tasks include:

RESPONSIBILITY I: Assess Needs, Resources, and Capacity for Health Education/Promotion

Competency 1.1: Plan assessment process for health education/promotion

Competency 1.2: Access existing information and data related to health

Competency 1.4: Analyze relationships among behavioral, environmental, and other factors that influence health

RESPONSIBILITY II: Plan Health Education/Promotion

Competency 2.1: Involve priority populations, partners, and other stakeholders in the planning process

Competency 2.2: Develop goals and objectives

Competency 2.3: Select or design strategies/interventions

Competency 2.4: Develop a plan for the delivery of health education/promotion

Competency 2.5: Address factors that influence implementation of health education/promotion

RESPONSIBILITY III: Implement Health Education/Promotion

Competency 3.3: Implement health education/promotion plan

RESPONSIBILITY IV: Conduct Evaluation and Research Related to Health Education/Promotion

Competency 4.1: Develop evaluation plan for health education/promotion

RESPONSIBILITY V: Administer and Manage Health Education/Promotion

Competency 5.3: Manage relationships with partners and other stakeholders

Competency 5.4: Gain acceptance and support for health education/promotion programs

Competency 5.5: Demonstrate leadership

Competency 5.6: Manage human resources for health education/promotion

RESPONSIBILITY VI: Serve as a Health Education/Promotion Resource Person

Competency 6.2: Train others to use health education/promotion skills

Competency 6.3 Provide advice and consultation on health education/promotion issues

RESPONSIBILITY VII: Communicate, Promote, and Advocate for Health, Health Education/Promotion, and the Profession

Competency 7.1: Identify, develop, and deliver messages using a variety of communication strategies, methods, and techniques

Competency 7.2: Engage in advocacy for health and health education/promotion

Competency 7.3: Influence policy and/or systems change to promote health and health education

Source: *A Competency-Based Framework for Health Education Specialists—2015*. Whitehall, PA: National Commission for Health Education Credentialing, Inc. (NCHEC) and the Society for Public Health Education (SOPHE). Reprinted by permission of the National Commission for Health Education Credentialing, Inc. (NCHEC) and the Society for Public Health Education (SOPHE).

Community organizing has been defined as "the process by which community groups are helped to identify common problems or change targets, mobilize resources, and develop and implement strategies to reach their collective goals" (Minkler & Wallerstein, 2012, p. 37). It is not a science but rather an art of building consensus within the democratic process (Ross, 1967). (See **Box 9.2** for definitions of related terms.) Although community organization may not be as "natural" as it once was, communities can still organize to analyze and solve problems through collective action. In working toward this end, those who assist communities with organizing must make several assumptions. Ross (1967, pp. 86–92) has stated these as follows:

1. Communities of people can develop the capacity to deal with their own problems.

2. People want to change and can change.

3. People should participate in making, adjusting, or controlling the major changes taking place in their communities.

<table>
<tr><td rowspan="2">BOX
9.2

Focus On</td><td colspan="2">**Terms Associated with Community Organizing**</td></tr>
<tr><td>Citizen Participation</td><td>The bottom-up, grassroots mobilization of citizens for the purpose of undertaking activities to improve the condition of something in the community.</td></tr>
</table>

Community Capacity	"Community characteristics affecting its ability to identify, mobilize, and address problems" (Minkler & Wallerstein, 2012, p. 45).
Community Development	"A process designed to create conditions of economic and social progress for the whole community with its active participation and the fullest possible reliance on the community's initiative" (United Nations, 1955, p. 6).
Empowerment	"Social action process for people to gain mastery over their lives and the lives of their communities" (Minkler & Wallerstein, 2012, p. 45).
Grassroots Participation	"Bottom-up efforts of people taking collective actions on their own behalf, and they involve the use of a sophisticated blend of confrontation and cooperation in order to achieve their ends" (Perlman, 1978, p. 65).
Macro Practice	The methods of professional change that deal with issues beyond the individual, family, and small group level.
Participation and Relevance	"Community organizing that 'starts where the people are' and engages community members as equals" (Minkler & Wallerstein, 2012, p. 45).
Social Capital	"The processes and conditions among people and organizations that lead to their accomplishing a goal of mutual social benefit, usually characterized by interrelated constucts of trust, cooperation, civic engagement, and reciprocity, reinforced by networking" (Last, 2007, p. 347)

4. Changes in community living that are self-imposed or self-developed have a meaning and permanence that imposed changes do not have.

5. A "holistic approach" can deal successfully with problems with which a "fragmented approach" cannot cope.

6. Democracy requires cooperative participation and action in the affairs of the community, and that the people must learn the skills that make this possible.

7. Frequently communities of people need help in organizing to deal with their needs, just as many individuals require help in coping with their individual problems.

▷ The Processes of Community Organizing and Community Building

There is no single unified model of community organizing or community building (Minkler & Wallerstein, 2012). In fact, Rothman and Tropman (1987, pp. 4–5) have stated, "We should speak of community organization methods rather than the community organization method." The early approaches to community organization used by social workers emphasized the use of consensus and cooperation to deal with community problems (Garvin & Fox, 2001). However, the best known categories of community organization were the three put forth by Rothman (2001) and include *locality development, social planning,* and *social action.* More recently, the strategies have been renamed *planning and policy practice, community capacity development,* and *social advocacy* (Rothman, 2007). At the heart of the *planning and policy practice* strategy are data. By using data, community/public health workers generate persuasive rationales that lead toward proposing and enacting particular solutions (Rothman, 2007).

The *community capacity development* strategy is based on empowering those impacted by a problem with knowledge and skills to understand the problem and then work cooperatively together to deal with the problem. Group consensus and social solidarity are important components of this strategy (Rothman, 2007). The third strategy, *social advocacy,* is used to address a problem through the application of pressure, including confrontation, on those who have created the problem or stand as a barrier to a solution to the problem. This strategy creates conflict (Rothman, 2007). Although each of these strategies has unique components, each of the strategies can be combined with the others to deal with a community problem. In fact, Rothman has offered a 3 × 3 matrix to help explain the combinations (Rothman, 2007). Regardless of whether one talks about the "old models" or the "new models," they all revolve around a common theme: The work and resources of many have a much better chance of solving a problem or meeting a goal than the work and resources of a few.

Minkler and Wallerstein (2012) have done a nice job of summarizing the newer perspectives of community organizing with the older models by presenting a typology that incorporates both needs- and strength-based approaches. That typology is presented in **Figure 9.1**. Their typology is divided into four quadrants with strength-based and needs-based on the vertical axis and consensus and conflict on the horizontal axis. Though this typology separates and categorizes the various methods of community organizing and building, Minkler and Wallerstein (2012) point out that when they

> ...look at primary strategies, we see that the consensus approaches, whether needs based or strengths based, primarily use collaboration strategies, whereas conflict approaches use advocacy strategies and ally building to support advocacy efforts. Several concepts span these

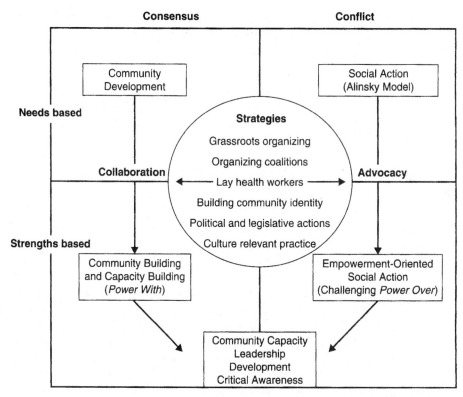

Consensus | **Conflict**

Community Development

Social Action (Alinsky Model)

Needs based

Strategies

Grassroots organizing

Organizing coalitions

Collaboration ← Lay health workers → **Advocacy**

Building community identity

Political and legislative actions

Strengths based

Culture relevant practice

Community Building and Capacity Building (*Power With*)

Empowerment-Oriented Social Action (Challenging *Power Over*)

Community Capacity Leadership Development Critical Awareness

▲ **Figure 9.1** Community Organization and Community-Building Typology

Source: Minkler, M., & Wallerstein, N. (2012). Improving health through community organization and community building: Perspectives from health education and social work. In M. Minkler (Ed.). *Community organizing and community building for health and welfare* (3rd ed., p. 43). New Brunswick, NJ: Rutgers University Press.

two strengths-based approaches, such as community competence, leadership development, and multiple perspectives on gaining power. Again, as with the Rothman model, many organizing efforts use a combination of these strategies at different times throughout the life of an organizing campaign and community building process (p. 44).

Because the purpose of this chapter is to provide an overview of the community organizing and community-building processes, and at the risk of oversimplifying the processes, we would like to present a very general or generic approach to community organizing and community building (see **Figure 9.2**). It does not include everything planners need to know about community organizing and community building, but it does present the basic elements.

For further information about community organizing, refer to any of several references (Minkler, 2012; Minkler et al., 2008; Ross, 1967; Rothman 2007; Snow, 2001) that are devoted entirely to the subject. Also, there are several works that deal specifically with the application of community organization to health promotion activities (Karwalajtys et al., 2013; Minkler, 2012; Minkler et al., 2008).

Before presenting the generic process for community organizing and community building, we would like to comment on the role of the planner in this process. For many years, the planner was seen as a "leader" of the community organizing effort. However, more often

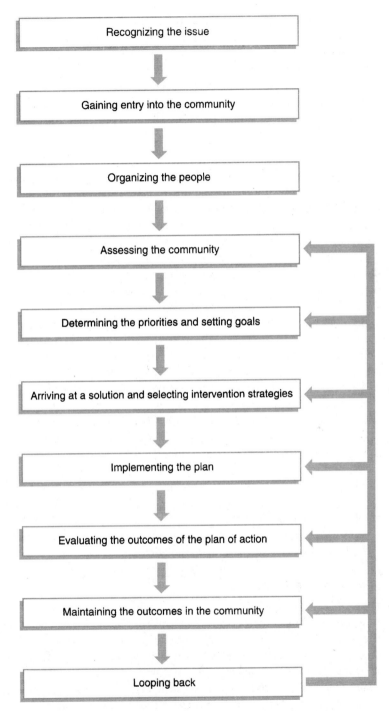

▲ **Figure 9.2** Summary of the Steps in Community Organizing and Building than not, the planner is an "outsider" with regard to the community being organized and, as such, has trouble gaining the credibility to serve as a leader. Yes, he or she may work in the community (remember that a community is often defined by something other than geographical boundaries) but often lives outside the community in which the organizing effort is needed. Thus, the role that the planner should take is that of a facilitator or assistant rather than the leader. Experience has shown that it is best if the leaders come from *within* the community. Keep this thought in mind as you read through the general model.

Recognizing the Issue

The processes of community organizing and building begin when someone recognizes that an issue exists in the community and that something needs to be done about it. This recognition may occur as a result of someone reviewing health data on the community and seeing a need (e.g., an unusually high number of teenage pregnancies), by someone actually observing a specific situation in the community that needs attention (e.g., injuries at a particular intersection), or as the result of a community crisis (e.g., lack of resources to deal with a natural disaster). "This person (or persons) is referred to as the initial organizer. This individual may not be the primary organizer throughout the community organizing/building process. He or she is the one who gets things started" (McKenzie & Pinger, 2015, p. 138). For the purposes of this discussion, assume that the concern is a health problem, but remember that the community organization process may be used with any type of problem found in a community. Concerns can be as specific as trying to get a certain piece of legislation passed or as general as advocating for a drug-free community.

The recognition of an issue can occur from inside or outside the community. A citizen or a church leader from within the community may identify the issue, or it may first be identified by someone outside the community, such as an employee of a local or state health department, a state legislator, a politically active group, or someone from a local voluntary health agency. However, the community organizing efforts that have been most successful have been those that are recognized from the inside. The primary reason for this is that those within the community are much more likely to take ownership of the effort. It is difficult for someone from the outside coming in and telling community members that they have problems or issues that need to be dealt with and they need to organize to take care of them. When there is internal recognition of the issue or concern, it is referred to as **grassroots**, **citizen-initiated**, or **bottom-up** organizing.

Gaining Entry into the Community

The second step of this generic process of community organizing and community building may or may not be needed. If the issue identified in the previous step is recognized by someone from within the community, then this step of the process will, more than likely, not be needed. We say "more than likely" because those within a community do not need to gain entry into it. But there may be some cases when someone from within a community may identify the issue but has not lived in the community long enough, lacks the political power, or does not know enough about the interactions of the community to proceed with the process. In these later cases, the person may be treated or feel like an "outsider" and may have to proceed as an outsider would.

If the issue is identified by someone from outside the community this becomes a most critical step in the process. Recognition of a concern does not mean that people should immediately set about correcting it. Instead, they should follow a set of steps to deal with it; gaining proper "entry" into the community is the first step. Braithwaite and colleagues (1989) have stressed the importance of tactfully negotiating entry into a community with the individuals who control, both formally and informally, the "political climate" of the community. These individuals are referred to as **gatekeepers**. The term infers that one must pass through the "gate" in order to get at the people in the community (Wright, 1994). These "power brokers" know their community, how it functions, and how to accomplish tasks within it. Longtime residents are usually able to identify the gatekeepers of their community. They may include people such as business leaders, education leaders, heads of law enforcement agencies, leaders of community activist groups, parent and teacher groups, clergy, politicians, and others. Their support is absolutely essential to the success of any attempt to organize a community.

Organizers must approach the gatekeepers on the gatekeepers' terms and "play" the gatekeepers' "game." However, before making this contact, organizers must first be familiar with the community with which they are working. "They must be *culturally sensitive* and work toward *cultural competence*. That is, they must be aware of the cultural differences within a community and effectively work with the cultural context of the community" (McKenzie & Pinger, 2015, p. 139). Tervalon and Garcia (1998) stress the need for *cultural humility*—openness to others' culture. In other words, community organizers must have a thorough knowledge of the community and the people living there before they try to enter the informal boundaries of the community (Braithwaite et al., 1989). Having a thorough understanding of the community and tactfully approaching its gatekeepers will help community organizers develop credibility and trust with those in the community, and, as noted earlier, it is not easy to bring a concern to the attention of those in the community. Few people are glad to know they have a problem, and fewer still like others to tell them they have a problem. Move with caution, and do not be too aggressive!

When people from outside the community are working to facilitate the organizing efforts, they will find it advantageous to enter the community through an already established, well-respected organization or institution in the community, such as a church, a service group, or another successful local group. If those who make up an existing organization/institution in the community can see that a problem exists and that solving the problem will improve the community, it can help smooth the way to gaining entry and achieving the remaining steps in the process.

Organizing the People

Obtaining the support of the community members to deal with the concern is the next step in the process. It is best to begin with those individuals who are already interested in addressing the concern. This is not the time to try to convert people to the cause or to make sure that all the key players of the community are involved. The initial group must be made up of those people most affected by the problem and who want to see change occur. For example, if the identified problem is teenage drug use, then teens needed to be included in the group. If the issue is housing for individuals with low-incomes, then those individuals need to be included. If the problem is something that a community agency or organization (e.g., the local health department or a social service agency) has dealt with for a period of time but is unable to solve, then this group should be involved. Or, if a group of parents, or another defined group, has been struggling with the problem without resolution, then its leaders should be invited to participate. More often than not, this core group will be small and consist of people who are committed to the resolution of the concern, regardless of the time frame. Brager and colleagues (1987) have referred to this core group as **executive participants**. From among the core group, a leader or coordinator must be identified. If at all possible, the leader should be someone with leadership skills, good knowledge of the concern and the community, and most of all, someone from within the community. One of the early tasks of the leader will be to help build group cohesion.

Not everyone is cut out to be an organizer or a leader. Researchers have found that good organizers are successful because of a combination of skills and attributes. These skills and attributes fall into three main areas: change vision attributes, technical skills, and interactional or experience skills. *Change vision attributes* are closely aligned with an organizer's view of the world political terms. These people see a need for change and are personally dedicated and committed to seeing the change occur—so much so that they are willing to put other priorities aside to see the project through (Mondros & Wilson, 1994).

Technical skills include two areas: those related to efficacy on issues and those related to organizational health and effectiveness. The former includes being able to analyze issues, opponents, and power structure; develop and implement change strategies; achieve goals; and possess outstanding communication and public relation skills. Organizational health and effectiveness skills include building structures for the recruitment and involvement of others, forming and maintaining task groups, and implementing skills of fundraising and organizational management (Mondros & Wilson, 1994).

The third characteristic of a good organizer is possessing *interactional* or *experience skills*. These include an ability to respond with empathy, to assess and intervene with individuals and groups, and to be able to identify, develop, educate, and maintain organizational members and leaders (Mondros & Wilson, 1994).

With the core group and leader in place, the next step is to expand the group to build support for dealing with the concern—that is, to broaden the constituency. Brager and colleagues (1987) have noted that other group participants will include *active, occasional*, and *supporting participants*. The **active participants** (who may also be executive participants) take part in most group activities and are not afraid to do the work that needs to be done. The **occasional participants** become involved on an irregular basis and usually only when major decisions are made. The **supporting participants** are seldom involved but help swell the ranks and may contribute in nonactive ways or through financial contributions. When expanding the group, look for others who may be interested in helping, and ask current group members for names of people who might be interested. Look for people who may already be dealing with the concern, affected by the problem through their present work, or who have resources to contribute. This search should include existing social groups, such as voluntary health agencies, agricultural extension services, religious organizations, hospitals, health care providers, political officeholders, policy makers, police, educators, lay citizens, or special interest groups. (See **Box 9.3** on tips for understanding the diversity in a working group.)

BOX

9.3

Focus On

Understanding Diversity

Members of a group come from many different backgrounds. Some members may be much older or much younger than other members; some may represent different cultural, racial, or ethnic groups; some may represent different educational levels and abilities. Extra awareness and flexibility are required for the facilitator and other group members to remain sensitive to different backgrounds. Below we suggest a few ways to improve your awareness of differences. In general, new information is acquired so that different perspectives can be understood and appreciated.

- Become aware of differences in the group by asking questions and getting involved in small group discussions.
- Seek involvement and input and listen to persons of different backgrounds without bias, and avoid being defensive.
- Learn the beliefs and feelings of specific groups about particular issues.
- Read about current and emerging issues that concern different groups, and read literature that is popular among different groups.
- Learn about the language, humor, gestures, norms, expectations, and values of different groups.
- Attend events that appeal to members of specific groups.
- Become attuned to cultural clichés, stereotypes, and distortions you may encounter in the media.
- Use examples to which persons of different cultures and backgrounds can relate.
- Learn the facts before you make statements or form opinions about different groups.

Source: Centers for Disease Control and Prevention, USDHHS, (no date), p. A2–15.

Over the last 50 years, in many communities the number of people interested in volunteering their time has decreased. Today, if you ask someone to volunteer, you may hear the reply, "I'm already too busy." There are two primary reasons for this response. First, there are many families in which both husband and wife work outside the home. Second, there are more single-parent households. (See **Box 9.4** for tips on working with volunteers.)

Sometimes these expanded community groups become *task forces* or *coalitions*. A **task force** has been defined as "a self-contained group of 'doers' that is not ongoing. It is convened for a narrow purpose over a defined timeframe at the request of another body or committee" (Butterfoss, 2013, p. 7). A **coalition** is "a formal alliance of organizations that come together to work for a common goal" (Butterfoss, 2007, p. 30)—often, to compensate for deficits in power, resources, and expertise. Coalitions "develop an internal decision-making and leadership structure that allows member organizations to speak with a united voice and engage in shared planning and implementation activities. Links to outside organizations and communication channels are formal. Member organizations are willing to pull resources from existing systems, as well as seek new resources to develop a joint budget. Agreements, benchmarks, roles, and assignments are often written" (Butterfoss, 2007, p. 30). The underlying concept behind coalitions is collaboration; for several individuals, groups, or organizations with their collective resources have a better chance of solving the problem than any single entity. "Building and maintaining effective coalitions have increasingly been recognized as vital components of much effective community organizing and community

Tips on Working with Volunteers

Volunteers work for self-satisfaction, personal growth, fun, and other intangible rewards. Each volunteer should be treated as a colleague and recognized as an official part of the team. However, offer volunteers more flexibility than you can to employees, and adjust your expectations accordingly. For example, because volunteers cannot contribute as much time as paid, full-time workers do, they cannot complete tasks as quickly. When scheduling activities, be realistic about how long a busy participant will need to complete it.

Get to know each volunteer personally so that you can learn about special abilities and limitations and match responsibilities to skills. Vary responsibilities as desired by volunteers.

Be sure to assign specific and clearly defined tasks and to explain procedures and expectations. Develop a work plan or job description for the volunteer to help ensure that roles and responsibilities are understood. Provide training and give credit for work done. Give lots of feedback, encouragement, and signs of appreciation. Be willing to change the placement of volunteers, if that seems appropriate, or even dismiss a volunteer if necessary.

Keep in mind the following key points of working with volunteers. They want to be:

- appreciated for the work that they do.
- busy with worthwhile and varied tasks.
- provided with clear communication about tasks and expectations.
- developed through training.

Source: Centers for Disease Control and Prevention (no date), p. A2–17.

building" (Minkler, 2012, p. 20). Much has been written about the importance and use of coalitions. Aitaoto, Tsark, and Braun (2009) found that the key to sustaining coalitions include having a champion, a supportive organizational home, and access to technical assistance and resources. Woods and colleagues (2014) presented a case study on the importance of training and technical assistance on coalition functioning and sustainability. Butterfoss (2009) has created a longer list of characteristics of successful coalitions (see **Box 9.5**), while Kegler and Swan (2011) have tested the community coalition action theory (CCAT) for consistency of its constructs with working community coalitions. Brown, Feinberg, and Greenberg (2012) have created a Web-based, self-report questionnaire that can be used to provide feedback to coalitions and technical assistance providers about coalition functioning. For those who want more information about coalition development, Butterfoss (2007, 2009, 2013), Butterfoss and Kegler (2012), and Goldstein (1997), provide nice overviews of the processes of building and sustaining coalitions.

Assessing the Community

Earlier in this chapter we noted that there were a number of strategies that have been used for community organizing. Many of those community organizing strategies operate "from the assumption that problems in society can be addressed by helping the community become better or differently organized, and each strategy perceives the problems and how or whom to organize somewhat differently" (Walter, 2005, p. 66). In contrast to those strategies

BOX

9.5

Focus On

Characteristics of Successful Coalitions

- Continuity of coalition staff, in particular the coordinator position
- Ownership of the problem by coalition members and the community
- Community leaders support the coalition and its efforts
- Active involvement of community volunteer agencies
- High level of trust and reciprocity among members
- Frequent and ongoing training for coalition members and staff
- Benefits of membership outweigh the costs
- Active involvement of members in developing coalition goals, objectives, and strategies
- Development of a strategic action plan rather than a project-by-project approach
- Consensus is reached on issues instead of voting
- Productive coalition meetings
- Large problems are broken down into smaller, solvable pieces
- Steering committee of elected leaders and staff guides coalition
- Task or work groups of members design and implement strategies
- Rules and procedures are formalized
- Local media are actively involved
- Coalition and its activities are evaluated continuously

Source: "Building and Sustaining Coalitions." F. D. Butterfoss, from *Community Health Education Methods: A Practical Guide*. R. J. Bensley and J. Brookins-Fisher (Eds.). Copyright © 2009 by Jones & Bartlett Learning. Reprinted with permission.

is *community building*. **Community building** "is an orientation to practice focused on community, rather than a strategic framework or approach, and on building capacities, not fixing problems" (Minkler, 2012, p. 10). Community building is intended to affirm strong community-rooted traditions, and to build on the good work already going on in communities (Kretzmann & McKnight, 1993). One of the major differences between community organization and community building is the type of assessment that is used to determine where to focus the community's efforts. In the community organization approach, the assessment is focused on the needs of the community, whereas in community building, the assessment focuses on the assets and capabilities of the community. A clearer picture of the community will be revealed, and a stronger base will be developed for change, if the assessment includes the identification of both the needs and assets, and involves those who live in the community.

You may recall (in Chapter 4) we outlined the procedures for conducting a needs assessment and described how the resulting needs could be placed on a map (i.e., *mapping*) to provide a visual representation of the needs of a community. **Figure 9.3** provides an example of such a map. However, an assessment that focuses entirely on needs/deficiencies presents only half of the information that is needed in community organizing and building (McKnight & Kretzmann, 2012). Organizers also need to know the capacities and assets. McKnight and Kretzmann (2012) point out "communities have never been built upon their deficiencies. Building community has always depended on mobilizing the capacities and assets of a people and a place" (p. 183).

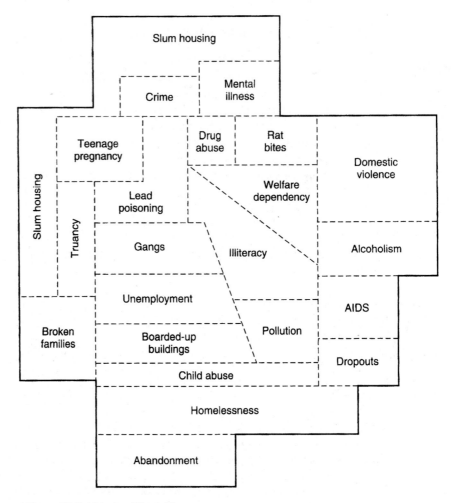

▲ **Figure 9.3** Neighborhood Needs Map

Source: Kretzman, John P. and John L. McKnight. "Figure 10.1: Neighborhood Needs Map," "Mapping Community Capacity" in *Community Organizing and Community Building for Health and Welfare*. Copyright © 2012 by Meredith Minkler. Reprinted by permission of Rutgers University Press.

In order to map community assets—a process referred to as **mapping community capacity**—McKnight and Kretzmann (2012) have categorized assets into three different groups based on their availability to the community and refer to them as *building blocks*. **Primary building blocks** are the most accessible assets (see **Figure 9.4**). They are located in the neighborhood and are largely under the control of those who live in the neighborhood. Primary building blocks can be organized into the assets of individuals and those of organizations or associations. (See **Box 9.6** for examples of each.) The next most accessible building blocks are **secondary building blocks**, which are assets located in the neighborhood but largely controlled by people outside. The least accessible assets are referred to as **potential building blocks**. They are resources originating outside the neighborhood and controlled by people outside. Figure 9.4 presents an example of an asset map using the three types of building blocks. Knowing both the needs and assets of the community, organizers can work to identify the true concerns of the community and the capacity to deal with them.

▲ **Figure 9.4** Neighborhood Assets Map

Building Blocks (Assets) of Communities

Primary Building Blocks

Individual assets

- Skills and abilities of residents
- Individual businesses
- Home-based enterprises
- Personal income
- Gifts of labeled (disabled) people

Organizational assets

- Associations of businesses (e.g., chamber of commerce)
- Citizens' associations (e.g., neighborhood watch)
- Cultural organization (e.g., Old West End Festival, British Club)
- Communications organizations (e.g., newspapers, TV, radio)
- Religious organizations
- Financial institutions

Secondary Building Blocks

Private and nonprofit organizations

- Higher education institutions
- Hospitals
- Social service groups (e.g., Rotary, Kiwanis)

Public institutions and services

- Public schools
- Police and fire departments
- Libraries
- Parks

Physical resources

- Vacant land, vacant commercial and industrial structures, vacant housing
- Energy and waste resources

Potential Building Blocks

   Welfare expenditures

   Public capital-information expenditures

   Public information

Source: "Mapping Community Capacity" by J. L. McKnight and J. P. Kretzmann from *Community Organizing and Community Building for Health,* Ed. M. Minkler. Copyright © 2005 by Rutgers, the State University Press.

Determining Priorities and Setting Goals

Once the community has been assessed, the community group is ready to develop its goals. The goal-setting process includes two phases. The first phase consists of identifying the priorities of the group—what the group wants to accomplish. The priorities should be determined through consensus rather than through formal voting. (See **Box 9.7** for tips on how to reach consensus.) The second phase consists of using the priority list to write the

BOX

9.7

Focus On

Reaching Consensus

Groups sometimes find it hard to reach a consensus, or general agreement. Remind participants of the following guidelines to group decision making.

- Avoid the "one best way" attitude; the best way is that which reflects the best collective judgment of the group.
- Avoid "either, or" thinking; often the best solution combines several approaches.
- A majority vote is not always the best solution. When participants give and take, several viewpoints can be combined.
- Healthy conflict, which can help participants reach a consensus, should not be smoothed over or ended prematurely.
- Problems are best solved when participants try to both communicate and listen.

If a group has trouble reaching consensus, consider using some special techniques such as brainstorming, the nominal group process, and conflict resolution.

Source: Centers for Disease Control and Prevention (no date), p. A2–12

goals. To help ensure that the ideals of community organization take hold, the stakeholders (those in the community who have something to gain or lose from the community organizing and building efforts) must be the ones to establish priorities and set goals. This may sound simple, but in fact it may be the most difficult part of the process. Getting the stakeholders to agree on priorities takes a skilled group facilitator because there is sure to be more than one point of view.

When working with coalitions and task forces, one is likely to face some challenges (Clark, Friedman, & Lachance, 2006). One challenge that may surface when determining priorities and setting goals is *turf struggles* (disagreements over the control of resources and responsibilities). Even though individuals or representatives of their organizations have come together to solve a problem, many people will still be concerned with finding specific solutions to the problems faced by their organization. For example, in the case of drug abuse in the community, consensus may indicate that the majority of people believe the solutions lie in the educational system, but people who work in drug treatment centers may believe that they lie in the treatment of drug abuse. The facilitator will need special skills to keep these treatment center people involved after the priority-setting process does not identify their concern as a problem the group will attack. One means of dealing with this is to have subgoals that can be worked on by special interest subcommittees. Such an arrangement will allow the subcommittee to have a feeling of **ownership** in the process.

Miller (2009) and Staples (2012) have identified criteria that community organizers need to consider when determining priorities and setting goals. The concern/issue/problem: must be winnable, ensuring that working on it does not simply reinforce fatalistic attitudes and beliefs that things cannot be improved; must be simple and specific so that any member of the organizing group can explain it clearly in a sentence or two; must unite members of the organizing group; and must involve them in a meaningful way in achieving concern/issue/problem resolution.

Arriving at a Solution and Selecting Intervention Strategies

To achieve the goals that it has set, the group will need to identify alternative solutions and—again, through consensus—choose a course of action. Most community problems/issues/concerns can be dealt with in any of several ways; however, each alternative has advantages and disadvantages. The group should examine the alternatives in terms of probable outcomes, acceptability to the community, probable long- and short-term effects on the community, and the cost of resources to solve the problem. Most of the intervention strategies discussed earlier (in Chapter 8) are means by which the group can address the problem/issue/concern.

Much of the work to identify the appropriate solution(s) can be accomplished through subcommittees. Subcommittees can complete specific tasks that will contribute to the larger plan of action. Their work should yield specific strategies that are culturally sensitive and appropriate for the community. The plan of action is usually written in a proposal format and will be given final approval at a meeting of the full committee or coalition. It is important to take care in putting together this proposal; as many as possible of the ideas of the various subcommittees should be included. This will help to ensure approval of the entire plan. In the end, the real test of the course of action selected is whether it can provide whatever it is the people are seeking (Brager et al., 1987).

Final Steps in the Community Organizing and Building Processes

The final four steps in community organizing and building processes include implementing the plan, evaluating the outcomes of the plan of action, maintaining (or sustaining) the outcomes in the community, and, if necessary, "looping" back to the appropriate point in the process to modify the steps and restructure the work plan. Implementation of the intervention strategy includes identifying and collecting the necessary resources for carrying out the solution and creating an appropriate time line for implementation. Often the resources can be found within a community and thus *horizontal relationships* (the interaction of local units with one another) are needed (Warren, 1963). Other times the resources must be obtained from units located outside the community and in this case *vertical relationships* (those where local units interact with extra-community systems) are needed (Warren, 1963). An example of this latter relationship is the interaction between a local chamber of commerce and its state affiliate. More detailed information on implementation is presented later (Chapter 12).

The evaluation step of the community organizing and building process includes two types of evaluation: *formative* and *summative evaluation*. Briefly, formative evaluation deals with the measurement of the process used to improve the quality of the effort, whereas summative evaluation focuses on comparing the outcomes of the process to the earlier stated goals (see Chapters 13 and 14 for more on evaluation). When reporting on the work of coalitions, Clark and her colleagues (2006) stated process evaluation (a form of formative evaluation) "was the easier type of assessment to conduct. Effective tools are more available, data collection is more immediate, and problems of association and correlation are less daunting than those associated with outcome evaluation. Outcome evaluation requires time, patience, and the willingness to accept that in complex community settings, definitive conclusions are elusive" (p. 152S).

Maintaining or sustaining the outcomes may be one of the most difficult steps in the entire process. Maintaining or sustaining the outcomes are challenged by (1) the energy and effort necessary to stay organized, (2) continuing the interest and involvement of the members (Clark et al., 2006), (3) the training and technical assistance provided (Woods et al., 2014),

(4) continuing need for funding to sustain the efforts, and (5) "ensuring the lasting impact of their work through policies, cross-facility agreements, standardized protocols, and so on" (Clark et al., 2006, p. 151S). At this point organizers need to seriously consider the need for long-term capacity for a lasting solution.

Through the steps of implementation, evaluation, and maintenance/sustainability of the outcomes, organizers may see a need to "loop back" to a previous step in the process to rethink or rework before proceeding onward in their plan. And finally, once the work of the group has been completed (that is, either the issue has been solved or community empowerment achieved), the group can either disband or reorganize to deal with other issues.

Summary

Community organization refers to various methods of intervention whereby individuals, groups, and organizations engage in planned collective action to deal with social concerns. The literature on community organizing and building is not distinct; it is often intertwined with such terms as *community-based, community empowerment, community participation, community partnerships,* and *systems change.* The process of community organization has been used for many years in the area of social work, but its history in the area of health promotion is much more recent. This chapter presented generic processes for community organizing and building, which should be an adequate introduction to the process.

Review Questions

1. What is meant by the term *community*?
2. How does community organization relate to community empowerment?
3. From which discipline did community organization originate?
4. What is the underlying concept of community organization?
5. What are some of the assumptions under which planners work when organizing a community?
6. What are the basic steps in the community organizing and building processes?
7. What is the difference between a task force and a coalition?
8. What is meant by the term *gatekeepers*?
9. What is the difference between a needs assessment and a capacities and assets assessment?
10. What is meant by *mapping community capacity?*
11. What are the differences among primary, secondary, and potential building blocks (assets)?

Activities

1. Assume that a core group of individuals have come together to deal with concern about the high rate of teenage pregnancy in a community. Identify (by job title/function) others who you think should be invited to be part of the larger group. In addition, provide a one-sentence rationale for inviting each. Assume that this community is large enough to have most social service organizations.

2. Provide a list of at least 10 different community agencies that should be invited to make up an antismoking coalition in your hometown. Provide a one-sentence rationale for including each.

3. Ask your professor if he or she is aware of any ongoing coalitions in the local community. If some exist, along with several of your classmates, select one of interest and contact the chairperson to see if it would be okay to attend a coalition meeting. After the meeting, write a two page paper that includes the following: (a) name of coalition, (b) purpose of the coalition, (c) goal(s) of the coalition, (d) list of coalition members, (e) strategies used to accomplish the goal(s), and (f) accomplishments of coalition to date. If you are missing any of this information after the meeting, stay after the meeting and ask the chairperson if he or she would provide such information.

4. Assume that you want to make entry into a community with which you are not familiar in order to help to organize and build the community. Describe such a community, and then write a two-page paper to tell what steps you would take to gain entrance into the community.

5. If you wanted to find out more about your community's resources regarding exercise programs, with whom would you network? Provide a list of at least five contacts, and provide a one-sentence rationale for why you selected each.

6. Ask your professor if he or she is aware of any community organizing or building efforts in a local community. If such exists, make an appointment along with some of your classmates to interview the organizers. Ask the organizers to respond to the following questions: (a) What concern is the group tackling? (b) Who identified the initial concern? (c) Who makes up the core group? How large is it? (d) Did the group complete an assessment? (e) What type of intervention is being used? and (f) What type of community organizing or building model was used?

7. To get a feel for the process of mapping community capacity, obtain a map of your college/university and "map" the health-related assets on your campus. Try to identify the assets in terms of primary, secondary, and potential building blocks for the campus as defined by McKnight and Kretzmann (2012). After your map is complete, analyze what you have found. Where are most of the assets located? Did the results surprise you? If your campus were going to increase its health capacity, what would you recommend? Why?

Weblinks

1. **http://www.abcdinstitute.org**

   Asset-Based Community Development (ABCD) Institute, Northwestern University

   The ABCD, a part of the Center for Civic Engagement, was founded by Jody Kretzmann and John L. McKnight. The Website provides a variety of information on community building including training videos and podcasts, a tool kit with templates for community mapping, and an overview of the research projects in which its staff is involved.

2. **http://ctb.ku.edu/en**

   The Community Tool Box (CTB), University of Kansas

   The CTB provides practical information to support work in promoting community health and development. This Website is maintained by the Work Group on Health

Promotion and Community Development at the University of Kansas in Lawrence, Kansas, and offers a list of chapters that provide step-by-step guidance for community-building skills. Within each chapter are a number of sections that include background information, examples, tools and checklists, and PowerPoint® slides. It also includes databases of best practices.

3. **http://here.doh.wa.gov/professional-resources/planning**

   Health Education Resource Exchange (H.E.R.E.), Washington State Department of Health

   H.E.R.E. is a Website of the Washington State Department of Health designed as an online clearinghouse of public health and health promotion materials, events, resources, and news. It is designed to assist individuals who perform population-based health promotion activities in a variety of settings. It includes a number of resources on community engagement and mobilization.

PART II IMPLEMENTING A HEALTH PROMOTION PROGRAM

The chapters in this section present information used in implementing a health promotion program. The chapters identify important components related to implementation and address the challenges one may face during the implementation process.

Identification and Allocation of Resources

Chapter Objectives

After reading this chapter and answering the questions at the end, you should be able to:

- Define *resources*.
- List the common resources used in most health promotion programs.
- Identify the tasks to be carried out by program personnel.
- Explain the difference between internal and external personnel.
- Explain how technical assistance, volunteers, teamwork, and cultural factors are related to program personnel.
- Define *culturally competent*.
- Explain what is meant by the term *canned health promotion programs*.
- Identify questions to ask vendors when they are selling their programs, products, and services.
- List and explain common means of financing health promotion programs.
- Identify and explain the major components of a grant proposal.
- Define *budget*.
- Explain what is meant by *direct* and *indirect costs*.

Key Terms

adjourning
budget
budget narrative
canned program
cultural competence
curriculum
direct cost
external personnel
flex time
forming
full-time equivalent (FTE)
gift
grant
grantsmanship
hard money
indirect cost
in-house materials
in-kind contributions
internal personnel
memorandum of understanding (MOU)

norming
peer education
performing
profit margin
proposal
reforming
request for applications (RFAs)
request for proposals (RFPs)
resources
SAM
seed dollars
sliding-scale fee
soft money
speakers' bureaus
storming
team
technical assistance
vendors
volunteers

F or a program to reach its identified goals and objectives, it must be supported with the appropriate resources. **Resources** include the "human, fiscal, and technical assets available" (Johnson & Breckon, 2007, p. 296) to plan, implement, and evaluate a program. The resources needed to plan, implement, and evaluate a program depend on the scope and nature of the program. Most resources carry a "price tag," which planners must take into account. Thus planners face the task of securing the financial resources necessary to carry out a program. However, several different resources are provided by organizations, mostly voluntary or governmental health organizations, that are free or inexpensive. This chapter identifies, describes, and suggests sources for obtaining the resources commonly needed in planning, implementing, and evaluating health promotion programs. **Box 10.1** identifies the responsibilities and competencies for health education specialists that pertain to the material presented in this chapter.

BOX

10.1

Responsibilities and Competencies for Health Education Specialists

This chapter focuses on identifying and allocating resources needed to plan, implement, and evaluate a program. Because resources are needed for all aspects of the program, Chapter 10 cuts across several different areas of responsibility. The responsibilities and competencies related to these tasks include:

RESPONSIBILITY I: Assess Needs, Resources, and Capacity for Health Education/Promotion

   Competency 1.1: Plan assessment process for health education/promotion

RESPONSIBILITY II: Plan Health Education/Promotion

   Competency 2.1: Involve priority populations, partners, and other stakeholders in the planning process

   Competency 2.4: Develop a plan for the delivery of health education/promotion

   Competency 2.5: Address factors that influence implementation of health education/promotion

RESPONSIBILITY III: Implement Health Education/Promotion

   Competency 3.1: Coordinate logistics necessary to implement plan

   Competency 3.3: Train staff members and volunteers involved in implementation of health education/promotion

RESPONSIBILITY IV: Conduct Evaluation and Research Related to Health Education/Promotion

   Competency 4.1: Develop evaluation plan for health education/promotion

   Competency 4.2: Develop a research plan for health education/promotion

RESPONSIBILITY V: Administer and Manage Health Education/Promotion

   Competency 5.1: Manage financial resources for health education/promotion programs

   Competency 5.2: Manage technology resources

   Competency 5.3: Manage relationships with partners and other stakeholders

   Competency 5.6: Manage human resources for health education/promotion programs

RESPONSIBILITY VI: Serve as a Health Education/Promotion Resource Person

   Competency 6.2: Train others to use health education/promotion skills

   Competency 6.3: Provide advice and consultation on health education/promotion issues

Source: *A Competency-Based Framework for Health Education Specialists—2015*. Whitehall, PA: National Commission for Health Education Credentialing, Inc. (NCHEC) and the Society for Public Health Education (SOPHE). Reprinted by permission of the National Commission for Health Education Credentialing, Inc. (NCHEC) and the Society for Public Health Education (SOPHE).

Box 10.2 lists the major categories of resources and accompanying questions that need to be answered in order to have the necessary resources to plan, implement, and evaluate a program. If you are currently planning a health promotion program, take a few minutes to read through the list and attempt to answer the questions as they pertain to the program you are planning *before* you read the rest of the chapter.

BOX

10.2

Application

What Resources Are Needed to Plan, Implement, and Evaluate a Program?

Personnel

- Who is needed to plan the program? Professionals? Advisory committee?
- Who is needed to implement the program? Facilitators? Support staff? Volunteers? Will you use a vendor?
- Who will evaluate the program? Someone associated with the program? Someone from outside?
- Is there a need for a partnership? If so, who would be appropriate partners?

Curriculum and other instructional resources

- What educational materials are needed to implement the program? Will the planners create them? Will they be purchased? Will they be donated? Can the materials be adopted or adapted from another program?
- Is there a need for a curriculum?
- Will a canned program be used?

Space

- What space is needed to implement the program? How will you obtain the space? Will there be a charge for the space? Will it be donated? If donated, are there hidden costs like paying for custodial services?

Equipment

- What equipment is needed to plan the program? Is office equipment such as computers and copy machines needed?
- Is equipment needed for implementation such as tables and chairs, instructional equipment (e.g., computer and projector), exercise equipment, etc.?

Supplies

- What supplies are needed for planning the program such as typical office supplies? Are postal and mailing supplies needed?
- What supplies are needed for implementation? Who will provide them? Planners? Participants? Outside group?
- What supplies are needed for evaluation? For example, supplies needed for data collection.

Financial resources

- How will the program be paid for? Will the planning group pay for it? Will the program participants pay for it? Will some third party pay for it (i.e., sponsoring group or agency, grant funded)? Or will it be paid for by a combination of sources?
- Who is responsible for creating and monitoring the budget?

▷ Personnel

The key resource of any program is the individuals needed to carry out the program. Instead of trying to identify all the individuals necessary to ensure a program's success (because many times the same person is responsible for several different program components), planners should focus on the tasks that need to be completed by the program personnel. These tasks include: planning; identifying resources; advertising; marketing; conducting the program, including having the necessary interpreters for those who speak a different language than the one in which the program is offered and accommodating those with disabilities; monitoring the program progress; evaluating the program; making arrangements for space and program materials; handling clerical work; and keeping records (for program sign-up, collection of fees, attendance, and budgeting).

In some cases, the program participants themselves constitute a program resource. For example, in the case of a worksite health promotion program, planners will need to find out whether the employees will participate on company time, on their own time before or after work hours, on a combination of company time and employee time, or on their own anytime during the work day as long as they put in their regular number of work hours. This last option is known as **flex time**. The current trend in worksite health promotion programs is to ask the employees to participate at least partially on their own time. The reasoning behind this trend is that this investment by the participant helps to promote a sense of program ownership ("I have put something into this program, and therefore I am going to support it") and thus build loyalty among participants.

Internal Personnel

When identifying the personnel needed to conduct a program, planners have three basic options. One, referred to as **internal personnel**, uses individuals from within the planning agency/organization or people from within the priority population to supply the needed labor. These individuals may be hired specifically to serve as program personnel or existing employees may be trained to handle specific tasks. An example of using internal personnel would be when a local health department was planning a health promotion program in a community, the employees of the health department might handle the planning, implementation, and evaluation of the program. If that same health department was planning a health promotion program for the faculty and staff of a school district, there would likely be many school employees (e.g., school nurse, health and/or physical education teacher, family and consumer science teacher) who have the expertise (knowledge and skills) to carry out much of the program. If the department was planning a worksite program, there would probably be some employees who would be qualified to conduct at least a portion of the program (for example, an employee who is certified to teach first aid or cardiopulmonary resuscitation).

Another internal resource that health promotion planners are using successfully in a variety of settings, especially in schools (from kindergarten to college), is **peer education**. The process is simple: Individuals who have specific knowledge, skills, or understanding of a concept help to educate their peers. For example, college students may work with other college students to help educate them about the dangers of drinking and driving. The major advantages of peer education are its low cost and the credibility of the instructor. Children, for example, are greatly influenced by slightly older peers.

External Personnel

Individuals from outside the planning agency/organization or priority population who would conduct part or all of the program make up a second source of personnel for a program. Such individuals are considered **external personnel**. Typically, these individuals are brought in when it is found that there is a gap between what can be provided internally and what ultimately must be provided to accomplish the program goals and objectives (Harris, 2001). Many companies now offer or sell programs, services, or consulting to groups wanting health promotion programs. These companies are referred to as **vendors**. Some vendors are for-profit groups—such as hospitals, consulting agencies, health promotion companies, or related businesses—whereas others are nonprofit organizations—such as voluntary health agencies, YMCAs, YWCAs, governmental health agencies, universities/colleges, extension services, or professional organizations. Planners must be careful when choosing vendors (see **Box 10.3**) because the quality of vendors can vary greatly.

Experts available through **speakers' bureaus** are often an untapped inexpensive source of personnel for health promotion programs. Most local offices of voluntary health agencies

---

BOX

10.3

Focus On

Selecting Health Promotion Vendors

Planners must be careful when selecting vendors because the quality of vendors can vary greatly. Harris, McKenzie, and Zuti (1986) created a checklist to help planners screen potential vendors to ensure they are a good match for the program being planned. Eight major areas to consider before selecting and entering into a contract with a vendor include:

1. Initial experience with the vendor—Was the vendor prepared for the first meeting? Can the vendor show how his/her product meets your needs? Did the vendor listen to you? Will the vendor provide a proposal? Does the vendor have a good reputation? Will the vendor provide the names of other customers?

2. Product quality—Does the vendor have evidence to show the effectiveness of the product? Will the vendor customize the product to fit your needs? Is the product up to date with regard to professional standards?

3. Professionals involved in service delivery—Are those who deliver the product qualified to do so? Are their credentials up-to-date? Are those who deliver the product evaluated?

4. Product/service delivery and satisfaction—Is the information about the product/service provided in a written document? Is there a contract to sign? Can the product/service be delivered as needed?

5. Vendor technological capability—Does the vendor have the technology to deliver the product/service as needed?

6. Evaluation and reporting—Does the vendor have the capability to collect, analyze, and report the data needed for the program?

7. Product cost and value—Is the cost competitive? Are there any hidden costs? Does the price per unit go down when more product/service is purchased?

8. General concerns—Does the vendor carry liability insurance? Is the vendor the best fit for the program?

Adapted from: "How to Select the Right Vendor for Your Company's Selecting Health Promotion Program." J. H. Harris, J. F. McKenzie, and W. B. Zuti, from *Fitness in Business 1.* Copyright © 1986 by American School Health Association. Reprinted with permission.

TABLE 10.1 **Advantages and Disadvantages of Using Internal and External Personnel**

	Advantages	Disadvantages
Internal Program Personnel	1. Reduced costs.	1. Limited by the interest and abilities of those on staff.
	2. Internal arrangements can be made to free needed personnel from their work schedules.	2. May have to train personnel or be limited by the expertise of those on staff.
	3. More control over those involved	3. Might spend more time developing the program than implementing it, thus reaching fewer people.
External Program Personnel	1. Known expertise.	1. Often more costly than using internal personnel.
	2. The responsibility for conducting the program becomes the work of another.	2. Subject to the limitations of any given vendor.
	3. Can request product (program) guarantees.	3. Sometimes less control over the program.
	4. Sometimes external personnel are more respected than internal personnel simply because they are from the outside.	
	5. Bring global knowledge to the program because they have worked with a variety of entities and cultures (Harris, 2001).	
	6. Have the resources for sophisticated tools and programs because they can spread the cost across many clients (Harris, 2001).	
	7. Can reach a priority population that is geographically dispersed (Harris, 2001).	

(e.g., American Cancer Society, American Heart Association), hospitals, and other health-related organizations maintain speakers' bureaus. The services of these experts are usually available at little or no cost to groups. With some inquiry and a little networking, it is not difficult for planners to identify organizations that have individuals available to speak on a variety of health-related topics, or health care organizations willing to send their medical experts into the community to share their knowledge. The speakers' bureau is a win-win concept for both the group offering the service and the one receiving it. Groups that take advantage of a speakers' bureau gain access to expert information, but those delivering the information gain in terms of public relations and recognition.

There are advantages and disadvantages connected with using either internal or external personnel to conduct health promotion programs. **Table 10.1** lists the pros and cons of each.

Combination of Internal and External Personnel

The third option for obtaining personnel to carry out a program is using a combination of internal and external personnel. This option is the most common because it allows program planners to make use of the advantages of the first two options, while avoiding many of the disadvantages.

Items Related to Personnel

In addition to determining the source of personnel for a program there are other personnel matters to which planners must attend. Four of these—technical assistance, volunteers, teamwork, and cultural factors—are discussed below.

TECHNICAL ASSISTANCE

Sometimes there are enough people willing and able to handle the tasks associated with planning, implementing, and evaluating a program but for whatever reason they do not have the capability (i.e., knowledge, skills, and know how) to carry out the tasks. Or personnel may have knowledge and skills but need help in completing the tasks more effectively. Such situations call for *technical assistance* to enhance group members' capacity to complete the work. **Technical assistance** (TA), also known as *technical support* or *capacity-building assistance* (CBA), can be defined as a relationship in which individuals with specific knowledge and skills share their expertise, via advice and training, with those who need it. TA often comes from consultants or may be a part of a support program offered by a funding agency. For example, it is not uncommon for the Centers for Disease Control and Prevention (CDC) to offer technical assistance to groups that receive CDC funding for their programs, or to state or local health departments that need to enhance their capabilities.

Technical assistance providers must be more than just experts. They must demonstrate that they are good listeners and effective helpers to the people who will be actually conducting the planning tasks (Butterfoss, 2007). For effective TA to take place there must be a collaborative working relationship between the two parties. TA is typically provided after some sort of needs assessment (i.e., completing a checklist or questionnaire) of those who need the assistance. Once the needs are known (e.g., priority setting, intervention planning and effectiveness, evaluation techniques) the actual TA can be planned and delivered. Delivery can be completed using a number of different training strategies and can range from providing information via a telephone call, to supplying written or self-help materials, to referring those in need to other resources, to pairing those in need with a peer group (i.e., another group of planners who have completed a similar project), to more elaborate face-to-face training sessions that may last from a few hours to a few days at one time.

VOLUNTEERS

There are times when paid staff members (i.e., professionals) are not available in sufficient numbers to carry out all the tasks necessary in planning, implementing, and evaluating health promotion programs. In such cases is not unusual to turn to volunteers for help. **Volunteers** are individuals who provide a service to others without being forced to do so. Volunteers do not get paid. Although volunteers are not paid they are not free of cost. There are costs associated with identifying, recruiting, selecting, training, and supervising volunteers (Shi & Johnson, 2014). In health promotion programs, common duties performed by volunteers include data collection for assessments and evaluation, facilitation of interventions, and clerical tasks. However, duties are only limited by the knowledge and skills of the volunteers. Often volunteers contribute services that otherwise would not be performed because of lack of funding.

As with other personnel, planners should create a job description that outlines the tasks that need to be performed before recruiting volunteers. (See **Box 10.4** for an example job description for a volunteer.) Do not reduce all the volunteer jobs to simply running errands;

some volunteers are happy doing that type of work but others want to be engaged and given meaningful tasks to complete (Fallon & Zgodzinski, 2012). Defining real jobs is very important (Wurzbach, 2002). "Volunteers that are not utilized quickly lose interest and find other outlets for their spare time" (Fallon & Zgodzinski, 2012, p. 116). In identifying the tasks to be completed by and creating job descriptions for volunteers, program planners need to remember that volunteers are motivated by different factors than those that motivate paid employees (Issel, 2014). The reasons vary. Some individuals are interested in volunteering as a means of giving back, sharing of their gifts and talents, or just helping others in the community. Others volunteer to gain experience or "get their foot in the door" of an organization where they hope to work some day. Some volunteer to do something worthwhile, stay active, or just for the social interaction (Van Der Wagen & Carlos, 2005). Still others may

---

BOX

10.4

Focus On

Sample Job Description for a Volunteer

Position Title:	Health Education Volunteer
Reports to:	Senior Health Education Specialist
Responsible for:	Distribution of health education materials at the patient education desk
Position Summary:	To assist patients of the Stonecrest Clinic in getting the education materials they need.
Duties:	• Greet all patients and significant others who approach the patient education desk.
	• Use materials available at the patient education desk to "fill" the patient education prescription provided by the health care providers in the Stonecrest Clinic.
	• Help obtain appropriate educational materials for use at the Stonecrest Clinic.
	• Monitor and maintain inventory; help to re-stock the education materials at the patient education desk, as needed.
	• Provide excellent customer service as outlined in the core values of the Stonecrest Clinic.
	• Answer the phone at the patient education desk.
Qualifications:	• Education
	—High school diploma or equivalent
	• Knowledge
	—Basic medical terminology
	• Skills
	—Communication: Good verbal and nonverbal skills
	—Computer: Typing speed of 40 wpm; able to search Internet; use word processing and database programs
	—Problem solving
Desirable:	• Health education experience
	• Customer service experience

volunteer to enhance their knowledge or learn a new skill. The key for planners is to match the potential volunteers' motivation to the volunteer opportunities.

Once a suitable job description has been created planners are ready to recruit volunteers. Depending on the how many and what type of individuals are needed, a variety of techniques can be used to recruit volunteers. The most traditional way of recruiting is via a mass media outlet (e.g., radio, television, and newspapers), but posting flyers in high-traffic areas where desired volunteers pass can be effective as well. In addition, viral recruiting can be used via social media or personal word-of-mouth invitations. Places where planners may find potential volunteers include religious organizations, community service organizations (e.g., Jaycees, Rotary), senior citizen centers, and colleges and universities. In fact, many educational institutions require community service or service learning as part of graduation requirements.

Potential volunteers should not be accepted automatically for a position; instead they should be interviewed, just as a prospective employee would be. It is important to make sure that the person is right for the job, and that the person's philosophy is consistent with that of the organization where they will volunteer (Wurzbach, 2002). After the interview process, planners may find that they have attracted good people but those individuals may not have all the knowledge and skills to complete the work. This makes training the volunteers particularly critical to the success of a health promotion program (Issel, 2014). In order to provide appropriate training, it is not uncommon to conduct a needs/assets assessment with the volunteers. This is something that can be completed as part of the interviewing process. With such data, a thorough training plan can be can be put together for new volunteers. Common topics for volunteer training sessions include: background information on the organization including goals, values, and organizational culture; human resource policies; privacy and confidentiality policies: HIPAA, GINA, and the Family Educational Rights and Privacy Act (FERPA); knowledge and skills to carry out volunteer tasks; and background on the attitudes, reactions, culture, and daily lives of those in the population being served (Shi & Johnson, 2014).

Once on the job, volunteers need to be supervised and periodically evaluated. The person to whom they report can handle this. If a program needs a large number of volunteers, it may be necessary to hire a volunteer coordinator (Wurzbach, 2002).

Good volunteers are not easy to find so every effort should be made to retain them. For the most part, if volunteers are happy and satisfied with the work they will continue. To increase the chances of this happening, include volunteers in staff meetings and functions when it is appropriate, and show appreciation for their help by saying thank you often, providing positive feedback, and publicly recognizing their achievements and service through newsletters, news releases, and/or recognition ceremonies (Wurzbach, 2002).

Before leaving our discussion of volunteers, we want you to be aware that volunteer help does not always work out as planned. Organizations have "the right to decide on the best placement of a volunteer, to express opinions about poor volunteer performance in a diplomatic way, and to release an inappropriate volunteer" (Van Der Wagen & Carlos, 2005, p. 180). And finally, when volunteers resign, always hold an exit interview with them to get their comments on the good and bad aspects of their volunteer work (Wurzbach, 2002) so that you can improve future volunteer experiences.

WORKING AS A TEAM

Because of the multiple tasks associated with planning, implementing, and evaluating health promotion programs and the need for a variety of resources to have effective programs, health education specialists often work as part of a group or team. Further, teamwork is becoming a preferred approach in many work settings because "organizational problems and issues are so complex today that no one person can grasp all the information nor have all the skills to adequately and thoroughly analyze and choose the best solutions. The complexity of problems also requires innovations and diversity of viewpoints to see all the options and consequences involved" (Kilingner et al., 2010, p. 224). A **team** had been defined as "a small group of people with complementary skills who are committed to a common purpose, a set of performance goals, and an approach for which they hold themselves mutually accountable" (Gomez-Mejia & Balkin, 2012, p. 384). Teams differ from working groups in that working group members are accountable for individual work but are not responsible for the output of the entire group (Gomez-Mejia & Balkin, 2012). Teams can vary in size and be as small as two people; however, the sizes of high-performing teams range between 5 and 12 members (Gomez-Mejia & Balkin, 2012).

In a 2009 study, Lovelace and colleagues found that health education specialists "participated in an average of four teams per individual; three of these were interorganizational teams. Moreover, 40% of the respondents participated in five or more teams" (p. 428). These authors further stated that in order to be effective, health education specialists "must be able to work collaboratively with community members and other professionals" (p. 429). "In fact, words like *boundary-spanning, collaborative public management, bridge building*, and *facilitative leadership* all attest to the way that contemporary work is conducted" (Kilingner et al., 2010, p. 224).

Team creation can come about in a couple of different ways. When teams are created within an organization, say within a local health department, member assignments may occur formally when a supervisor or manager organizes a team based on the people and their skills. If interorganizational teams are assembled, typically the team is composed of whomever each organization assigns to the team. This is a more informal means of team composition in that no one individual selects team members for their individual knowledge and skills. Whichever way is used, each team will need a leader or leaders to guide the work of the team.

"Teams are not instantly functional and effective" (Butterfoss, 2007, p. 164); they take time to develop. Understanding how teams develop and what stage a team is in can help planners be more efficient in the planning process. To help explain the development, Tuckman (1965) identified the development sequence of small groups and created a model to explain it (Tuckman, 2001). The original model included four stages—*forming, storming, norming*, and *performing*. Several years later, Tuckman and Jensen (1977) added a fifth stage—*adjourning*. More recently, the fifth stage has been called *mourning* (Butterfoss, 2007) or *reforming* (UNRCE, 2003). Over time, the "stages of group development" terminology has changed a bit and the five stages are now associated with team development.

The first stage, **forming**, can be thought as an orientation stage. As such, little real work is accomplished. In this stage members are introduced, meet, and get to know each other. During this stage the ground rules for the group are established, such as defining the purpose of the team, team structure (e.g., roles and responsibilities), logistics for operation (e.g., procedures, meeting times), and expectations (Gomez-Mejia & Balkin, 2012). As such, "two important things must be accomplished in this first stage: members must feel welcome and included and have a sense that their opinions will be respected; and they need to develop a consensus, or group agreement, about the basic mission or goal they are working toward" (Butterfoss, 2007, p. 164). In the second stage, **storming**, members will have different opinions about team goals, assigned tasks and responsibilities, and procedures (Gomez-Mejia & Balkin, 2012). The conflict may be uncomfortable, turf wars can occur, and some members may feel frustrated. Good teams with good leadership will be able to work through this stage, but if the conflict is too great and cannot be resolved, teams may disband.

The teams that emerge will enter into stage three, **norming**. In this stage, "team members finally understand their roles and establish closer relationships, intensifying the cohesion and interdependence of members" (Gomez-Mejia & Balkin, 2012, p. 390). In the fourth phase, **performing**, teams are involved in "constructive action" (Tuckman, 1965); they are working toward the team goals. "This is the stage where a great deal of work can occur, and the team may become creative. As new tasks emerge, members confidently tackle them. The whole team works together or may delegate work to task groups and individuals" (Butterfoss, 2007, p. 165). After the performing stage, teams may enter into the **adjourning** (or *mourning*) stage or decide to move to **reforming**. In the former, the team has reached its goal, thus completing its work. As such it may decide to disband. However, the disbanding may not be easy, thus the term *mourning*. In the latter, reforming, the team may continue on by refocusing its efforts on other tasks or problems.

There is no single prescription for creating effective working teams; however, several authors have identified characteristics that are important. Gomez-Mejia and Balkin (2012) have identified five behavioral characteristics of effective teams: (1) cohesiveness, (2) selecting high-performance norms, (3) cooperation, (4) exhibiting interdependence, and (5) trusting one another. Getha-Taylor (2008) asserts that there are three factors associated with collaborative competencies that set exemplars apart from average performers. Those factors include interpersonal understanding, teamwork and understanding, and team leadership. In identifying these three factors Getha-Taylor indicated that interpersonal understanding is the most important and only comes about through time and experience.

CULTURAL FACTORS

Regardless of who is involved in planning, implementing, and evaluating a health promotion program, there is a need to be aware of the importance of cultural factors. Cultural factors arise from guidelines (both explicit and implicit) that individuals "inherit" from being a part of a particular society, racial or ethnic group, religious community, or other group. In order for planners to be effective, they need to strive to be culturally competent (Davis & Rankin, 2006; Luquis, Pérez, & Young, 2006; Pérez & Luquis, 2014; Selig, Tropiano, & Greene-Moton, 2006). **Cultural competence** is "a developmental process defined as a set of values, principles, behaviors, attitudes, and policies that enable health professionals to work effectively across racial, ethnic, and linguistically diverse populations" (Joint Committee on Health Education and Promotion Terminology, 2012, p. 16). Luquis and Pérez (2003) and Martinez-Cossio (2008) have discussed some of the issues surrounding cultural competence and some strategies by which planners can become more culturally competent. One strategy is becoming familiar with Standards for Culturally and Linguistically Appropriate Services (CLAS) in Health and Health Care (Office of Minority Health, 2013) (see Weblinks at the end of this chapter for the Website). The National CLAS Standards were created to advance health equity, improve quality, and help eliminate health care disparities by establishing a blueprint for individuals and organizations to implement culturally and linguistically appropriate services (OMH, 2013). In addition, if planners are not familiar with the culture of those in the priority population we would recommend that they work with indigenous health workers and/or those who are well trained and are bilingual and bicultural.

▷ Curricula and Other Instructional Resources

Earlier (in Chapter 8), the word **curriculum** was defined as a "planned set of lessons or courses designed to lead to competence in an area of study" (Gilbert et al., 2015, p. 437). When it comes to selecting the curriculum and other instructional materials that will be used to present the content of the program, planners can proceed in four ways: (1) by developing their own materials (in-house) or having someone else develop custom materials for them; (2) by purchasing or obtaining various instructional materials from outside sources; (3) by purchasing or obtaining entire "canned" programs from outside vendors; or (4) by using any combination of in-house materials, materials from outside sources, and canned program materials.

Developing **in-house materials** or having someone else develop custom materials has the major advantage of allowing the developers to create materials that very closely match the needs of the priority population. The more "unique" the priority population, the more important this approach may be—especially if the priority population possesses cultural differences. Materials must be relevant and culturally appropriate to the priority population (Luquis, 2014). However, a serious drawback is the time, money, and effort necessary to develop an original curriculum and other instructional materials. The exact amount of time necessary would obviously depend on the scope of the program and the expertise of those doing the work. No matter who does the work, however, the commitment of time and resources is sure to be considerable. In putting together an in-house program, planners should be aware of several different sources from which they can obtain free or inexpensive materials to supplement the ones they develop. Planners might also find that there is no need to create in-house materials because of the wide array of materials available. For example, most voluntary and governmental health agencies have up-to-date pamphlets on a variety of subjects that they are willing and eager to give away in quantity. Also, most communities have a public library with a video/DVD section that includes some health videos and DVDs. If the public library does not carry health videos and DVDs, almost all local and state health departments offer such a service. Planners who are working in K–12 school settings will want to use the Health Education Curriculum Analysis Tool (HECAT) (CDC, 2013) that can be used to identify a curriculum that best meets the needs of the children being served (see Weblinks at the end of this chapter for the Website). Planners who are unsure about what sources of information are available in their community can begin by checking the Yellow Pages of the local telephone directory or the Internet.

Planners need to remember that just because a piece of instructional material exists does not mean it is appropriate for the priority population with which they are working. To help ensure that materials are suitable for the priority population, we would recommend the use of **SAM:** a suitability assessment of materials instrument (Doak, Doak, & Root, 1996) (see **Figure 10.1**). This validated instrument "was originally designed for use with print material and illustrations, but it has also been applied successfully to video- and audiotaped instructions. For each material, SAM provides a numerical score (in percent) that may fall in one of three categories: superior, adequate, or not suitable" (Doak et al., 1996, p. 49). Here are the steps for using SAM (Doak et al., 1996):

1. Read through the SAM factor list and the evaluation criteria.

2. Read the material (or view the video) you wish to evaluate and write brief statements as to its purpose(s) and key points.

2 points for superior rating

1 point for adequate rating

0 points for not suitable rating

N/A if the factor does not apply to this material

FACTOR TO BE RATED	SCORE	COMMENTS
1. CONTENT		
(a) Purpose is evident	_____	_____
(b) Content about behaviors	_____	_____
(c) Scope is limited	_____	_____
(d) Summary or review included	_____	_____
2. LITERACY DEMAND		
(a) Reading grade level	_____	_____
(b) Writing style, active voice	_____	_____
(c) Vocabulary uses common words	_____	_____
(d) Context is given first	_____	_____
(e) Learning aids via "road signs"	_____	_____
3. GRAPHICS		
(a) Cover graphic shows purpose	_____	_____
(b) Type of graphics	_____	_____
(c) Relevance of illustration	_____	_____
(d) List, tables, etc. explained	_____	_____
(e) Captions used for graphics	_____	_____
4. LAYOUT AND TYPOGRAPHY		
(a) Layout factors	_____	_____
(b) Typography	_____	_____
(c) Subheads ("chunking") used	_____	_____
5. LEARNING STIMULATION, MOTIVATION		
(a) Interaction used	_____	_____
(b) Behaviors are modeled and specific	_____	_____
(c) Motivation—self-efficacy	_____	_____
6. CULTURAL APPROPRIATENESS		
(a) Match in logic, language, experience	_____	_____
(b) Cultural image and examples	_____	_____

Total SAM score: _____

Total possible score: _____ , Percent score: _____ %

▲ **Figure 10.1** SAM Scoring Sheet

Source: *Teaching Patients with Low Literacy Skills, 2nd Edition*. C. C. Doak, L. G. Doak, & J. H. Root. Copyright © 1996 by J. B. Lippincott Company. Reprinted with permission of the authors.

3. For short materials, evaluate the entire piece. For long materials, select samples that are central to the purpose of the document to evaluate.

4. Evaluate and score each of the 22 SAM items, rating them as "superior" and assigning a score of two, "adequate" and assigning a score of one, "not suitable" and assigning a score of zero, or marking an item "N/A" if the factor does not apply to the material.

5. Calculate the total suitability score by summing the scores from the rated items and dividing by the total number of items rated. Do not include the items marked N/A. Multiply the score by 100 to get a percentage.

> 70–100% = superior material
>
> 40–69% = adequate material
>
> 0–39% = not suitable material

6. Decide on the impact of deficiencies of the material and what action to take about whether to use or not use the material.

Purchasing or obtaining entire canned programs from vendors has the advantage of saving the time and money needed to create programs. A **canned program** is one that has been developed by an outside group and includes the basic components and materials necessary to implement a program. Because some vendors are for-profit groups whereas others are nonprofit organizations, the cost of these programs can range from literally nothing at all to thousands of dollars. For example, there are both not-for-profit (e.g., American Cancer Society and American Lung Association) and for-profit organizations that have created canned programs for smoking cessation.

Most canned programs have five major components:

1. A participant's manual (printed material that is easy to follow and read and is handy for participants)

2. An instructor's manual (a much more comprehensive document than the participant's manual, which includes the program content, background information, and lesson and unit plans with ideas for presenting the material)

3. Audiovisual materials that help present the program content (usually including videotapes/DVDs and audiotapes, PowerPoint® presentations, charts, or posters)

4. Training for the instructors (a concentrated experience that prepares individuals to become instructors)

5. Marketing (the "wrapping" that makes the program attractive to both the participants and the planners who will purchase it to market to the participants)

The advantages and disadvantages of canned programs are just the opposite of those for materials developed in-house. No time is spent on development; however, the program may not fit the needs or the demographic characteristics of the priority population. For example, using the same canned smoking cessation program with middle-aged adults who realize the long-term hazards of cigarettes and with teenagers who are required to attend a smoking cessation program for disciplinary reasons may not be advisable. Most adults who enter smoking cessation programs are there because they do not want to smoke. Obviously, this is not the case with teenagers who have been caught smoking. The approaches taken with these two programs would have to be very different if both are to be successful. Another example of when use of a canned program would not be advisable is use of a program that was designed for upper-middle-class suburban adults in a program for low-income inner-city populations. The lifestyles of the two groups are just too different for the same program to be appropriate in both situations. Because of the possible mismatch between the needs and peculiarities (i.e., age, culture, ethnicity, norms, race, sex, socioeconomic status) of a particular priority population, planners are urged to move with caution when deciding on the use of a canned program

Canned programs often come attractively packaged and seemingly complete, but this does not mean that they are well-conceived and effective programs. Before using canned programs, planners should consider the following seven questions:

1. Is the program based on best practices? If not, why not?

2. Is there evidence to show the program is effective?

3. Does the program include a long-term behavior modification component? There are no "quick fixes" with regard to many health behavior changes. If behavior modification is used, it should be based on sound health behavior practice over an appropriate time frame.

4. Is the program educationally sound? Not only should the program be based on sound psychological and sociological theory but it should also be based on valid educational theory.

5. Is the program motivational? Health behavior change is not easy to accomplish, and so all programs need to include activities that motivate people to get and stay involved.

6. Is the program enjoyable? Planned programs should be enjoyable. Some people like hard work, but it is difficult to sustain hard work for a long time without some enjoyment.

7. Can the program be modified (i.e., adapted—see Chapter 8 for information on adapting an intervention) to meet the specific needs and peculiarities of the priority population? As mentioned earlier, not all populations have the same needs, beliefs, traditions, and ways of approaching a problem.

▷ Space

Another major resource needed for most health promotion programs is sufficient space—a place where the program can be held. Depending on the type of program and the intended audience, space may or may not be readily available. For example, an employer may make space available for a worksite program, or a school system may furnish space for a school program. If space is a problem, planners may be able to locate inexpensive space in local schools, colleges and universities, religious facilities, and in "community service rooms" (rooms that are available free of charge to community groups as a community service) of local businesses. In addition, planners may find educational institutions and local businesses that are willing to co-sponsor programs and thus contribute the space necessary to conduct the program. It may also be possible to obtain space by trading for it. For instance, a planner might trade expertise, such as serving as consultant for a program, in return for the use of suitable space. Or it might be possible to trade one space for another, such as trading the use of school classrooms for time in the local YMCA/YWCA pool.

One final note of caution about space: Even if space is provided free of charge for a program, make sure to ask if there are any associated costs for the "free space." It is not uncommon for an organization offering the space (e.g., a school district) to do so with the obligation for the users to pay for the custodial time to clean up the space once it has been used. Thus, a charge such as two hours of overtime pay for the custodial staff may be an obligation in order to use the free space.

▷ Equipment and Supplies

Most health promotion programs will need both equipment and supplies in order to be planned, implemented, and evaluated. Though often the words *equipment* and *supplies* are used to mean the same thing, from planning and budgeting perspectives they are usually considered two different types of commodities, and not all organizations define the words the same. Some organizations define equipment and supplies by costs. That is, equipment may be anything costing more than $500, whereas supplies are anything costing between $1 and $499. Thus, a computer may be equipment, while paper or even a chair may be a supply. These same organizations usually have a dollar amount definition for major equipment items (sometimes referred to as *capital expenditures* or *capital equipment*) as anything costing more than so many thousands of dollars depending on the nature of the organization. Other organizations may define equipment and supplies based on the "life" of the commodity. For example, equipment may be anything that will last three years or more, and supplies anything that lasts fewer than three years. Thus, under this type of classification a computer may be considered a supply. Or, an organization may define equipment as something that is not consumable, like a desk, and a supply to be something that is consumable like photocopy paper. It is not so important how the words are defined, but planners need to know how they are defined and work within those parameters.

Some programs may require a great deal of equipment and supplies. For example, first aid and safety programs need items such as CPR mannequins, splints, blankets, bandages, dressings, and video equipment. Other programs, such as a stress management program, may need only paper, pencils, and a CD player. Whatever the kinds and amounts of equipment and supplies required, planners must give advance thought to their needs so as to:

- Determine the necessary equipment and supplies, in the correct amount/number, to facilitate the program
- Identify the sources where the equipment and supplies can be obtained
- Find a way to pay for the needed equipment and supplies

▷ Financial Resources

To hire the individuals needed to plan, implement, and evaluate a health promotion program and to pay for the other resources required, planners must obtain appropriate financial support. Most programs are limited by the financial support available. In fact, few programs are financed at such a level that planners would say they have all the money they need. Because of this, the planners are often faced with making decisions about how to allocate the funds that are available. Some typical financial questions that planners generally must address are the following:

- Is it better to run an adequately financed program for a few people or to run a poorly financed program for more people?

- If funds are limited where could cuts be made?
- Should a program be started knowing funding will fall short, or should the program be delayed until appropriate funding is available?
- Is it better to have fewer instructors or to make do with fewer supplies?

Programs can be financed in several different ways. Some sources of financial support are very traditional, whereas others may be limited only by the creativity and imagination of those involved. Following are several established ways of financing programs.

Participant Fee

This method of financing a program requires the participants to pay for the cost of the program. Depending on whether the program is offered on a profit-making basis, this fee may be equal to expenses or may include a **profit margin**. Participant fees not only are a means by which programs can be financed but they also help motivate participants to stay involved in a program. If people pay to participate in a program, then they may be more likely to continue to participate because they have made an investment—that is, a commitment. This concept has also been referred to as *ownership* (see the discussion on behavioral economics in Chapter 8). Many participants who pay a fee feel like they are part "owners" of the program. However, it should be noted that not everyone shares in the ownership concept. There are some participants who still would prefer a free or almost free program that has been paid for by others. An example of the ownership and cost issue is the participant fees associated with smoking cessation programs. If planners were looking for vendors of smoking cessation programs, they would find that the costs of such programs range from zero (e.g., American Cancer Society's *FreshStart* program) to modest (e.g., American Lung Association's *Freedom from Smoking* program) to expensive (e.g., those offered by private health promotion companies).

Deciding to finance a program through a participant fee may sound easy, but planners need to give serious thought to how much they will charge and who will be charged. Often, those most in need of a health promotion program are the least able to pay. Planners do not want to create a barrier to program participation by charging a fee or setting the fee too high. If a fee is necessary, then planners should consider creating a fee structure on "ability to pay." One form of this is a **sliding-scale fee**—that is, the less one's income, the lower the participant fee. Or, planners may want to consider offering "scholarships" to those unable to pay.

Third-Party Support

Most individuals are familiar with insurance companies' acting as third-party payers to cover the costs of health care. Although health insurance is not often used to pay for health promotion programs, others can be third-party payers. Third-party means that someone other than participants (the first-party) or planners (the second-party) is paying for the program. Third-party payers that may cover the cost of health promotion programs are:

- Employers that pick up the cost for employees, as is often the case in worksite health promotion programs

- Agencies other than the groups sponsoring the program—for example, when local service or civic groups "adopt" a pet program
- A professional association or union that financially supports a program

The money used by third-party payers can be generated from a special fund-raising event, from sale of concessions, or with money saved from reduced health care costs, absenteeism, or the remodeling of employee benefit plans.

Cost Sharing

A third means of financing a program involves a combination of participant fee and third-party support. It is not unusual to have an employer pay 50% to 80% of a program's costs and have employees pay the remaining 50% to 20%. Or, an employer may have a reimbursement policy for program participation. With such policies, employees are responsible for paying the participation fee, and then based on either attendance at the program (e.g., the employee must attend at least 80% of the program sessions) or completion of the program (e.g., employee must produce a certificate of completion), the employer reimburses the employee for either all or a portion of the participant fee. Such arrangements have the advantages of both ownership and a fringe benefit.

Cooperative Agreements

There are times when two parties (e.g., groups, organizations, individuals, agencies) establish agreements that offer mutual benefits to both parties when they share resources and work together to offer a program or service. Often these agreements do not involve the transfer of money from one party to the other (though they may), but rather access to and sharing of resources (Fertman et al., 2010). For example, one agency may be willing to provide educational literature to another agency in return for space to present a program or the use of an employee's time. It is not uncommon for such agreements to be spelled out in a written document and signed by an individual of each agency with authority to do so. The written document may be a *letter of agreement*, which once signed by both parties becomes legally binding, or something less formal (i.e., not legally binding) like a memorandum of understanding (MOU) or memorandum of agreement (MOA). A **memorandum of understanding** is defined as "a document that describes the general principles of an agreement between parties, but does not amount to a substantive contract" (Dictionary .com, 2015). It is not unusual for such an MOU or MOA to help support a grant proposal (see the discussion of grants below).

Organization/Agency Sponsorship

Many times, the sponsoring organization/agency bears the cost of the program as a part of its programming or operating budget. In such cases, the source of the money to fund a program would depend on how the agency is funded. For example, many health promotion programs are offered or sponsored by governmental (i.e., public) health agencies. The primary source of funding of governmental health agencies is tax dollars. As such, many governmental health agency programs are free or relatively inexpensive compared to similar programs offered by for-profit groups for those who live in the jurisdiction of the agency. Depending on which agency is offering the program, tax dollars to pay for it could come from multiple levels. For example, in local (i.e., city or county) health departments (LHD) in the United States it would not be unusual for two-thirds to three-fourths the department's revenue to come from a combination of local, state, and federal tax dollars. The remainder of a LHD's revenue would come from several sources including fees (e.g., for birth and death certificates), fines (e.g., for failure to implement policy such no smoking ordinance), insurance payments (e.g., health insurance for health care provided), and private foundations.

In the case of a voluntary health agency being the sponsoring organization/agency the source of the funding would be primarily donations that have been made to the agency. For example, the American Cancer Society offers a program called Reach To Recovery® to help people with breast cancer free of charge. Program materials are provided free and an American Cancer Society volunteer conducts the program. The program is paid for with the society's community service funds.

Grants and Gifts

Another means of financing health promotion programs is through grants and gifts from other agencies, foundations, groups, and individuals. A **grant** is an award of financial assistance, the principal purpose of which is to transfer a thing of value from the grantor to a recipient to carry out a specific purpose, whereas a **gift** (or *contributions*) can be sums of money or non-monetary items that are given voluntarily without compensation in return. Nonmonetary gifts are known as **in-kind contributions** and include such things as materials, equipment, supplies, training, donated space, or other services that are used to operate programs. Both grants and gifts are often referred to as *external money*, or **soft money**. The term *soft money* refers to the fact that grants and gifts are usually given for a specific period of time and at some point will no longer be received. This is in contrast to **hard money**, which is an ongoing source of funds that is part of the operating budget of an organization from year to year.

Grant money has become an important source of program funding, especially for those working in voluntary or governmental health agencies. It thus becomes necessary for planners to develop adequate **grantsmanship** skills. These skills include (1) discovering where the grant money is located, (2) finding out how to get (apply for) the money, and (3) writing a proposal requesting the money.

LOCATING GRANT MONEY

There are four basic types of grant makers: foundations, corporations, voluntary agencies, and government. These grant makers are found at three different levels: local, state, and national. They are not the only grant makers, however. Planners may also find a variety of local organizations (such as service groups like the Lion's Club or the Jaycees, or a community group like the United Way) that may be willing to support specific local causes through a grant. Philanthropic foundations are not-for-profit organizations that award grants to serve the public interest. A number of large national foundations support health promotion (e.g., Robert Wood Johnson Foundation, Rockefeller Foundation, W. K. Kellogg Foundation), but planners may find state and local foundations as well.

Not all corporations have giving programs, but many do as a part of a community service or public relations program. Planners will need to contact the corporations to "ask who is in charge of charitable giving, what subjects they consider for grants, and how the company giving program operates" (Guyer, 1999, p. 1). Library or Internet searching will possibly help answer these questions.

Voluntary health agencies also have grant programs. Though most grants from voluntary organizations at the national level are specified for research efforts, planners may find the local or state offices of these organizations are willing to provide **seed dollars** (start-up dollars) or *in-kind* contributions (such as providing free materials or other resources) for local programs.

Government is the largest grant maker. Government, at all three levels—local, state, and federal—makes grants for many purposes. With the other three grant makers (foundations, corporations, and voluntary agencies), planners can ask them to fund any project. However, with the government, only grants that are in one of the subjects specified by the government have a chance of being funded.

When looking for grant makers, planners need to look for a pattern in giving by asking key questions: Has this funder made grants in the past for programs like mine? In my geographic area? In the amount I need? For the things I need funded? (Guyer, 1999) The answers to these questions, often found at Internet Websites of the grant makers, will indicate whether it is a good idea to contact the funder. After doing this initial "research," planners should call or email funding sources to ask questions and to obtain any guidelines, grant request forms or applications, and printed material about their grant making. This contact will also help establish a relationship with the funder. Planners not only can obtain needed information but they can also introduce their organization to the funder. This can be done by sending publications about the planners' organization, making personal contacts, and staying in touch (Guyer, 1999).

Planners can identify possible funding sources in several different ways. The first is by networking with others who have been successful in obtaining grant funding in the past. Because seeking grant funding is a competitive process, planners may have to network with others who are not seeking funding from the same grant maker. A second means of identifying funding sources is through "research." A variety of books on grants may be found online or in college and university libraries as well as many larger public libraries. For example, there are directories of grant makers for foundations and corporations, and there is usually a directory that lists grant funders that are specific to a state. Most of these books are indexed by subject area.

Three good places to begin searches for government grants are the *Catalog of Federal Domestic Assistance* (CFDA), the *Federal Register*, and Grants.Gov. (See the Weblinks at the end of the chapter.) The CFDA, which is updated biweekly, is an online catalog database of all Federal programs available to state and local governments (including the District of Columbia); federally-recognized Indian tribal governments; territories (and possessions) of the United States; domestic public, quasi-public, and private profit and nonprofit organizations and institutions; specialized groups; and individuals. The CFDA allows planners to search the database for programs meeting their needs and for which they are eligible. However, to apply for one of the programs, planners need to contact the office that administers the program they are interested in.

The *Federal Register* is the official daily publication for rules, proposed rules, and notices of Federal agencies and organizations, as well as executive orders and other presidential documents. It would list the latest grant opportunities. *Grants.Gov* is a Website where planners can find and apply for federal government grants. The site was created in 2002 to improve government services associated with grants. At this Website planners will find over 1,000 grant programs from 26 federal grant-making agencies.

A third way of identifying funding sources is through the Internet. There are several advantages to using the Internet for seeking grant makers: convenience, time saving, and being able to reach several grant makers at the same time. In addition, some Websites permit an applicant to complete one form for grant consideration at several different funders (Breen, 1999).

The fourth way of identifying grant makers is the least difficult—identifying requests for proposals or requests for applications. **Request for proposals (RFPs)** or **request for applications (RFAs)** are issued by organizations/agencies in order to solicit for services to complete a specific project. A RFP or RFA outlines the specific services that are needed, the process for applying, the timeline for applying, the terms of the contract when awarded, and how the proposal/application should be presented. For example, a state health department may issue a RFP to solicit proposals to train lay personnel to deliver immunization education programs in the community. Those who feel qualified to deliver the training could submit a proposal for review.

SUBMITTING GRANT PROPOSALS

As noted in the previous section, most funding agencies have specific guidelines outlining who is qualified to submit a proposal (perhaps only nonprofit groups can apply, or only practitioners who hold certain certifications) and the format for making an application. Those seeking money can request or apply for the money by writing a proposal. A **proposal** can be thought of as a written document that represents a request for money. A good proposal is one that is well written and explains how the group wishing to receive the money can meet the needs of the funding agency. To increase their chances of writing a good proposal, planners should call the funding agency first and speak with the grant officer to find out specifically what he or she is looking for and the format desired.

Because there is a great deal of competition for grant money, it is more than likely that proposals will be read by a busy, impatient, skeptical person who has no reason to give any one proposal special consideration and who is faced with many more requests than he or she can grant, or even read thoroughly. Such a reader wants to find out quickly and easily the answers to these seven questions:

1. What do you want to do, how much will it cost, and how much time will it take?
2. How does the proposed project relate to the sponsor's interests?
3. What will be gained if this project is carried out?
4. What has already been done in the area of the project?
5. How do you plan to do it?
6. How will the results be evaluated?
7. Why should you, rather than someone else, conduct this project?

The Components of a Grant Proposal

1. *Title (or cover) page.* When writing the title, be concise and explicit; avoid words that add nothing.
2. *Abstract or executive summary.* Provides a summary of the proposed project. May be the most important part of the proposal. Should be written last and be about 200–300 words long.
3. *Table of contents.* May or may not be needed, depending on the length of the proposal. It is a convenience for the reader.
4. *Introduction.* Should begin with a capsule statement, be comprehensible to the informed layperson, and include the statement of the problem, significance of the program, and purpose (or aims) of the program.
5. *Background.* Should include the proposer's previous related work and the related literature.
6. *Description of proposed program.* Should include the objectives, description of intervention, evaluation plan, and time frame.
7. *Description of relevant institutional/agency resources.* Should identify the resources the proposer's organization will bring to the project.
8. *List of references.* Should include references cited in the proposal.
9. *Personnel section.* Should include the biographical sketch (i.e., biosketch), curriculum vitae, or résumés of those who are to work with the program.
10. *Budget and Narrative.* Should include financial needs for personnel (salaries and wages), equipment, materials and supplies, travel, services, other needed items, and indirect costs, as well as an explanation for the amounts needed and how the amounts were calculated.

As noted, funding agencies request proposals/applications in a variety of different forms. However, several components are contained in most proposals no matter what the funding agency. **Box 10.5** presents these components.

Combining Sources

It should be obvious that planners should not be limited to any single source for financing a health promotion program. In fact, it is more than likely that most programs will be funded via a variety of sources—that is, any combination of the sources listed previously.

Preparing and Monitoring a Budget

Simply put, a **budget** is a statement of the estimated revenues and expenditures with an itemized listing of the nature of each (Johnson & Breckon, 2007; Last, 2007) for a program. A budget represents the decision makers' intentions and expectations by allocating funds to achieve desired outcomes (program goals and objectives) (Fallon & Zgodzinski, 2012).

A budget can be prepared for any length of time. When programs are planned, budgets are usually created for the entire length of the program. However, when a program is projected to last longer than a year, the overall program budget is typically broken down into 12-month periods.

Developing a budget is an essential and critical step of the planning process (Johnson & Breckon, 2007; Fallon & Zgodzinski, 2012). Typically, those planning the program and any other key decision makers who control resources that will be used in the program develop a program budget. The process begins by examining the financial objective of the program. From a financial standpoint, programs can make money (a profit), lose money, or break even. If a program must make money, the revenue will have to be greater than the expenditures, and the intended profit (profit margin) will need to be included in the budgeting process. **Figure 10.2** presents a sample budget sheet that lists line items that are often included in health promotion program budgets.

Revenue and Support	Amount
Contribution from sponsors	_____
Gifts	_____
Grants	_____
Participant fee	_____
Sale of curriculum material	_____
Total income	_____
Expenditures	
Direct Costs	
Personnel	
Salary & wages	_____
Fringe benefits	_____
Consultants	_____
Supplies	
Instructional materials	_____
Incentives	_____
Meeting costs	_____
Equipment	_____
Travel	_____
Postage	_____
Advertising	_____
Total of direct costs	_____
Indirect costs (includes rent, insurance, telephone, & other utilities)	_____
Total of indirect costs	_____
Total expenditures	_____
Balance	_____

▲ **Figure 10.2** Sample Budget Sheet

Once the financial objective of the program is known, planners can then turn their attention to the estimated revenues of the program. In other words, from where will the income come? If a program is being paid for by a grant, gift, or contributions from sponsors, the planners may know exactly how much money they will have to work with. However, if the revenue for a program is coming, either in part or whole, from participant fees, an estimate will have to be made of how many participants are expected to take part. At this point budgeting becomes a bit more complicated. Hopefully, there may be some history from previous programs to guide planners in estimating participation and thus estimate revenue, but sometimes planners may have to make decisions based on "best guesses." Whether revenue is estimated based on previous programs or best guesses, it is not uncommon to see a budget line in the revenue portion of the budget for participants' fees as X number of participants times the cost of participation. For example 22 participants @ $50 each = $1,100.

After the revenue for the program has been determined, planners need to estimate what expenditures are necessary for the program. An expenditure is a cost incurred while planning, implementing, or evaluating a program. The labels given to the various categories of expenditures (e.g., personnel, instructional materials, equipment) and the detail to which the expenditures are listed in a budget will vary based on the accounting practices of the organization. The two types of costs that are most often found in budgets are *direct costs* and *indirect costs*. A **direct cost** is the portion of cost that is directly expended in providing a product or service (VentureLine, 2015) and is expressed in a budget as the actual number of dollars expected to be spent. Included would be things like wages, salaries, and supplies. An **indirect cost** is the portion of cost that is indirectly expended in providing a product or service (VentureLine, 2015). The purpose of indirect cost is to capture overhead costs incurred by an organization that offers several programs and whose administrative costs cannot be connected directly to a program. Items covered in indirect costs include things such as the cost of telephones, other utilities, insurance, space, and equipment maintenance. An example would be an organization running several different programs at the same time but using just one telephone line to service all of the programs. So what percent of the telephone bill should be associated with each program? To handle this situation in the budget it is typical to determine the indirect costs as a percentage of the direct costs. The actual percentage used varies depending on the practices of the organization; however the percentage typically ranges between 10% and 50%. Thus, a budget that has direct costs of say $50,000 and an indirect cost rate of 30% would enter $15,000 in the budget for indirect costs.

In putting a budget together many of the direct cost items' dollar value is pretty straightforward. For example, if it is estimated that 20 500-page reams of photocopy paper are needed to conduct a program and a ream paper costs $4.00, the cost of paper in the budget will be $80 (20 × $4.00). A direct cost that is not as straightforward to calculate is the cost of personnel to carry out a program. For example, when planners are calculating personnel costs they need to account for salaries or wages, Social Security taxes, and fringe benefits (e.g., health and disability insurance, vacation days, sick days). While the exact dollar amount may be known for the salary or wages based on number of hours worked and for the Social Security taxes based on the prevailing rate, it is more difficult to put an exact value on the costs of the fringe benefits. Instead, the cost of fringe benefits is calculated for a budget as a percentage of an employee's salary or wage. Thus, a fringe benefit line of a budget may read: 0.30 of $30,000 = $9,000. This means that the person preparing the budget estimates that the value of providing fringe benefits to a full-time employee making $30,000 per year is an additional $9,000. Another complicating factor in calculating personnel expenditures for a program is that a person may not be dedicated full time to a program, but the program is just one of many duties assigned to the employee.

The term used to quantify the number of people working on a program is *full-time equivalent* (FTE). A **full-time equivalent** is a unit of measurement that is calculated by dividing the average number of hours a person works per week by the average number of hours worked by a full-time employee per week. Thus, a person who works full-time is counted as 1.0 FTE. If a full-time employee averages 40 hours per week and a part-time employee works 20 hours per week, the part-time employee would count as 0.5 FTE. FTEs can also express the amount of time a person works on a program. For example, an FTE of say 0.40 would indicate that a person is working 40% of his or her time on the program. Therefore in a budget, it is not uncommon to see a salary budget line presented as: 0.20 FTE of $40,000 = $8,000. This means that 20% of a full-time equivalent (FTE) employee who makes $40,000 a year is being charged to the program. Regardless of the format used to create a budget, the budget should be put together in sufficient detail so that all revenue and expenditures are accounted for.

Depending on the source of funding for a program, planners may also be required to include a budget narrative (or budget justification) along with their budget. This is especially true if the funding is coming from a grant, but many organizations require a budget narrative as part of the annual budgeting process. A **budget narrative** is a statement that explains the need for the costs in a budget and how the costs were estimated. Although, often the format for a budget narrative is provided by the organization providing the funding, there are two basic ways of structuring a budget narrative. One option is to place the budget narrative on the budget sheet, inserting a brief explanation under each item (Grant Central Station, n.d.). "Another option is to number items in the left margin or attach footnote-style numbers to each line and to follow the numeric budget with: 'Notes to the Budget.' Regardless of the format, the categories in the narrative should use budget headings, follow the exact order in which the items are listed in the numerical budget, and include semi-totals" (Grant Central Station, n.d., para. 8). Here is an example line item in a budget and the budget narrative that follows.

> Consultant – Program Evaluator: $100/hour × 2 hours/week × 52 weeks = $10,400.
> The program evaluator will be responsible for designing and implementing an evaluation to determine program effectiveness and user satisfaction. In addition, the evaluator will be responsible for creating written bi-monthly reports to be shared with all stakeholders.

After a program is up and running, the budget must be monitored. This duty often falls to the person who oversees the financial resources of those planning the program. It may be one of the program planners, but will more than likely be a person who has financial responsibilities for the planning organization. This person may be responsible for both preparing and distributing the financial reports. At a minimum, those receiving the reports should include the decision makers and those responsible for the day-to-day operation of the program. The financial reports are usually generated and distributed on a regular basis (i.e., monthly, bimonthly, quarterly), and each report usually includes actual revenue and expenditures for the period, year-to-date totals on actual revenue and expenditures, and year-to-date budgeted revenue and expenditures. Such data allows decision makers and planners to know exactly where they are with regard to financial resources (see **Figure 10.3**).

Note: 3 months = 25% of budget	Total Budget	Ytd 3/31/16	Percent of Budget	Budget Balance
Revenue & Support				
Contributions	1,747.50	1,247.00	71.35%	500.50
Grant #0428	1,000.00	0.00	0.00%	1,000.00
Grant #1205	62,000.00	23,000.00	37.10%	39,000.00
Grant #1107	120,000.00	60,000.00	50.00%	60,000.00
Participant fees	4,500.00	3,505.00	77.89%	995.00
Interest income	100.00	27.98	23.98%	72.02
Total revenue & Support	189,347.50	87,779.98	46.36%	101,567.52
Expenditures				
Personnel				
Salary & Wages—Administration	10,000.00	2,400.00	24.00%	7,600.00
Salary & Wages—Educators	70,000.00	18,000.00	25.71%	52,000.00
Salary & Wages—Clerical	30,000.00	7,600.00	25.33%	22,400.00
Subtotal salary & Wages	110,000.00	28,000.00	25.45%	82,000.00
Payroll taxes	19,000.00	5,000.00	26.32%	14,000.00
Health insurance	15,500.00	3,500.00	22.58%	12,000.00
State unemployment taxes	8,000.00	2,000.00	25.00%	6,000.00
Workers comp. insurance	500.00	125.00	25.00%	375.00
Subtotal personnel	153,000.00	38,625.00	25.25%	114,375.00
Operating expenses				
Supplies	1,300.00	600.00	46.15%	700.00
Instructional materials	2,500.00	2,000.00	80.00%	500.00
Incentives	750.00	200.00	26.67%	550.00
Meeting costs	1,200.00	400.00	33.33%	800.00
Equipment—copier lease	1,200.00	400.00	33.33%	800.00
Travel	4,000.00	1,800.00	45.00%	2,200.00
Postage	300.00	125.00	41.67%	175.00
Advertising	400.00	150.00	37.50%	250.00
Subtotal operating expenses	11,650.00	5,675.00	48.71%	250.00
Total direct costs	164,650.00	44,300.00	26.91%	5,975.00
Total indirect costs (rate=15%)	24,697.50	6,646.10	26.91%	18,051.40
Total expenditures	189,347.50	50,946.10	26.91%	138,401.40
Net surplus or (deficit)	-.—	36,833.88	-.—	-.—

▲ **Figure 10.3** Example First-Quarter Budget Report

Summary

This chapter identified and discussed the most often used resources for health promotion programs: personnel, curriculum and other instructional materials, space, equipment and supplies, and funding. In addition, information was presented on how to secure and allocate resources, how to obtain funding, and how to create and monitor a budget.

 ## Review Questions

1. What are the major categories of resources that planners need to consider when planning a health promotion program?
2. What are the advantages and disadvantages of using internal personnel? External personnel?
3. How are technical assistance, volunteers, teamwork, and cultural factors associated with program personnel?
4. Define the terms *ownership, flex time, vendor,* and *canned programs.*
5. What are some key questions that planners should ask vendors when they try to sell their product?
6. How might program planners obtain free or inexpensive space for a program?
7. What is the SAM? What is it used for?
8. List and explain the different means by which health promotion programs can be funded.
9. What is meant by the term *profit margin?*
10. What is a budget? What are the major components of a budget?
11. What is the difference between direct and indirect costs? How is each calculated?

 ## Activities

1. Identify and describe the resources you anticipate needing to carry out a program you are planning. Be sure to answer the following questions that apply to your program:
   a. What personnel will be needed to carry out the program? List the individuals and the duties to be carried out.
   b. What curriculum or educational materials will you use in your program? Why did you select it or them?
   c. What kind of space allocation will your program require? How will you obtain the space? How much will it cost?
   d. What equipment and supplies do you anticipate using? How will you obtain them?
   e. How do you anticipate paying for the program? Why did you select this method?
   f. What would be the major sources of income and expenses that would be associated with the program you are planning? Prepare a one-year budget sheet for the program.

2. Visit the local office of a voluntary agency and find out what type of resources it makes available to individuals planning health promotion programs. Ask for a sample of the materials. Also, ask if the agency offers any canned programs. If it does, find out as much as you can about the programs and ask for any available descriptive literature.

3. Through the process of networking and using the Internet and/or local telephone book, find where in your community there is free or inexpensive space available for health promotion programs.

4. Call three different voluntary agencies and one hospital in your community and find out if they have a speakers' bureau. If they do, find out how to use the bureaus and what topics the speakers can address.

5. Prepare a mock grant proposal for a program you are planning. Make sure it includes all the components noted in Box 10.5.

6. Using the outline provided below, create a job description for a volunteer position that could assist in a program you are planning.

   a. Position title:

   b. Reports to:

   c. Responsible for:

   d. Position summary:

   e. Duties:

   f. Qualifications:
       – Required:
       – Preferred:

Weblinks

1. **http://www.cancer.org/**

   American Cancer Society (ACS)

   The ACS Website presents the most up-to-date information on cancer including treatment and prevention. The site also provides information about the ACS and the resources it can provide for cancer survivors and program planners. [Note: The ACS Website is the only Website of a voluntary health agency listed in the Weblinks of this chapter. Be aware that most all other voluntary health agencies have similar resources available at their Website.]

2. **http://www.welcoa.org**

   Wellness Councils of America (WELCOA)

   WELCOA's Website provides a variety of resources for those interested in worksite wellness programs.

3. **http://www.cdc.gov/HealthyYouth/HECAT/**

   Centers for Disease Control and Prevention, Adolescent and School Health

   This page at CDC's Website provides an overview the Health Education Curriculum Analysis Tool (HECAT) and links to many documents that can help planners use the tool.

4. **http://www.aarp.org**

   AARP

   AARP is a nonprofit membership organization dedicated to addressing the needs and interests of persons 50 years of age and older. The organization's Website provides information that is applicable to those planning programs for seniors. This site also has a special section on health.

5. **http://www.nih.gov**

   National Institutes of Health (NIH)

   The NIH's Website not only includes information about NIH and links to all the institutes, centers, and offices but also includes health information, grant opportunities, and scientific resources.

6. **http://www.cdc.gov/learning/**

   Centers for Disease Control and Prevention (CDC)

   This page at CDC's Website provides a wealth of information about various products and resources developed by CDC and CDC partners for the public health community.

7. **http://www.healthfinder.gov**

   healthfinder

   Of all the Weblinks provided in this chapter, the healthfinder Website offers information on the greatest variety of health topics. It includes information on prevention, wellness, diseases, health care, and alternative medicine. It also includes medical dictionaries, an encyclopedia, journals, and more.

8. **http://www.grants.gov**

   Grants.gov

   This Website allows planners to electronically find and apply for competitive grant opportunities from all federal grant-making agencies. The site provides all the information planners need to apply for a grant and walks them through the process, step-by-step to their preferred practice setting.

9. **http://www.minorityhealth.hhs.gov**

   Office of Minority Health (OMH)

   The OMH Website presents information on cultural competence. The OMH was mandated by the U.S. Congress in 1994, via P.L. 101–527, to develop the capacity of health care professionals to address the cultural and linguistic barriers to health care delivery and increase access to health care for limited English-proficient people. This site provides many different resources including, but not limited to, standards, materials, minority population profiles, grant opportunities, and links to other websites to assist health professionals in becoming more culturally competent.

Marketing

Developing Programs That Respond to the Wants and Needs of the Priority Population

<table>
<tr><td colspan="2">

Chapter Objectives

After reading this chapter and answering the questions at the end, you should be able to:

- Define *market*, *marketing*, and *social marketing*.
- Explain the exchange process.
- Describe the segmentation process.
- List and explain the factors that are used to segment an audience.
- Explain the relationship between a needs assessment and a social marketing program.
- Explain the marketing mix or four Ps of marketing.
- Explain the six elements that make the social marketing approach unique.

</td></tr>
</table>

Key Terms

barriers	marketing mix
benefit	place
competition	pretesting
consumer-based	price
consumer orientation	product
exchange	promotion
market	segmentation
marketing	social marketing

As you read each chapter in this text, you are learning how to develop, implement, and evaluate health promotion interventions that will influence behavior and ultimately improve individual and community health status. In this chapter you will learn how you can use social marketing as a planning approach to develop **consumer-based** programs and interventions. In other words, how to design programs that are based on a priority population's wants, needs, desires, preferences, and so forth. **Box 11.1** identifies the responsibilities and competencies for health education specialists that pertain to the material presented in this chapter.

▷ Marketing and Social Marketing

Social marketing uses marketing principles to design programs that facilitate voluntary behavior change for the purpose of improved personal or societal well-being (Andreasen, 1995; Kotler & Zaltman, 1971). In contrast, commercial **marketing** is defined by the American Marketing Association as a set of processes for creating, communicating, and delivering value to customers. It is concerned with outcomes, typically financial, that benefit

Responsibilities and Competencies for Health Education Specialists

The content of this chapter includes information on several tasks that occur during the social marketing process. These tasks are related to four areas of responsibility for the health education specialist and are centered on involving the priority population, collecting data, and designing a strategy.

RESPONSIBILITY I: Assess Needs, Resources, and Capacity for Health Education/Promotion

Competency 1.3: Collect primary data to determine needs

RESPONSIBILITY II: Plan Health Education/Promotion

Competency 2.1: Involve priority populations partners, and other stakeholders in the planning process

Competency 2.3: Select or design strategies/interventions

RESPONSIBILITY IV: Conduct Evaluation and Research Related to Health Education/Promotion

Competency 4.4 Collect and manage data

Competency 4.5: Analyze data

Competency 4.7: Apply findings

RESPONSIBILITY VII: Communicate, Promote, and Advocate for Health, Health Education/Promotion, and the Profession

Competency 7.1: Identify, develop, and deliver messages using a variety of communication strategies, methods, and techniques

Source: *A Competency-Based Framework for Health Education Specialists—2015*. Whitehall, PA: National Commission for Health Education Credentialing, Inc. (NCHEC) and the Society for Public Health Education (SOPHE). Reprinted by permission of the National Commission for Health Education Credentialing, Inc. (NCHEC) and the Society for Public Health Education (SOPHE). AAHE (2015).

the organization or its stakeholders. Regardless of the intended outcome, the key marketing principles that ensure success are the same for marketing and social marketing. This chapter will focus on social marketing's unique contribution to health promotion by examining six key areas that make this approach unique from other planning approaches: consumer orientation, audience segmentation, exchange theory, the marketing mix, competition, and continuous monitoring (Thackeray & McCormack Brown, 2005).

When people hear the word *marketing*, what often comes to mind are images such as highway billboards, humorous television commercials aired during the Super Bowl, or colorful advertisements in their favorite magazines. While these communication materials are an important part of a marketing strategy, they represent only the promotion piece of the marketing mix (also referred to at the 4Ps—see **Table 11.1**). Marketing, as it relates to health promotion programs, is really a consumer-based planning approach (Neiger, Thackeray, Barnes, & McKenzie, 2003).

A consumer-based planning approach is one of several approaches for developing interventions (see Chapter 8). When using a social marketing approach to design interventions, planners make it easy and convenient for the priority population to do a behavior. They do this by providing the priority population with opportunities and choices, also known as *products*, or tangible items and services (Rothschild, 1999). This approach is in contrast to educational or communication campaigns or other persuasion techniques to facilitate the behavior change. It is also different than advocating for and enacting laws and policies to coerce people to change behavior. Although these are all viable intervention methods, and often a multifaceted approach is needed to effectively address a community health problem,

TABLE 11.1 **The Marketing Mix/4Ps for Social Marketing**

Behavior: Purchase and install one LED blub in a recessed can light.

4Ps	Definition	Example
Product (tangible item or service)	What the planners are offering meets the consumers' needs, makes it easy and convenient to do the behavior, and provides a benefit that consumers value	LED lightbulbs
(core)	Benefits that are associated with using a product or service	Protect the environment Save money on electrical bill
Price	What it costs the consumer to obtain the product and its associated benefits	$20USD Effort to install
Place	Where the consumer has access to the product	Events at local Home Depot and Costco stores during October
Promotion	The communication strategy, including the message and associated visuals or graphics as well as the channels, used to let the priority population know about the product, how to obtain or purchase it, and the benefits they will receive	In-store signage Flyers in customer bags Direct mail postcards Email notifications to energy customers Sticky notes on newspapers

Source: Adapted from Schultz, et al., 2015.

BOX
11.2

Application

Different Intervention Approaches to a Carbon Emissions Reduction Program

Social Marketing: Provide recycling bins at low cost to all neighborhood homes, making it easy and convenient to conserve energy.

Education: Teach school-aged children the benefits of saving energy though a series of five interactive lessons

Communications: Conduct a media campaign using channels of television, radio, and social media to encourage people to take public transportation as a way to reduce a person's carbon footprint

Law Policy: Develop a policy that requires people who exceed their allotment of energy each month to pay higher prices for the excess electricity they consume

Source: Categories based on Rothschild, 1999.

---

a social marketing-based intervention focuses on providing products to make it easy to do a behavior. **Box 11.2** compares social marketing with other intervention approaches to protect the environment through reducing carbon emissions.

▷ The Marketing Process and Health Promotion Programs

Exchange

The marketing process operates on the underlying concept of exchange theory (Bagozzi, 1975). That is, there are buyers who have needs and sellers who have products that can fill those needs. In order for the exchange between the buyer and the seller to be successful the seller has to offer a product to the buyer that meets a need at a price he or she is willing to pay. The product benefits must be greater than what it costs the buyer to obtain the product. Additionally, the benefits must be outcomes that are important and of value to the buyer.

In health promotion, the priority population is the buyer, also called the *consumer, target audience*, or *market*. Kotler and Clarke (1987, p. 108) define **market** as "the set of all people who have an actual or potential interest in a product or service." In this chapter we will use the terms *consumer* and *priority population* interchangeably. In health promotion, the seller (i.e., program planner) has a product, which is either a tangible item or service that meets consumers' needs, provides a benefit that they value, and will help support their efforts to make a positive behavior change. The seller's goal is to make it possible for consumers to get the product and the associated benefits at a reasonable cost and with minimal effort. This process is referred to as the **exchange**.

For example, a women's health program may have as one of its impact objectives to increase the number of working women who breastfeed their children (behavior). To help women to do this behavior, the program offers a breast pump rental service (product). The program is offering the breast pumps in exchange for women paying a small rental fee (the cost). This provides women with the benefit of providing the highest-quality nutrition to their children while continuing to work.

Consumer Orientation

To successfully facilitate a product exchange, planners must have an understanding of the consumers. This **consumer orientation** means that all marketing-related program decisions—including the type of product that is developed, how it is offered, how much it will cost, how it is promoted, and the benefits promised—are based on what planners know about the priority population and their preferences. If planners are making decisions without knowing who is in the priority population, including things such as how they see the world, what makes them tick, how they spend their time, and what is important to them, then planners are not practicing marketing.

In the above breastfeeding example, it would be important for planners to know that women consider the opportunity to bond with their children as a key benefit to breastfeeding (Lindenberger & Bryant, 2000). This benefit is of greater importance than the health benefits program planners often promote, such as "your baby will be healthier," or "breastfeeding will cost less money." Although those health benefits are true, what matters most to women is "bonding with my child."

The process of knowing and understanding the priority population is part of the formative research process (see Chapter 3). This formative research may be included as part of the needs assessment process (see Chapter 4). However, while similar data collection methods are used for gathering primary and secondary data, the focus of formative research as performed in social marketing is a bit different than that of a traditional needs assessment for a program. The types of data planners try to uncover in formative research are, as described in the SMART model (see Chapter 3), related to consumer analysis (wants, needs, and preferences of the priority population, barriers and facilitators to behavior change, as well as using the product), market analysis (identifying competing behaviors, messages, and programs), and channel analyses (communication preferences). Planners conducting formative research may want to consider asking questions such as those as outlined in **Table 11.2**.

TABLE 11.2 **Types of Questions to Ask During Formative Research**

Topic	Questions
Behavior	• What is keeping members of the priority population from doing the desired behavior?
Needs	• What needs do members of the priority population have?
Competition	• What are the members of the priority population choosing to do right now to fill their needs? • What do they see as the benefits of that choice?
Product	• What type of products would help the priority population make behavior changes? • What would make it easy for the priority population to obtain the product?
Benefits	• What benefit does the priority population want as a result of doing the desired behavior? • What benefit does the priority population think the product provides?
Barriers	• What would make it difficult for or keep the priority population from using the product? • What makes it difficult for or keeps the priority population from doing the desired behavior?
Price	• What would the priority population be willing to give up or pay to obtain the product and accompanying benefits?
Place	• Where would the priority population like the product offered?
Promotion	• What is the best way to communicate information to the priority population about the product?

COMPETITION

People always have choices for how they are going to fill a need. These alternative choices are the **competition**. Knowing what the priority population perceives is the competition and the benefits that they get from choosing that option can help planners make strategic decisions about products to offer that will provide a greater benefit at a lower cost than the competitive option. In addition to helping planners make product related decisions, understanding the competition also helps planners to know how to price products and how to frame messages for a promotional campaign. Planners should identify the competition during the formative research phase.

For example, if people need to quench their thirst, they can drink water, milk, soda pop, or fruit juice. If people need new running shoes, they can choose different brands such as Nike, Adidas, or New Balance, and so forth. In social marketing, people have choices for what behaviors they will participate in and products they will use to fulfill their needs. For instance, if people have a desire or need to lose weight so that they can wear a new swimsuit during their summer vacation, they could choose from two behaviors to lose weight: (1) eat fewer calories and/or (2) engage in more physical activity. There are several tangible products that could help them do this behavior, including purchasing a book that outlines a specific diet plan, attending a weight management class offered by the local community center, hiring a personal trainer, buying a gym membership, using a pedometer to keep track of steps

> BOX
>
> **11.3**
>
> ## Warm Embrace as an Example of Competition
>
> Jane Chen and the social enterprise group Embrace discovered that newborn infants in developing countries were dying due to the lack of access to incubators. As part of their formative research they interviewed women, health care providers, and other people in the community. The data revealed that women lived too far from the hospital and an incubator was too expensive for villages to purchase. Researchers found that as an alternative choice (the competition) parents were engaging in unsafe and ineffective behaviors including putting their babies under a light bulb or using a water bottle to keep them warm. The solution to this problem that met the parents' need to keep their infants alive was a new product called the Warm Embrace. The Warm Embrace is an infant-sized sleeping bag equipped with meltable wax that keeps the baby's body at a constant temperature for four to six hours. It costs less than 1% of a regular incubator and is saving lives.
>
> Source: Adapted from http://embraceglobal.org/

walked each day, and so forth. Each of these alternative behavioral choices and tangible products comes with both costs and benefits.

On another level, competition can come from other programs or services that are offering similar programs or products or that are sending messages that are in conflict with the behaviors program planners are trying to promote (Wayman et al., 2007). For weight loss, competitive messages might come from fast food restaurants advertising low-cost, convenient foods (products) that are high in fat and calories. Competing programs would be any number of different organizations or agencies that offer similar weight loss classes. Competing products would include ways, other than a pedometer, to track physical activity such as a smartphone app.

Box 11.3 is an example of competition as it relates to choices for keeping newborns warm when there is no incubator available.

Segmentation

Program planners may think that everyone can benefit from health promotion interventions, so they should try to reach everyone. However, not everyone is interested in responding, or even ready or willing to respond. Additionally, motivations for responding to interventions vary by individuals. **Segmentation** is a way to divide the priority population into smaller, more homogeneous or similar groups. The goal of segmentation is to create groups of people who share similar characteristics or qualities who will respond in a similar way to the intervention.

There are several advantages to segmenting the priority population. Segmentation helps planners to narrow the focus of the marketing strategy. It is more likely that the right product will be developed to meet the specific needs and desires of the priority population, thus greatly increasing the chances for an exchange between the two parties. It helps planners to be more effective and efficient with limited resources because they are able to identify groups of the priority population who have similar needs and will respond to the marketing strategy in a similar way. Segmentation also helps planners to make the best decisions in terms of where to offer a product, how to make the price affordable, and how to tailor the promotional strategy including messages and communication channels to the priority population.

For example, a segmentation process discovered that among women who did not regularly receive mammograms, a lack of knowledge about how often they should get a mammogram was a key factor. One group did not know that they should have an annual mammogram, while the other one did (Forthofer & Bryant, 2000). Therefore, each segment of the population needed a unique marketing strategy. For those who already knew about the importance of an annual mammogram, the strategy might include providing a mobile mammography screening unit in places that are convenient for the women, such as their workplace. The marketing strategy for the segment who were not aware that they need an annual mammogram may include a promotional strategy with messages to first increase awareness that annual mammograms are recommended for women of their age and then offer mobile mammography screening units at their workplace.

Planners developing an alcohol prevention program discovered three different segments among youth (Dietrich, Rundle-Thiele, Leo, & Connor, 2015). The first segment included both males and females. They had low intentions to drink alcohol and their attitudes toward binge drinking of alcohol were considered low-risk. Segment number two were primarily males who had high-risk attitudes toward drinking and intentions to drink. The final segment were females who had low-risk attitudes towards binge drinking and had neutral intentions about whether or not they would drink. Interventions could be developed for these three groups that reflect their attitudes and behaviors toward alcohol and binge drinking.

Planners can segment groups of people using information gathered from secondary data such as literature and epidemiological data (*a priori*) or after collecting primary data using focus groups, interviews, and surveys (*a posteriori*). In this chapter you will learn a simple process that you can use as a framework for conducting audience segmentation that begins with a priori segmentation.

Factors or variables on which to base segmentation include demographics, geographics, geodemographics, lifestyle/psychographics, benefits sought, and behavior (readiness to change, knowledge, attitudes, beliefs, or behaviors) (see **Box 11.4**). Planners will need to experiment with several variables to determine what works best for them.

Planners most often start the segmentation process by using secondary data that include demographic variables such as age, gender, income, marital status, occupation, religion, ethnicity, and socioeconomic status. Nevertheless, just because people share similar demographics does not mean that they will engage in the same behaviors. So while these data are usually the most accessible and may describe who is at greatest risk, these data do not always explain why people engage in behaviors or predict whether they will respond to the marketing efforts. Variables related to consumers' motives, personality attributes, and lifestyles can be "the most powerful segmentation variables in social marketing" (Slater, Kelly, & Thackeray, 2006, p. 171). For example, one segmentation study found that the most important factor that influenced the number of hours a person spent watching television was the lifestyle of eating dinner in front of the television (King et al., 2010). Demographic factors such as ethnicity or where they lived in the country did not make a difference. Knowing this information would help planners to create interventions to increase physical activity and reduce screen time.

Before beginning the segmentation process planners should have completed the needs assessment process (see Chapter 4), selected a priority topic, and written a goal statement (see Chapter 6). In addition, planners should have conducted formative research, as noted earlier, to gain an understanding of the priority population, including who is most affected

BOX

11.1

Focus On

Example of Segmentation Categories and Variables

Demographic

Age: 25 to 29; 30 to 34; 35 to 39; 40 to 44; 45 to 49; 50 to 54; 55 to 59; 60 to 64; 65 to 69; 70 to 74; 75 years or greater

Gender: Male; female

Educational attainment: GED or high school graduate; some college; associate's degree; bachelor's degree; master's degree; professional degree; doctoral degree

Income: <10,000; 10-19,999; 20-29,999; 30-39,999; 40-49,999; 50-59,999; 60-69,999; 70-79,999; 80,000 or greater; or high, medium, low income; or below poverty line, at poverty line, above poverty line

Religion: Catholic; Protestant; Mormon; Jehovah Witness; Jewish; Buddhist; Hindu; Muslim

Race/Ethnicity: White; Black; Asian; Pacific Islander; Hispanic/Latino

Geographic

There could be several segmentation levels based on where people live including: country; province; state; counties; neighborhoods; census tracks; zip codes

Behavioral

Perceived risk: High at risk, medium risk, low risk, not at risk

Health status: Excellent, very good, good, fair, poor

Frequency of behavior: Daily, few times a week, once a week, 2–3 times a month, monthly

Psychosocial Variables

Intrinsic motivation*

Self-efficacy*

Social support*

Perceived barriers to doing the behavior (*depends on target behavior*)

Perceived benefits from doing behavior (*depends on target behavior*)

Stage of readiness to change: Pre-contemplation, contemplation, preparation action, maintenance

Attitude toward behavior: Positive, neutral, negative

Knowledge level: High, medium, low

* The classification for these variables could be based on how they are measured. For example the variable could be measured on a Likert or similar scale ranging from high to low, or present to non-existent.

and the associated risk factors. This information provides the foundation and will be used in decision making throughout the segmentation process.

Ideally, planners use multiple variables to identify audience segments. This often requires use of statistical software programs that can analyze data and create clusters or groups of people based on shared characteristics. For example, in segmenting Hispanic consumers, researchers used variables including language preference, generation (1st, 2nd, 3rd), length of time in the United States, education, income, identification with American way of life and Hispanic heritage, and attitudes toward family. Using statistical tests to cluster the groups they discovered four distinct segments. The primary differences between the groups were language preference, identification with American culture or Hispanic heritage, and generation (Alvarez, Dickson, & Hunter, 2014). However, even without statistical tests simple segmentation using primary and secondary data is still possible as described in the following five steps.

The first step in segmentation is to review the formative research data to identify behaviors that influence whether people experience morbidity or mortality associated with the health topic. For example, if a program is focused on reducing diabetes-related morbidity, planners would review the secondary data and determine which behaviors influence whether someone experiences diabetes-related illnesses. They may find out that daily monitoring of blood glucose, regular physical activity, eating five servings of fruits and vegetables a day, and visits to the doctor for an annual eye exam are all behaviors that reduce the risk for diabetes complications.

Second, once planners have identified all the possible behaviors, program staff and other stakeholders must decide which behavior will be the program's focus. This will become the impact objective. Questions to consider when choosing between the possible behaviors include:

1. Is the behavior modifiable?

2. What is the relative impact that changing the behavior will have on the health status or risk factor; in other words, does the literature suggest that changing one behavior will result in greater outcomes than another behavior?

3. What are the current rates of the behavior in the priority population?

4. Is it possible to create a product that will make it easy or convenient to change the behavior, or are education or laws and policies more effective approaches?

The third step is to again review the data and literature, this time to identify which segmentation factors (see **Box 11.4**) are associated with and influence whether people participate in that particular behavior. If the behavior is a visit to the health care provider for an annual eye exam, planners may discover that having health insurance, making less than $25,000 dollars a year, being of Hispanic ethnicity, and a belief that eye exams are not important are all associated with whether or not someone receives an annual eye exam.

The fourth step is to group people together who share similar characteristics as it relates to the behavior. There is no right or wrong way to identify population segments. Planners will want to choose factors that distinguish how the priority population will respond to the marketing strategy. The segmentation process planners develop for the priority population must be useful to the organization and relevant for program planning decisions. If planners have used statistical methods to create clusters then groups are naturally created. If planners are using primary and secondary data, they can simply group people by one or two variables that most influence or are associated with the behavior.

In one study, researchers were interested in creating segments of the population for a global warming engagement campaign (Maibach, Leiserowitz, Roser-Renouf, & Mertz, 2011). The variables they used to create their segments were global warming motivations (including beliefs about the issue and degree of involvement), behaviors, and policy preferences.

The segmentation process revealed six distinct segments of the population with varying levels of beliefs about whether global warming is actually happening and if it is a problem, steps they are personally taking to reduce global warming, and what actions they think the government, businesses and individuals should take.

At this point, planners may decide that they need to have additional information about these potential audience segments so they collect primary data. These data may include psychographics (attitudes, values, and lifestyle), risk factors, health history, or personal health behaviors. Additional a posteriori segmentation could be completed after the primary data are collected and analyzed.

Lastly, once planners have identified potential segments, they have to choose one segment to focus on. There is no right or wrong, or simple and easy, way to choose between segments. Planners must weigh the data against the organization's abilities and its goals or what they are trying to achieve, then make the best decision. One approach to take—once all the possible segments are identified—is to review the segments by considering the extent to which segments exhibit each of the following five criteria (Kotler & Keller, 2016):

1. *Measurable.* With this criterion planners consider how many people are in the segment and whether important characteristics (or factors) can be measured. For example, can you measure readiness to change among the population?

2. *Substantial.* This criterion includes whether the segment is large enough and profitable enough, meaning will enough people be reached with the intervention to make a difference. Will the efforts be effective and efficient? The segmentation process for mammography discussed earlier actually resulted in seven segments, but they found that the majority of the population was in only two of the segments (Forthofer & Bryant, 2000).

3. *Accessible.* This criterion assesses whether or not planners will be able to reach the segment and then deliver the services. Perhaps the product is a mobile mammography unit. One segment identified is located in a remote area of the state. Due to time and distance factors program staff are not able to reach them to deliver the service.

4. *Differentiable.* Are the segments unique or different enough so that each segment responds in its own way to the marketing strategy? If the segments will respond the same, then they are really not unique groups. In developing a program to increase use of folic acid by women of childbearing age, planners found that women 18–24 were not receptive to messages about pregnancy whereas older women were more amenable to discussing the possibility of becoming pregnant (Lindsey et al., 2007). A marketing strategy for these two groups would be unique.

5. *Actionable.* Here planners decide whether programs can be developed that will attract and serve segments. Because of segment characteristics or organizational abilities, planners may not be able to create a product that adequately meets a segment's needs or provides benefits its members want. Planners in the United Kingdom learned that one of the main reasons that low-income people smoked was that smoking was a way to cope with stress and anxiety and it was one of their only pleasures in life (MacAskill, Stead, MacKintosh, & Hastings, 2002). In evaluating this segment, planners would have to decide whether they could develop a smoking cessation intervention that would be appealing and provide a benefit that helped people cope with stress and gave them greater pleasure.

Another alternative to choose between segments is to use the criteria suggested by Andreasen (1995) that share similar items: segment size, problem incidence, problem

BOX

11.5

Application

Segmentation for Preconception Health Care

Planners at the Centers for Disease Control and Prevention conducted a segmentation study to identify women for a campaign focused on increasing the number of women who practiced healthy behaviors prior to becoming pregnant (e.g., get a flu shot every year, take a multivitamin with 400 micrograms of folic acid, get screening and treated for HIV/AIDS, and so forth). They used multiple data sources, including surveys and previous literature to create a profile of these women. Segmentation variables included age, whether or not they were intending to become parents in the next 12 months (intenders/non-intenders), awareness of preconception health practices, health insurance status prior to pregnancy, receptivity to preconception health terminology and motivation for practicing preconception health behaviors. The planners identified two initial segments (intenders and non-intenders). They then described differences between the two groups based on other variables; for example, intenders were 14% of women ages 18–44 and non-intenders were 86%. For intenders, motivating factors to practice preconception health behaviors were desires to be pregnant, to have a healthy pregnancy, and to have a healthy baby. For non-intenders, motivating factors were personal health and well-being. A social marketing strategy to promote behaviors among these two segments would be clearly different.

Source: Adapted from Lynch, et al, 2014

severity, defenselessness, reachability, general responsiveness, incremental costs, response to marketing mix, and organizational capability.

Box 11.5 spotlights the results of the segmentation process conducted by the Centers for Disease Control and Prevention related to women and pre-conception health care practices.

Marketing Mix

Once audience segments are selected, planners are ready to make strategic decisions related to four marketing variables: product, price, place, and promotion—the four Ps. These variables are what planners use to design interventions that will help achieve their objective(s) and are referred to as the **marketing mix** (see **Table 11.1**). To realize the greatest effect in a marketing strategy there must be a combination of all market mix components, not just promotion (Belch & Belch, 2015).

PRODUCT

The **product** is what the planners are offering that will meet the consumers' needs, make it easy and convenient to do the behavior, and provide a benefit that consumers value. Products can be either tangible items or services and are sometimes referred to as *augmented products*. See **Box 11.6** for examples of social marketing–related products. These products provide the priority population with choices to help them change their behavior.

The benefits that are associated with using a product or service are called *core products* or the bundle of benefits (Lee & Kotler, 2016). People choose to buy certain products for the value or **benefit** the product provides. A common illustration of this point is the person who goes to a home improvement store and buys a drill; what he or she is really purchasing is the benefit of using that drill to have a hole in the wall. Similarly, a person who buys a hotel room is purchasing a restful night's sleep. The products or services provided by planners as part of a social marketing program must also provide a value that is of benefit to the priority

---

BOX

11.6

Focus On

Products (Tangible Items and Services) in Social Marketing Programs

Insecticide treated nets

Contraceptives

Nutritional supplements

Food

Battery collection cage

Bike helmet

Clay pot

Glasses

Hand-washing facilities/containers

Medicine

Mosbar soap

Recycling container

Software program

Water disinfectant

Testings or screenings

Exams

Source: *Adapted from* Thackeray, Fulkerson, & Neiger (2012).

---

population. Those values are determined during the formative research process. These core benefits are one of the most important things to discover, as they will become the motivation for people using the products to help them change behavior. These core benefits will also become part of the promotional strategy, discussed later in this chapter. See **Box 11.7** for examples of core products in social marketing campaigns.

The following two social marketing case studies illustrate products and their associated benefits. The Road Crew offered a transportation service to young males in rural Wisconsin to encourage them to not drive after a night of drinking alcohol (Rothschild, Mastin, & Miller, 2006). The Road Crew used older luxury vehicles to provide transportation for the men to and from the town as well as between bars during the night. The price for this service was $15 per night. The benefits that it provided the men included a fun way to get around town, the opportunity to have a last drink while going home, and less worry about getting a ticket or being in a crash as a result of drinking, all things that were important to the priority population.

In Florida, program planners were concerned with reducing eye injuries among local citrus workers while harvesting fruit. They discovered that among the barriers that kept the workers from wearing protective eyewear was a belief that most workers expected the glasses would reduce their productivity and therefore reduce their income. Their solution was to provide safety goggles that were comfortable and did not fog up or fall off while being worn. The core benefit they provided was "pick rapidly without fear of daily irritation" (Monaghan et al., 2008, p. 80).

PRICE

Price is what it costs the priority population to obtain the product and its associated benefits. It is what they have to "give up." In other words, price is the sum of costs the consumer must accept to engage in the exchange process (Neiger & Thackeray, 1998). The cost to the priority population may be financial, but often with health promotion interventions the

Example of Benefits or Core Products in Social Marketing Studies

"Don't lose your dreams"

"Have iron. Have power"

Makes us healthy

Avoid costly fines and penalties from noncompliance

Close loving bond; emotional benefits

Crew dependability on fire scene

Avoidance of HIV infections

Keep the family healthy and energetic; women charming; children more intelligent

Don't worry about getting home at end of the evening; continue to enjoy themselves; a way to have more fun during an evening out

Enhance women's beauty and health; decreased anemia

Financial savings; health and energy to spend with children and grandchildren; more fit, so able to do leisure activities

Find and develop relationships

Harvest without fear of injury or daily irritation

Hope and peace of mind

Maintain pride and self-esteem as they earn WIC benefits and learn about nutrition and other ways to help their families

Well-being; energy; ability to perform their roles better

Opportunity to keep their relationship (family) intact by ending the violence toward their partner

Peace of mind and life-saving benefit of early detection

Protect individual health; sense of altruism; information provision

Reduce traffic congestion; defer need to build road infrastructure; reduce environmental consequences of car use; increase physical activity and health outcomes; increase use of walking and cycling infrastructure and public transport

Safety of family or workers, financial concerns, impact of debilitating injuries

Spending time with friends, playing, having fun, have opportunity to be active with parents, recognition from peers and adults, opportunity to discover and explore world around them

Source: Adapted from Thackeray, Fulkerson, & Neiger (2012).

costs are nonfinancial, that is, they involve social, mental, emotional, behavioral, or psychological costs. For example, if a program focused on getting Hispanic women with diabetes to regularly check their glucose, a low-cost glucometer could be offered to the priority population. In order to get this product and the associated benefit of a peace of mind that their blood sugar is in range so they will be less likely to damage their eyesight, the women would have to pay a certain amount of money. In addition to this financial cost, the women would have to give up time to go purchase the glucometer and learn how to use it. They would also have to take time every day to check their blood glucose.

As discussed earlier with the exchange process, in designing a marketing strategy, planners must make sure that the benefits the priority population receives are greater than what it costs them to obtain the product. Even if the costs are not actually less, planners have to make them appear less than what they are getting in return. Likewise, as part of the promotional strategy, planners must convey how the benefits received are much greater than what they cost. For example, for a mother to bring her child in to be immunized might cost her time away from other tasks, time to drive to the clinic, the effort to get to the clinic, and being willing to put up with a cranky baby for a few hours after the immunization is received. In communicating about this product (immunizations), the health education specialist has to convey that the benefits of knowing that her child is safe from childhood diseases are greater than a few minor inconveniences (her cost).

Price is not the same thing as barriers. **Barriers** are what keep people from responding to an intervention or doing a behavior. The cost or price of the product may be one factor that keeps people from obtaining it and using it to make a desired behavior change. But there may be other factors as well. In addition to price, barriers to using LED light blubs (see Table 11.1) were being unfamiliar with options, having the product available, and uncertainty about the benefits of using LED lights.

Researchers have found that among young people, barriers to getting tested for sexually transmitted infections are access to testing services, stigma associated with the infections and fear of results (Friedman et al., 2014). Thus interventions had to address these barriers in order to increase the number of youth screened.

In another example, when planners asked people about what would keep them from attending a nutrition education class, they said that the major reasons were that they lacked transportation and there was nobody to babysit their children (John, Kerby, & Landers, 2004). These are barriers but not costs: the people do not have to give up transportation or childcare to participate in the exchange. However, either thing will keep them from obtaining the product. They would have to give up money for transportation or to pay a sitter. In designing the product or intervention, planners have to make sure that they reduce the barriers and lower the cost—both for the same purpose—to make it easy for people to obtain the product or service and engage in the desired behavior. In this case, the planners may want to offer a baby-sitting service at the same location where the class is being held.

From an economic standpoint, *price* refers to charging the appropriate amount for the product being provided. Planners who were promoting the use of LED light bulbs found that price was a barrier to people wanting to purchase the bulbs (Schultz et al., 2015). Therefore, their pricing strategy included providing a rebate with bulb purchase, reducing the price range from US$20–US$59 to US$2–US$21. Offering the bulbs at an affordable price increased sales.

There are many ways to finance a program (see Chapter 10). The price must match the consumer's ability and willingness to pay and should not be so high that it becomes a barrier to them using the product or service. When considering the amount to be charged for a product, planners should answer seven questions:

1. Who are the clients?
2. What is their ability to pay?
3. Are co-payers involved?
4. Is the program covered under an insurance program?
5. What is the mission of the planner's agency?
6. What are competitors charging?
7. What is the demand for the program or product?

The price of a program and who pays for it help determine how a program should be marketed. Whether the program is intended to make a profit will have a great impact on the price. Does the program have to make money? Break even? Or can it lose money? It is a real art not to overprice or underprice the program. Demand and location (*place*) will also influence price. If a program is in high demand, obviously the price can be raised. For example, a stress-management program in a large metropolitan area may be able to command a higher price than one located in a small rural area.

Not only do the demand and the location influence the amount one might charge for a program, but so can the psychological mindset of those in the priority population. Some individuals would not participate in a free or inexpensive program because they question how such a program could be any good. They may believe they have to spend a lot of money to get anything of worth. Also, sometimes when programs are offered free of charge, people are less likely to attend regularly because they have not invested financially in the program. On the other hand, there are some people who, if given the choice of a free program versus one with a cost, will always take the free program, even if they are financially able to pay. Being able to segment the priority population with regard to these economic issues can help set the right price.

PLACE

The third marketing variable is **place**, which can be thought of as where the priority population has access to the product. When considering place, planners make sure that it easy for the consumer to obtain the product or service. In addition, it is important to avoid areas where people do not normally go or places where they would not feel comfortable or safe. For example, in New Mexico, the HABITS for Life program discovered that barriers to annual health screenings and eye exams were time, cost, and easy access (Brown-Connolly, Concha, & English, 2014). To address these barriers they provided mobile screening units at worksites, faith-based programs, senior centers, and health fairs. Another example is a partnership between bar owners and public health researchers who aimed to make it easier for people to get a taxi ride home, thereby discouraging drinking and driving. They provided cab drivers with a special spot to wait (which also guaranteed them passengers). The area was well-lit, covered, and in a generally safe place, all important things to the customers (Bhatt, 2006).

When a product is offered it is closely associated with its place. If the priority population has to go to a specific location to obtain the product, planners might think about when it will be most convenient for the priority population to do so. For example, if consumers have to come to the local health department to have their car seat checked to ensure that it is properly installed, making the service available at times that are convenient for the priority population will reduce a barrier and make it more likely that consumers will take action to use this service. If it is a program, then planners might consider the optimum time of day to offer the program. If a worksite program is offered in the evening, so that the workers have to return to the worksite after dinner, that probably would not be much different from driving across town from work to attend a program. Offering a program right after a shift or on a lunch hour would probably be much more appealing to most workers. Obviously, planners should be concerned about placing their program in a desirable locale (where they are wanted and needed) at the best possible time.

PROMOTION

The fourth marketing variable is **promotion**. As mentioned at the beginning of this chapter, promotion is what most people think of when they hear the word *marketing*. But promotion is just one component of the overall marketing mix. Promotion is the communication strategy, including the message and associated visuals or graphics as well as the channels, used to let the priority population know about the product, how to obtain or purchase it, and the benefits they will receive. Promotion is not about a general awareness campaign or related health communication intervention strategies. Promotion, also referred to as marketing communications, has four primary purposes (McDonald & Wilson, 2011):

1. **Inform**—increase product awareness or inform consumers
2. **Persuade**—convince people to purchase the product
3. **Reinforce**—remind them that the product exists
4. **Differentiate**—position the product as being different from the competition

There are various tools and associated channels that planners can use to achieve these purposes. Traditionally, promotional tools have included advertising, direct marketing, digital communications, sales promotion, personal selling, and publicity/public relations (Belch & Belch, 2015; McDonald & Wilson, 2011). The following section gives a general overview of these tools.

Advertising is marketing communication that is paid and nonpersonal, meaning it is not trying to reach one person but rather large groups of people. Common channels for advertising have included broadcast media (television and radio), print media (newspapers and magazines), outdoor media (billboards, bus wraps, and so forth). The national 5-a-day campaign used point-of-purchase advertising in grocery store produce departments to remind people to eat five servings of fruits and vegetables. Local coalition members developed a summer VERB program where they increased the number of places in the community for tweens to be active. They developed a card on which tweens could keep track of places they went to be physically active. Advertising space was paid for in the local newspaper, in a local family magazine, and on the radio. In addition, they got free publicity from the local media outlets and word of mouth from program partners and coalition members (Courtney, 2004). The National Bone Health Campaign used advertising including print ads and 30-second radio spots (Lefebvre, 2006).

Direct marketing involves communicating directly with consumers about a product with the purpose of getting them to purchase the product or service (Belch & Belch, 2015). Common channels for direct marketing include direct mail, internet, interactive television, or telemarketing. Tobacco companies use direct mail to provide coupons and other incentives with the purpose of encouraging people to try tobacco products (Brown-Johnson, England, Glantz, & Ling, 2014). One of the more recent applications of direct marketing in public health and health care is that of direct-to-consumer genetic tests (Liang & Mackey, 2011). Health planners may use direct marketing to reach specific groups who might be at high risk and in need of the programs. For example, direct marketing has been identified as a way to get people connected with treatment for mental health and substance abuse interventions (Becker, 2015). Other direct marketing approaches could include emailing recent heart attack patients about a program on the need to eat in a heart healthy manner, or distributing inserts about upcoming wellness program events with employee paychecks.

Personal selling refers to person-to-person interaction intended to persuade the customer to buy the product. Personal selling is used regularly in health care marketing. Pharmaceutical companies have representatives who meet one-on-one with health care providers for the purpose of convincing them to use a certain prescription drug. Another example of personal selling is the use of lay health workers, or promotoras. In rural South Carolina, promotoras were used to give information, assistance, and referrals to services (Sherrill et al., 2005). One way these lay health workers could engage in personal selling is by going to individual homes and encouraging people with diabetes to attend the health clinic screening and have their blood glucose tested.

Sales promotions are incentives that entice consumers to try the product. Types of sales promotion include coupons, premiums (e.g., prizes with purchase), contests and sweepstakes, rebates, or samples (Clow & Baack, 2014). In Japan, coupons for free cervical cancer screenings were sent to women between the ages of 20–40 as a way to increase screening rates. (Ueda, et al., 2015). Other examples include providing a coupon for a free bike helmet or a reduced fee at the local fitness center.

Public relations, also called publicity, represents both internal and external marketing communications. The news media coverage that external public relations activities generate is typically not paid for by the organization (as compared with advertising). Typical public relations tools include the use of ongoing news media outreach and sponsorship of large events that draw attention and exposure such as a special kickoff, countdown, ribbon-cutting, or health party to get a program started. Public relations activities can also be used to increase awareness about new products. The health care organization Kaiser Permanente uses social media as a public relations tool to disseminate information and engage with their stakeholders (Hether, 2014). These social media public relations activities help them to communicate with customers about the services they provide and to clear up any misunderstandings that may have resulted from media coverage.

Finally, there is digital communication. In recent years, the availability of the Internet has increased the options available for planners to use these traditional tools across a spectrum of channels. This form of promotion can generate a great deal of interest in the product for a relative low cost and in a short period of time. The availability of electronic media in addition to the Internet, including cell phones, has expanded promotional alternatives. For example, social marketers can use podcasts and other downloads to promote their products. Websites are probably the most common channel for Internet promotion. For example, advertising can now be part of a home page or social networking site, or included as a banner ad in an online newspaper. The National Bone Health Campaign developed a Website specifically for teen girls (Lefebvre, 2006), and they placed banner ads on other Websites that the priority population often visited.

There are several factors to consider when deciding which of the promotional tools and channels to use. Two of the most critical are the communication objectives and the communication preferences for the priority population. If the objective is to increase awareness of a product, the tools and channels are different than if the purpose is to demonstrate how to use the product, or to illustrate key attributes, or provide in-depth details about the product features. The priority populations' communication preferences are also critical. For example, formative research for a disaster preparedness campaign in Vietnam found that the majority of respondents owned a radio, fewer people owned a television, and almost nobody had subscriptions to the newspaper or magazines (Ramaprasad, 2005). Therefore, in selecting a promotional strategy and materials, planners probably would not place an advertisement in the newspaper, but might consider a radio spot. The National Bone Health Campaign found that the most common ways for girls grades 6–12 to stay in touch with their friends was through text messages, instant messaging, and cell phones. In addition, the most popular magazines were *Seventeen* and *Teen People* (Lefebvre, 2006). For the Hispanic segments mentioned earlier, one segment (bi-cultural) preferred marketing materials to be in English, while the other two segments (retainers and non-identifiers) preferred Spanish language materials (Alvarez, Dickson, & Hunter, 2014).

Additional questions that planners may want to ask when selecting a promotional tool and channel include:

1. What are the costs of each tool or channel versus the benefits?
2. Can the tool's or channel's capability build on or multiply the effects of another tool or channel?
3. Will the message reach a significant portion of the priority population?
4. Can the message be sent through several different channels?
5. Through how many intermediaries must the message travel to reach the priority population?
6. Can a tool be overused to the point that it will "turn off" the priority population to the message?

Messages include the words and graphics that are used to convey information about the product, where to obtain it and the benefits it will provide. The process for developing appropriate messages is both an art and a science. Many communication theories and models can be used to develop effective messages. A good place to start is with consumer-based health communications as described in the National Cancer Institute's (NCI) book *Making Health Communication Programs Work* (NCI, n.d.), otherwise known as the "Pink Book" (See http://www.cancer.gov/publications/health-communication /pink-book.pdf) In order to develop effective messages, planners must know what is motivating the priority population. This is learned while conducting formative research. They must know how to frame the message so that it will cut through the clutter, capture the priority population's attention, and motivate them to action. Key parts of the message should be that the product will offer a benefit that the priority population desires, that the product costs less than the benefits it provides, and how they can obtain the product.

For example, after performing formative research related to diet and physical activity among a group of public employees, planners learned that preferences for message content included "helping employees understand that the desired changes could be inexpensive, fun and easy, and that changes would require only a minimal amount of time." Based on these preferences, messages through email, public announcements, posters, and direct supervisor contacts (all preferred channels) were successfully used to recruit a large group of participants in a successful intervention (Neiger et al., 2001).

Another example of this concept was the segmentation process that resulted from focus groups conducted with teenage girls as part of a physical activity project (Staten, Birnbaum, Jobe, & Elder, 2006). The process resulted in seven main segments that described the girls:

athletic, preppy, quiet, rebel, smart, tough, and other. In addition, they discovered preferences for the types of images that would be best for communication materials.

> Respondents provided the following suggestions: (a) for athletic girls, pictures should show girls participating in organized, competitive activities; (b) for preppy girls, pictures might show girls cheerleading, well-dressed individuals, groups of friends being active, girls being active with boys watching (with positive affect, not leering or jeering), and organized sports with "cute" uniforms; (c) for quiet girls, pictures should show girls alone or in small groups doing activities (don't focus on competitive sports); (d) for rebel girls, pictures might include girls on skateboards, perhaps with some visible body piercing, girls wearing dark clothes, images implying dancing to punk rock music; and (e) for smart girls, pictures should show girls who are not too muscular or strong being active in small groups, and positive attitudes and neat but not trendy dress may be appealing. Small group images that show some smart girls and some preppy girls being active together may be appealing. And (f) for tough girls, pictures might show girls doing stepping or hip-hop dance or girls playing basketball (not necessarily in uniform; show street games, pick-up games). Images of girls should not be conservative. Groups of friends would be appealing. (p. 76)

WORKING WITH CREATIVE TEAMS TO HELP EXECUTE THE PROMOTIONAL STRATEGY

Depending on the agency and the available budget, planners may be responsible for developing and executing the promotional strategy or they may hire a marketing or public relations firm to do some of the creative work including creating messages, materials, or brand logos and tag lines. If planners are working with a creative agency, the following suggestions will help ensure that the process is successful. Keep in mind that the actual process may vary depending on the creative team and their agency policies. At all phases of the process, planners should make sure to have open and honest communication with the creative team. It is important to trust their creative skills and abilities, but planners need to make sure that they are on track with the program objectives.

The first step is to identify a public relations or marketing agency. The organization that a planner works for may require all outside work to be solicited through a specific procurement or bid process. In other instances, planners may be able to work directly with an agency of choice. In either circumstance, the first step is to identify a list of possible agencies. Consider getting recommendations from other health promotion programs or health-related organizations that have hired creative agencies. Ask the agency for samples of their previous health-related campaigns.

Once an agency has been selected, hold a meeting with members of the program planning team and the creative team. This is sometimes referred to as a *discovery meeting*. At this meeting the creative team will assess what needs to be accomplished. Planners should bring to this meeting all the research about the priority population and the program goals and objectives. A concise way to convey this information is by using a creative brief, which is a synopsis that describes the priority population, the benefits they seek, the barriers they face, the purpose of the communication, and potential communication channels. (See **Box 11.8** for an outline of a creative brief.)

After the discovery meeting, the creative team will come back to the agency with recommendations for how to proceed, including the type of appeal (e.g., humor, slice of life) and the type of communication materials. They should also provide a cost estimate for how many person-hours it will take to develop the materials and the cost of material production.

Outline of the Creative Brief for a Promotional Strategy

1. Background (overview about the topic and project):
2. Priority Population/Segment (concise description of the priority population):
3. Purpose of Promotion (increase awareness of product, remind them product exists, or encourage them to act):
4. Core Benefit to Highlight:
5. Place (where the people will access the product):
6. Price (both tangible and intangible):
7. Communication Preferences (tools and channels):

The next step is to sign an estimate agreement. Before doing so, planners need to make sure that they agree with the creative team's recommendations. That is, does the recommended approach on strategy correspond to program goals and communication objectives? At this point planners want to clarify what work and deliverables are included in the fees.

Once the agreement is signed, the creative team will begin their work. Based on the budget, they will flesh out a limited number of concepts, also known as *draft ideas*. After reviewing the concepts, planners can choose which one(s) they want to be part of their campaign. A limited number of modifications (sometimes just one) is included in the original cost estimate. Other major changes beyond that may require another fee. Knowing that several modifications can increase the cost of a promotional campaign is one reason that the discovery meeting is so important and why planners want to be prepared with formative research about the priority population. Planners should also make sure to build in time and money for pretesting materials and messages with the priority population, as discussed in the next section.

Pretesting

Though planners conduct formative research and learn as much about consumers as they can prior to developing the marketing strategy, planners need to make sure that they are still on track with consumer preferences before offering products or launching the promotional campaign. The process of getting this feedback is called **pretesting**. Pretesting ensures that planners have developed program components in response to, and are reflective of the priority population's needs, wants, and expectations.

Ideally, planners should test all components of the marketing strategy including products, messages, materials, and selected promotional tools. However, the breadth and depth of pretesting is usually determined by the budget. It is important to include in the project time line, as well the budget, adequate time and financial resources to complete pretesting.

Pretesting can be completed in two phases, both of which occur during the development process when products and promotional materials are in draft form, before ideas are finalized or any promotional materials are produced. Phase one involves testing the product concepts. Think of concepts as a prototype or draft form of products and services. For example, you are considering offering a service where people can take a photo of a mole or other mark on their skin and send it to the dermatologist for analysis. You want to know what people think about this service and if they would use it. Pretesting concepts gives planners the opportunity to get feedback on the design of the product as well as the product-related benefits. The topics planners would want to receive feedback on when pretesting the product or service may include:

- How likely they would be to use the product
- What they see as benefits to using the product
- What they see as the barriers; what factors would keep them from using it
- What products features they like
- What product features they would change, and why
- If the places selected to offer the product are convenient
- If the product price is reasonable
- If the benefits associated with product use are believable
- If the product functions as designed
- If instructions for how to use the product are clear

The second pretesting phase is testing the promotional strategy messages and materials. It is best to test messages and materials separately because planners will not know if the priority population is responding to the message or the material. For instance, you test a message and brochure together and find that the message is not very motivating. Is this because of the content of the message? Or is it because the brochure design influenced how they understood the message? **Box 11.9** outlines aspects of the promotional messages and materials about which planners may want to get feedback during the pretesting process.

Pretesting allows planners to identify red flags or, in other words, parts of the strategy that may reduce the chances of success. However, positive feedback from the priority population during the pretesting phase cannot indicate the degree to which the consumers will like the product or service, or how successful the promotional messages and materials will be at influencing people to use the product or service. The inability to generalize pretesting results to a larger population is due to a small sample size and selection methods (see Chapter 5).

The methods planners can use for pretesting depend on what aspect of the marketing strategy is being tested, the topics being explored, the amount of money available for pretesting, and the timeline. In general, focus groups (see Chapter 4) and central location intercept interviews are common pretesting methods. Focus groups have the advantage of group discussion and brainstorming from several people at once. But sometimes group discussion can sway people's opinions so you may want to use individual interviews. Central location intercept interviews requires going to a place where the priority population can be easily found (e.g., young mothers at pediatrician offices) and then asking if people would be willing to spend 10-15 minute answering some questions. These qualitative methods are preferred because they allow the planners to interact with the priority population, get in-depth reactions to products, messages and materials, and follow up with clarifying questions or probes. You can also use surveys, administered in-person, through the internet, or the mail (see Chapters 4 and 5 for more information about survey questionnaires). A survey will allow you to get feedback from more respondents but it limits the planner's ability to probe for additional feedback. Factors to consider when using each of these methods for pretesting are presented in **Table 11.3**.

Pretesting should always be completed with members of the priority population. Planners can use probability or nonprobability (also called purposive) samples (see Chapter 5) to select the participants. In addition, planners may want to obtain reviews from subject matter experts

Topics for Message and Material Pretesting

Show a copy of draft messages and ask:

What is the main idea that you get from this message?
What do you think they want you to know?
What do you think they want you to believe?
What action do you think they want you to take?
What image comes to mind when you hear this message?
What emotions do you feel as you hear this message?
Where is the best place to reach you with this message?
Where would you most likely notice it and pay attention to it?
What words are confusing or hard to understand?

Describe what type of person this message is trying to reach.

The main purpose of this message is to persuade you and people like you to [describe action related to the product].

How likely is it that you would take action based on this message? *(Note: Use a Likert scale here to measure response.)*
What about this message is motivating?
What about this message is not motivating?

Show a draft of a promotional material and ask:

What do you like about this [material]?
What don't you like about this [material]?
What stands out to you?
How attention-getting is this [material]? *(Note: Use a Likert scale here to measure response.)*

Source: Adapted from Lee & Kotler (2016); National Cancer Institute (n.d.).

or gatekeepers. Subject matter experts are people who have advanced knowledge about the health topic. Having subject matter expert review ensures that the promotional messages are factually and technically correct, thereby reducing the chance of conveying false information. Gatekeepers are people who control whether messages, materials, or products reach the priority population. Gatekeeper review enables the planners to get buy-in from individuals who are influential in distributing the product or disseminating promotional materials. Examples of gatekeepers are nurses at doctors' offices, radio station owners, newspaper editors, or individuals whom the priority population identifies as community leaders.

Continuous Monitoring

Continuous monitoring conducted as part of a marketing strategy is somewhat analogous to aspects of both formative and process evaluations (see Chapter 14). What makes continuous monitoring unique is its focus on getting reaction and comment from the priority population about all aspects of the program during the implementation phase. The monitoring function determines if things are going as planned, if the program is operating below expectations, and whether changes noted indicate that the program is moving in the right

TABLE 11.3 **Factors to Consider When Choosing Pretesting Methods**

Factor	Potential Options	Example	Preferred Pretesting Method
1. What part of the social marketing strategy is being tested?	Promotional messages	Postcard to be received in the mail	Survey; intercept interview; focus group
	Promotional materials based on messages	Brochure, flyer, Website banner,	Intercept interview; focus group
	A product prototype or sample	Text message service	Intercept interview; focus group
2. What type of responses do you want from the priority population	Ratings	"Rate on a scale of 1-5 how likely would you be to take action after seeing this message."	Survey; intercept interview
	A long list of ideas from group brainstorming	"Tell me about the places you might see messages like this in your neighborhood."	Focus group
	In-depth reactions. You want to be able to ask follow-up questions based on their responses	"Tell me about the type of person this message is talking to." "Tell me about how they spend their time." "Tell me about what makes you think it is for women only."	Intercept interview; focus group
3. What do you want the priority population to do?	See a message, material, or product in-person	Show them a poster with the message and then ask questions.	Intercept interview; focus group
	Read a message	Provide a copy of the message in writing	Survey; intercept interview; focus group
	Hear a message	Ask them to listen to a radio spot	Survey; intercept interview; focus group
	Touch a product or material	Hold the product in their hands	Intercept interview; focus group
	Try out a product	Ask them to use the Website to contact their health care provider	Intercept interview; focus group
4. Would the priority population talk about this product or message in a group setting?	Behaviors that are considered socially undesirable or sensitive may not be discussed as openly in a group setting	Drinking and driving; intravenous drug use; sexually transmitted infections	Survey; intercept interview

direction (Andreasen, 1995). This continuous monitoring provides program planners with data regarding level of program acceptance by the priority population, reach of messages, product distribution sites, and in general, what is working and what is not working. Overall, continuous monitoring improves the effectiveness of the program by continually integrating feedback from the priority population.

Summary

An important aspect of any health promotion program is being able to design a product that will attract the priority population initially and keep them involved once they have begun a new behavior. All products must provide a benefit or outcome that the priority population values. Using marketing principles can help planners develop successful programs. Understanding the priority population, including their wants and needs, is at the heart of the marketing process. An important step in the process is identifying segments that share similar characteristics. The marketing mix should take into account the four Ps of marketing: product, price, place, and promotion. These elements together become the basis for the marketing strategy that will facilitate the exchange between the program planner as the marketer and the priority population as the customer. Before launching the program, products, messages, and materials should be pretested with the priority population. After the program starts, continuous monitoring and getting feedback from the priority population will help keep the program on track.

Box 11.10 is a template that planners can use to write a one-page summary of their social marketing strategy.

Review Questions

1. Define the following terms: *market, marketing,* and *social marketing.*
2. What is the relationship between formative research and needs assessment?
3. How does segmenting your priority population help you in planning?
4. What are some factors to use when segmenting your priority population? Which ones are most important?

BOX	**One Page Social Marketing Summary**

11.10

Application

In order to help _____ [priority population segment] _____

To do _____ [behavior] _____

We will offer _____ [product] _____

Which will help overcome _____ [barriers] _____

And provide _____ [benefits] _____

For this _____ [price] _____

At _____ [location] _____

We will let the priority population know about this product by using _____ [promotional strategies] _____

We will pretest our strategy by _____ [pretesting methods] _____

We will measure our success by _____ [continuous monitoring] _____

5. What has to happen in order for an exchange to take place between a planner and the priority population?

6. Describe the six elements that make a social marketing approach unique from other planning approaches?

7. What are the four Ps of marketing? Explain each one.

8. Describe how to best work with a creative team to execute a promotional strategy.

9. What are the purposes of pretesting?

10. What are factors to consider when choosing pretesting methods?

 ## Activities

1. Respond to the following statements/questions with regard to a program you are planning. Make sure to explain the rationale on which you based your decision.

   a. Describe your product (i.e., tangible item or service).

      a1. How will the product make it easy and convenient for the priority population to do the behavior and receive the associated benefits?

      a2. How will the product help to reduce barriers to, and/or the cost of the behavior you want the priority population to engage in.

      a3. What is the core product (or bundle of benefits) that they will receive if they purchase and use the product?

   b. Describe your segmented priority population. What segmentation factors did you use to identify segments?

   c. What will the priority population have to "give-up," or "pay" to receive the augmented product and the bundle of benefits? Consider both financial and non-financial costs.

   d. Describe where priority population will access the augmented product. In other words, where will the product be available or distributed to the priority population. What is your reason for placing it this way? If you have a service product, when will it be offered (location, days, and time)?

   e. What promotional tools will you use to promote your program? How, when, and where will you let the priority population know about the item or service?

2. Detail a pretesting plan for your marketing strategy.

   a. Identify which components of the marketing strategy you will test (product, messages, materials). Include rationale for the choice of those components for pretesting. That is, why is it important to pretest those aspects?

   b. Describe what specific components of the product, message or materials will be tested. For example, are you going to test the color of the print for the materials? The appeal of the message? If people understand the main message?

   c. Write out the questions that you would ask during pretesting,

   d. Describe when (dates) and where (geographic locations) the data will be collected and who will participate (the sample) in the pretesting.

3. Using Box 11.10, create a one-page summary of your social marketing strategy.

4. Create a promotional piece that could be used to promote your product through advertising, direct marketing, personal selling, or sales promotions. This promotional piece should include both text and graphics and highlight the core benefit being offered.

5. Survey members of the priority population to find out what would motivate them to begin a specific health behavior. Make sure to ask about products and services that would help them make that change. See Chapter 5 about survey layout and design.

 # Weblinks

1. **http://www.marketingpower.com**

   American Marketing Association

   The American Marketing Association is one of the largest professional associations for marketers. This Website provides best practices related to marketing strategies, including marketing tools and templates and marketing services directories.

2. **http://www.cbsm.com/public/world.lasso**

   Fostering Sustainable Behavior and Community-Based Social Marketing

   This Website highlights how social marketing is used in the areas of energy, water, transportation, and the environment. On this Website there are articles, case studies, discussion forums, and other resources.

3. **http://www.europeansocialmarketing.org/**

   European Social Marketing Association

   The European Social Marketing Association is primarily for connecting social marketers in Europe. On their Website you will find news, job announcements, events, and networking opportunities.

4. **http://www.i-socialmarketing.org/**

   International Social Marketing Association

   The International Social Marketing Association's mission is to "advance social marketing practice, research, and teaching through collaborative networks of professionals, supporters and enthusiasts." On the Website you will find jobs, events, networking opportunities, webinars, social marketing news, and other resources. Some content is available for member's only.

5. **http://www.toolsofchange.com/en/programs/social-marketers/**

   Tools of Change

   This Website is based on social marketing work in Canada. Here you will find case studies, planning guides, and list of webinars and workshops available through Tools of Change.

6. **http://ctb.ku.edu/en/sustain/social-marketing/overview/main**

   Community Tool Box

   This Website provides excellent resources on promoting participation and social marketing. Topic sections include step-by-step instruction, examples, checklists, and related resources.

7. http://www.social-marketing.com

Weinreich Communications

This Website contains social marketing-related articles, resources, conference calendar, and extensive lists of links to pertinent sources of information.

8. http://www.thensmc.com/

National Social Marketing Centre (NSMC)

The NSMC is a center for excellence in behavior change and social marketing located in the United Kingdom. This Website provides tools and resources for designing social marketing programs as well as case studies from around the world.

9. LISTPROC@LISTPROC.GEORGETOWN.EDU

Georgetown Social Marketing Listserv

This is an active social marketing listserv with discussions centering on a variety of social marketing topics. Subscribers can elect to receive a daily digest of emails or receive each one as it is posted. To subscribe, send an email message to the URL listed above. In the body of the message write "SUBSCRIBE SOC-MKTG [insert your own name]."

Implementation
Strategies and Associated Concerns

Chapter Objectives

After reading this chapter and answering the questions at the end, you should be able to:

- Define and explain a logic model.
- Define *implementation*.
- Identify the different phases for implementing health promotion programs.
- Define *management*.
- Identify and briefly explain the major resources that must be managed during implementation.
- Identify major pieces of federal legislation that impact human resource management.
- List and briefly describe the concerns that need to be addressed before implementation can take place.

Key Terms

accounting	internal audit
act of commission	logic model
act of omission	management
anonymity	negligence
audit	news hook
beneficence	nonmaleficence
confidentiality	outcomes
critical path method	outputs
disability	PERT
ethical issues	phased in
external audit	pilot testing
financial management	program kick off
fiscal accountability	program launch
fiscal year	program monitoring
Gantt chart	program rollout
HIPAA	prudent
implementation	task development
implementation	time line
science	technical resources
informed consent	Type III errors
inputs	

Earlier (in Chapters 1–10) we discussed the steps necessary to plan a solid health promotion program, and presented information (in Chapter 11) that would assist planners in marketing the program they planned. With the planning and marketing processes complete, planners need to focus on implementation. There are many things that need attention in the implementation process that are critical to a successful program. The eventual impact of a program will be judged not only by the effectiveness of the interventions but also by the quality of the implementation (Parcel, 1995). In fact, Timmreck (2003) has stated "implementation is the most critical part of the planning process; a plan that is not implemented is no plan at all" (p. 171). In this chapter, we present the key phases in implementing a program and identify the many concerns that must be addressed as implementation unfolds. **Box 12.1** identifies the responsibilities and competencies for health education specialists that pertain to the material presented in this chapter.

BOX

12.1

Responsibilities and Competencies for Health Education Specialists

This chapter focuses on program implementation. Because implementation is a culmination of all the preparation and planning that has come before it, several of the responsibilities and competencies for health education specialists apply. The responsibilities and competencies related to these tasks that are associated with implementation include:

RESPONSIBILITY II: Plan Health Education/Promotion

Competency 2.4: Develop a plan for the delivery of health education/ promotion

Competency 2.5: Address factors that influence implementation of health education/promotion

RESPONSIBILITY III: Implement Health Education/Promotion

Competency 3.1: Coordinate logistics necessary to implement a plan

Competency 3.2: Train staff members and volunteers involved in implementation of health education/promotion

Competency 3.3: Implement health education/promotion plan

Competency 3.4: Monitor implementation of health education/ promotion

RESPONSIBILITY V: Administer and Manage Health Education/Promotion

Competency 5.1: Manage financial resources for health education/ promotion programs

Competency 5.2: Manage technology resources

Competency 5.3: Manage relationships with partners and other stakeholders

Competency 5.6: Manage human resources for health education/ promotion programs

RESPONSIBILITY VI: Serve as a Health Education/Promotion Resource Person

Competency 6.2: Train others to use health education/promotion skills

Competency 6.3: Provide advice and consultation on health education/ promotion issues

RESPONSIBILITY VII: Communicate, Promote and Advocate for Health, Health Education/ Promotion, and the Profession

Competency 7.1: Identify, develop, and deliver messages using a variety of communication strategies, methods, and techniques

Competency 7.2: Engage in advocacy for health and health education/ promotion

Competency 7.3 Influence policy and/or systems change to promote health and health education

Source: *A Competency-Based Framework for Health Education Specialists—2015.* Whitehall, PA: National Commission for Health Education Credentialing, Inc. (NCHEC) and the Society for Public Health Education (SOPHE). Reprinted by permission of the National Commission for Health Education Credentialing, Inc. (NCHEC) and the Society for Public Health Education (SOPHE).

▷ Logic Models

Before discussing the various phases of implementation and the issues related to them, we feel it is important to present information on logic models because of their usefulness in the implementation process. While logic models can be created and used at various times during the planning, implementing, and evaluating processes, they are especially useful at this stage of program development because they can help identify the steps that must be taken to implement and manage successful programs. A **logic model** is a systematic and visual way for planners to share and present their understanding of the relationship among the resources they have to operate a program, the activities they plan to implement, and the outputs and outcomes they hope to achieve (CDC, 2008b; WKKF, 2004); "that is the logic of the program" (Lando, Williams, Sturgis, & Williams, 2006, p. 2). Simply put, a logic model is a road map (Goldman & Schmalz, 2006) showing the connections among the key components of a program.

Logic models can take many different shapes (linear, circular, lists) and be presented in various levels of detail (simple, complex) but all depict the relationship and linkages of various components in a graphic display of boxes and arrows. "Program-level logic models are often meta-summaries of complex processes; as a result, additional logic models may be needed to 'unpack' each component in the original model so that more details can be articulated" (Helitzer et al., 2009, p. 64). In its most basic form a logic model includes four components: *inputs* (or resources), *activities* (or interventions or strategies), *outputs* (or evidence of activities), and *outcomes* (or results or effects). (See **Figure 12.1** for the basic logic model.) The **inputs** in a logic model are the resources (or infrastructure) that are used to plan, implement, and evaluate a program. They often include human resources (and related items like training, technical assistance, volunteers), partnerships, funding sources, equipment, supplies, materials, and community resources (e.g., space, gifts). The **activities** in a logic model are the interventions or strategies used in a program to bring about change. The **outputs** are the direct results of the activities and include things such as products (e.g., curricula, educational DVDs, new software, data collection tools), services (e.g., in-service trainings, screenings, counseling, events), and new components of infrastructure (e.g., structure, capacity, process, and relationships).

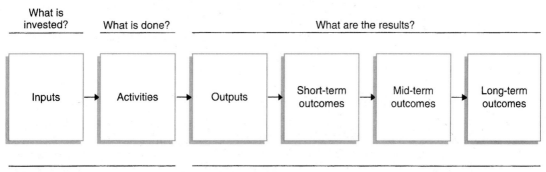

Planned work · Intended results

▲ **Figure 12.1** Basic Logic Model

The **outcomes** in a logic model are the intended results and are broken into *short-term* (or immediate) (e.g., changes in awareness, attitudes, knowledge, skills), *mid-term* (or medium) (e.g., changes in behavior or the environment), and *long-term* (e.g., risk reduction, change in health status, or quality of life). Some logic model experts have a step after outcomes called *impact*, which they define as the fundamental intended or unintended change occurring in organizations, communities, or systems as a result of program. While, others (CDC, 2010b; Goldman & Schmaltz, 2006; The Pell Institute, 2015; University of Kansas, 2015; WKKF, 2004) have suggested that logic models can also include (1) the purpose or mission of the program; (2) the context, conditions, or situations under which the program will be offered; (3) assumptions associated with the planned program; (4) external factors that could influence the success of the program; and (5) a description of the evaluation of the proposed program. There is no one right way to create a logic Model (CDC, 2010b). "Ideally a logic model is contained within a single page with enough detail that it can be explained fairly easily and understood by other people" (Schmidtz & Parsons, 1999, para. 6). Although most logic models are created and read from right to left, they do not have to be configured that way. Part of the usefulness of a logic model is that it is created with a series of "if...then" statements. So starting from the left hand side of the schematic the first statement may read—"If we have these resources then we will be able to create and deliver these activities." The second statement might then read—"If we conduct these activities then we should expect these outputs." A third statement might read—"If the planned activities deliverer the outputs that were expected, then the health of the program participants will be improved." Good "if...then" statements create the "links in the chain of reasoning" (Schmidtz & Parsons, 1999, para. 11) that take planners from the program resources to the expected program outcomes. "If at any point, as you read through the logic model and the reasoning does not follow, it could mean one or more elements of the planned work in the program design does not strategically lead to an element or elements in the intended program results" (The Pell Institute, 2015, para. 2) **Box 12.2** provides an example of a logic model that was used as part of the planning process for a program aimed at reducing the incidence of colon cancer.

▷ Defining Implementation

In the simplest terms, implementation means to carry out. Timmreck (1997) defined **implementation** as "the act of converting planning, goals, and objectives into action through administrative structure, management activities, policies, procedures, regulations, and organizational actions of new programs" (p. 328). Whereas Bartholomew and colleagues (2011) indicated that implementation is one of the three stages of program diffusion, with the other two being *adoption* and *sustainability*. Let's look now at the phases in the implementation process.

▷ Phases of Program Implementation

The phases of implementation that we present here are a combination of some of our own ideas with those of Parkinson and Associates (1982), Bartholomew and colleagues (2011), and Johnson and Breckon (2007). It should be noted that the resulting generic phases presented are flexible in nature and can be modified to meet the many different situations and circumstances faced by planners.

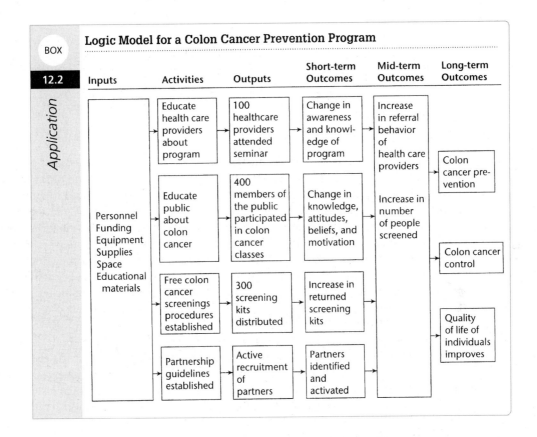

BOX

12.2

Application

Logic Model for a Colon Cancer Prevention Program

Inputs	Activities	Outputs	Short-term Outcomes	Mid-term Outcomes	Long-term Outcomes
Personnel Funding Equipment Supplies Space Educational materials	Educate health care providers about program	100 healthcare providers attended seminar	Change in awareness and knowledge of program	Increase in referral behavior of health care providers	Colon cancer prevention
	Educate public about colon cancer	400 members of the public participated in colon cancer classes	Change in knowledge, attitudes, beliefs, and motivation	Increase in number of people screened	Colon cancer control
	Free colon cancer screenings procedures established	300 screening kits distributed	Increase in returned screening kits		Quality of life of individuals improves
	Partnership guidelines established	Active recruitment of partners	Partners identified and activated		

Phase 1: Adoption of the Program

Because the adoption process was presented at length earlier (in Chapter 11), we will not repeat it here. However, we do want to remind planners that great care must go into the marketing process to ensure that a relevant product (i.e., the health promotion program) is planned so that those in the priority population will want to participate in it.

Phase 2: Identifying and Prioritizing the Tasks to Be Completed

In order for a program to be implemented, planners will need to identify and prioritize a number of smaller tasks. Even though many of these tasks are small in nature, they cannot be overlooked if planners want a smooth implementation. Reserving space where the program is to be held, making sure audiovisual equipment is available when requested, ordering the correct number of participant education packets or manuals, and arranging for interpreters when working with a diverse population are examples of tasks that are important to the success of a program. Other implementation tasks are presented later in this chapter in the section titled "Concerns Associated with Implementation."

Appoint committee	Determine the purpose and scope	Gather data	Analyze data	Identify risk factors linked to health problem	Identify problem focus	Validate the need

▲ **Figure 12.2** Sample Basic Time Line for a Needs Assessment

To assist with identifying and prioritizing these tasks, it is recommended that planners use some form of a planning timetable or time line. Planning timetables and time lines can graphically represent the dates, time span, and sequence of events involved in a program (Issel, 2014). They can also aid in monitoring program progress "so that midcourse corrections can be made, if needed" (McDermott & Sarvela, 1999, p. 72). Planning timetables that are commonly used include basic time lines, task development time lines (TDTLs) (Anspaugh, Dignan, & Anspaugh, 2000), Gantt charts, PERT charts, and the critical path method (CPM). A basic time line is the simplest of the tools. It places the key activities or tasks on a line in the order that they will be completed. It may or may not include an estimate of the dates when the activities or tasks will take place, and the time allocated to complete them (see **Figure 12.2**).

Task development time lines and Gantt charts are very similar. They are both composed of rows and columns. The rows on the left-hand side of the chart represent the tasks or activities to be completed, while the columns represent periods of time. In the examples presented in **Figures 12.3** and **12.4**, the columns represent months, but they could just as easily represent weeks or for that matter days if the chart were being used for a short-term project. The major difference between a TDTL and a Gantt chart is in the detail presented. A **task development time line** identifies the tasks that need to be completed and the time frame in which the tasks will be completed (Anspaugh et al., 2000). A **Gantt chart**, developed in 1917 by Henry Gantt as a production control tool (TechTarget, 2007–2015a), does the same plus provides an indication of the progress made toward completing the task by using different size lines to distinguish between the projected time frame for a task and the progress toward completing the task. In addition, a Gantt chart uses a marker above the columns to indicate the current date (Timmreck, 2003). (See the check mark above the month of August in Figure 12.4.) Thus, when using a Gantt chart, planners would update their progress regularly on the chart.

PERT is an acronym for program evaluation and review technique. PERT charts are more complex than Gantt charts and have not been used as much with health promotion programs (Timmreck, 2003). PERT charts are composed of two components, a diagram and a timetable (Minelli & Breckon, 2009). The diagram presents a visual representation of the relationship between and among the tasks to be completed. The diagram also indicates the order of completion by sequentially numbering the tasks. This means that tasks identified with lower numbers must be completed prior to taking on tasks identified with higher numbers (TechTarget, 2007–2015b). The timetable of a PERT chart is similar to the key activity chart but also includes three estimates of time for each task. Included in the estimates are an optimistic, pessimistic, and a probabilistic time frame. The complexity of PERT puts a detailed explanation beyond the scope of this textbook. If readers are interested in learning more about it, we recommend referring to business management textbooks.

Tasks Year 1	Months											
	J	F	M	A	M	J	J	A	S	O	N	D
Develop program rationale	✔	✔										
Conduct needs assessment			✔									
Develop goals and objectives				✔								
Create intervention					✔							
Conduct formative evaluation						✔						
Assemble necessary resources						✔						
Market program						✔	✔					
Pilot test program								✔				
Refine program									✔			
Phase in intervention #1										✔		
Phase in intervention #2											✔	
Phase in intervention #3												✔

Tasks Year 2	Months											
	J	F	M	A	M	J	J	A	S	O	N	D
Phase in intervention #4	✔											
Total implementation		✔	✔	✔	✔	✔	✔	✔	✔	✔	✔	✔
Collect and analyze data for evaluation			✔									
Prepare evaluation report				✔								
Distribute report					✔							
Continue with follow-up for long-term evaluation						✔	✔	✔	✔	✔	✔	✔

▲ **Figure 12.3** Sample Task Development Time Line for Program Planning, Implementation, and Evaluation

Date
√

	Mar.	April	May	June	July	Aug.	Sept.	Oct.	Nov.	Dec.
Hire and train program facilitators	▬▬▬	▬▬▬								
Pilot test program			▬▬▬	▬▬						
Revise program based on pilot					▬▬▬					
Promote the program					▬▬▬	▬				
Prepare for program "kick off"						▬▬				
Phase in program							▬▬▬			
Full implementation								▬▬▬	▬	
Evaluate program									▬▬▬	▬
Write final report										▬▬

▬▬▬ = planned time frame

───── = completed

▲ **Figure 12.4** Sample Gantt Chart for Program Implementation and Evaluation

The last planning timetable to be presented is the **critical path method** (CPM). CPM charts are similar to PERT charts and are sometimes referred to as PERT/CPM. Like all the other planning timetables presented here, the CPM provides a graphical view of the project and predicts the time required to complete the project. But what is unique to CPM is that it focuses on time by showing which tasks are critical to maintaining the planning schedule and which are not (NetMBA, 2002–2010). Thus, the critical path is indicated and consists of the set of dependent tasks (each dependent on the preceding one) that together take the longest time to complete. The tasks on the path are critical because any delay in their completion will lengthen program implementation unless appropriate action is taken (NetMBA, 2002–2010).

Phase 3: Establishing a System of Management

Once all the tasks have been identified and the timetable for completing them has been developed, planners can turn their attention to how the program will be managed. **Management** has been defined as "the process of working with and through others to achieve organizational or program objectives in an efficient and ethical manner" (Shi & Johnson, 2014, p. 658). Typically, the sets of resources include human, financial, and technical resources (Johnson & Breckon, 2007). Management is an important part of the program implementation process. "The efficient, satisfactory management of a health promotion program is vital to its long-term success" (Anspaugh et al., 2000, p. 124). Yet, management is both challenging and necessary (Hitt et al., 2012). It is challenging because the large number of responsibilities (e.g., planning, organization, coordination, and control) associated with the task of managing and because of change, both expected and unexpected, throughout the life of a program. Thus, good management is needed to ensure that programs are both effective and efficient (Gomez-Mejia & Balkin, 2012). Effective programs are ones that meet stated goals and objectives.

They are efficient when the best possible use is made of program resources. Good managers can go a long way in making this happen. Hitt and colleagues (2012) have identified three types of skills needed by managers—technical, interpersonal, and conceptual. "Technical skills involve having specialized knowledge about procedures, processes, and equipment, and include knowing how and when to use that knowledge" (p. 19). Interpersonal skills include such qualities as sensitivity, persuasiveness, and empathy, while conceptual skills, sometimes called cognitive ability or cognitive complexity, include such skills as logical reasoning, judgment, and analytical abilities.

Depending on the type of program being planned, the management process could range from consuming a small portion of a single planner's time and resources, such as when a smoking cessation program is being planned for 10 people, to needing several people working full-time to manage a large community-wide program. Many of the tasks associated with the management phase of implementation are presented later in this chapter. In the space below we will provide an overview of the management of the three major resources.

HUMAN RESOURCES MANAGEMENT (HRM)

There are four fundamental functions associated with HRM. "These functions, designated by the acronym PADS, are planning, acquisition, development, and sanction" (Klingner et al., 2010, p. 4). Personnel planning (the P of PADS) refers to the work that must be completed in order to be able to determine what positions are needed to carry out a program and how to fill them (Dessler, 2012), whether they are filled with employees or volunteers. (See Chapter 10 for more information on volunteers.) Thus knowing: (1) what tasks that must be completed by the personnel of a program, (2) what knowledge and skills the personnel need to complete the tasks, (3) how many people will be needed to complete the tasks, (4) how to describe the jobs (see Box 10.4 for a sample job description), and (5) how much compensation (pay and benefits) is appropriate for the jobs are all part of planning.

Once the planning for personnel is complete and job descriptions are in place, program managers can then focus on acquisition (the A of PADS) of personnel; that is, the recruitment and selection of the personnel. The process used in the acquisition of personnel in organizations is usually governed by specific procedures, rules, and laws (Shi & Johnson, 2014). This process begins by generating a pool of candidates for the jobs through recruitment. This is typically handled through advertising via the job posting at various sites (e.g., newspapers; online on Webpages or recruiting job boards; professional organization job lines or newsletters; at job fairs, employment agencies or career centers) where viable candidates will find the information (Dessler, 2012). Job postings not only describe the positions that need to be filled, needed qualifications, and salary range, but also include information about the application process. It is not unusual to have applicants provide a letter of application, complete an application form, submit a résumé, and provide either letters of recommendation or the names of references to be contacted later. With the formal applications in hand, candidates must be screened (which in addition to looking for the appropriate qualifications may include testing for knowledge and skills, background checks, physical exams, and drug testing), decisions must be made on how and when to interview them, and finally the best candidates must be selected, and their services secured.

The D in PADS stands for development. Development includes the orientation, training, performance appraisal, and professional growth or development opportunities to increase the personnel's willingness and competencies to perform well (Dessler, 2012; Klingner et al., 2010). Orientation (often called *onboarding*) has two major purposes: (1) to provide background information to perform the job satisfactorily, and (2) to socialize new personnel to the work environment (i.e., culture of the organization) by instilling the attitudes, standards, values, and patterns of behavior that are expected (Dessler, 2012). Training involves providing personnel with the knowledge and skills needed to be successful in the position. Much training today revolves around building capacity and teamwork. (See Chapter 10 for more on these topics.) Performance appraisal and professional development opportunities frequently go hand in hand. Performance appraisal often includes some informal appraisal in which feedback is provided as needed and a more formal evaluation that is conducted on either a semi-annual or annual basis. The results of these appraisals can be used to plan additional training to deal with deficiencies or plan professional development opportunities to expand staff abilities and competencies. Such development opportunities are important for two reasons. One, employee growth/development leads to greater job satisfaction, improved morale, reduced turnover and enhanced performance. And two, organizations benefit from a staff with enhanced skills, knowledge, and attitudes (Shi & Johnson, 2014).

Because of the ever-changing work environment (e.g., new technology, economic conditions, and increased accountability), every organization needs a line item in its budget for professional development and each employee needs a professional development plan that includes specific skills and personal growth components (Shi & Johnson, 2014). Professional growth opportunities can come in many different forms (i.e., training, education, mentoring) but they need to be planned and updated regularly. (See **Box 12.3** for a sample professional development plan.)

BOX

12.3

Application

Sample Template for a Professional Development Plan

Employee Name: Year:

Current position:

Directions: Parts A, B, C, and D of this form should be completed and returned to your supervisor after your annual review meeting. Parts E and F should be completed at the end of the year and are your report of your professional development. Bring the completed form to your next annual review meeting with your supervisor. (Note: SMART objectives are specific, measurable, achievable, realistic, and time phased.)

Part A: Assessment

1. Self-assessment (Knowledge and skills you believe you need to learn more about; consider strengths, weaknesses, opportunities, and threats [SWOT])
2. Supervisor assessment (Knowledge and skills your supervisor believes you need)

Part B: Learning objectives (Using SMART objectives, state what you plan to accomplish next year.)

Part C: Proposed learning activities (State what you will do to meet your learning objectives; consider education, training, mentoring.)

Part D: Budget (Identify the cost of items to meet the objectives.)

Part E: Completed learning activities (State what you did during the year to meet your learning objectives.)

Part F: Evaluation (Indicate what has changed as a result of your professional development experiences during the past year.)

The final fundamental function in HRM is sanction. Sanction (the *S* of PADS) deals with maintaining the expectations and obligations program personnel and their program manager have to one another through appropriate compensation, promotion, discipline/grievances, health and safety, and personnel rights (Klingner et al., 2010).

Much of the work of program managers as related to HRM is guided by laws and legal decisions. **Box 12.4** includes a list of a number of the important pieces of federal legislation that impact the management of human resources. Note that most of the legislation presented in Box 12.4 applies to all employees and most employers but not all. In certain situations specific requirements must be met for the legislation to apply. For example, the Family and Medical Leave Act (FMLA) only applies in work settings with 50 or more employees. Also note that in addition to the federal legislation individual states may also have laws that impact human resources. An example is the "state-by-state laws that establish insurance plans to compensate employees injured on the job" (Gomez-Mejia & Balkin, 2012, p. 286).

FINANCIAL MANAGEMENT

Financial management "is the process of developing and using systems to ensure that funds are spent for the purposes for which they have been appropriated" (Klingner et al., 2010, p. 88). Financial management begins after funds have been obtained and the program budget has been created. (See Chapter 10 for more information on sources of funding and budgets.) Thus, it is the program manager who is responsible for ensuring that program funds are spent on the things for which they were appropriated. This process begins with a system to record the transactions that take place over the life of a program. These transactions include funds coming into, the income (e.g., grant money, gifts, participant fees), and going out, the expenditures (e.g., paying for salaries and wages, and the purchase of materials, supplies, and equipment) of the program. The process of recording and summarizing these transactions and interpreting their effects on the program budget is referred to as **accounting** (Fallon & Zgodzinski, 2012). Each organization has an accounting process and depending on the size of the organization, responsibility for the accounting process may fall on the program manager or if the organization is large enough it may fall to an accounting department.

The accounting process generates financial statements. "Financial statements can be prepared at any point in time and can cover any period of time" (Fallon & Zgodzinski, 2012, p. 60). Most organizations work on a **fiscal year** (or funding year) (i.e., FY) running from either January 1st to December 31st or July 1st to June 30th. The United Stated federal government uses a FY that begins October 1 and ends September 30. However, it is common for financial statements to be created at regular intervals (i.e., weekly, monthly, quarterly, semi-annually, or annually) during the fiscal year. (See Figure 10.3.) Each "organization selects a reporting period and prepares financial statements at the end of the designated reporting period" (Fallon & Zgodzinski, 2012, p. 61). The statements usually include "actual revenue and expenses for the period, year-to-date actual, and year-to-date variance" (Johnson & Breckon, 2007, p. 180). It is then the responsibility of the person in charge of program finance to determine the status of the budget and compare the financial statement to the program budget. Armed with such information, the program manager can make the necessary financial decisions. **Fiscal accountability** "refers to the need for sound accounting, careful documentation of expenses, and tracking or revenues" (Issel, 2014, p. 340).

Audits are conducted to ensure that the accounting process within an organization is being handled properly. An **audit** is a "review and confirmation that financial reports

BOX

12.4

Focus On

Important Pieces of Federal Legislation Impacting Human Resources

Year	Legislation	Topic
1935*	Social Security Act	Retirement system for workers
1938	Fair Labor Standards Act	Prescribes standards for wages and overtime pay
1959	Labor-Management Reporting and Disclosure Act (LMRDA)	Deals with the relationship between a union and its members
1963	Equal Pay Act	Prohibits discrimination in pay based on gender
1964**	Civil Rights Act	Prohibits discrimination based on race, color, religion, gender, or national origin
1967	Age Discrimination Employment Act	Prohibits discrimination against a person 40 or older because of age
1970	Occupational Safety and Health (OSH) Act	Workplace Safety
1973	Vocational Rehabilitation Act	Prohibits discrimination against qualified individuals with handicaps
1974	Vietnam Era Veterans' Readjustment Assistance Act	Requires affirmative action in employment for veterans of the Vietnam War era
1974	Employee Retirement Income Security Act	Regulates employers who offer pension or welfare benefit programs for their employees
1978	Pregnancy Discrimination Act	Prohibits discrimination in employment against pregnant women, or related conditions
1985	Consolidated Omnibus Budget Reconciliation Act (COBRA)	Provides opportunity to allow employee pay for continued health insurance coverage after termination
1988	Drug-Free Workplace Act	Employers must implement certain policies to restrict employee drug use
1990***	Americans with Disability Act (ADA)	Prohibits employment discrimination based on ability
1993***	Family and Medical Leave Act (FMLA)	Time off for medical issues for self and family
1996	Health Insurance Portability and Accountability Act (HIPAA)	Health insurance and privacy
2008	Genetic Information Nondiscrimination Act (GINA)	Prohibits discrimination in health coverage and employment based on genetic information
2010	Affordable Care Act (ACA)	Identifies the responsibilities of both employers to provide and employees to have health insurance

*Amended numerous times
**Amended in 1991
***Amended in 2008
Source: Created from Dessler (2012); Fallon & Zgodzinski (2012); Gomez-Mejia & Balkin (2012); Grudzien (2009); Johnson & Breckon (2007); Klingner et al., (2010); and USDOL (n.d.).

are accurate and that standard accounting procedures were used to prepare the reports" (Johnson & Breckon, 2007, p. 288). The main purpose of an audit "is to determine if fraud or other undesirable practices are occurring" (Johnson & Breckon, 2007, p. 292). Further, audits can be either external or internal. An **external audit** is one that is conducted by a qualified independent accountant usually just once a year, whereas an **internal audit** is a frequent and ongoing audit conducted by an employee of the organization not responsible for the accounting practices (BusinessDictionary.com, 2015a).

TECHNICAL RESOURCES MANAGEMENT

Technical resources (also referred to as *other resources*) include all other resources besides human or financial. Included in this category of resources are communication (both internal and external to the organization), equipment (e.g., computers), expertise, information, materials, partnerships, relationships, space, and supplies. (See Chapter 10 for discussion on technical assistance.) This may be the most difficult category of resources to manage because sometimes it is difficult to quantify the amount of a technical resource like personnel and funding needed for a program. For example, how are external communication and relationships quantified?

Phase 4: Putting the Plans into Action

Parkinson and Associates (1982) suggested three major ways of putting plans into action: by using a piloting process; by phasing them in, in small segments; and by initiating the total program all at once. These three strategies are best explained by using an inverted triangle, as shown in **Figure 12.5**. The triangle represents the number of people from the priority population who would be involved in the program based on the implementation strategy chosen. The wider portion of the triangle at the top would indicate offering the program to a larger number of people than is represented by the point of the triangle at the bottom.

These three different implementation strategies exist in a hierarchy. It is recommended that all programs go through all three of the strategies, starting with piloting, then phasing

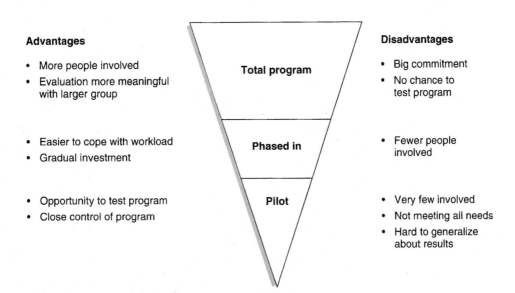

▲ **Figure 12.5** Putting Plans Into Action

in, and finally implementing the total program. However, keep in mind that limited time and resources may not always allow planners to work through all three strategies. In addition, if the priority population is relatively small it may not make sense to use all three strategies. In such cases the phasing in strategy would probably not be used.

PILOT TESTING

Pilot testing (or *piloting* or *field testing*) a program is a crucial step. Even though planners work hard to bring a program to the point of putting it into action, it is important to try to identify any problems with the program that might exist. Pilot testing allows planners to work out any bugs before the program is offered to a larger segment of the priority population, and also to validate the work that has been completed up to this point. For the most meaningful results, a newly developed program should be piloted in a similar setting and with people as much like those who will eventually use the program as possible. Use of any other group may fail to identify problems or concerns that would be specific to the priority population. As an example of the piloting process, take the case of a hospital developing a worksite health promotion program that will be marketed to outside companies. It would be best if the program were piloted on a worksite group before it was marketed to worksites in the community. The hospital could look for a company that might want to serve as a pilot group, or it might use its own employees.

As part of piloting the program, planners should check on the following four areas:

1. The intervention strategies were implemented as planned. This is known as *fidelity*.
2. The intervention strategies worked as planned.
3. Adequate resources were available to carry out the program.
4. Participants in the pilot group had an opportunity to provide feedback about the program.

It is important to have the program participants critique such aspects of the program as content, approaches used, facilitator's effectiveness, space, accommodations, and other resources used. Such feedback will help planners determine if they need to revise the program, and if so how to revise it. If many changes are made in the program as a result of piloting, planners may want to pilot it again before moving ahead. (This evaluation process during the piloting phase is part of formative evaluation and will be discussed further in Chapter 13.)

PHASING IN

Once a program has been piloted and revised, the program should, if applicable, be **phased in** rather than implemented in its entirety. This is especially true when there is a very large priority population. Phasing in allows the planners to have more control over the program and helps to protect planners and facilitators from getting in over their heads. There are four ways in which to phase in a program by: (1) different program offerings; (2) limiting the number of participants; (3) choice of location; or (4) participant ability

Say a comprehensive health promotion program was being planned for Blue Earth County, Minnesota. To phase in the program by different offerings, planners might offer stress-management classes the first six months. During the next six-month period, they could again offer stress management but also add smoking cessation programs. This process would continue until all offerings are included.

If the program were to be phased in by limiting the number of participants, planners might limit the first month's enrollment to 25 participants, expand it to 35 the second month, to 45 the third month, and so on, until all who wanted to participate were included.

To phase in the program by location, it might initially be offered only to those living in the southwest portion of the county. The second year, it might expand to include those in the southeast, and continue in the same manner until all were included. A program planned for a college town might be offered first on campus, then off campus to the general public. A program phased in by participant ability might start with a beginning group of exercisers, then add an intermediate group, and finally include an advanced group.

TOTAL IMPLEMENTATION

Implementing the total program all at once, in most situations, would be a mistake. Rather, planners should work toward total implementation through the piloting and phasing in processes. The only exceptions to this might be "one-shot" programs, such as programs designed around a single lecture, possibly screening programs, or programs that have been offered before to the same population, but even then piloting would probably help.

FIRST DAY OF IMPLEMENTATION

No matter what program is being planned, there will be a "first day" for the program. The first day of the program, also referred to as the **program launch, program rollout**, or **program kickoff**, is just an extension of the fourth P of marketing: promotion (see Chapter 11). The focus of promotion is on creating and sustaining demand for a product. The creation of the demand for the product leads to the initiation of the program. As such, some special planning needs to take place for the first day of implementation. First, decide on a day when the program is to be rolled out. Consider launching the program to coincide with other already-occurring events or special days that can help promote the program. Examples include starting a weight loss program at the beginning of the calendar year to coincide with New Year's resolutions, beginning a smoking cessation program on the third Thursday of November (the day each year for the American Cancer Society's Great American Smokeout), having immunization programs and physical examinations for children prior to the beginning of a new school year, launching a skin cancer prevention program on a college campus prior to the annual spring break, or rolling out the community-wide exercise program at the beginning of February, Heart Health month.

Second, kick off the program in style. This is important to bring attention to the program, and to create momentum and enthusiasm for the program (Chapman, 2006). Planners should consider having a first day that includes some special event such as a ribbon cutting, health screening, health fair, contest, appearance by a celebrity, or some other event that starts the program on a positive note. Celebrities need not be individuals with national or international recognition, but may be individuals such as an executive or supervisor of the organization for which the program is being planned (e.g., chief executive officer [CEO] or executive director), a visible or well-known person from the community (e.g., the mayor or a coach), or a common person who has been affected by the health problem on which the program will focus.

Third, consideration should be given to obtaining news coverage (print and/or broadcast) for the first day to further publicize the program. If it is decided to seek such coverage, you should (CDC, 2003):

- Inform appropriate media representatives of your plans
- Make arrangements to meet the media representatives at the designated time and place

- Prepare the following and have them ready for the day:
  - Press releases
  - Video news releases
  - Spokespersons trained to respond to inquires from media representatives

To get news coverage it might be useful to use a **news hook** to interest the media in the program being launched. By news hook, we mean something that will make the media want to cover the launch. The planners' organization may have newsworthy data or information related to the health problem being targeted by the program, or there may be a related news event that is receiving media attention that would help bring attention to the new program (CDC, 2003). For example, if a new program is aimed at reducing teen pregnancy and new state legislation has been proposed to assist in such efforts or an event related to teen pregnancy is currently an important news item, then linking the new program with those timely events can make it more newsworthy (CDC, 2003). Human-interest stories also make for good news hooks. For example, if you are starting a smoking cessation program, getting former quitters to talk about how quitting changed their lives can be of interest to others. Or, if your program is aimed at teaching children what to do in an emergency situation, and you know of a child who has completed a similar program and was able to put the education to use in helping someone, many people would like to know about that. Planners should even consider linking the launch of the program with some important date in history to make it newsworthy. Linking the influenza epidemic of 1918–19 to launch the countywide flu shot program may make it more newsworthy.

MONITORING IMPLEMENTATION

Once a program is up and running it must be monitored. **Program monitoring** "is an essential function in program implementation" (Schiavo, 2014, p. 401) and it involves the ongoing collection and analysis of data and other information to determine if the program is operating as planned. It is a form of process evaluation (see Chapter 13). One way to approach program monitoring is to ask the question "Who is doing what, when, where, and how often and with what resources" (USDJ, n.d., para 1). Basic monitoring data and information for a program has the following utilities (USDJ, n.d.):

- It provides operating and descriptive data and information for funders and overseers of the program, other stakeholders, and most importantly for program staff and administrators.
- It provides the basic information for comparing outcomes to the program objectives. Such a process may lead to the refinement of an objective or changes to an intervention.
- It provides educational information about many aspects of the program for all involved in the program even if unexpected surprises result.
- Monitoring data serve as a preventive maintenance function by tracking indicators of critical elements which, if they deviate too much from the expected, may signal a program problem.

Typically, the responsibility for monitoring a program falls to the administrator or manager of a program. However, if it is a large program with many different components, certain aspects of monitoring may be assigned to individuals other that the administrator or manager. For example, in a large program the personnel in the accounting office may handle the financial monitoring. Although primary monitoring functions include the collecting and analyzing the data, successful monitoring is not complete unless the findings of such efforts are integrated into the decision-making processes about the program (USDJ, n.d.).

Phase 5: Ending or Sustaining a Program

The final phase of the implementation process is to determine how long to run a program. For some programs the answer will be simple: If the program met its goals and objectives and the priority population has been served to the fullest extent necessary, then the program can be ended. For example, a worksite health promotion program may have a goal to certify 50% of the workforce in CPR. If that goal is reached, then the program's resources could be used on other health promotion programming. However, a greater concern facing most planners is how to sustain a needed program for a longer period of time when the goals and objectives have not been met (e.g., only half of those who were expected to get flu shots got them), or goals and objectives of the program are long-term in nature (e.g., providing food and shelter for the homeless). This is especially difficult when original program funding and other types of resources and support may end or be withdrawn. Financial sustainability is a real concern with grant-funded programs. Today many funders want potential grantees to include a sustainability plan as part of the initial grant proposal. Earlier (in Chapter 11), we presented information on how to maintain interest in program participants, but here we are referring to the maintenance and institutionalization of a program or its outcomes. Techniques that have been used by planners to sustain programs include: (1) working to institutionalize the program (see Chapter 2; Goodman & Steckler, 1989; and Goodman et al., 1993); (2) seeking feedback from program participants and evaluating the program in order to generate evidence to show its worth (Sleet & Cole, 2010); (3) advocating for the program (see Chapter 8 for a discussion of advocacy); (4) partnering with other organizations/agencies with similar missions to share resources, expenses, and responsibilities; (5) revisiting and revising the rationale used to create the program initially (see Chapter 2); and (6) establishing a resource development committee to create business and marketing plans aimed at sustainability (Doll, Bonzo, Mercy, & Sleet, 2007).

▷ Implementation of Evidence-Based Interventions

While most of the concepts presented so far in this chapter apply to all health promotion programs, especially those that are being created for the first time, there are some special considerations that must be addressed when adopting or adapting an evidence-based intervention. With the movement toward evidence-based practice, more researchers (e.g., Jones-Webb, Nelson, McKee, & Toomey, 2014; Rosati et al., 2012; Wiecha, Hannon, & Meyer, 2013) have been engaged in implementation science. The focus of **implementation science** is to study how interventions, which have been shown to be effective in one setting, can be applied to sustain improvements to population health (Lobb & Colditz, 2013).

Tomioka and Braun (2013) created a four-step fidelity assurance protocol that was used with the adaptation of evidence-based health promotion programs for seniors. We think that their protocol could be useful to others adopting and adapting evidence-based programs.

Step one of the protocol has planners deconstructing the program into its components (i.e., marketing, recruiting participants, identifying staff, training, implementing, and evaluating) noting exactly how it was implemented in its original setting. Also as a part of step one the planners prepare a step-by-step plan for program replication in the new setting. An important component to consider in this step is to ensure that the program adaptation includes adaptation to the culture of the new population (Rosati et al., 2012). In step two, planners need to identify agencies that are ready to replicate the intervention including providing the necessary training to staff who will deliver and coordinate the new program. Step three of the protocol has planners closely monitoring the fidelity of the program by using standardized checklists to ensure that the primary components of the intervention are being delivered. This third step also includes a rating (i.e., above standard, meets standards, and needs improvement) of those implementing the intervention. The fourth, and final, step of the protocol has planners using the evaluation tools of the program in order to track program participants' progress and be able to compare the collected data to the expected outcomes. The results of such analysis are then shared with staff members so that, if needed, adjustments can be made.

▷ Concerns Associated with Implementation

Many matters of detail must be considered before and during the implementation process. Although we believe all the topics presented in this section are important, we feel that the topics of safety and medical concerns and ethical issues are the most important. That is why these topics are presented first.

Safety and Medical Concerns

The ultimate goal of most health promotion programs is to maintain or improve the health of its participants. As such, planners in no way want to put the health of participants in danger. Therefore, planners must give attention to the safety and medical concerns associated with health promotion programs. To ensure the safety of participants, planners need to inform participants about the program they are considering joining. Only after they understand what the program is all about should they agree to participate. This concept is referred to as informed consent. More formally, **informed consent** means: (1) making the participants fully aware of the relevant information about the program; (2) making sure the participants comprehend the information provided; and (3) obtaining the participants voluntary agreement, free of coercion and undue influence, to participate.

As a part of the process of obtaining informed consent from participants, program facilitators should take seven steps:

1. Explain the nature and purpose(s) of the program.
2. Inform program participants of any inherent risks or dangers associated with participation and any possible discomfort they may experience.
3. Explain the expected benefits of participation.
4. Inform participants of alternative programs (procedures) that will accomplish the same thing.
5. Indicate to the participants that they are free to discontinue participation at any time.

6. Allow the participants to ask questions about the program and make sure that their questions are fully answered.

7. When appropriate have participants sign informed consent forms. For example, it would be prudent to have participants of an exercise program complete an informed consent form, but not when a population-based media campaign is being conducted to improve safety belt use.

Program planners must be aware that informed consent forms (sometimes called *waiver of liability* or *release of liability*) do not protect them from being sued. There is no such thing as a waiver of liability. If you are negligent, you can be found liable. However, informed consent forms do make participants aware of special concerns. Further, because people must sign the forms, they may not consider legal action even if they have a case, feeling that they were duly warned. **Box 12.5** presents a sample consent form.

Once participants have agreed to participate in a program, if the act of participating in the program puts anyone at medical risk (e.g., cardiovascular exercise programs), then these individuals need to obtain medical clearance before participating. Some organizations that conduct such programs on a regular basis will have a medical clearance form that will need to be completed. Typically, a physician who is familiar with the person's health history must sign the form. If such a form is not available, then steps need to be taken to create one and have it reviewed by a lawyer to make sure it includes all the necessary information.

After participants have medical clearance and are enrolled in a program, steps must be taken to ensure the safety and health of all associated with the program (i.e., participants

---

BOX

12.5

Application

Sample Informed Consent Form

Consent to Perform Cholesterol Screening

I hereby grant permission to the Institute for Health Promotion personnel to perform a cholesterol screening on me. I am engaging in this screening voluntarily. I have been told this screening will provide an analysis of total blood cholesterol and that a trained employee will take my blood from a finger stick sample. This finger stick may be uncomfortable. I understand that the results of this screening are considered to be preliminary in nature and in no way conclusive. Results of a blood cholesterol screening like this can be affected by a number of factors including, but not limited to, smoking, stress level, amount of exercise, hormone levels, food eaten, heredity, and pregnancy. I also understand that my physician can perform a more complete blood lipid (fat) analysis for me, if I so desire.

Further, I have been told that all the information related to this screening is considered confidential.

I have read the above statement and understand what it means. I have also had an opportunity to ask questions about the screening, and all my questions have been answered to my satisfaction.

Participant's Signature	Date	Signature of Witness

NOTE TO PROGRAM PLANNERS: To ensure this form meets all related organizational policies and local and state laws, this form should be submitted to legal counsel before use.

Checklist of Items to Consider When Developing an Emergency Care Plan

1. Duties of program staff in an emergency situation are defined.
2. Program staff is trained (CPR and first aid) to handle health emergencies.
3. Program participants are instructed what to do in an emergency situation (e.g., medical, natural disaster).
4. Participants with high-risk health problems are known to program staff.
5. Emergency care supplies and equipment are available.
6. Program staff has access to a telephone.
7. Standing orders are available for common emergency problems.
8. There is a plan for notifying those needed in emergency situations.
9. Responsibility for transportation of ill/injured is defined.
10. Injury (incident) report form procedures are defined.
11. Universal precautions are outlined and followed.
12. Responsibility for financial charges incurred in the emergency care process are defined.
13. The emergency care plan has been approved by the appropriate personnel.
14. The emergency care plan is reviewed and updated on a regular basis.

and staff members). Providing a safe program includes: finding a safe program location (e.g., low-crime area), providing appropriate security at the location; ensuring that all building codes are met at the location, and ensuring that the classroom, locker rooms, laboratories, and any other facilities used are free of hazards. In addition to a safe environment, programs need qualified instructors (i.e., appropriately trained and certified), and planners need to be prepared for emergency situations by supplying the appropriate first-aid supplies and equipment, and developing an emergency care plan. **Box 12.6** provides a checklist of items that should be considered when creating an appropriate emergency care plan.

Ethical Issues

"Ethical issues permeate almost every decision and action undertaken in health education" (Goldsmith, 2006, p. 33), including many of the decisions associated with program planning. By **ethical issues** we mean situations in which competing values are at play and program planners need to make a judgment about what is the most appropriate course of action. For example, planners may want to create an intervention that includes an economic incentive for a priority population that, for the most part, is composed of individuals with a low socioeconomic status. Because of the socioeconomic status of those in the priority population, the ethical issue that faces the planners is deciding at what dollar value does the incentive cross over from encouraging people to participate in a program to manipulating their participation in the program?

What guides ethical decision making? Most often, these decisions are compared to a standard of practice that has been defined by other professionals in the same field. For health promotion planners, the standard of practice is outlined in the *Code of Ethics for the Health Education Profession* developed by the Coalition of National Health Education Organizations

(CNHEO, n.d.) (see the Appendix for a copy of the Code). The preamble of the *Code* states: "Health Educators are responsible for upholding the integrity and ethics of the profession as they face the daily challenges of making decisions. Health Educators value diversity in society and embrace a multiplicity of approaches in their work to support the worth, dignity, potential, and uniqueness of all people" (CNHEO, n.d., para. 1). For program planners this means having integrity, and being honest, loyal, and accountable. Unethical practice leads to professional suicide; planners who act unethically damage their professional reputation and integrity (Bensley, 2009).

Many of the ethical issues that program planners will face revolve around the three fundamental principles of *The Belmont Report: Ethical Principles and Guidelines for the Protection of Human Subject Research* (National Commission for Protection of Human Subjects of Biomedical and Behavioral Research, 1979). These principles include: (1) respect for persons, (2) beneficence, and (3) justice. Here are some examples of the application of these principles to program planning. The principle of *respect for persons* acknowledges the dignity and autonomy (i.e., freedom) of individuals, and requires that people with diminished autonomy (e.g., children, mentally disabled, and people with severe illnesses) be provided special protection (USDHHS, 2015e). It is not unusual for health education specialists to be working with program participants who have values, behavior, including health behavior, and goals that are different than their own. Even though they are different, it is important to respect them. For example, health education specialists working in a family planning clinic may see clients choose a course of action that may be different than what they personally would select, but clients have the right to choose a course of action and it must be respected.

The principle of *beneficence* requires program planners to protect participants by maximizing anticipated benefits and minimizing harms. This principle dates back to the Hippocratic Oath written by the famous Greek physician Hippocrates who lived from about 460 B.C.E. until 377 B.C.E. (Cottrell et al., 2015). The principle embodies two concepts: doing good, **beneficence**, and not causing harm, **nonmaleficence**. The Hippocratic maxim "do no harm" has long been a fundamental principle of medical ethics, but also applies to the work of health education specialists. The concepts associated with this principle seem to be common sense, but well-intending health education specialists who may not be as well informed on best practices (see Chapter 8 for a discussion of best practices) could put participants at risk without knowing they are doing so. For example, much attention has been given to the public health issue of youth violence. Evidence shows that a number of well-meaning approaches to dealing with youth violence at all three levels of prevention—primary (e.g., holding youth back a grade in school), secondary (e.g., redirecting youth behavior or shifting peer group norm programs), and tertiary (e.g., "boot camps" for delinquent youths)—can bring harm to the youth (USDHHS, 2001).

When dealing with the principle of beneficence, health education specialists may need to make ethical decisions revolving around the "benefit-harm ratio." For example, should a health education specialist be barred from releasing information about a person without his or her consent, even if it will benefit that person? Consider a high school sophomore who approaches the health teacher with confidential information that she is pregnant. Should the health teacher tell anyone else, such as the girl's parents?

The principle of *justice* requires that program planners treat participants fairly. For example, the question of fairness may have ethical implications when it comes to charging a registration fee for a program. Because of the policies of the organization conducting the program, the program may need to turn a profit, but those in need of the program may not be able to afford the cost of registration. Other ethical issues of justice and fairness can arise from issues of sexism, racism, and other cultural biases.

The opportunities for dealing with ethical issues are many, and planners need to be prepared to handle them.

Legal Concerns

Legal liability is on the mind of many professionals today because of the concern over lawsuits. With this in mind, all personnel connected with the planned health promotion program, no matter how small the risk of injury to the participants (physical or mental), should make sure that they are adequately covered by liability insurance. In addition, program personnel should have an understanding of negligence and how to reduce one's risk of liability.

NEGLIGENCE

Negligence is failing to act in a **prudent** (reasonable) manner. If there is a question whether someone should or should not do something, it is generally best to err on the side of caution. Negligence can arise from two types of **acts: omission** and **commission**. An act of omission is not doing something when you should, such as failing to warn program participants of the inherent danger in participation. An act of commission is doing something you should not be doing, such as leading an exercise class when you are not trained to do so.

REDUCING THE RISK OF LIABILITY

When professional service (i.e., a health promotion program) is provided there is always the chance that disputes may arise between those offering the service (program planners) and those (program participants) receiving it or other (third) parties, such as a vendor. Such disputes may lead to the professionals being held legally liable for their actions. Although this is not a common occurrence as a result of health promotion activities, program planners should nonetheless take the appropriate steps to reduce their risk of liability. At the heart of reducing the risk of legal liability is to perform quality work with professional competence. In addition, program planners should:

1. Be aware of anything for which you are legally responsible, for example, protecting private health information.
2. Be aware of any professional standards associated with the services you are providing, for example, *Exercise During Pregnancy and the Postpartum Period* (ACOG, 2009).
3. Keep your professional knowledge and skills up-to-date.
4. Maintain any professional certification (e.g., CHES, MCHES, CPH) and make sure others associated with the program are appropriately certified for the service they are providing and for emergency care procedures.
5. Require participants to have the appropriate "clearances" prior to participation, such as a medical clearance for participation in an exercise class.
6. Provide a safe environment for all program activities.
7. Purchase adequate liability insurance for all (i.e., staff members and volunteers) who have responsibilities associated with the program.

With regard to item 7 in the preceding list, planners should check on the availability of liability insurance through their employer or special coverage from a professional organization. Liability insurance may also be available through one's homeowner's or renter's insurance.

Program Registration and Fee Collection

If the program you are planning requires people to sign up and/or pay fees, you will need to establish registration procedures. Program registration and fee collection may take place before the program (preregistration), by mail, online, in person, via an indirect method like payroll deduction, or at the first session. Planners should also give thought to the type of payment that will be accepted (cash, credit card, or check) and plan accordingly. Though it may seem obvious, some thought also must be given to the security of the money received. That is, how it will be handled, transported, and deposited or otherwise secured.

Procedures for Record Keeping

Almost every program requires that some records be kept. Items such as information collected at registration, medical information, data on participant progress, and evaluations must be accounted for. The importance of privacy for those planners working in health care settings was further emphasized in 2003 with the enactment of the *Standards for Privacy of Individually Identifiable Health Information* section (the Privacy Rule) of the Health Insurance Portability and Accountability Act of 1996, officially known as Public Law 104–191 and referred to as **HIPAA**. The Rule sets national standards that health plans, health care clearinghouses, and health care providers who conduct certain health care transactions electronically must implement to protect and guard against the misuse of individually identifiable health information. Failure to implement the standards can lead to civil and criminal penalties (USDHHS, OCR, n.d.).

The two terms associated with protecting the privacy of participants are anonymity and confidentiality. **Anonymity** exists when no one, including the planners, can relate a participant's identity to any information pertaining to the program. Thus information associated with a participant may be considered anonymous when such information cannot be linked to the participant who provided it. In applying this concept, planners need to ensure that collected data had no identifying information attached, such as the participant's name, social security number, or any other less common information.

Confidentiality exists when planners are aware of the participants' identities and have promised not to reveal those identities to others. When handling confidential data, planners need to take every precaution to protect the participants' information. Often this means keeping the information "under lock and key" while participants are active in a program, then destroying (e.g., shredding) the information when it is no longer needed.

Procedural Manual and/or Participants' Manual

Depending on the type and complexity of a program, there may be a need to develop a program procedural manual and/or participants' manual. If a program is very involved (e.g., has several interventions or a very detailed curriculum) and/or may have a number of different people facilitating the program (i.e., one that will be used in a number of locations like an educational program of a voluntary health agency), there is probably a need to create a program procedural manual. The purposes of a program procedural manual (also sometimes referred to as a *training manual*) are to: (1) ensure that all who are associated with the program understand the program and its parameters, (2) standardize the intervention so it can be replicated and to avoid what Basch and colleagues (1985) referred to as **Type III errors**—failure to implement the health education intervention properly (see Chapter 15 for a discussion of Type I and II errors), (3) provide ideas for facilitation, (4) provide additional background information on the topic, and (5) provide citations for additional resources.

Participants' manuals may also be needed and/or useful for several reasons. First, they may be a good way of getting all program information into participants' hands at one time, including the educational materials and program procedures and guidelines. Second, they can help participants organize information they receive and keep it all in one place, especially if they are set up as loose-leaf notebooks or folders. Third, they can serve as a reference or resource for the participants. And fourth, if participants frequently use their manual as part of the program and become familiar with it, they may be more inclined to refer to it outside of the program sessions.

If a program is being developed in-house and manuals are needed, they will more than likely need to be developed in-house as well. Developing either type of manual—procedural or participant—in-house is a major task; therefore, adequate resources and time need to be given to developing the manuals. If a canned program is obtained from another organization (e.g., a voluntary health agency) or is being purchased from a vendor, it should more than likely include manuals.

Program Participants with Disabilities

A special situation for program planners during not only the implementation phase, but in all phases of program planning is ensuring that the programs being planned meet the needs of program participants with disabilities. From legal, benefit, and social program perspectives, **disability** is "often defined on the basis of specific activities of daily living, work and other functions essential to full participation in community-based living" (USDHHS, 2005, p. 4). Disability can range from sensory problems (e.g., seeing and hearing) to problems resulting from cognitive impairment, neuromuscular disorders, serious injury, and intellectual and developmental disabilities. However, "disability is not an illness. The concept of health means the same for persons with or without disabilities: achieving and sustaining an optimal level of wellness—both physical and mental—that promotes a fullness of life" (Krahn, 2003, as stated in USDHHS, 2005, p. 3). The number of people with disabilities in the United States are estimated to be about 12.6% (~38+ million) (Erickson, Lee, & von Schrader, 2015). As such, program planners must be prepared to work with individuals who have disabilities. Because most program planners have not received training developing programs for people with disabilities, Drum and colleagues (2009) have put forth useful guidelines and criteria. We have presented a list of their guidelines, criteria, and key questions (see **Box 12.7**) that need to be answered to ensure programs meet the needs of these individuals.

Training for Facilitators

An important part of the implementation process is to make sure that the program intervention is implemented as planned, as noted earlier this is referred to as *fidelity*. There are a couple reasons for this. First, as you are now aware, a great deal of effort goes into adoption,

BOX

12.7

Focus On

Guidelines, Criteria, and Issues to Consider When Implementing Programs for Individuals with Disabilities

Operational Guidelines for Health Promotion Programs for People with Disabilities

Criterion 1. Health promotion programs for people with disabilities should have an underlying conceptual or theoretical framework.

Issues:

1. Does the program use theories and concepts drawn from a wide variety of disciplines such as health promotion, disability studies, and/or education?
2. Does the program integrate appropriate theories and concepts into all aspects of the health promotion program (i.e., in planning, implementation, and evaluation)?

Criterion 2. Health promotion programs should implement process evaluation.

Issues:

1. Does the program include process evaluation measures for people with disabilities and their families or caregivers, including rating their satisfaction with the program?
2. Does the program make changes based on participant feedback?
3. Does the program have mechanisms for obtaining process feedback using appropriate methods such as the use of readers or interpreters?
4. Does the program record intervention-related expenses such as cost of materials, recruitment, equipment, space, and personnel?

Criterion 3. Health promotion programs should collect outcomes data using disability-appropriate outcomes measures.

Issues:

1. Does the program collect data on outcomes of health promotion activities?
2. Are the outcomes measures appropriate for people with disabilities (e.g., not penalizing for functional limitations)?

Participation Guidelines for Health Promotion Programs for People with Disabilities

Criterion 4. People with disabilities and their families or caregivers should be involved in the development and implementation of health promotion programs for people with disabilities.

Issues:

1. Did people with disabilities and their families or caregivers participate in the development of the program by identifying program outcomes or reviewing program content before implementation?
2. Are people with disabilities and their families or caregivers involved in implementing the program?

Criterion 5. Health promotion programs for people with disabilities should consider the beliefs, practices, and values of its target groups, including support for personal choice.

BOX

12.7

continued

Issues:

1. Are the beliefs, practices, and values of people with disabilities reflected in the program's mode of delivery, training materials, and written materials?
2. Does the program support participants in identifying and achieving personal health goals?

Accessibility Guidelines for Health Promotion Programs for People with Disabilities

Criterion 6. Health promotion programs should be socially, behaviorally, programmatically, and environmentally accessible.

Issues:

1. Does the program consider social and behavioral and programmatic barriers that reduce participation among people with disabilities?
2. Does the program consider environmental barriers that reduce participation among people with disabilities, including environmental accessibility of the program site (e.g., physical and signage)?
3. Is the program site available via accessible public transportation?
4. Do the program materials (training materials and handouts) lend themselves to being translated into alternative formats?
5. Are process and outcomes measures produced in a variety of other formats, including but not limited to Braille, large print, and computer disk?
6. Are such accommodations provided when requested?

Criterion 7. Health promotion programs should be affordable to people with disabilities and their families or caregivers.

Issues:

1. Does the program maintain reasonable participant fees?
2. Does the program ensure low-cost transportation for participants?

Source: "Guidelines and Criteria for the Implementation of Community-Based Health Promotion Programs for Individuals With Disabilities" by C. E. Drum, J. J. Peterson, C. Culley, G. Krahn, T. Heller, T. Kimptron, J. McCubbin, J. Rimmer, T. Seekins, R. Suzuki, and G. W. White from *American Journal of Health Promotion*. Copyright © 2009 by the *American Journal of Health Promotion*. Reprinted with permission.

---

adapting, or creating an intervention for the specific priority population, possibly even tailoring the intervention; that effort should not be wasted. And second, appropriate implementation is necessary to be able to evaluate and document the effectiveness of an intervention. To ensure that a program is implemented as planned, the program facilitators need to be familiar with the intervention. This familiarity may come about by participating in the planning of the intervention or through a training session. If those who implement the intervention are also the ones who planned the intervention, then a brief review of the steps in the intervention may be all that is needed. If those who will be facilitating the intervention are brought in specifically for that task and are not familiar with the intervention more in-depth training will be needed. Also, regardless of how familiar the intended facilitators are with an intervention, if multiple facilitators are going to be used for implementation (e.g., the same program being implemented at different sites at the same time) then implementation training would be useful to ensure there is a standardized delivery of the program. Without standardization of the intervention through training, the actual intervention delivered can deviate from what was intended depending on the personal preferences of those facilitating the intervention (Issel, 2014). "This has serious implications for achieving the desired outcomes and, subsequently, for ensuring the long-term sustainability of the program" (Issel, 2014, p. 255).

A qualified instructor should conduct the actual training sessions. That instructor may be internal to the organization offering the program or it may be necessary to hire a vendor or consultant to conduct the training. It may also mean sending the people to be trained to other training classes outside the organization to become qualified facilitators. Finally, if the intervention being implemented needs a specially qualified person (e.g., certified or licensed) to facilitate it, such a person must be used. Do not assume some knowledgeable person who is not formally qualified to facilitate a program can do it because that places those who appoint/hire the facilitators in a high-liability situation. For example, if you are planning an exercise program for a group of people and someone comes to you and indicates he wants to lead the classes because he has been a participant in such a program for two years and knows just as much as past instructors but is not certified or licensed to facilitate the program, he should not be permitted to do so.

Dealing with Problems

With the program up and running, the task of the planners is to anticipate and deal with problems that might arise and to do so in a constructive manner. Even if a program has been piloted and phased in prior to total implementation problems can still arise. Astute and effective planners must anticipate the possibility of things going wrong (Timmreck, 2003). "If problems are anticipated, they can be resolved more easily should they occur in the implementation process" (Timmreck, 2003, pp. 182–183). The problems that could be encountered can range from petty concerns to matters of life and death. Problems might involve logistics (room size, meeting time, or room temperature), participant dissatisfaction, or a personal or medical emergency. Whatever the problem, it should be worked out as much as possible to the satisfaction of all concerned. If there is a question of whether to accommodate a program participant or the program personnel, 99% of the time the participants should be satisfied. They are the lifeblood of all programs. As a part of this implementation concern, it might be a good idea to conduct an early evaluation, say after one month, asking questions similar to the ones asked in the piloting evaluation.

Documenting and Reporting

Throughout the implementation process there are various times when program planners may need to collect data or information to document program activities and ongoing progress. Planners need to decide what types of data and information need to be collected to best serve and protect their program. Documentation can range from keeping track of program registration and attendance to the use of program resources (e.g., personnel and financial records) to the collection of data for an evaluation. Good documentation can: (1) assist planners in monitoring program implementation; (2) provide feedback on whether things are working properly (Shi & Johnson, 2014); (3) help identify where changes need to be made in a program; (4) provide feedback on participant satisfaction with a program; and (5) if ever needed, provide evidence if there is a legal challenge to any aspect of implementation.

In addition to appropriate documentation, planners should keep the stakeholders informed about the progress of the program for several different reasons, including: (1) accountability associated with the delivery of the product and the use of program resources, (2) public relations for the program and organization, and (3) participant motivation, satisfaction, and recruitment. The procedures for documenting and reporting will vary by organization, but "can be integrated in to daily routines and may require coordination among various units and sites in order to provide meaningful data for future planning" (Shi & Johnson, 2014, p. 492). And finally, depending on the sensitivity of the data and information collected, organizations need to identify a secure location for their storage (Fallon & Zgodzinski, 2012)

 ## Summary

A great deal of work goes into developing a program before it is ready for implementation. The process used to implement a program may have much to say about its success. This chapter presents five phases planners can follow in implementing a program: (1) adoption of the program, (2) identifying and prioritizing the tasks to be completed, (3) establishing a system of management, (4) putting the plans into action, and (5) ending or sustaining a program. Also presented in this chapter are matters that need to be considered and planned for prior to and during implementation.

 ## Review Questions

1. What are logic models? Why are they used? What are the major components of logic models?

2. What is meant by the term *implementation*?

3. Name and briefly describe the five phases of implementation presented in this chapter.

4. Briefly describe how each of the following planning timetables can be used:
   a. Basic time line
   b. Task development time line
   c. Gantt chart
   d. PERT chart
   e. Critical path method

5. What is meant by the term *management*?

6. What are the three major categories of resources that need to be managed during implementation?

7. Why is professional development so important to human resource management?

8. What are three strategies from the modified model of Parkinson and Associates (1982) for implementing health promotion programs?

9. What are some techniques planners can use to enhance the first day of implementation? What does it mean to kick off a program? What is included in monitoring a program?

10. What is meant by the term *informed consent*?

11. What is meant by implementation science? What is its relationship to evidence-based interventions?

12. What can program planners do to ensure the health and safety of program participants?

13. What is an ethical issue? What are the three ethical principles associated with the *Belmont Report*?

14. Where can you find the *Code of Ethics for the Health Education Profession*?

15. What is negligence? What is the difference between an act of omission and an act of commission?

16. How can program planners reduce their risk of liability?

17. What implications does HIPAA have for planners?

18. What is the difference between anonymity and confidentiality?

19. What are procedural and participant manuals? When should they be used?

20. Why is it important that those who implement planned interventions be trained well to do so?

 # Activities

1. Using the guidelines presented in this chapter, create a logic model for a program you are planning.

2. Create two different types of planning timetables for the program you are planning.

3. Explain how you would implement a program you are planning using a pilot study, phasing in, and total implementation. Also explain what you plan to do to kick off the program.

4. Using the template presented in Box 12.3, create a professional development plan for yourself that covers the next 12 months.

5. In a one-page paper, identify what you see as the biggest ethical concern of health promotion programming, and explain your choice.

6. Select one of the pieces of legislation listed in Box 12.4 to learn more about. Once selected, locate a U.S. government Website that includes information about the legislation and then write a one-page paper that describes why the legislation is important to human resources management.

7. Visit the Community Tool Box Website (http://ctb.ku.edu/en/tablecontents /sub_tools_1165.aspx) and review the information presented in the sample informed consent forms. After reviewing the information, create a consent form that could be used with the collection of primary data via a written questionnaire for a program you are planning.

Weblinks

1. **http://www.hhs.gov/ocr/privacy**

   U.S. Department of Health and Human Services (USDHHS)

   At this page of the USDHHS Website you can get more information about the National Standards to Protect the Privacy of Personal Health Information.

2. **http://www.history.com/this-day-in-history**

   This Day in History

   This commercial Webpage allows you to input a specific date to find out what historical events took place that day. It can be of use to planners when trying to make the kick off of the program newsworthy by linking it to a historical event.

3. **http://www.cnheo.org**

   Coalition for National Health Education Organizations (CNHEO)

   You can find both the short and long versions of the *Code of Ethics for the Health Education Profession* at the CNHEO Website.

4. **http://asq.org/learn-about-quality/project-planning-tools/overview/gantt-chart.html**

   American Society for Quality (ASQ)

   The ASQ Webpage provides information on how to create a Gantt chart.

5. **http://www2a.cdc.gov/phlp/?source=govdelivery**

   Centers for Disease Control and Prevention (CDC)

   This page at the CDC Website presents the Public Health Law Program. The site was created in 2000 and has as its goals to: (1) improve the understanding and use of law as a public health tool, (2) develop CDC's capacity to apply law to achievement of its Health Protection Goals, and (3) develop the legal preparedness of the public health system to address all public health priorities.

6. **http://www.dol.gov/opa/aboutdol/lawsprog.htm**

   United States Department of Labor (USDOL)

   The USDOL Website presents a summary of the major laws associated with labor. You'll find brief descriptions of many of the principal statutes most commonly applicable to businesses, job seekers, workers, retirees, contractors, and grantees.

PART III **EVALUATING A HEALTH PROMOTION PROGRAM**

The chapters in this section present an overview of the evaluation process, including how to plan an evaluation, how to analyze and interpret data, and how to report evaluation results.

Evaluation

An Overview

Performing adequate and appropriate evaluation is necessary for any program regardless of size, type, or duration. While it is true that program resources, namely the proportion of the budget that can be devoted to evaluation, as well as the evaluation expertise of program staff and partners, will influence the type and quality of the evaluation performed, every effort should be made to address the two most critical and basic purposes of program evaluation: (1) assessing and improving **quality**, and (2) determining **effectiveness**.

As displayed in **Box 13.1**, conducting evaluation and research is a major area of responsibility for health education specialists who must demonstrate both knowledge of and the capacity to develop evaluation plans and collect and analyze related data (NCHEC & SOPHE, 2015). Your credibility as a planner and evaluator will often be directly linked to your ability to perform these important tasks. Those who neglect evaluation also risk losing all or part of their program funding.

This chapter presents an overview of evaluation and introduces evaluation terminology; the basic purposes of evaluation, including distinctions between formative and process

BOX

13.1

Responsibilities and Competencies for Health Education Specialists

Responsibilities and competencies that are connected with the content in this chapter include:

RESPONSIBILITY IV: Conduct Evaluation and Research Related to Health Education

            Competency 4.1: Develop an evaluation plan for health education/ promotion

            Competency 4.4: Collect and manage data

            Competency 4.5: Analyze data

            Competency 4.6: Interpret results

            Competency 4.7: Apply findings

Source: *A Competency-Based Framework for Health Education Specialists—2015*. Whitehall, PA: National Commission for Health Education Credentialing, Inc. (NCHEC) and the Society for Public Health Education (SOPHE). Reprinted by permission of the National Commission for Health Education Credentialing, Inc. (NCHEC) and the Society for Public Health Education (SOPHE).

evaluation, as well as summative, impact, and outcome evaluation; the process of conducting an evaluation; problems or barriers in conducting program evaluation; and other issues to consider when conducting an evaluation.

▷ Basic Terminology

In general, **evaluation** can be defined as the process of determining the value or worth of a health promotion program or any of its components based on predetermined criteria or standards of success identified by stakeholders. Two broad *categories* of evaluation correspond to the two basic *purposes* of evaluation—improving quality and determining effectiveness. **Formative evaluation** relates to quality assessment and program improvement, whereas **summative evaluation** pertains to determining effectiveness.

Formative evaluation begins when programs are conceived and developed (or are forming). Though it continues through the implementation phase and usually ends when the program is concluded, it is particularly important and most relevant during the early stages of program development and implementation. The purpose of formative evaluation is to improve the *quality* of a program or any of its components before the program concludes (Fink, 2015).

Another type of evaluation closely associated with formative evaluation is **process evaluation**, which assesses the implementation process in general, and tracks and measures what went well and what went poorly and how these factors contributed to the success or failure of a particular program. It also measures fidelity, or how closely program implementation followed existing standards or protocol. Process evaluation is not focused on improving the quality of a program while it is in process. Rather, it measures how well program implementation occurred. While this represents a process of looking backward after the program concludes, data are collected throughout the implementation process. Process evaluation also measures how many products were distributed or how many services were offered as well as how many people participated in the program (i.e., the extent of a program's reach). An occasional criticism leveled at health promotion is that programs sometimes limit their assessment to process evaluation (e.g., the number of program participants, etc.) and do not adequately address summative evaluation (the degree to which actual changes occurred as a result of the program). While process evaluation is important, it should not be performed in lieu of formative or summative evaluation.

In professional practice, formative and process evaluations are often used interchangeably and have become somewhat synonymous. However, commonly accepted features serve to distinguish the two, at least in theory. For example, formative evaluation attempts to enhance program components before and during implementation so the very best products and services are offered to the priority population. Formative evaluation includes pretesting program components (e.g., curriculum, video clips, public service announcements, language for potential policy change, etc.) as well as pilot testing (testing the complete program with a small segment of the priority population before broad implementation). Though both formative and process evaluations are related to implementation, formative evaluation focuses on improving the quality of the program and its components while they are being implemented, whereas process evaluation measures the degree to which the program was successfully implemented and generally applies lessons learned in subsequent versions or implementations of the program. (Specific components of both formative and process evaluation, which will more clearly distinguish the two, are presented in Chapter 14.)

The purpose of summative evaluation on the other hand, is to assess the *effectiveness* of the intervention and the extent to which awareness, attitudes, knowledge, behavior, the environment, or health status changed as a result of a particular program. Summative evaluation requires the measurement and establishment of a baseline value (the starting point or status of a health indicator prior to the implementation of an intervention) as well as measurement of the same health indicator after the program is concluded (i.e., a posttest). Accordingly, summative evaluation occurs after a program is finished.

Closely associated with summative evaluation are both **impact** and **outcome evaluations**. While summative evaluation is more generally an umbrella term associated with effectiveness, impact evaluation tends to focus on intermediate measures such as behavior change or changes in attitudes, knowledge, and awareness, whereas outcome evaluation tends to measure the degree to which end points such as diseases or injuries actually decreased. Collectively speaking, at least in health promotion practice, impact and outcome evaluations together constitute summative evaluation.

To summarize, in formative evaluation the quality of program components is measured and improved prior to or during program implementation. In process evaluation the mechanics and results of program implementation are assessed. In summative evaluation, program outcomes are measured including impact evaluation (e.g., behavior change) and outcome evaluation (e.g., disease). Without evaluation, claims related to program quality and effectiveness can rarely, if ever, be made.

Both historical and more contemporary supporting definitions for *formative, summative, process, impact, and outcome evaluation* are presented below.

- **Formative evaluation:** "Any combination of measurements obtained and judgments made before or during the implementation of materials, methods, activities or programs to control, assure or improve the quality of performance or delivery" (Green & Lewis, 1986, p. 362). Data derived from formative evaluation help assess the feasibility of program implementation and interventions, the acceptability of program methods and materials, and the potential to produce short-term results (Windsor, 2015). Formative evaluation focuses on the current status of a program and provides regular feedback to administrators and those delivering the program (Spaulding, 2014).

- **Summative evaluation:** "Any combination of measurements and judgments that permit conclusions to be drawn about impact, outcome, or benefits of a program or method" (Green & Lewis, 1986, p. 366). Summative evaluation determines whether results have met stated goals (Chen, 2015) and assesses impact, outcome, and benefits (Perrin, 2015).

- **Process evaluation:** "Is used to monitor and document program implementation and can aid in understanding the relationship between specific program elements and program outcomes" (Saunders, Evans, & Joshi, 2005, p. 134). The central purposes for process evaluation are to "identify the key components of an intervention that are effective, to identify for whom the intervention is effective, and to identify under what conditions the intervention is effective" (Steckler & Linnan, 2002, p. 1). It also evaluates the "extent to which a program is being implemented as planned" (Harris, 2010, p.207). In summary, it examines all aspects of implementation including the environment surrounding the implementation (Perrin, 2015).

- **Impact evaluation:** Focuses on "the immediate observable effects of a program, leading to the intended outcomes of a program; intermediate outcomes" (Green & Lewis, 1986, p. 363). Most notably, impact evaluation is associated with intermediate or long-term changes in behavioral impact (Windsor, 2015).

- **Outcome evaluation:** Focuses on "an ultimate goal or product of a program or treatment, generally measured in the health field by mortality or morbidity data in a population, vital measures, symptoms, signs, or physiological indicators on individuals" (Green & Lewis, 1986, p. 364). Outcome evaluation is long-term in nature and generally takes more time and resources to conduct than impact evaluation. Ultimately, it makes a determination of the effect of a program or policy on its beneficiaries (Harris, 2010).

▷ Purpose of Evaluation

Beyond improving the quality of programs and their components and measuring effectiveness, stakeholders will determine which factors will be measured to determine the worth or value of the program. While the outcome of any health promotion program should relate in some way to improved health, a number of factors leading to this outcome can be measured in the evaluation process. These include how broadly and successfully a program was implemented and the degree to which the program influenced knowledge, attitudes, confidence, abilities, and behaviors.

An evaluation can also assess less tangible benefits deemed important by stakeholders. These benefits may include outcomes such as the degree of good will or organizational presence produced by a program, the amount of social capital or community cohesiveness created, or the extent to which consumers are satisfied with a program for reasons other than improved health status. Ultimately, stakeholders will determine the worth of a program based on criteria unique and important to them.

In the most basic sense, programs are evaluated to gain information and make decisions. The information gained through evaluation may be used by planners during the implementation of a program to make immediate improvements (i.e., formative evaluation) as well as improvements to the implementation process in subsequent versions of the program (i.e., process evaluation). In other words, you do not want to continue indefinitely with a bad program. Evaluation may also be used to see if certain immediate outcomes—such as knowledge, attitudes, skills, environment, and behavior change—have occurred (i.e., impact evaluation). It may also be used over time to determine whether long-term program goals and objectives associated with disease outcomes and improved health status have been met (i.e., outcome evaluation). Capwell, Butterfoss, and Francisco (2000) identified six general reasons why stakeholders may want programs evaluated:

1. *To determine achievement of objectives related to improved health status.* In other words, evaluation can measure the scope of a program's effects, the duration of outcomes and the extent of its influence in improving health (Fink, 2015). Probably the most common reason for program evaluation is to determine the degree to which program objectives related to improved health conditions were met. In this sense, evaluation may also be used to determine which of several programs was most effective in achieving a given objective. You should always attempt to link and limit the scope of evaluation (and the degree to which your personal or program performance is assessed) to program goals and objectives. For this reason, it is important to ensure that goals and objectives are specific, measurable, attainable, realistic and time-phased.

2. *To improve program implementation.* Planners should always be interested in improving a program. Program evaluation can help planners understand why a particular intervention worked (Valente, 2002) or did not work, and thus, weak elements can be identified, removed, and replaced (Green & Lewis, 1986). This is most closely associated with process evaluation. In other words, evaluation can help ensure that implementation is completed in timely and organized ways (Perrin, 2015). With respect to implementation, evaluation can also monitor staff performance and improve staff skills (Windsor, 2015).

3. *To provide accountability to funders, the community, and other stakeholders.* Many stakeholders are interested in the value of a program to a community, or if the program is worth its cost. Perhaps more importantly, stakeholders will want information to improve the program and to determine if the program worked and if it should be continued (Chen, 2015).

4. *To increase community support for initiatives.* The results of an evaluation can increase community awareness of a program. Positive evaluation data channeled through proper communication channels can generate backing for a program, which in turn may lead to additional funding. So, data produced by appropriate evaluation can be used by funders to determine continued support, but also by consumers to assess continued interest (Fink, 2015). Evaluation can also promote positive public relations and community awareness (Windsor, 2015).

5. *To contribute to the scientific base for community public health interventions.* Program evaluation can provide findings that can lead to new hypotheses about human behavior and individual or community change, which in turn may lead to new and better programs. According to Spaulding (2014) and Windsor (2015), one of the key purposes of applied research is to inform practice and contribute to the science-evidence base of programs, or to help ensure that only effective or promising approaches are used.

6. *To inform policy decisions.* Program evaluation data can be used to impact policy within the community. For example, studies on passive or secondhand smoke have been the impetus for many states and local communities to pass laws or ordinances prohibiting indoor smoking. Evaluation can also be useful in investigating potential political ramifications and sustainability of a particular program or initiative (Perrin, 2015).

▷ Framework for Program Evaluation

In 1999, the Centers for Disease Control and Prevention (CDC, 1999a) published an evaluation framework for public health programs. The framework was developed by a working group that included evaluation experts, public health program managers and directors, state and local public health officials, teachers, researchers, U.S. Public Health Service agency representatives, and CDC staff members. This framework has stood the test of time and is still very robust.

The framework (see **Figure 13.1**) is composed of six steps that can be helpful in any evaluation, regardless of type (formative, summative, etc.) or setting. However, this framework probably has more application for what has been described earlier as impact evaluation (i.e. measuring changes in behavior as well as knowledge, attitudes, and awareness, etc.) than any other evaluation type. These steps are not a prescription; rather, they are starting points for tailoring the evaluation. The early steps provide the foundation, and all steps should be finalized before moving to the next step:

- *Step 1—Engaging stakeholders.* This step begins the evaluation cycle. Stakeholders must be engaged to ensure that their perspectives are understood. "Stakeholders are much more likely to support the evaluation and act on results and recommendations if they are involved in the evaluation process (CDC, 2011c, p.14)." This engagement must occur

▲ **Figure 13.1** CDC Framework for Program Evaluation
Source: CDC (1999c), p. 4.

early in the planning process to determine how stakeholders will gauge the success of the program and to build this information into goals and objectives. Otherwise, planners and evaluators open themselves up to criticism or resistance later when results are reported to stakeholders and are inconsistent with predetermined values. The three primary groups of stakeholders are (1) those involved in the program operations, (2) those served or affected by the program, and (3) the primary users of the evaluation results. While the scope and level of stakeholder involvement will vary with each program being evaluated, it is important to focus on stakeholders who can increase the credibility of your evaluation and program or those who will advocate for or authorize funding for your program (CDC, 2011c).

- *Step 2—Describing the program.* "A comprehensive program description clarifies all the components and intended outcomes of the program, thus helping you focus your evaluation on the most central and important questions (CDC, 2011c, p. 21)." This step sets the frame of reference for all subsequent decisions in the evaluation process. At a minimum, the program should be described in enough detail that the mission, goals, and objectives are understood. Also, the program's capacity to affect change, its stage of development, and how it fits into the larger organization and community should be known. Usually, a logic model is used in this step to display a sequence of program events (see Chapter 12 for a discussion of logic models) and the relationship among inputs, activities, and outputs or outcomes. Logic models have been used for several years in health promotion practice to graphically display the relationship between a program's activities and its intended outcomes and the role evaluation plays in describing these relationships (CDC, 2011c). As intended outcomes are established in this step, it is important to set targets for success that are meaningful without being unreasonable or unattainable. Stakeholders will be invaluable in helping make these decisions.

- *Step 3—Focusing the evaluation design.* Among the items to consider in this step are: stating the reason for the evaluation (e.g., improve the quality of programs as in formative evaluation or assess effects, including behavior change and changes in health status, as in impact and outcome evaluation, etc.). This step also includes formulating research questions and/or hypotheses, determining the specific type of evaluation design that will be used, selecting participants and related sample sizes, deciding on the types of statistical analyses that will be used, and recruiting evaluation participants. Again, these decisions relate back to stakeholders and are made in the context of who will use the evaluation results and how evaluation results will be used (CDC, 2011c).

- *Step 4—Gathering credible evidence.* During this step, evaluators decide on measurement indicators [i.e., specific, observable, and measurable outcomes that describe exactly what evaluators are looking for (CDC, 2011c)], sources of evidence, quality and quantity of evidence, and logistics for collecting the evidence. This step also involves organizing data including specific processes related to coding, filing, and cleaning. In this step, evaluators make arrangements to have questionnaires copied or available electronically. They make arrangements for space if paper/pencil (in-person) surveys or face-to-face surveys etc. are conducted. Program partners need to be assigned dates and times to administer evaluation methods, including how to collect and store data.

- *Step 5—Justifying conclusions.* This step includes the comparison of the evidence against the standards of success (i.e., analyzing and synthesizing data); interpreting those comparisons; judging the worth, merit, or significance of the program; and creating recommendations for actions based on the results of the evaluation. In essence, evaluators compare their data or evidence against the measures of success that were developed in previous steps to determine effectiveness, and ultimately, the value of the program. Part of this analysis will assess the fidelity of the evaluation process itself, or how carefully steps were taken to follow appropriate evaluation protocol to reduce bias. Evaluators must make every effort to increase objectivity and decrease subjectivity. "When agencies, communities, and other stakeholders agree that the conclusions are justified, they will be more inclined to use the evaluation results for program improvement (CDC, 2011c, p. 74)."

- *Step 6—Ensuring use and sharing lessons learned.* This step focuses on the use and dissemination of the evaluation results. This is a time when a decision can be made to modify, continue, or discontinue the intervention(s) based on data. This is sometimes referred to as the evaluation feedback loop. Stakeholders will also determine the format of the data report (e.g. PowerPoint (R) slides, a data report, an executive summary, or a paper submitted to a peer-review journal, etc.). Specific aims of sharing evaluation results include: demonstrating that allocated resources are justified and are making a difference in terms of improved health outcomes; retaining or increasing funding associated with the program; enhancing the image of the program; identifying training and technical assistance needs; and suggesting different, perhaps more reasonable, outcomes, etc. (CDC, 2011c).

In addition to these six steps, the framework uses four **standards of evaluation**, which are displayed in the box at the center of Figure 13.1. These standards provide practical guidelines for the evaluators to follow when having to decide among evaluation options. For example, these standards help evaluators avoid evaluations that may be accurate and feasible but not useful or those that would be useful and accurate but not feasible (CDC, 1999a). The four standards are:

1. "Utility standards ensure that information needs of evaluation users are satisfied" (CDC, 1999a, p. 27). This includes determining who needs the evaluation results and ensuring that the evaluation will provide relevant information in a timely manner to appropriate audiences (CDC, 2011c).

2. "Feasibility standards ensure that the evaluation is viable and pragmatic" (CDC, 1999a, p. 27). In other words, the evaluation is realistic and affordable given the time, resources and expertise available (CDC, 2011c).

3. "Propriety standards ensure that the evaluation is ethical (i.e., conducted with regard for the rights and interests of those involved and effected)" (CDC, 1999a, p. 27). In addition to ensuring the welfare of those involved and affected by the evaluation, propriety helps ensure that the evaluation is engaging those in the community most directly affected by a particular health problem (CDC, 2011c).

4. "Accuracy standards ensure that the evaluation produces findings that are considered correct" (CDC, 1999a, p. 29). This means findings are both valid and reliable, or that what is reported is not only accurate but consistent with the data that were collected, and that similar findings can be repeated over time As used here, accuracy also requires an adequate number of community participants engaged with the program and its evaluation (CDC, 2011c).

▷ Practical Problems or Barriers in Conducting an Evaluation

Several authors have identified practical problems or barriers to effective evaluation. Some of the more common problems or barriers that remain consistent over time are presented below.

1. Planners either fail to build evaluation in the program planning process or do so too late (Koelen et al., 2001; Solomon, 1987; Timmreck, 2003; Valente, 2002).

2. Adequate resources (e.g., personnel, time, money) may not be available to conduct an appropriate evaluation (Jacobs et al., 2010; NCI, n.d.; Robinson et al., 2006; Solomon, 1987; Valente, 2002).

3. Organizational restrictions on hiring consultants and contractors may prohibit evaluation efforts (Datta & Petticrew, 2013; Lobo et al., 2014; NCI, n.d.).

4. Effects are often hard to detect because changes are sometimes small, come slowly, or do not last (Glasgow, 2002; Koelen et al., 2001; Solomon, 1987; Valente, 2002).

5. Length of time allotted for the program and its evaluation is not realistic given the nature of behavior change or the interval that is necessary to measure mortality or morbidity (NCI, n.d.).

6. Restrictions (i.e., policies, ethics, lack of trust in the evaluators) that limit the collection of data among the priority population (NCI, n.d.).

7. It is difficult to make an association between cause and effect (Robinson et al., 2006; Solomon, 1987).

8. It is difficult to separate the effects of multiple interventions within a program (Glasgow et al., 1999), or multiple programs within a community, or to isolate program effects on the priority population since evaluators/researchers cannot control all the influences of real-world phenomena (Datta & Petticrew, 2013; NCI, n.d.).

9. Discrepancies arise between professional standards and actual practice (Lobo et al., 2014; Solomon, 1987) with regard to appropriate evaluation design, particularly among novice evaluators.

10. Sometimes evaluators' motives to demonstrate success introduce bias (Datta & Petticrew, 2013; Lobo et al., 2014; Solomon, 1987; Valente, 2002).

11. Stakeholders' perceptions of the evaluation's value may vary too drastically (NCI, n.d.; Robinson et al., 2006).

12. Intervention strategies are sometimes not delivered as intended (i.e., Type III error) (Glasgow, 2002), or are not culturally specific (NCI, n.d.; Valente, 2002).

Examples of these problems in health promotion programs may occur by not collecting initial information from participants because evaluation plans were not in place, failing to budget for the cost of the evaluation (e.g., printing questionnaires, additional staff, postage), or conducting the evaluation prematurely before a change can occur (e.g., changes in cholesterol level) or too long after program completion (e.g., posttest effects of a smoking cessation program). Those without evaluation expertise may conduct an evaluation without a sound design, such as not using appropriate sampling techniques or comparison groups. Lack of capacity or inability to conduct an evaluation may be one of the most significant barriers to meaningful evaluations in general (Lobo et al., 2014). Additionally, program managers who are motivated to make their programs cost-effective may minimize costs and unwittingly jeopardize the integrity of an evaluation.

Awareness of these problems and development of strategies to deal with them will improve the value of program evaluation. The remainder of this chapter discusses strategies that can help minimize problems with evaluation, such as including evaluation in the early stages of program planning, accounting for ethical considerations, determining who will conduct the evaluation, carefully considering the evaluation design, increasing objectivity, and developing a plan to use the evaluation results.

▷ Evaluation in the Program Planning Stages

Evaluation design must reflect the goals and objectives of the program (see Chapter 6). In turn, the results of the evaluation will determine whether the goals and objectives were met. To be most effective, the evaluation must be planned in the early stages of program development and should be in place before the program begins. Results from evaluations conducted early in the program planning process can assist in improving the program (i.e., formative evaluation). Having a plan in place to conduct an evaluation before the end of a program will make collecting data related to program outcomes much easier and more reliable.

Discussion on how evaluation plans can be included in program planning will focus on examples of formative and summative evaluations. The formative evaluation should provide feedback to the program administrator, with program monitoring beginning in the early stages. Collecting information and communicating it to the administrator quickly allows for the program to be modified and improved.

Data reflecting the initial status or interests of the participants—**baseline data**—or something like qualitative data from focus groups can be used to assess participant satisfaction. Additional information from the formative evaluation may indicate that the necessary number of staff members has been hired, program sites are available, materials have been printed, participants are satisfied with the times the programs are offered, and classes are offered with the needs of the prospective participants in mind.

Initial data regarding the program should be analyzed promptly to make any necessary adjustments to the program. This type of evaluation can improve both new and existing programs. Information from the formative evaluation can also be useful in answering questions such as whether the programs are provided at convenient locations for the community members, whether the necessary materials were available on time, and whether people are attending the workshops at all the various times they are offered. If the answer to any of these questions is "no," specific program attributes needing quality improvement can be identified and addressed.

By developing the summative evaluation plan at the beginning of the program, planners can ensure that the results will be less biased. Early development of the summative evaluation plan ensures that the questions answered relate to the original objectives and goals of the program. This type of evaluation can provide answers to many questions, such as whether the group approach or the individual approach was more effective in reducing tobacco use among the participants in a smoking cessation program, whether the participants in a weight loss program actually lost weight and/or maintained the weight loss, and how many people in the priority population increased their knowledge, changed their attitudes, or reduced their risks.

▷ Ethical Considerations

Always remember that evaluation or research should never cause mental, emotional, or physical harm to those involved. Nor should it cause a delay in products or services that could potentially improve health among those being evaluated/researched. Evaluation participants should always be informed of the purpose and potential risks of any evaluation and should always give their consent before participating. Generally, evaluators assure the confidentiality and anonymity of evaluation responses. Although evaluation data are reported in the aggregate, no individual should ever have his or her personal information revealed in any setting or circumstance.

Because evaluations may have ethical considerations for the individuals involved, most colleges, universities, school systems, and large health organizations have boards to review the evaluation design and potential risk to participants. These groups are most often referred to as **institutional review boards** (IRBs) or human subjects committees (Cottrell & McKenzie, 2011). These boards serve to safeguard the rights, privacy, health, and well-being of those involved in the evaluation/research. Before conducting any evaluation or research involving human subjects, make sure to get IRB approval.

▷ Who Will Conduct the Evaluation?

At the beginning of the program, planners must determine who will conduct the evaluation. The program evaluator must be as objective as possible and should have nothing to gain personally from the results of the evaluation. The evaluator may be someone associated with the program or someone from outside.

If an individual trained in evaluation and personally involved with the program conducts the evaluation, it is called an **internal evaluation**. For example, a local health department may assign one of its own employees to evaluate its programs. An internal evaluator would have the advantage of: (1) being more familiar with the organization and the program history, (2) knowing the decision-making style of those in the organization, (3) being present to remind others of results over time, and (4) being able to communicate technical results more frequently and clearly (Fitzpatrick, Saunders, & Worthen, 2004). Conducting an internal evaluation is also less expensive than hiring additional personnel to conduct the evaluation. The major drawback, however, is the possibility of evaluator bias or conflict of interest. Someone closely involved with the program has an investment in the outcome of the evaluation and may not be completely objective. After all, a positive evaluation of the program may result in future funding that would enhance the positions of the staff members.

An **external evaluation** is one conducted by someone who is not connected with the program. Often an external evaluator is referred to as an **evaluation consultant**. Having a researcher from a university or some other type of research institute conduct evaluations for a local health department would be an example of an external evaluator. External evaluators are somewhat isolated, often lacking knowledge of and experience with the program that the internal evaluator possesses. Evaluation of this nature is also more expensive, since an additional person must be hired to carry out the work. However, an external evaluator: (1) can often provide a more objective review and a fresh perspective, (2) can help to ensure an unbiased evaluation outcome, (3) brings a global knowledge of evaluation having worked in a variety of settings, and (4) "typically brings more breadth and depth of technical expertise" (Fitzpatrick et al., 2004, p. 23). When selecting an external evaluator, planners should look for someone with formal training in evaluation methods.

Whether an internal or external evaluator conducts the program evaluation, the main goal is to choose someone with credibility who values objectivity. The evaluator must have a clear role in the evaluation design and accurately report the results regardless of the findings. **Box 13.2** presents characteristics of good evaluators.

Characteristics of a Good Evaluator

- Experience in the type of evaluation needed
- Comfortable with quantitative data sources and analysis
- Able to work with a wide variety of stakeholders, including representatives of target populations
- Can develop innovative approaches to evaluation while considering the realities affecting a program (e.g., a small budget)
- Incorporates evaluation into all program activities
- Understands both the potential benefits and risks of evaluation
- Educates program personnel in designing and conducting the evaluation
- Will give the staff full findings (i.e., will not gloss over or fail to report certain findings)

Source: Centers for Disease Control and Prevention (2011c), p. 11.

▷ Evaluation Results

The question of who will receive the evaluation results is also an important consideration. The evaluation can be conducted from several vantage points, depending on whether the results will be presented to the program administrator, the funding source, the organization, or the public. These stakeholders may all have different sets of questions they would like answered. The evaluation results must be disseminated to groups interested in the program. Different aspects of the evaluation can be stressed, depending on the group's particular needs and interests. An administrator may be interested in which program approach was more successful, the funding source may want to know if all objectives were reached, and a community member may want to know if participants felt the program was beneficial.

The planning process associated with the evaluation should include a determination of how the results will be used. It is especially important in formative evaluation to implement the findings rapidly to improve the program. However, a feedback loop and action plan are needed in summative, impact, and outcome evaluation to ensure that results and lessons learned are used to determine how to proceed with health promotion programs.

Summary

Evaluation can be thought of as a way to make sound decisions regarding the value and effectiveness of health promotion programs, to compare different types of programs, to eliminate weak program components, to meet requirements of funding sources, or to provide information about programs. The evaluation process takes place before, during, and after program implementation. If the evaluation is well designed and conducted appropriately, the findings can be very beneficial to program stakeholders.

Review Questions

1. What are the two basic purposes of program evaluation?

2. What are the two broad categories of evaluation and how do they relate to the two basic purposes of program evaluation?

3. List and describe the six steps in CDC's framework for program evaluation.

4. List and describe the four evaluation standards in CDC's framework for program evaluation.

5. Give an example of a question that could be answered in a process evaluation, impact evaluation, and outcome evaluation.

6. What are some of the more common problems associated with or barriers to effective evaluation?

7. What different types of information could an evaluation provide for the various stakeholders (planners, funding source, administrators, and participants)?

8. Why is it important to begin the evaluation process in the program planning stages?

9. Explain how feedback from an evaluation can be used in program planning.

10. In what type of situation would an internal evaluation be more appropriate than an external evaluation?

11. What are the desirable characteristics of an external evaluator (evaluation consultant)?

Activities

1. Describe potential roles and results of formative and summative evaluations in a program related to an HIV needle-exchange program.

2. Describe how process, impact, and outcome evaluation could be used in a stress management program for college students.

3. Write a rationale to a funding source for hiring an external evaluator (evaluation consultant).

4. Review the evaluation component from a health promotion program in your community and/or discuss an evaluation plan with a planner or evaluator. Look for the planning process used, the rationale for the data collection method, and how the findings were reported. To what extent did the program follow CDC's framework for evaluation?

5. Assume you are responsible for selecting an evaluator for a health promotion program you are planning. Would you select an internal or an external evaluator? Explain your rationale. If you select an external evaluator (evaluation consultant), where do you think you could find such a person?

Weblinks

1. **http://www.eval.org**

   American Evaluation Association (AEA)

   The AEA is an international professional association of evaluators devoted to the application and exploration of program evaluation, personnel evaluation, technology, and many other forms of evaluation.

2. http://www.evaluationcanada.ca/

   Canadian Evaluation Society (CES)

   The CES is a professional association of evaluators dedicated to the advancement of evaluation theory and practice. Information at this Website is available in both English and French.

3. http://ctb.ku.edu/en/default.aspx

   Community Tool Box

   This Website has long provided technical assistance to health professionals on a number of tasks related to planning and evaluation in health promotion. With respect to evaluation, a general search for evaluation will present a number of specific links including introduction to evaluation, operations in evaluating community interventions, methods for evaluating comprehensive community initiatives, and using evaluation to understand and improve the initiative.

4. http://www.cdc.gov/mmwr/preview/mmwrhtml/rr4811a1.htm

   CDC Framework for Program Evaluation in Public Health

   This is CDC's evaluation framework described earlier in this chapter published in *Morbidity and Mortality Weekly Report.* This document describes in detail the six steps related to the framework.

5. http://www.cdc.gov/eval/guide/cdcevalmanual.pdf

   Introduction to program evaluation for public health programs: A self-study guide

   This is an excellent evaluation resource from the CDC that provides additional information and training on CDC's evaluation framework as well as information on evaluation in general.

6. http://www.rand.org/pubs/technical_reports/TR101.html

   Getting to Outcomes: Promoting Accountability through Methods and Tools for Planning, Implementation, and Evaluation

   An excellent evaluation resource related to establishing and measuring evidence-based program oucomes.

7. http://whqlibdoc.who.int/hq/2000/WHO_MSD_MSB_00.2e.pdf

   Process Evaluations

   This is a document on process evaluations from the World Health Organization. It is a good resource for designing and conducting process evaluations.

Evaluation Approaches and Designs

Key Terms

accountability
adjustment
approaches
blind
capacity
comparison group
confounding variables
consumer orientation
context
control group
cost-benefit analysis
cost-effectiveness analysis
cost-identification analysis
deductive
designs
dose
double blind
evidence
experimental design
experimental group
external validity
fidelity
generalizability

inclusion
inductive
interaction
internal validity
justification
multiplicity
nonexperimental design
pilot testing
posttest
pretest
pretesting
qualitative method
quantitative method
quasi-experimental design
reach
recruitment
resources
response
satisfaction
summative evaluation
support
triple blind

This chapter focuses on evaluation approaches and designs. The term **approaches** refers to formative, process, and summative evaluation and suggests these types of evaluation are distinct. **Designs** are diagrams that display steps or associations between elements in the evaluation process, often including specific and unique notations. For the purpose of this chapter, designs relate exclusively to summative evaluation. Whereas formative and process

BOX

14.1

Responsibilities and Competencies for Health Education Specialists

This chapter describes evaluation approaches including formative, process, and summative evaluations (including impact and outcome evaluations), elements of formative and process evaluations, and evaluation designs associated with summative evaluation. Responsibilities and competencies connected with this chapter include:

RESPONSIBILITY IV: Conduct Evaluation and Research Related to Health Education/
Promotion

Competency 4.1: Develop an evaluation plan for health education/
promotion

Competency 4.4: Collect and manage data

Competency 4.5: Analyze data

Competency 4.6: Interpret results

Competency 4.7: Apply findings

Source: *A Competency-Based Framework for Health Education Specialists—2015*. Whitehall, PA: National Commission for Health Education Credentialing, Inc. (NCHEC) and the Society for Public Health Education (SOPHE). Reprinted by permission of the National Commission for Health Education Credentialing, Inc. (NCHEC) and the Society for Public Health Education (SOPHE).

evaluations are typically defined with descriptions of strategies, summative evaluations are generally associated with experimental, quasi-experimental, and non-experimental designs. **Box 14.1** identifies the responsibilities and competencies for health education specialists that pertain to the material presented in this chapter.

▷ Formative Evaluation

At its core, formative evaluation focuses on the quality of program content and program implementation. Some elements of formative evaluation occur before the start of the implementation phase and help ensure that a program and its elements have been conceptualized and developed appropriately. Formative evaluation collects data and informs stakeholders of important findings that could potentially improve a program or its delivery, and allows for appropriate changes before the program is fully implemented and completed. Although a formative evaluation can be used to improve a program between implementation cycles (i.e., an evaluator identifies various issues that need to be addressed before the program is implemented again), it is usually better to allow a formative evaluation to inform and guide the development and implementation of a program as it unfolds. In cases where a program's implementation is ongoing, the distinction between formative and process evaluation is not as clear or relevant as long as programs are being improved based on feedback collected in the evaluation process.

Table 14.1 displays the elements of a comprehensive formative evaluation. The degree to which these elements are used will be determined by many factors including the preferences of stakeholders. However, all 15 elements are important and have a bearing on program quality, which, in turn, leads to program effectiveness as measured in summative evaluation.

Formative evaluation occurs from the time of program inception through implementation. By nature, certain elements of formative evaluation are more applicable at the time of program inception. This is when planners either begin developing a new program or decide to use an existing program and adapt it to their priority population. For example, addressing

TABLE 14.1 **Elements of a Comprehensive Formative Evaluation**

Element	Description
Justification	Degree to which a program, service, or activity is mandated or approved by relevant stakeholders and justified by needs assessment data and analysis
Evidence	Degree to which the program, service, or activity is evidence-based (i.e., documented evaluation results in the literature suggest the program is effective or at least promising)
Capacity	Extent to which professionals have adequate knowledge, skills, and abilities to design and implement a program, service, or activity or the degree to which they can access or contract with other organizations and professionals to provide the same program, service, or activity
Resources	Adequacy of resources (e.g., budget, community resources or assistance, assets, time, etc.)
Consumer-Orientation	Degree to which the program, activity, or service is tailored to the priority population (i.e., culturally appropriate and based on consumer preferences)
Multiplicity	Degree to which multiple components (i.e., intervention strategies) are built into the program, service, or activity (e.g., education, communication, policy, environmental change, etc.)
Support	Degree to which a support component is built into a program, service, or activity (e.g., a hotline/quit line for a tobacco media campaign, development of walking paths for a community physical activity campaign)
Inclusion	Extent to which an adequate range and number of appropriate partners or organizations are involved with the program, service, or activity
Accountability	Extent to which internal staff and external partners are fulfilling their responsibilities as planned and are communicating needs appropriately
Adjustment	Degree to which programs, services, or activities are modified based on feedback received from participants, partners, or other stakeholders
Recruitment*	Degree to which members of the priority population are adequately recruited through appropriate communication channels and places consistent with cultural and other unique characteristics
Reach*	Proportion of the priority population given the opportunity to participate in the program, activity, or service
Response*	Proportion of the priority population actually participating in the program, activity, or service
Interaction	Quality of interactions (e.g., customer service; interpersonal, counseling, and presentation skills; clarity of instructions) between professionals (those providing programs, services, and activities) and participants
Satisfaction	Degree to which the needs of participants are being met, how satisfied they are with the program, service, or activity, and their belief that a positive impact is being made in their lives

*These items relate to formative evaluation as they help ensure that an adequate number of people are participating in the program. But they also relate to process evaluation as an evaluation of the implementation process itself would naturally measure not only how many people had the opportunity to participate in the program, but more importantly, how many people actually participated.

the elements termed **justification** and **evidence** provides assurance that programs are supported by key stakeholders and are evidence-based. It is easy to make assumptions about these issues during a planning process. But addressing these key elements initially will influence planners to make careful assessments about other program and evaluation components. In this regard, formative evaluation can be beneficial before much, if any, time and effort are applied to the program.

Three additional elements displayed in Table 14.1 relate to issues that should be addressed early in the formative evaluation process. Assessing **capacity** requires evaluators to carefully examine the abilities and competency of those who are designing and implementing a program. This can be somewhat challenging if those performing the evaluation are the same professionals designing and implementing the program. Despite this potential challenge, planners and evaluators should identify the strengths and weaknesses of the internal staff and external partners and either invest in training or contract for external providers as necessary.

Resources relate to adequate internal or external funding and/or assistance from partner organizations. Although it is easy to underestimate program costs, evaluators performing a formative evaluation should match the projected costs with available resources to determine whether the program can be realistically implemented. Closely related to the concept of resources are three types of cost analyses that can help guide planners in the selection of specific interventions. **Cost-identification analysis** (or cost-feasibility analysis) is used to compare different interventions available for a program, often to determine which intervention would be the least expensive. With this type of analysis, evaluators identify various items (e.g., personnel, facilities, materials, curriculum, etc.) associated with a given intervention, determine a cost for each item, total the costs for that intervention, and then compare total costs across interventions. For example, if a health department is interested in providing a tobacco prevention and control program for a school district, it could conduct a cost-identification analysis on three different interventions: (1) teacher led, (2) peer-to-peer, and (3) voluntary agency provided. Costs for each of these interventions—such as staff time, staff benefits, curriculum materials, and volunteer training—would be identified, compared, and analyzed. While cost-identification analysis provides good data on cost variation, it does not include the benefit of each program alternative or option as in cost-benefit analysis or cost-effectiveness analysis (Dedhia et al., 2011).

Cost-benefit analysis yields the dollar benefit received from the dollars invested in the program. "Because cost-benefit analysis compares program alternatives in monetary terms, the evaluator documents whether a method has economic benefits exceeding costs" (Windsor, 2015, p. 293). **Cost-effectiveness analysis** relates to how much it costs to produce a certain effect. For example, based on the cost of a program, the effect of years of life saved, number of smokers who stop smoking, or morbidity or mortality rates can be determined. Cost-effectiveness analysis generally assesses program alternatives or options to determine which approach is more likely to provide the greatest yield per unit cost, thus providing planners with useful data to make resource allocation decisions (Windsor, 2015). In summary, cost-benefit analysis measures how much money you will save for every dollar spent (e.g., for every dollar spent on this program, taxpayers will save three dollars, etc.) and cost-effectiveness analysis measures how much change you will derive for every dollar spent (e.g., every dollar spent on this program will result in X pounds of weight loss per participant, etc.).

As displayed in Table 14.1, evaluators must also ensure that **consumer orientation**, or the degree to which programs are adapted to the needs of the priority population, is adequately addressed. Professionals commonly assume that members of the priority population hold the same understanding and value for programs as those who design and implement the programs. Data from social marketing studies indicate this is not the case

(Neiger & Thackeray, 2002; Thackeray, Neiger, & Keller, 2012). Assuring that programs are tailored to the values, wants, and needs of the priority population is an important component of a formative evaluation and helps ensure that programs are more readily accepted by the priority population and that intended outcomes occur.

Two elements displayed in Table 14.1 relate to the development and content of a program. The term **multiplicity** relates to a concept in health promotion where, compared with single-component programs (i.e.,one intervention strategy), multiple-component programs cater more effectively to the varied needs of consumers and tend to be accepted more readily. For example, the Truth Campaign in Utah offered a multidimensional approach to preventing and controlling tobacco use among both youth and adults. Program components involved educational materials including a comprehensive guide for schools, media resources, models for policy and legislation, materials for health care professionals, and a quit line to assist smokers in cessation efforts (Utah Department of Health, 2011). **Support**, a closely related concept to multiplicity, assures that programs have appropriate built-in reinforcement components to assist participants with the expected level of involvement and/or behavior change. For example, a well-baby program that promotes prenatal care through a media campaign cannot responsibly broadcast messages without an infrastructure that can actually support prenatal care. In addition, a well-baby program of this nature should also be prepared to make referrals based on a variety of demographic variables within the priority population, including the ability to pay for services.

Certain elements in formative evaluation relate to key components of program implementation and ensure that: the right people and organizations are participating in the delivery of the program; partners are doing what they're assigned to do; and necessary changes are being made based on feedback from both participants and partners.

Inclusion ensures that the right partners are involved with the program. The natural inclination of most professionals or organizations is to include as many partners as possible to bear the burden of a program's cost and implementation. Care should be taken, however, to ensure that only those organizations and individuals that share similar values and commitment are included as program partners. This is not to suggest that organizations should not seek diverse or nontraditional partners. However, ideally, all partners should bring a similar level of vision and energy to the program development and implementation process. While partners will be those who actively participate in the program, other agencies, programs, or individuals can be classified as sponsors or supporters.

Accountability ensures that each partner organization performs its work as previously arranged. For this reason, it is important for partners to meet regularly, report on progress and identify ways to improve performance. **Adjustment**, perhaps the most critical element of formative evaluation, is the process whereby planners make necessary changes to the program or its implementation based on feedback from participants and partners. In this regard, those who develop and implement programs must collect data (or information) on what needs to change and then ensure that appropriate changes are made. **Recruitment**, **reach**, and **response** pertain to promoting a program and ensuring that people in the priority population are aware of the program, have the opportunity to participate in the program, and that an adequate number actually do participate in the program. Obviously, the budget, among other factors, influences the proportion of the priority population that has access to the program. Evaluators must develop projections for participation early and then match projections with actual participation. Furthermore, evaluators must determine whether methods for recruitment or promotion are appropriate based on communication capabilities and preferences of the priority population. For example, social media approaches will not work if members of the priority population do not use their devices to download information planners want to send them. Similarly, newspaper advertisements will do little good if word-of-mouth communication is a preferred channel within the priority population.

Interaction and **satisfaction** address the degree to which practitioners effectively work and communicate with program participants and how satisfied participants are with the program in general or with specific components. For example, an evidence-based curriculum for weight loss among adults may be appealing to participants, theoretically grounded, and technically sound in every way but not resonate with participants because of an ineffective instructor. A formative evaluation can identify this problem and generate necessary recommendations or adjustments (e.g., a new instructor). Likewise, data regarding participant satisfaction may produce important modifications during program implementation or in future applications of the program.

In contrast to formative evaluation, a process evaluation looks back on the implementation process and measures what went well and what went poorly. While data from process evaluation can certainly inform subsequent versions of a program, its main objectives are to describe how closely the program implementation followed protocols; how successful it was in recruiting and reaching members of the priority population; how many people participated or how many products or services were distributed; and what other factors may have competed with or confounded program results.

Elements of process evaluation are displayed in **Table 14.2**. **Fidelity** ensures that programs are implemented either as intended or as per protocol. Because the results of effective programs may be published in scientific journals or other reporting venues, methods sections should provide a sequential order or step-by-step description of how the program was implemented. Other practitioners may then rely on this information to replicate the

TABLE 14.2 **Elements of a Process Evaluation***

Element	Description
Fidelity	Extent to which the program, activity, or service was delivered as planned or as per protocol including the use of Gantt charts (i.e., time lines) and logic models
Dose	Number of program units delivered (e.g., presentations, products, services, messages etc.)
Recruitment*	Degree to which members of the priority population are adequately recruited through appropriate communication channels and places consistent with cultural and other unique characteristics.
Reach*	Proportion of the priority population given the opportunity to participate in the program, activity, or service
Response*	Proportion of the priority population actually participating in the program, activity, or service
Context	External factors that may influence program results (e.g., competing programs, conflicting messages, other confounders)

*Adapted from Steckler & Linnan (2002); and Saunders, Evans, & Joshi (2005).

program. In addition, programs should routinely include some type of procedures outline or protocol that guides implementation. In this regard, process evaluation can assure that appropriate procedures are followed throughout implementation.

Dose is a measurement of how many products, services, or other program components were delivered to the priority population (e.g., number of educational sessions presented, number of nicotine devices distributed, number of car seats on loan, number of times a public service announcement was aired, etc.). Often, process evaluation is associated with dose. In other words, the practitioner tracks and reports how many products were distributed and equates this with the quality of a program. Although dose is an important element of process evaluation, it should not be the sole focus of the evaluation. As an independent measurement, dose cannot fully represent process evaluation nor should it be used as a proxy measure to describe the quality, value, or effectiveness of a program.

As described in formative evaluation, recruitment, reach, and response are also measured in process evaluation since an evaluation of the implementation process itself would naturally measure fairness and adequacy of recruiting practices, how many members of the priority population had the opportunity to participate in the program, and most importantly, how many people actually participated.

Finally, **context** assesses the presence of any confounding factors, or naturally occurring events in the same environment that may affect program participation and results. For example, participation in a school-based alcohol/drug-free graduation celebration may be diminished by alternative activities that appeal more directly to the intended participants. Negative aspects of the physical environment or location of a program may have a negative effect on program participation or retention. A television program documenting disabling aspects of cancer aired at the same time a cancer screening program is initiated may scare potential program participants and impact their involvement.

Strategies for conducting formative evaluations, and to some extent process evaluations, are displayed and briefly described in **Table 14.3**. Although no single strategy is inherently superior to another, the element being evaluated (see Tables 14.1 and 14.2) will largely influence the selection of the appropriate strategy. For example, a key informant interview would generally be appropriate if an evaluator is measuring capacity or resources. In this scenario, the key informant would probably be an administrator with adequate information about the skill sets of his or her staff and the type of budget that would be dedicated to the program. On the other hand, assessing fidelity in a process evaluation can be accomplished with a protocol checklist. Certain elements can be addressed by one of many strategies or a combination of strategies. For example, assessing interaction or satisfaction can be accomplished by focus groups, in-depth interviews, or surveys.

Each of the strategies listed in Table 14.3 has a specific protocol to guide its use. Evaluators must ensure that these strategies are used appropriately and that data are not extrapolated or projected beyond their natural or appropriate function. (For further explanation on specific strategies, see Chapter 4 for information on focus groups, survey methods, interviews, use of forms or existing records, and observations, etc.)

Two additional strategies, pretesting and pilot testing, commonly associated with formative evaluation, are presented here as ways to assess the quality of distinct components of a program and to assess the overall quality of a program before full implementation occurs. Although the two terms are often used interchangeably, certain distinctions are important to make and understand.

TABLE 14.3 **Procedures Used in Formative Evaluation**

Procedure	Description
Focus Groups*	Qualitative research wherein a trained moderator uses an interview or moderator's guide to ask questions about new programs, products, services, ideas, or topics to determine the attitudes, opinions, and preferences of a group of 6–12 individuals from a subgroup of the priority population (see Chapter 4).
Surveys	The collection of data, generally through questionnaires, from a representative sample of the priority population that allows evaluators to draw general conclusions about the entire priority population. May involve face-to-face interviews or written questionnaires, mailed questionnaires, telephone interviews, electronic questionnaires, etc. An intercept survey attempts to approach consumers in their natural environments (e.g., grocery stores, malls, community events) for a brief face-to-face interview (see Chapter 4).
In-Depth Interviews*	Formal interviews with program participants generally lasting a half hour or longer with the use of an interview guide and related probes. Allows evaluators to observe body language and facial expressions as prompts for additional questions and information.
Informal Interviews	Brief interviews with program participants that may take the form of a conversation rather than a formal interview.
Key Informant Interviews	Qualitative, in-depth interviews with individuals who understand the priority population and can represent their attitudes, values, and opinions to evaluators. Key informants are often people of influence within the priority population (see Chapter 4).
Direct Observation	A process wherein evaluators immerse themselves in the program and assess the interactions between professionals and other participants, the general reactions and behaviors of the participants, and any problems or issues associated with program content and delivery. Use of this procedure sometimes involves concealing the observer from the program participants (see Chapter 4).
Expert Panel Reviews	A process wherein a small group of professionals, not associated with the program but who have expertise related to the program, volunteer or are contracted to collect data, analyze the program, draw conclusions about its strengths and weaknesses, and make recommendations.
Quality Circles	A qualitative approach wherein internal staff from the same program or work area meet regularly to discuss the strengths and weaknesses of a product, program, service, or activity and make recommendations for improvement. As an alternative to quality circles, evaluators may choose to interview program staff directly.
Protocol Checklist	A linear or sequential list of tasks or procedures that allows evaluators to compare how a program is being implemented compared with how it was originally intended to be implemented, or compared with what has been done elsewhere and reported in published studies or reports. Use of logic models may be used in lieu of the protocol checklist.
Gantt Chart	A type of bar or line chart that displays a program's time line or project schedule. Whereas protocol checklists or logic models are not usually time phased, Gantt charts display the start and finish dates of key program elements (e.g., program objectives or key activities and tasks) (see Chapter 12).
Program and Evaluation Forms	Program forms collected prior to program implementation may provide relevant information to evaluators (e.g., factors that have motivated participation, identification of goals, previous participation). Data from forms compiled during the program may reveal information helpful to program improvement (e.g., strengths, barriers, risks). Evaluation forms are generally administered at the conclusion of a program to measure the awareness, knowledge, attitudes, skills and behaviors, and general levels of satisfaction as well as feedback on specific program components.

*Responses are recorded, transcripted, coded, and analyzed to identify themes and draw conclusions. (Note: see Chapter 4 for types of data collection.)

Pretesting

Pretesting can be defined in at least two ways: (1) testing components of a program (e.g., strategies and materials), services, and products with the priority population prior to implementation (Grier & Bryan, 2005); and (2) collecting baseline data prior to program implementation that will be compared with posttest data to measure the effectiveness of programs. The type of pretesting that relates to formative evaluation pertains to the first definition—testing components of a program prior to program implementation. This type of pretesting is often associated with social marketing and health communication. When applied to health communication, pretesting has been defined as an evaluation that involves systematically collecting intended-audience reactions to messages and materials before the messages and materials are produced in final form (NCI, n.d.).

Pretesting, however, can be applied to any component of a program (e.g., specific sessions of an educational curriculum, a video clip to be used in a presentation, a participant manual, draft language for a legislative bill, the visual presence and structural layout of a booth that will be used in a health fair, a planned location and structure of a community exercise path, etc.).

Pretesting assumes that program components have already been reviewed for evidence. That is, the component is demonstrated to be evidence-based in the literature or through some other reporting mechanism. Pretesting also assumes that practitioners have prepared program components in nearly final form. In other words, it is not appropriate for practitioners to take short cuts and present materials with the mindset that members of the priority population will correct any flaws.

Many of the same strategies displayed in Table 14.3 are used to pretest program components. The most common strategies involve focus groups, in-depth interviews, and surveys (NCI, n.d.). Practitioners would be well advised to receive training in these strategies before attempting to conduct them. Otherwise, it is prudent to contract for services with professionals who have appropriate experience and expertise. In addition, it has been proposed that if practitioners want to reliably predict the effectiveness of interventions during a developmental phase such as pretesting, experimental research methods should also be applied (Whittingham, Ruiter, Zimbile, & Kok, 2008).

Pilot Testing

Whereas pretesting focuses on specific program components, **pilot testing** (also referred to as *field testing* or *alpha testing*) generally presents the entire program to a limited and manageable number of members of the priority population so necessary modifications can be made before the program is implemented to a larger segment of the priority population.

Pilot testing allows for "dry runs" to assess and measure the overall quality of a program. Occasionally, pilot testing may be associated with shorter durations of time compared with actual implementation time, but this is generally not advisable. Implementing the entire program to a limited number of people in the actual time frame is helpful for evaluators to discover important issues related to timing, spacing, and duration of interventions. (See Chapter 12 for more information on this application.) Pilot testing offers evaluators a wide angle or broad view of the program to assess how the entire program impacts participants.

Conducting a pilot test generally involves collecting data from participants. It is advisable to use the same data collection instruments that will be used in the actual implementation of the program to make adjustments to the instruments (e.g. a questionnaire) and program components simultaneously. (The specific methodologies associated with summative evaluation are addressed later in this chapter and in Chapter 15. Chapter 5 also provides useful information on measurement, data collection, and sampling.)

▷ Summative Evaluation

If a program accounts for the elements displayed in Table 14.1 and adequately monitors and improves quality through formative evaluation, practitioners can assume that the collective efforts of stakeholders in designing and implementing a high-quality program will result in the accomplishment of program goals and objectives related to changes in behaviors and disease indicators. These expected outcomes are the focus of **summative evaluation**, which is any combination of measurements that permit conclusions to be drawn about impact, outcome, or benefits of a program (Green & Lewis, 1986).

By way of review, summative evaluation includes both impact evaluation, which focuses on intermediate indicators such as awareness, knowledge, attitudes, skills, environment, and most importantly, behaviors, as well as outcome evaluation, which focuses on long-term program measures such as mortality, morbidity, or disability. Indicators used in summative evaluation might include years of potential life lost (or saved), prevalence of tobacco use, reductions in diabetes mortality, a decreased incidence of HIV/AIDS, reduced absenteeism (as often measured in worksite settings), number of pounds lost, and health care costs saved due to health promotion programs. As in formative and process evaluations, the list of potential indicators in summative evaluation can be extensive.

Although many types of indicators and outcomes may be related to summative evaluation, the process itself is usually associated with the development of designs. This is particularly true of impact evaluation, which requires a thoughtful design, appropriate data collection procedures, valid and reliable questionnaires or other instruments, and proper analysis and data reporting. Outcome evaluation related to communities or large populations often involves analysis of vital statistics and trend data with the evaluator trying to measure the effectiveness of a program or intervention over time while accounting for **confounding variables**, or additional influences not part of an intervention which, nonetheless, have some type of impact on results (Sullivan, 2008). Impacts due to confounding variables or "confounding" can be positive or negative. In other words, community-wide programs often have great difficulty identifying, with any precision, the degree to which the programs themselves had an impact when the priority population was exposed to many other influences simultaneously. As described earlier, confounding variables relate to the element of context as measured in process evaluation.

An evaluation design is used to organize a summative evaluation and to provide for planned, systematic data collection, analysis, and reporting. A well-planned evaluation design helps ensure that the conclusions drawn about the program will be as accurate as possible. The design is developed during the early stages of program planning and focuses on program goals and objectives. CDC's Framework for Program Evaluation (1999a) (discussed in Chapter 13) suggests the study design should be addressed in Step 3, only after engaging stakeholders and describing the program. As designs are developed, evaluators must consider the audience and/or stakeholders who will read the results of the evaluation. In other words, the design must produce information that will answer the evaluation questions of stakeholders.

▷ Selecting an Evaluation Design

There are no perfect evaluation designs, because no situation related to program design and implementation is ideal, and there are always constraining factors, such as limited resources. The challenge is to devise an *optimal* evaluation—as opposed to an *ideal* evaluation (CDC, 1999a). Planners should give much thought to selecting the best design for each situation. The following questions may be helpful in the selection of a design for summative evaluation:

- How much time do you have to conduct the evaluation?
  - Do stakeholders want basic results or do they want a more sophisticated analysis?
  - What indicators are stakeholders most interested in tracking (e.g. costs, attitudes, knowledge, awareness, behavior change, decreases in disease, etc.)?
- What financial or budgetary resources are available to conduct the evaluation?
- How many participants can be included in the evaluation?
- Are you more interested in qualitative or quantitative data?
- Do you have data analysis skills or access to statistical consultants?
- Is it important to be able to generalize your findings to other populations?
- Are the stakeholders concerned with validity and reliability?
- Do you have the ability to randomize participants into experimental and control groups?
- Do you have access to a comparison group?

Dignan (1995) presented four steps in choosing an evaluation design. These four steps are outlined in **Figure 14.1.**

The first step is to orient oneself to the situation. The evaluator must identify resources (time, personnel), constraints, and hidden agendas (unspoken goals). During this step, the evaluator must determine what is to be expected from the program and what can be observed.

The second step involves defining the problem—determining what is to be evaluated. During this step, definitions are needed for independent variables (what the sponsors think makes the difference), dependent variables (what will indicate a difference, e.g., awareness, knowledge, attitudes, skills, environmental change, behaviors, disease prevalence), and confounding variables (what the evaluator thinks could be impacting the results in addition to or in place of the program under investigation).

The third step involves making a decision about the design—that is, whether to use qualitative or quantitative methods of data collection or both. The **quantitative method** is **deductive** in nature (applying a generally accepted principle to an individual case), so that the evaluation produces numeric (hard) data, such as counts, ratings, scores, or classifications. Examples of quantitative data include the posttest scores on a nutrition knowledge test, a decrease in percent of body weight from pretest to posttest, and reduction of mortality rates related to cancer. This method is suited to programs that are well defined and compares outcomes of programs with those of other groups or the general population. It is the method most often used in evaluation designs.

The **qualitative method** is an **inductive** method (individual cases are studied to formulate a general principle) and produces narrative data, such as words and descriptions. This is a good method to use for programs that emphasize individual outcomes or in cases where

▲ **Figure 14.1** Steps in Selecting an Evaluation Design

Source: *Measurement and Evaluation of Health Education*. M. B. Dignan. Copyright © 1995 by Charles C. Thomas Publisher, Ltd. Reprinted with Permission.

other descriptive information from participants is needed. That is, qualitative data provide depth of understanding, study motivation, enable discovery, are exploratory and interpretive, and allow insights into behavior and trends. Conversely, quantitative data measure levels of occurrence, provide proof, and measure levels of actions and trends (NCI, n.d.). **Box 14.2** provides a summary of various qualitative methods.

Patton (1988) produced a checklist to determine whether qualitative data might be appropriate in a particular program evaluation. Collecting qualitative data may be a good strategy if there is a need to describe individual outcomes, to understand the dynamics and process of the programs, to obtain in-depth information on certain clients or sites, or to gather information to improve the program during process evaluation.

The fourth step in selecting an evaluation design includes choosing how to measure the dependent variable, deciding how to collect the data (these components were discussed in Chapter 4) and how the data will be analyzed, and determining how the results will be reported. (These components are discussed in Chapter 15.)

▷ Experimental, Control, and Comparison Groups

As in research studies, when evaluating a health promotion program, the group of individuals who receive the intervention is known as the **experimental group** (or treatment group). The evaluation is designed to determine what effects the program has on these participants. To ensure the effects are caused by the program and not due to some other

BOX

14.2

Focus On

Qualitative Methods Used in Evaluation

- *Case studies:* In-depth examinations of a social unit, such as an individual, family, household, work site, community, or any type of institution as a whole.
- *Content analysis:* A systematic review identifying specific characteristics of messages.
- *Delphi techniques:* A process that generates consensus through a series of questionnaires. (See Chapter 4 for an in-depth discussion of the Delphi technique.)
- *Ethnographic studies:* A variety of techniques (participant-observer, observation, interviewing, and other interactions with people) used to study an individual or group.
- *Films, photographs, and videotape recording (film ethnography):* Includes the data collection and study of visual images.
- *Focus group interviewing:* Interviews used to obtain information about the feelings, opinions, perceptions, insights, beliefs, misconceptions, attitudes, and receptivity of a group of people concerning an idea or issue. (See Chapter 4 for an in-depth discussion of focus group interviewing.) See also Table 14.3.
- *Historical analysis:* A review of historical accounts that may include an interpretation of the impact on current events.
- *In-depth interviewing:* Formal interviews with program participants. Allows evaluators to observe body language and facial expressions as prompts for additional questions and information. See also Table 14.3.
- *Nominal group process:* A highly structured process in which a few knowledgeable representatives of the priority population are asked to qualify and quantify specific needs. (See Chapter 4 for an in-depth discussion of the nominal group process).
- *Participant-observer studies:* Those in which the observers (evaluators) also participate in what they are observing.
- *Quality circle:* A group of internal program people who meet at regular intervals to discuss problems and to identify possible solutions. See also Table 14.3.
- *Unobtrusive techniques:* Data collection techniques that do not require the direct participation or cooperation of human subjects and include such things as unobtrusive observation, review of archival data, and study of physical traces.

Source: *Health Education Evaluation and Measurement: A Practitioner's Perspective.* Robert McDermott and Paul Sarvela. Copyright © 1999 by McGraw-Hill.

factor, a **control group** should be used. The control group should be as similar to the experimental group as possible, but the members of this group do not receive the program (intervention or treatment) that is to be evaluated.

Without the use of a properly selected control group, the apparent effect of the program could actually be due to a variety of confounding variables. Ideally, participants should be randomly selected, then randomly assigned to one of two groups, and finally it should be randomly determined which group becomes the experimental group and which becomes the control group. Theoretically, randomization evenly distributes the characteristics of the participants and increases the credibility of the evaluation by controlling for confounding variables.

It is not always possible, practical or ethical to assign participants to a control group, especially in population-based programs, or if doing so would mean that individuals would be denied a necessary, or even critical program or service. For example, a health promotion program could be designed for individuals with hypertension. Individuals diagnosed with hypertension could be referred by a physician into a health promotion class focused on reducing the risk factors associated with this disease. Denying some individuals access to the program in order to form a control group would clearly be unethical.

One way to deal with this problem is to provide the control group with an alternative program or to offer the regular program to the group at a later time (if a delay is not potentially harmful). Another alternative is to compare two programs (e.g., offer an innovative program to some participants and continue the conventional program for others). Because the main purpose of social programs is to help individuals, the individuals' viewpoints should be the primary concern. It is important to keep this in mind when considering ethical issues in the use of control groups. When participants cannot be randomly assigned to an experimental or control group, a nonequivalent group may be selected. This is known as a **comparison group**. It is important to find a group that is as similar as possible to the experimental group, such as two classrooms of students with similar characteristics or a group of residents in two comparable cities. Factors to consider include participants' age, gender, education, location, socioeconomic status, and experience, as well as any other variable that might impact program results.

▷ Evaluation Designs

Measurements used in evaluation designs can be collected at three different times: after the program; both before and after the program; and several times before, during, and after the program. *Measurement* is defined as the quantitative data or numbers that come from applying an instrument (e.g., a questionnaire) to attributes about a person or people (Windsor, 2015).

Figure 14.2 presents evaluation designs commonly used in health promotion. In the figure, the letter *O* refers to measurement or observations involving data derived from questionnaires, tests, interviews, observations, or other methods of gaining information. When multiple measurements are taken, the subscript number beside each *O* indicates the order in which the measurements are made. Measurement before the program begins is known as the **pretest**, and measurement after the completion of the program is known as the **posttest**. The letter *X* represents the program (intervention, or independent variable); the relative positions of the two letters in the table indicate when measurements are made in relation to when the program is provided. The figure also shows which groups receive the program and when participants are randomly assigned to groups [(R)].

Windsor (2015) differentiates between experimental and quasi-experimental designs. **Experimental design** offers the greatest control over confounding variables that may influence the results of an intervention and its evaluation. It involves random assignment to experimental and control groups with pretest and posttest measurement of both groups. This evaluation design produces the most reliable evidence of effectiveness. **Quasi-experimental design** results in interpretable and supportive evidence of program effectiveness, but usually cannot control for all factors that affect the validity of the results. There is no random assignment to the groups, and comparisons are made between experimental and comparison groups. A **nonexperimental design** (referred to by Windsor, 2015, as a pre-experimental design) also uses pretest and posttest measurements among one

I. Experimental design

1. Pretest-posttest design

— Experimental group	(R)	O_1	X	O_2			
— Control group	(R)	O_1		O_2			

2. Posttest-only design

— Experimental group	(R)		X	O			
— Control group	(R)			O			

3. Time series design

— Experimental group	(R)	O_1	O_2	O_3	X	O_4	O_5 O_6
— Control group	(R)	O_1	O_2	O_3		O_4	O_5 O_6

II. Quasi-experimental design

1. Pretest-posttest design

— Experimental group	O_1	X	O_2			
— Comparison group	O_1		O_2			

2. Time series design

— Experimental group	O_1	O_2	O_3	X	O_4	O_5 O_6
— Comparison group	O_1	O_2	O_3		O_4	O_5 O_6

III. Nonexperimental design

1. Pretest-posttest design

— Experimental group	O_1	X	O_2

2. Time series design

— Experimental group	O_1	O_2	O_3	X	O_4	O_5 O_6

Key: (R) = Random assignment
    O = Measurement/Observation
    X = Program/Intervention

▲ **Figure 14.2** Evaluation Designs

group of participants without a control or comparison group. This approach has little control over confounding variables and bias that affect the validity and interpretation of results.

The most powerful design is the experimental design, in which participants are randomly assigned to the experimental and control groups. The difference between designs I.1 and I.2 in Figure 14.2 is the use of a pretest to measure the participants before the program begins. Use of a pretest would help ensure that the groups are similar and provide baseline measurement. Random assignment should equally distribute any of the variables of the participants (such as age, gender, and race) between the different groups. Potential disadvantages of the experimental design are that it requires a relatively large group of participants and the intervention may be delayed for those in the control group.

A design more commonly found in evaluations of health promotion programs is the quasi-experimental pretest-posttest design using a comparison group (II.1 in Figure 14.2). This design is often used when a control group cannot be formed by random assignment. In such a case, a comparison group (a nonequivalent control group) is identified, and both groups are measured before and after the program. For example, a program on healthy eating for two ninth-grade classrooms could be evaluated by using a food inventory instrument at pretest and posttest. Two other ninth-grade classrooms not receiving the program could serve as the comparison group. Similar pretest scores between the comparison and experimental groups would indicate that the groups were equal at the beginning of the program and comparisons of posttest scores could indicate the differences between the groups at the conclusion of the program. However, without random assignment, it would be impossible to be sure that other variables (e.g., a unit on meal preparation in a family and consumer science course, a reality television show related to weight loss, changes made by the primary meal preparer at home, etc.) did not influence the results.

Sometimes participants cannot be assigned to a control group and no comparison group can be identified. In such cases, a nonexperimental pretest-posttest design (III.1 in Figure 14.2) can be used, but the results are of limited significance, because changes could be due to the program or to some other event. An example of this type of design would be the measurement of safety belt use after a community program on that topic. An increase in use might mean that the program successfully motivated individuals to use safety belts; however, it could also reveal the impact of increased enforcement of a mandatory safety belt law, a traffic fatality in the community, or a social media campaign related to safety.

A time series evaluation design (I.3, II.2, III.2 in Figure 14.2) can be used to examine differences in program effects over time. Random assignment to groups (I.3) offers the most control over factors influencing the validity of the results. The use of a comparison group (II.2) offers some control; without a control group or comparison group (III.2), it is possible to determine changes in the participants over time, but one cannot be sure that the changes were due only to the program.

In the time series design, several measurements are taken over time both before and after a program is implemented. This process helps to identify other factors that may account for a change between the pretest and posttest measurements and is especially appropriate for measuring delayed effects of a program. A time series design could be used in a weight loss program to indicate the amount of participants' weight loss over time and their ability to maintain a desired weight. This is especially important since most change will generally be more prominent at the immediate conclusion of a program. But stakeholders may want to investigate results over time (e.g. three months and six months) to ensure change is lasting.

Another design that may be used is the staggered treatment design (see **Figure 14.3**), which is used to determine the effects of a program over time by including several measurements after the end of the program. It also indicates the effects of testing, since not all groups in this design receive a pretest. The staggered treatment design can also be used in quasi-experimental and nonexperimental designs, although with the limitations of not using a control group or comparison group.

Experimental group 1	(R)	X	O_1		O_2		O_3		O_4	
Experimental group 2	(R)		O_1	X	O_2		O_3		O_4	
Experimental group 3	(R)				O_1	X	O_2		O_3	
Experimental group 4	(R)							X	O_1	

Key: (R) = Random assignment
    O = Measurement/Observation
    X = Program/Intervention

▲ **Figure 14.3** Staggered Treatment Design

▷ Internal Validity

The **internal validity** of evaluation is the degree to which change that was measured can be attributed to the program and allows evaluators to speak with more confidence that the program itself actually made a difference (Issel, 2014). Many factors can threaten internal validity, either singly or in combination, making it difficult to determine if the outcome was brought about by the program or some other cause(s). Cook and Campbell (1979) identified common threats to internal validity which have come to be known as the Campbellian validity typology (Chen, 2015). Campbell's typology is still supported today (Chen, 2015; Fink, 2015; Sharma & Petosa, 2014) and is summarized as follows:

- *History* occurs when unanticipated events happen between the pretest and posttest that are not part of the health promotion program being evaluated. An example of history as a threat to internal validity is having a national antismoking campaign coincide with a local smoking cessation program.

- *Maturation* occurs when the participants in the program show pretest-to-posttest differences due to growing older, wiser, or stronger as a function of time. For example, in tests of muscle strength in an exercise program for junior high students, an increase in strength could be the result of muscular development and not the effect of the program.

- *Testing* occurs when the participants become familiar with the test format due to repeated testing. For example, participants in a job training program may perform better in job interviews as a result of past interviews compared with the effect of the program itself (Chen, 2015). Pretest measurements may also change the perceptions or knowledge of participants thus making their responses on posttests less accurate (Sharma & Petosa, 2014).

- *Instrumentation* occurs when there is a change in measurement between pretest and posttest, such as the observers becoming more familiar with or skilled in the use of the testing format over time. Instrumentation bias can also occur when evaluators themselves change or when there is inconsistency between evaluators (e.g., evaluators making direct observations of people practicing relaxation techniques and measuring outcomes differently).

- *Statistical regression* is when extremely high or low scores (which are not necessarily accurate) on the pretest naturally move closer to the mean or average on the posttest. This might be relevant if an evaluator is trying to assess a certain risk factor and those surveyed in the pretest include a disproportionately large number of high risk individuals (i.e. people who score high on the risk factor). Results from the posttest may reflect statistical regression compared with the effect of the program itself.

- *Selection* reflects differences in the experimental and comparison groups, generally due to lack of randomization. For example, people who are very motivated to change in a particular way may self-select to the experimental group whereas people who have more neutral feelings may self-select to the comparison group. Selection can also interact with other threats to validity, such as history, maturation, or instrumentation, which may appear to be program effects.

- *Attrition* (originally referred to as mortality by Cook and Campbell, 1979) refers to participants who drop out of the program between the pretest and posttest. For example, if most of the participants who drop out of a weight loss program are those with the least (or the most) weight to lose, the group composition is different at the posttest. Attrition occurs for various reasons (e.g. sickness, loss of interest, relocation to a different city or state, etc.).

- *Interaction* (originally referred to as diffusion or imitation of treatments by Cook and Campbell, 1979) results when participants in the control or comparison group interact and learn from the experimental group. Students randomly assigned to an innovative drug prevention program in their school (experimental group) may discuss the program with students who are not in the program (control or comparison group), biasing the results.

- *Compensatory equalization of treatments* occurs when the program or services are not available to the control or comparison group and there is an unwillingness to tolerate the inequality. For instance, the control or comparison group from the previous example (students not enrolled in the innovative drug prevention program) may complain, since they are not able to participate.

- *Compensatory rivalry* is when the control or comparison group is seen as the underdog and is motivated to work harder.

- *Resentful demoralization of respondents receiving less desirable treatments* occurs among participants receiving the less desirable treatments compared to other groups, and the resentment may affect the outcome. For example, an evaluation to compare two different smoking cessation programs may assign one group (control) to the regular smoking cessation program and another group (experimental) to the regular program plus an exercise class. If the participants in the control group become aware that they are not receiving the additional exercise class, they may resent the omission, and this may be reflected in their smoking behavior and attitude toward the regular program.

The most significant way in which threats to internal validity can be controlled is through *randomization*. By random selection of participants, random assignment to groups, and random assignment of types of intervention or no intervention to groups, any differences between pretest and posttest can be interpreted as a result of the program. When random assignment to groups is not possible and quasi-experimental or nonexperimental designs are used, the evaluator must make all threats to internal validity explicit and then rule them out one by one.

▷ External Validity

The other type of validity that should be considered is **external validity**, or the extent to which the program can be expected to produce similar effects in other populations. This is also known as **generalizability** which is most closely associated with program evaluations that involve large sample sizes and are found to be internally valid (Harris, 2010). However, the more a program is tailored to a particular population, the greater the threat to external validity, and the less likely it is that the program can be generalized to another group.

As with internal validity, several factors can threaten external validity. They are sometimes known as *reactive effects*, since they cause individuals to react in a certain way. The following are several types of threats to external validity:

- *Social desirability* occurs when individuals give a particular response to try to impress or satisfy the wants of the evaluator (Sharma & Petosa, 2014). An example would be children who tell their teacher they brush their teeth every day, regardless of their actual behavior.

- *Expectancy effect* or Pygmalion effect (Sharma & Petosa, 2014) is when attitudes projected onto individuals cause them to act in a certain way. For example, in a drug abuse treatment program, the facilitator may feel that a certain individual will not benefit from the treatment; projecting this attitude may cause the individual to behave in self-defeating manners.

- *Hawthorne effect* refers to a behavior change because of the special status of those being tested (Sharma & Petosa, 2014) or when behavior changes as participants become more aware they are being studied (Fink, 2015).
- *Placebo effect* causes a change in behavior due to the participants' belief in the treatment.

Cook and Campbell (1979) discussed the threats to external validity in terms of statistical interaction effects. These include interaction of selection and treatment (the findings from a program requiring a large time commitment may not be generalizable to individuals who do not have much free time); interaction of setting and treatment (evaluation results from a program conducted on campus may not be generalizable to the worksite); and interaction of history and treatment (results from a program conducted on a historically significant day may not be generalizable to other days).

Conducting the program several times in a variety of settings, with a variety of participants can reduce the threats to external validity. Threats to external validity can also be counteracted by making a greater effort to treat all subjects identically. In a **blind** study, the participants do not know whether they have been assigned to the experimental group or the control group. In a **double blind** study, the type of group participants are in is not known by either the participants or the planners. In a **triple blind** study, this information is not available to the participants, planners, or evaluators.

It is important to select an evaluation design that provides both internal and external validity. This may be difficult, because lowering the threat to one type of validity may increase the threat to the other. For example, tighter evaluation controls make it more difficult to generalize the results to other situations. There must be enough control over the evaluation to allow evaluators to interpret the findings while sufficient flexibility in the program is maintained to permit the results to be generalized to similar settings.

Summary

This chapter focused on evaluation approaches, design elements, and strategies for conducting a comprehensive evaluation. Distinctions between formative and process evaluation were made and key issues related to summative evaluation were outlined.

The steps for selecting an evaluation design were also presented with a discussion about quantitative and qualitative methods. Evaluation design should be considered early in the planning process. Evaluators need to identify what measurements will be taken as well as when and how. In doing so, a design should be selected that controls for both internal and external validity.

Review Questions

1. List the elements of a comprehensive formative evaluation and describe when in the design and implementation process they are most appropriately applied.
2. What are the fundamental differences between formative and process evaluations?

3. What is the difference between cost-benefit analysis and cost-effectiveness analysis? Which is more appropriate for use in health promotion programs?

4. What is the difference between quantitative and qualitative evaluations? When would one method be more appropriate than the other? How could they be combined in an evaluation design?

5. Name at least five different qualitative methods of evaluation and describe each.

6. What are the advantages of using a control group? What types of evaluation design do not use control groups? What is the difference between a control group and a comparison group?

7. What is the difference between experimental, quasi-experimental, and nonexperimental designs?

8. What is the difference between internal validity and external validity?

9. What are some considerations in the selection of an evaluation design presented in this chapter? What considerations can you add to this list?

 Activities

1. Interview the manager of a health promotion program of your choice about how he or she measures quality. How many elements of formative evaluation can you detect?

2. Look at an evaluation of a health promotion program that has been conducted in your community. Identify the evaluation approach that it most closely follows. Discuss your view with the program evaluator.

3. Develop an evaluation design for a program you are planning. Explain why you chose this design, and list the strengths and weaknesses of the design.

4. If you were hired to evaluate a weight loss program in a community, what evaluation design would you use and why? Assume you have all the resources you need to conduct the evaluation.

5. Explain what evaluation design you would use in evaluating the difference between two social media approaches. Why would you choose this design?

 Weblinks

1. **https://www.wmich.edu/evaluation/checklists**

   Evaluation Center at Western Michigan University (WMU)

   The Evaluation Center at WMU Website provides evaluation specialists and users with refereed checklists to improve the quality and consistency of evaluations. The site's purpose is to improve evaluation capacity through the promotion and use of high-quality checklists targeted to specific evaluation tasks and approaches. Visitors to this site can download a number of checklists and information on how to create them.

2. **http://oerl.sri.com/**

   Online Evaluation Resource Library (OERL)

   Funded by the National Science Foundation (NSF), OERL was developed for professionals seeking to design, conduct, document, or review project evaluations. OERL's resources include instruments, plans, and reports from evaluations that have proven to be sound and representative of current evaluation practices.

3. **http://www.eric.ed.gov/**

   Educational Resources Information Center (ERIC)

   The ERIC Clearinghouse on Assessment and Evaluation Website offers a variety of resources and seeks to provide balanced information concerning educational assessment, and resources to encourage responsible test use.

4. **http://www.socialresearchmethods.net/kb/destypes.php**

   Web Center for Social Research Methods

   This site addresses the basic types of evaluation designs and reinforces the material covered in this chapter including information on experimental, quasi-experimental, and nonexperimental designs as well as random selection and threats to validity.

5. **http://whqlibdoc.who.int/hq/2000/WHO_MSD_MSB_00.2e.pdf**

   World Health Organization

   This is a link to WHO's document on process evaluation that supplements material in this chapter. It describes why a process evaluation should be performed and how to do a process evaluation.

6. **http://www.rand.org/pubs/technical_reports/TR101/**

   Rand Organization—Getting to Outcomes

   This document, which focuses on substance abuse, provides an excellent explanation of promoting accountability through methods and tools for planning, implementation, and evaluation. One focus of the document is how to get to outcomes that justify prevention programs in general.

Data Analysis and Reporting

Chapter Objectives

After reading this chapter and answering the questions at the end, you should be able to:

- Define data management.
- List examples of univariate, bivariate, and multivariate analyses and explain how they can be used in evaluation.
- Differentiate between descriptive and inferential statistics.
- Differentiate between parametric and non-parametric data.
- Explain the difference between the null hypothesis and the alternative hypothesis in significance testing.
- Define level of significance, Type I error, and Type II error.
- Define independent variable and dependent variable.
- Describe guidelines for presenting data, and ways to enhance an evaluation report.
- Discuss ways to increase the use of evaluation findings.

Key Terms

alpha level
alternative hypothesis
analysis of variance (ANOVA)
bivariate data analysis
chi-square
correlations
data management
dependent variables
descriptive statistics
independent variables
inferential statistics
level of significance
mean
measures of central tendency
measures of spread or variation
median
mode

multiple regression
multivariate data analysis
non-parametric tests
null hypothesis
parametric tests
program significance
range
statistical significance
t-tests
Type I error
Type II error
univariate data analysis
variable

Like other aspects of evaluation, the type of data analysis used in an evaluation should be determined in the pre-planning stage. Basically, the analysis will help determine what, if any, impact was made by the program. The evaluator then draws conclusions and prepares reports and/or presentations. The types of analyses used and how the information is presented are determined by the evaluation questions as well as the needs of the stakeholders.

This chapter describes different types of analyses commonly used in evaluating health promotion programs. To present them in detail or to include all possible techniques is

BOX

15.1

Responsibilities and Competencies for Health Education Specialists

This chapter describes managing data collected in evaluations or other research; types of data analyses; applications of data analyses; interpreting data; reporting the results of evaluation, including designing written reports and how and when to present evaluation reports; and increasing the use of evaluation results. Responsibilities and competencies related to the content in this chapter include:

RESPONSIBILITY IV: Conduct Evaluation and Research Related to Health Education/Promotion

Competency 4.5: Analyze data

Competency 4.6: Interpret results

Competency 4.7: Apply findings

Source: *A Competency-Based Framework for Health Education Specialists—2015*. Whitehall, PA: National Commission for Health Education Credentialing, Inc. (NCHEC) and the Society for Public Health Education (SOPHE). Reprinted by permission of the National Commission for Health Education Credentialing, Inc. (NCHEC) and the Society for Public Health Education (SOPHE).

beyond the scope of this text. If you need more information, refer to statistics textbooks, research methods and statistics courses, or statistical consultants. **Box 15.1** identifies the responsibilities and competencies for health education specialists that pertain to the material presented in this chapter.

Evaluations affected by methodological problems are not likely to inspire confidence. A common problem in this regard is inadequate documentation of methods, results, and data analysis. The evaluation should be well designed and implemented and the data report itself should contain a complete background and description of the program, a thorough explanation of methodology including information about the instrumentation, the program participants and their selection, evaluation design and statistical analysis, as well as an objective interpretation of facts, and a discussion of features of the study that may have influenced the findings. Attention to these details will help ensure a more accurate assessment of program effectiveness as well as enhance the credibility of planners/evaluators among stakeholders. In addition, this level of professionalism will also increase the likelihood that evaluation reports can be translated to peer reviewed publications and contribute to the research and knowledge base of health promotion in general.

▷ Data Management

Once data have been collected (see Chapter 4 for data collection methods), they must be organized in such a manner that they can be analyzed in order to interpret related findings. To do this, the data, whether quantitative or qualitative, must be coded, cleaned, and organized into a usable format. These steps are collectively referred to as **data management**. By coded, we mean that the data are assigned labels so they can be read and processed by a computer. Evaluators often create codebooks that include descriptions of all the questions, codes, and variables associated with a survey or any other method used to collect data (Fink, 2015). For example, if the answer to a question on an instrument is yes, yes answers may be coded as the number 1 when entered into the computer, whereas no answers may be coded as a number 2. In addition to creating the coding scheme for raw data, a coding system also establishes rules for dealing with coding problems such as when respondents circle both yes and no for their answer to a question, or when neither yes nor no is circled but rather the space between the yes and no is circled.

Once the data have been coded, they must be cleaned before being entered into a computer system. Data cleaning entails checking for errors associated with data entry and may involve searching for missing values or discarding certain data that are indecipherable or incomplete (Sharma & Petosa, 2014; Fink, 2015). For example, if the possible range of answers for a particular question is 1 to 3 and the frequency distribution identifies some 4s, those response forms with the 4s must be identified and checked to determine if the person completing the instrument made an error or if there was an error made by the person coding the data. If it was a data coding error, it should be corrected. If the person completing the data collection instrument made an error, it would be treated as no response to that question or as missing data (Cottrell & McKenzie, 2011). Once data have been cleaned, the appropriate data analysis can begin.

▷ Data Analysis

Once data have been cleaned, the goal of data analysis is to apply the correct statistical tests or procedures to the data to answer evaluation or research questions or to test hypotheses. Regardless of the type of data analysis to be used, the process begins with the identification of the variables of interest. A **variable** is a characteristic or attribute that can be measured or observed (Creswell, 2002). In program evaluation, variables are generally classified as independent or dependent variables. **Independent variables** are those that are either controlled by the evaluator or cause or exert some influence, whereas the **dependent variables** are the outcome variables being studied. In other words "independent variables influence dependent variables" (Valente, 2002, p. 165). Examples of independent variables include exposure to an intervention, gender, race, age, education, income, and so on, while dependent variables may include awareness, knowledge, attitudes, skills, and behaviors.

Statistics are used to analyze variables. **Descriptive statistics** are used to organize, summarize, and describe characteristics of a group. Descriptive statistics are generally displayed as frequency distributions (e.g. tables and graphs) or presented as measures of central tendency (e.g. a mean score or mathematical average) (Sharma & Petosa, 2015) and answer basic questions related to: who; what; where; when; and how much. **Inferential statistics** test relationships between variables and attempt to explain causality in order to make generalizations (or inferences) about a larger population based upon findings from a sample. When one variable is analyzed, it is called **univariate data analysis**. Analysis of two variables is called **bivariate data analysis** and analysis of more than two variables is referred to as **multivariate data analysis**. Box 15.2 contains examples of the types of evaluation questions that can be answered by using different types of data analyses.

The type of analysis selected is based on the evaluation questions, the type of data collected, and the audience that will receive the results (Newcomer & Wirtz, 2004). For some types of analysis in evaluation, descriptive data are all that stakeholders want and need, and techniques might be selected to create simple frequencies only. Other evaluation questions are designed to test a hypothesis about relationships between variables; in such cases, more elaborate statistical techniques are needed.

The level of measurement (i.e., nominal, ordinal, interval, or ratio) (discussed in Chapter 5) is also an important factor in selecting the type of analysis to be used. For example, after you have identified the level of measurement related to the data you have collected, you apply either parametric or non-parametric tests. **Parametric tests** assume a normal distribution curve

BOX

15.2

Application

Examples of Evaluation Questions Answered Using Univariate, Bivariate, and Multivariate Data Analysis

Univariate Analysis

- What was the average score on the cholesterol knowledge test?
- How many participants at the worksite attended the healthy lifestyle presentation?
- What percentage of the participants in the corporate fitness program met their target goal?

Bivariate Analysis

- Is there a difference in smoking behavior between the individuals in the experimental and control groups after the healthy lifestyle program?
- Is peer education or classroom instruction more effective in increasing knowledge about the effects of drug abuse?
- Do students' attitudes about bicycle helmets differ in rural and urban settings?

Multivariate Analysis

- Can the risk of heart disease be predicted using smoking, exercise, diet, and heredity?
- Can mortality risk among motorcycle riders be predicted from helmet use, time of day, weather conditions, and speed?
- Which of the following most accurately predict successful management of stress among program participants: physical activity, diet, meditation, anger management, yoga, or deep breathing?

while **non-parametric tests** assume the distribution curve is skewed (i.e. not normal as in negatively or positively skewed).

A more basic distinction between parametric and non-parametric tests is that if your measurement scale is nominal or ordinal then you use non-parametric statistics. If you are using interval or ratio scales, then use parametric statistics. Parametric data are considered to be more powerful since they use more information in their calculations (though there is at least one non-parametric test that is equivalent to each parametric test). Examples of inferential statistical tests associated with parametric data include: t-tests; analysis of variance (ANOVA); and Pearson's correlation. Examples of inferential statistical tests associated with nonparametric data include: chi-square; Mann-Whitney U test; Wilcoxon Signed-Ranks test; and Spearman's Rank-Order Correlation.

The issue of who will receive the final evaluation report should also be considered when selecting the type of analysis. Evaluators want to be able to present the evaluation results in a form that can be understood by stakeholders. With regard to this issue, it is probably best to err on the side of too simple an analysis rather than one that is too complex. Finally, regardless of the type of analysis selected for an evaluation, the method should be identified early in the evaluation process and put in place before the data are collected.

Univariate Data Analyses

Univariate data analyses examine one variable at a time. It is common for univariate analyses to be descriptive in nature. As noted earlier, descriptive statistics are used to describe, classify, and summarize data. Summary counts (frequencies) are totals, and they are the easiest type of data to collect and report. Summary counts can be used in process evaluation—for example, to count the number of participants in blood pressure screening programs at various sites. The information would assist the planners in publicizing sites with low attendance or adding additional personnel to busy sites. Other examples of frequencies, or summary counts, are the number of participants in a workshop, those who scored above 80% on a knowledge posttest, or the number of individuals wearing a safety belt.

Measures of central tendency are other forms of univariate data analyses. The **mean** is the arithmetic average of all the scores. The **median** is the midpoint of all the scores, dividing scores ranked by size into equal halves. The **mode** is the score that occurs most frequently. These are all useful in describing the results, and reporting all three measures of central tendency will be especially helpful if extreme scores are found.

Measures of spread or variation refer to how spread out the scores are in the data set. **Range** is the difference between the highest and lowest scores. For example, if the high score is 100 and the low score is 60, the range is 40. Measures of spread or variation—such as range, standard deviation, or variance—can be used to determine whether scores from groups are similar or spread apart.

Bivariate Data Analyses

Bivariate data analyses are used to study two variables simultaneously and determine how they relate to one another. When using bivariate analyses, it is common to state evaluation questions in the form of hypotheses. The **null hypothesis** holds that there is no observed difference between groups. The **alternative hypothesis** states there is a difference between groups. For example, a null hypothesis might state there is no difference between two groups, for example men and women, in knowledge about cancer risk factors, while the alternative hypothesis states there is a difference in their knowledge.

Statistical tests are used to determine if the relationships or differences between groups are statistically significant. **Statistical significance** "is a statement regarding the likelihood that observed variable values happened by chance" (Sharma & Petosa, 2014, p. 281). In other words, statistical tests are used to determine whether the null hypothesis is rejected (meaning a relationship between the groups probably does exist) or whether it fails to be rejected (indicating that any apparent relationship between groups is due to chance).

There is the possibility that the null hypothesis can be rejected when it is, in fact, true; this is known as **Type I error**. There is also the possibility of failing to reject the null hypothesis when it is, in fact, not true; this is a **Type II error**. The probability of making a Type I error is reflected in the alpha level. The **alpha level**, or **level of significance**, is established before the statistical tests are run and is generally set at 0.05 or 0.01. This indicates that the decision to reject the null hypothesis is incorrect 5% (or 1%) of the time; that is, there is a 5% probability (or 1% probability) that the outcome occurred by chance alone.

When a smaller alpha level is used (0.01 or 0.001), the possibility of making a Type I error is reduced; at the same time, however, the possibility of a Type II error increases. An example of a Type I error is the adoption of a new program due to higher scores on a knowledge test, when, in reality, increases in knowledge occurred by chance and the new program is not more effective than the existing program. An example of a Type II error is not adopting the new program when it is, in reality, more effective.

Bivariate analyses that are commonly used in program evaluation include chi-square, t-tests, analysis of variance, and correlations. **Chi-square** is a statistical test "that measures the association between two nominal and/or ordinal variables" (Valente, 2002, p. 170).

An example of this type of analysis would be measuring the association of grade levels (e.g., third and fifth grades) with the attitudes of children toward the use of bicycle helmets (i.e., strongly agree, agree, disagree, and strongly disagree).

While chi-square is used to study nominal and/or ordinal variables (as with non-parametric tests described earlier), **t-tests** and **analysis of variance (ANOVA)** are statistical tests used to study group differences when the dependent variables involve interval or ratio data (e.g., as with parametric tests described earlier). There are several situations in which a t-test could be used. The most common use of a t-test is to determine whether a variable changed significantly in one group at two different points in time, such as between baseline before the intervention (pretest) and at follow-up after the intervention (posttest). This type of t-test is called a dependent t-test. A second common use of a t-test is to study the differences between two groups at a single point in time. An example of such a situation is the comparison of scores on nutrition practices after two groups have been exposed to different nutrition education interventions. This type of t-test is called an independent t-test.

ANOVA is a statistical test that can be used to study differences between two groups just like a t-test, but is more commonly used to study differences between more than two groups. For example, an ANOVA could be used to determine if there was a difference in the test scores of three groups (i.e., different age groups like 15–24, 25–45, and 46–65 year olds) on a physical activity assessment following exposure to a single health promotion intervention.

While the bivariate analyses discussed so far are used to determine if differences exist between groups, **correlations** are used to study the extent to which two variables are related to each other such that the changes in one variable are accompanied by changes in another variable (Furlong, Lovelace, & Lovelace, 2000). Correlations are expressed as values between +1 (a positive correlation) and -1 (a negative correlation), with a 0 indicating no relationship between the variables. Larger absolute values that are either positive or negative indicate stronger relationships (Furlong et al., 2000).

Correlation between variables indicates only a relationship; this technique does not establish cause and effect. An example of the use of correlation would be to determine the relationship between safety belt use and age of the driver. If older people were found to wear their safety belts more often than younger people, that would constitute a positive correlation between age and safety belt use. If younger people wore their safety belts more often, it would be a negative correlation. If age made no difference in what population wore safety belts more frequently, the correlation would be 0.

Multivariate Data Analyses

Multivariate data analyses are used to study three or more variables simultaneously. Examples of multivariate analyses include multiple regression, discriminant analysis, and factor analysis. Of these, the one that tends to be used most commonly in health promotion evaluation is **multiple regression**. Though the procedures and applications for various types of regression differ (e.g. stepwise regression, logistic regression, and general linear regression), they are "useful in exploring relationships among variables or in exploring the independent effects of many variables on one dependent variable" (Fitzpatrick et al., 2004, p. 359). An example of the latter would be trying to predict the risk of heart disease (the dependent variable) using the independent variables of smoking, cholesterol, lack of exercise, high stress, etc.

Applications of Data Analyses

Many evaluation concepts have been presented. Therefore, a few examples here will help you see how to move from a program goal to an intervention to an evaluation design to data analysis. To illustrate these concepts, a few statistics have been selected that are commonly used with health promotion programs: chi-square and t-tests.

Case #1

Program goal: Reduce the prevalence of smoking in the priority population

Priority population: The 140 employees of Company X who smoke

Intervention (independent variable): Two different smoking cessation programs

Variable of interest (dependent variable): Smoking cessation after six months

Evaluation design:

$$R \quad A \quad X_1 \quad O_1$$
$$R \quad B \quad X_2 \quad O_1$$

where:

R	=	random assignment
A	=	group A
B	=	group B
X_1	=	method 1
X_2	=	method 2
O_1	=	self-reported smoking behavior

Data collected: Nominal data; quit yes or no

	Smoking Employees	
	Group A Method 1	Group B Method 2
Quit	24%	33%
Did not quit	76%	67%

Data analysis: A chi-square test of statistical significance can be used to test the null-hypothesis that there is no difference in the success of the two groups.

Case #2

Program goal: Increase knowledge of HIV/AIDS within the priority population

Priority population: The 3,200 incoming freshmen at University X

Intervention (independent variable): A two-hour lecture-discussion program presented during the freshmen orientation program

Variable of interest (dependent variable): Knowledge of HIV/AIDS

Evaluation design: $\quad O_1 \quad X \quad O_2$

where:

O_1	=	pretest scores
X	=	two-hour program at freshman orientation
O_2	=	posttest scores

Data collection: Ratio data; scores on 100-point-scale test

	Test Results	
	Pretest	**Posttest**
Number of students	3,200	3,200
Mean score	69.0	78.5

Data analysis: A dependent *t*-test of statistical significance can be used to test the null hypothesis that there is no difference between the pre- and posttest means on the knowledge test.

Case #3

Program goal: To improve the testicular self-examination skills of the priority population

Priority population: All boys enrolled in the eighth grade at Junior High School X

Intervention (independent variable): Two-week unit on testicular cancer

Variable of interest (dependent variable): Score on testicular self-exam skills test

Evaluation design:

$$A \quad O_1 \quad X \quad O_2$$
$$B \quad O_1 \quad \quad O_2$$

where:

A	=	eighth-grade boys at Junior High School X
B	=	eighth-grade boys at Junior High School Y
O_1	=	pretest scores
X	=	two-week unit on testicular cancer
O_2	=	posttest scores

Data collected: Ratio data; scores on 100-point skills test

	Test Results	
	Junior High X **($n = 142$)**	**Junior High Y** **($n = 131$)**
Pre	62	63
Post	79	65

Data analysis: An independent *t*-test of statistical significance can be used to (1) test the null hypothesis that there is no difference in the pretest scores of the two groups be cause the groups were not randomly assigned, and (2) test the null hypothesis that there is no difference in the posttest scores of the two groups.

▷ Interpreting the Data

With the data analyses completed, attention turns to interpreting the data. By interpretation we mean attaching meaning to the analyzed data and drawing conclusions. "Interpretation should be characterized by careful, fair, open methods of inquiry." (Fitzpatrick et al., 2004, p. 364.)

To ensure that the interpretation is fair and as objective as possible, it is recommended that the interpretation not be the sole responsibility of the evaluator or, for that matter, any other single person. Earlier, when we began our discussion of evaluation, we spoke of the importance of making sure that the evaluation process is a collaborative process that includes representation from all of the stakeholders (see Chapter 13). That principle applies not only to the planning of the evaluation but also to the interpretation of the data. It is advisable to bring stakeholders and evaluators together in one or more meetings to systematically review evaluation findings. Such meetings take advantage of the diverse perspectives of the stakeholders, as well as allowing for a discussion of the implications of various interpretative conclusions.

There is no single method used to interpret data. In fact, a number of different methods could be used. Fitzpatrick and colleagues (2004) have identified eight methods:

1. "Determining whether objectives have been achieved;
2. Determining whether laws, democratic ideals, regulations, or ethical principles have been violated;
3. Determining whether assessed needs have been reduced;
4. Determining the value of accomplishments;
5. Asking critical reference groups to review the data and to provide their judgments of successes and failures, strengths, and weaknesses;
6. Comparing results with those reported by similar entities or endeavors;
7. Comparing assessed performance levels on critical variables to expectations of performance or standards;
8. Interpreting results in light of evaluation procedures that generated them" (p. 364).

Given this list, it becomes clear that there is a difference between what is termed statistical significance and **program significance**. Program significance measures the meaningfulness of a program (based on stakeholder preferences) compared with statistical significance determined by statistical testing. It is possible—especially when a large number of people are included in the data collection—to have statistically significant results that indicate gains in performance that are not meaningful in terms of program goals. For example, if the mean scores on a knowledge test of two groups are 70 and 69 (out of 100 points) and the groups are large enough, it would be possible that the difference in the scores (i.e., 1 point) could be statistically significant. But in practical terms, the group with a mean score of 70 compared with 69 will likely not have more knowledge that will translate to anything meaningful. Thus, spending extra dollars on the program that generated the mean score of 70 versus the less expensive program that generated a mean score of 69 would not be cost-effective. Statistical significance is similar to reliability in that they are both measures of precision. In addition, while program results may not be considered statistically significant, stakeholders may feel the program should be continued for various reasons (e.g., goodwill is being developed in the community or the organization is receiving a lot of positive attention that is drawing more clients to other programs, etc.).

▷ Evaluation Reporting

The results and interpretation of the data analyses, as well as a description of the evaluation process, are incorporated into a final report that is presented to stakeholders. The report itself generally follows the format of a research report, including an introduction, methodology, results, and discussion, including conclusions and recommendations.

Some may see the creation of an evaluation report as a nonessential step in the larger process of evaluation; however, an evaluation report is essential for several reasons (Wurzbach, 2002). An evaluation report can provide:

- The impetus "to help you critically analyze the results of the evaluation and think about any changes you should make as a result
- A tangible product for your agency
- Evidence that your program or materials have been carefully developed—to be used as a sales tool with gatekeepers (e.g., television station public service directors)
- A record of your activities for use in planning future programs
- Assistance to others who may be interested in developing similar programs or materials
- A foundation for evaluation activities in the future (e.g., it is easier to design a new questionnaire based on one you have previously used than to start anew)" (p. 590)

The number and type of reports required are determined at the beginning of the evaluation based on the needs of the stakeholders. For a formative evaluation, reports are needed early and may be provided on a weekly or monthly basis. Related feedback may be formal or informal, ranging from scheduled presentations to informal telephone calls but must be submitted in a timely manner in order to provide immediate feedback so that program modifications can be made before program implementation has progressed too far. For a summative evaluation, the report is generally more formal and may resemble a scientific paper that can be submitted to a journal for publication. In fact, it is advisable in many circumstances to recommend to stakeholders that the evaluation report take the form of such a paper so that publication is an option. In this regard, successful programs can be shared with the larger profession of health promotion. Ultimately, stakeholders will determine the format of the report (technical report, journal article, news release, meeting, presentation, press conference, letter, or workshop, etc.) as well as the criteria that will define program success. Often, an oral presentation will accompany the submission of a final evaluation report and at times, more than one method is selected in order to meet the needs of all stakeholders. For example, following an innovative worksite health promotion program, the evaluator might prepare a story for the worksite newsletter, a letter of findings to all staff who participated, a technical report for the funding source, and an executive summary for the administrators.

Evaluators must be able to communicate to all audiences when presenting the results of the evaluation. The reaction of each audience—participants, media, administrators, funding sources—must be anticipated in order to prepare the necessary information. In some cases, technical information must be included; in other cases, anecdotal information may be appropriate. The evaluator must fit the report to the audience as well as prepare for a negative response if the results of the evaluation are not favorable. This involves looking critically at the results and developing responses to anticipated reactions.

Designing the Written Report

As previously mentioned, the evaluation report follows a similar format to that used in a scientific or research report. The evaluation report generally includes the following sections:

- *Abstract or executive summary:* This is a summary of the total evaluation including goals and objectives, methods, results, and discussion, including conclusions and recommendations. It is a concise presentation of the evaluation because it may be the only portion of the report that some of the stakeholders read. Most abstracts/executive summaries range in length from 200 to 500 words.

- *Introduction:* This section of the report contains a complete description of the program including background information as well as rationale or justification for the program and its evaluation. Goals and objectives of the program are listed, as well as the evaluation questions to be answered.

- *Methods/procedures:* This section includes information on the evaluation design, priority populations, instruments used, and how the data were collected and analyzed.

- *Results:* This section is the most critical component of the report. It includes the findings from the evaluation, summarizing and simplifying the data and presenting them in a clear, concise format. Data are presented for each evaluation or research question. If null and alternative hypotheses were developed as part of the evaluation or research, they are also explained and answered as part of this section.

- *Discussion:* This section interprets the results (presented in the previous section) to determine significance and provide explanations for what was found. Conclusions and recommendations are included in this section and may be based on findings from other studies, other literature previously published, or related theories.

Box 15.3 summarizes what is included in the evaluation report.

Presenting Data

The data that have been collected and analyzed are presented in the evaluation report. Data presentation should be simple and straightforward. Graphic displays and tables may be used to illustrate certain findings; in fact, they are often a central part of the report. They also often make it easier for the readers of a written report or the audience of an oral report to understand the findings of the evaluation. Graphic displays should be self-explanatory. In fact, it is usually ill-advised to describe in the text too much of what is already displayed in a table or figure. When presenting the data in graphic form it is often helpful to include a frame of reference—such as a comparison with national, state, local, or other data—and explain any limitations of the data. If graphic displays are used in a report, it is recommended (USDHHS, CDC, n.d.) that such displays are appropriate for the results:

- Use horizontal bar charts to focus attention on how one category differs from another.
- Use vertical bar charts to focus attention on a change in a variable over time.
- Use cluster bar charts to contrast one variable among multiple subgroups.
- Use line graphs to plot data for several periods and show a trend over time.
- Use pie charts to show the distribution of a set of events or a total quantity.
- Use brownie pans (i.e. colored charts in rectangular or square form that display proportional amounts of data, similar to a pie chart) to show proportions of data (i.e. large versus medium versus small data amounts).
- Use pictographs (or pictograms) to show pictorial representations of data.

BOX

15.3

Focus On

What to Include in the Evaluation Report

Abstract/executive summary	Overview of the program and evaluation
	General discussion of results, conclusions, and recommendations
Introduction	Purpose of the evaluation
	Rationale or justification for the evaluation
	Program and participant description (including staff, materials, activities, procedures, etc.)
	Goals and objectives
	Evaluation questions
Methods/procedures	Design of the evaluation
	Priority population
	Instrumentation, including information on validity and reliability
	Sampling procedures
	Data collection procedures
	Pilot study results
	Data analyses procedures
Results	Description of findings from data analyses
	Answers to evaluation questions
	Explanation of findings
	Charts and graphs of findings
Discussion	Interpretation of results
	Conclusions about program effectiveness
	Limitations
	Program recommendations
	Determining if additional information is needed

If many tables or graphs are included, only the most relevant should be inserted in the text of the report with the remainder placed in an appendix. In addition, it should not be necessary to describe or explain elements of tables or graphs in detail in an evaluation report. In other words, these displays should be self-explanatory.

How and When to Present the Report

Evaluators must carefully consider the logistics of presenting the evaluation findings and should discuss this with the stakeholders involved in the evaluation. An evaluator may be in the position of presenting negative results, encountering distrust among staff members, or submitting a report that will never be read. Following are several suggestions for enhancing the evaluation report:

- Give key stakeholders advance information on the findings; this increases the likelihood that the information will be processed most appropriately. Avoid releasing any information to media outlets until all stakeholders have had an opportunity to read and discuss findings.
- Maintain anonymity (i.e. responses cannot be linked to a specific individual) and confidentiality (i.e. personal information of respondents is not released). Be sensitive to cultural norms in reporting data and ensure that individuals and populations involved in the evaluation study are not portrayed unfairly or unreasonably.
- Choose ways to report the evaluation findings so as to meet the needs of diverse stakeholders, and include information that is relevant to each group.

▷ Increasing Utilization of the Results

Far too often an evaluation will be conducted and a report submitted to the stakeholders without the recommendations being implemented. This occurs for a variety of reasons. Evaluators may not use findings because they are conducting the evaluation only to fulfill the requirements of the funding source, to serve their own self-interest, or to gain recognition for a successful program. If decision makers do not press those responsible for the program to make improvements, those implementing the program may not feel inclined to go to the trouble of making the necessary changes. Those who are given the evaluation results for their program may find that they are unable to make sense of the report due to language and concepts that are unfamiliar to them. Weiss (1984) developed the following guidelines to increase the chances that evaluation results will actually be used:

1. Plan the study with program stakeholders in mind and involve them in the planning process.
2. Continue to gather information about the program after the planning stage; a change in the program should result in a change in the evaluation.
3. Focus the evaluation on conditions about the program that the decision makers can change.
4. Write reports in a clear, simple manner and submit them on time. Use graphs and charts within the text and include complicated statistical information in an appendix.
5. Base the decision on whether to make recommendations on how specific and clear the data are, how much is known about the program, and whether differences between programs are obvious. A joint interpretation between evaluator and stakeholders may be best.
6. Disseminate the results to all stakeholders, using a variety of methods.
7. Integrate evaluation findings with other research and evaluation as they relate to the program focus.
8. Provide high-quality research.

Summary

Evaluation questions developed in the early program planning stages can be answered once the data have been analyzed. Descriptive statistics can be used to summarize or describe the data, and inferential statistics can be used to generate or test hypotheses and infer and transfer findings to the broader population. These statistics are generated by applying the appropriate univariate, bivariate, and/or multivariate analyses. Evaluators then interpret the data and present the results to the stakeholders via a formal or informal report.

Review Questions

1. What issues should be addressed to ensure an accurate evaluation?
2. What is meant by the term *data management*?
3. What is the difference between descriptive statistics and inferential statistics?
4. What is the difference between parametric data and non-parametric data?
5. What are some types of univariate data analyses used in evaluation? When would these be used?
6. How are bivariate and multivariate data analyses used in evaluation?
7. Explain the concepts of hypothesis testing, level of significance, Type I error, and Type II error.
8. What are the roles of evaluators and stakeholders in interpreting program results and making recommendations?
9. What is the difference between statistical significance and program significance?
10. What information is included in the written evaluation report? How is the information modified for various audiences?
11. What are some guidelines for presenting data in an evaluation report?
12. How can the evaluation report be enhanced?
13. How can the evaluator increase the likelihood of utilization of the evaluation findings?

Activities

1. Obtain an actual report from a program evaluation (perhaps in a data-based article in a scientific journal pertaining to health promotion). Look for the type of statistical tests used, level of significance, independent and dependent variables, interpretation of the findings, recommendations, and format for the report.
2. Discuss evaluation with a decision maker from a health agency. Find out what types of evaluation the agency conducted, who conducted them, what the findings were, whether the findings were implemented, and how the information was reported.
3. Compare an evaluation report with a research report (e.g., perhaps a peer-reviewed journal article). What are the similarities and differences? How could you improve the report?
4. Using data that you have generated or data presented by your instructor, create one table and one graph.

Weblinks

1. http://www.astho.org/

Association of State and Territorial Health Officials (ASTHO)

ASTHO is the national nonprofit organization representing the state and territorial public health agencies of the United States, the U.S. territories, and the District of Columbia. ASTHO's members are the chief health officials of these jurisdictions. At this site you can link to all the state and territorial public health agencies where you can find various examples of the presentation of health data using charts, graphs, and tables.

2. http://www.cancercontrol.cancer.gov/index.html

National Cancer Institute (NCI)

NCI's Website provides information on cancer control and population sciences, including evaluation/research reports on a number of cancer-related programs.

3. https://developers.google.com/chart/?hl=en

Google Charts

Google charts provides users with interactive charts and other data tools to represent evaluation elements described in this chapter.

4. http://www.cdc.gov/Learning/

Centers for Disease Control and Prevention (CDC Learning Connection)

This is a CDC Webpage where you can access information related to concepts described in this chapter.

5. http://www.cdc.gov/nchs/

National Center for Health Statistics (NCHS)

This Website is a rich source of information about America's health and provides many examples of the presentation of health data.

6. http://www.nhtsa.gov/

State Traffic Safety Information (STSI)

This is NHTSA's National Center for Statistical Analysis Website. STSI presents a state-by-state profile of traffic safety data and information including crash statistics, economic costs, legislation status, funding programs, and more. Here you will find examples of the presentation of health data using charts, graphs, and tables.

CODE OF ETHICS FOR THE HEALTH
EDUCATION PROFESSION

Preamble

The Health Education profession is dedicated to excellence in the practice of promoting individual, family, group, organizational, and community health. Guided by common goals to improve the human condition, Health Educators are responsible for upholding the integrity and ethics of the profession as they face the daily challenges of making decisions. Health Educators value diversity in society and embrace a multiplicity of approaches in their work to support the worth, dignity, potential, and uniqueness of all people.

The Code of Ethics provides a framework of shared values within the professions in which Health Education is practiced. The Code of Ethics is grounded in fundamental ethical principles including: promoting justice, doing good, and avoidance of harm. The responsibility of each health educator is to aspire to the highest possible standards of conduct and to encourage the ethical behavior of all those with whom they work.

Regardless of job title, professional affiliation, work setting, or population served, Health Educators should promote and abide by these guidelines when making professional decisions.

Article I: Responsibility to the Public

A Health Educator's responsibilities are to educate, promote, maintain, and improve the health of individuals, families, groups and communities. When a conflict of issues arises among individuals, groups, organizations, agencies, or institutions, health educators must consider all issues and give priority to those that promote the health and well-being of individuals and the public while respecting both the principles of individual autonomy, human rights, and equality.

Section 1

Health Educators support the right of individuals to make informed decisions regarding their health, as long as such decisions pose no risk to the health of others.

Section 2

Health Educators encourage actions and social policies that promote maximizing health benefits and eliminating or minimizing preventable risks and disparities for all affected parties.

Source: The Coalition of National Health Education Organizations, Ethics Task Force, September 30, 2015. www.cnheo.org /ethics.html. Reprinted by permission.

Section 3

Health Educators accurately communicate the potential benefits, risks, and/or consequences associated with the services and programs that they provide.

Section 4

Health Educators accept the responsibility to act on issues that can affect the health of individuals, families, groups, and communities.

Section 5

Health Educators are truthful about their qualifications and the limitations of their education, expertise, and experience in providing services consistent with their respective level of professional competence.

Section 6

Health Educators are ethically bound to respect, assure, and protect the privacy, confidentiality, and dignity of individuals.

Section 7

Health Educators actively involve individuals, groups, and communities in the entire educational process in an effort to maximize the understanding and personal responsibilities of those who may be affected.

Section 8

Health Educators respect and acknowledge the rights of others to hold diverse values, attitudes, and opinions.

Article II: Responsibility to the Profession

Health Educators are responsible for their professional behavior, for the reputation of their profession, and for promoting ethical conduct among their colleagues.

Section 1

Health Educators maintain, improve, and expand their professional competence through continued study and education; membership, participation, and leadership in professional organizations; and involvement in issues related to the health of the public.

Section 2

Health Educators model and encourage nondiscriminatory standards of behavior in their interactions with others.

Section 3

Health Educators encourage and accept responsible critical discourse to protect and enhance the profession.

Section 4

Health Educators contribute to the profession by refining existing and developing new practices, and by sharing the outcomes of their work.

Section 5

Health Educators are aware of real and perceived professional conflicts of interest, and promote transparency of conflicts.

Section 6

Health Educators give appropriate recognition to others for their professional contributions and achievements.

Section 7

Health educators openly communicate to colleagues, employers and professional organizations when they suspect unethical practice that violates the profession's Code of Ethics.

Article III: Responsibility to Employers

Health Educators recognize the boundaries of their professional competence and are accountable for their professional activities and actions.

Section 1

Health Educators accurately represent their qualifications and the qualifications of others whom they recommend.

Section 2

Health Educators use and apply current evidence-based standards, theories, and guidelines as criteria when carrying out their professional responsibilities.

Section 3

Health Educators accurately represent potential and actual service and program outcomes to employers.

Section 4

Health Educators anticipate and disclose competing commitments, conflicts of interest, and endorsement of products.

Section 5

Health Educators acknowledge and openly communicate to employers, expectations of job-related assignments that conflict with their professional ethics.

Section 6

Health Educators maintain competence in their areas of professional practice.

Section 7

Health Educators exercise fiduciary responsibility and transparency in allocating resources associated with their work.

Article IV: Responsibility in the Delivery of Health Education

Health Educators deliver health education with integrity. They respect the rights, dignity, confidentiality, and worth of all people by adapting strategies and methods to the needs of diverse populations and communities.

Section 1

Health Educators are sensitive to social and cultural diversity and are in accord with the law when planning and implementing programs.

Section 2

Health Educators remain informed of the latest advances in health education theory, research, and practice.

Section 3

Health educators use strategies and methods that are grounded in and contribute to the development of professional standards, theories, guidelines, data, and experience.

Section 4

Health Educators are committed to rigorous evaluation of both program effectiveness and the methods used to achieve results.

Section 5

Health Educators promote the adoption of healthy lifestyles through informed choice rather than by coercion or intimidation.

Section 6

Health Educators communicate the potential outcomes of proposed services, strategies, and pending decisions to all individuals who will be affected.

Section 7

Health educators actively collaborate and communicate with professionals of various educational backgrounds and acknowledge and respect the skills and contributions of such groups.

Article V: Responsibility in Research and Evaluation

Health Educators contribute to the health of the population and to the profession through research and evaluation activities. When planning and conducting research or evaluation, health educators do so in accordance with federal and state laws and regulations, organizational and institutional policies, and professional standards.

Section 1

Health Educators adhere to principles and practices of research and evaluation that do no harm to individuals, groups, society, or the environment.

Section 2

Health Educators ensure that participation in research is voluntary and is based upon the informed consent of the participants.

Section 3

Health Educators respect and protect the privacy, rights, and dignity of research participants, and honor commitments made to those participants.

Section 4

Health Educators treat all information obtained from participants as confidential unless otherwise required by law. Participants are fully informed of the disclosure procedures.

Section 5

Health Educators take credit, including authorship, only for work they have actually performed and give appropriate credit to the contributions of others.

Section 6

Health Educators who serve as research or evaluation consultants maintain confidentiality of results unless permission is granted or in order to protect the health and safety of others.

Section 7

Health Educators report the results of their research and evaluation objectively, accurately, and in a timely fashion to effectively foster the translation of research into practice.

Section 8

Health Educators openly share conflicts of interest in the research, evaluation, and dissemination process.

Article VI: Responsibility in Professional Preparation

Those involved in the preparation and training of Health Educators have an obligation to accord learners the same respect and treatment given other groups by providing quality education that benefits the profession and the public.

Section 1

Health Educators select students for professional preparation programs based upon equal opportunity for all, and the individual's academic performance, abilities, and potential contribution to the profession and the public's health.

Section 2

Health Educators strive to make the educational environment and culture conducive to the health of all involved, and free from all forms of discrimination and harassment.

Section 3

Health Educators involved in professional preparation and development engage in careful planning; present material that is accurate, developmentally and culturally appropriate; provide reasonable and prompt feedback; state clear and reasonable expectations; and conduct fair assessments and prompt evaluations of learners.

Section 4

Health Educators provide objective, comprehensive, and accurate counseling to learners about career opportunities, development, and advancement, and assist learners in securing professional employment or further educational opportunities.

Section 5

Health Educators provide adequate supervision and meaningful opportunities for the professional development of learners.

Approved by the Coalition of National Health Education Organizations February 8, 2011

Task Force Members:
Michael Ballard
Brian Colwell
Suzanne Crouch
Stephen Gambescia
Mal Goldsmith, Chairperson
Marc Hiller
Adrian Lyde
Lori Phillips
Catherine Rasberry
Raymond Rodriquez
Terry Wessel

HEALTH EDUCATION SPECIALIST PRACTICE
ANALYSIS (HESPA 2015)—RESPONSIBILITIES,
COMPETENCIES AND SUB-COMPETENCIES

The Seven Areas of Responsibility contain a comprehensive set of Competencies and Sub-competencies defining the role of the health education specialist. These Responsibilities, Competencies, and Sub-competencies were verified by the 2015 Health Education Specialist Practice Analysis (HESPA) project.

Coding:

No asterisk = Entry-level Sub-competency

* = Advanced–1 level Sub-competency

** = Advanced–2 level Sub-competency

Area I: Assess Needs, Resources, and Capacity for Health Education/Promotion

1.1 Plan assessment process for health education/promotion

1.1.1   Define the priority population to be assessed

1.1.2   Identify existing and necessary resources to conduct assessments

1.1.3   Engage priority populations, partners, and stakeholders to participate in the assessment process

1.1.4* Apply theories and/or models to assessment process

1.1.5   Apply ethical principles to the assessment process

1.2 Access existing information and data related to health

1.2.1   Identify sources of secondary data related to health

1.2.2* Establish collaborative relationships and agreements that facilitate access to data

1.2.3   Review related literature

1.2.4   Identify gaps in the secondary data

1.2.5   Extract data from existing databases

1.2.6   Determine the validity of existing data

1.3 Collect primary data to determine needs

1.3.1   Identify data collection instruments

1.3.2   Select data collection methods for use in assessment

1.3.3   Develop data collection procedures

1.3.4   Train personnel assisting with data collection

1.3.5   Implement quantitative and/or qualitative data collection

1.4 Analyze relationships among behavioral, environmental, and other factors that influence health

1.4.1   Identify and analyze factors that influence health behaviors

1.4.2   Identify and analyze factors that impact health

1.4.3   Identify the impact of emerging social, economic, and other trends on health

1.5 Examine factors that influence the process by which people learn

1.5.1   Identify and analyze factors that foster or hinder the learning process

1.5.2   Identify and analyze factors that foster or hinder knowledge acquisition

1.5.3   Identify and analyze factors that influence attitudes and beliefs

1.5.4   Identify and analyze factors that foster or hinder acquisition of skills

1.6 Examine factors that enhance or impede the process of health education/promotion

1.6.1   Determine the extent of available health education/promotion programs and interventions

1.6.2   Identify policies related to health education/promotion

1.6.3   Assess the effectiveness of existing health education/promotion programs and interventions

1.6.4   Assess social, environmental, political, and other factors that may impact health education/promotion

1.6.5   Analyze the capacity for providing necessary health education/promotion

1.7 Determine needs for health education/promotion based on assessment findings

1.7.1* Synthesize assessment findings

1.7.2   Identify current needs, resources, and capacity

1.7.3   Prioritize health education/promotion needs

1.7.4   Develop recommendations for health education/promotion based on assessment findings

1.7.5   Report assessment findings

Area II: Plan Health Education/Promotion

2.1 Involve priority populations, partners, and other stakeholders in the planning process

2.1.1   Identify priority populations, partners, and other stakeholders

2.1.2   Use strategies to convene priority populations, partners, and other stakeholders

2.1.3   Facilitate collaborative efforts among priority populations, partners, and other stakeholders

2.1.4   Elicit input about the plan

2.1.5   Obtain commitments to participate in health education/promotion

2.2 Develop goals and objectives

2.2.1   Identify desired outcomes using the needs assessment results

2.2.2   Develop vision statement

2.2.3   Develop mission statement

2.2.4   Develop goal statements

2.2.5   Develop specific, measurable, attainable, realistic, and time-sensitive objectives

2.3 Select or design strategies/interventions

2.3.1*   Select planning model(s) for health education/promotion

2.3.2*   Assess efficacy of various strategies/interventions to ensure consistency with objectives

2.3.3*   Apply principles of evidence-based practice in selecting and/or designing strategies/interventions

2.3.4   Apply principles of cultural competence in selecting and/or designing strategies/interventions

2.3.5   Address diversity within priority populations in selecting and/or designing strategies/interventions

2.3.6   Identify delivery methods and settings to facilitate learning

2.3.7   Tailor strategies/interventions for priority populations

2.3.8   Adapt existing strategies/interventions as needed

2.3.9*   Conduct pilot test of strategies/interventions

2.3.10*   Refine strategies/interventions based on pilot feedback

2.3.11   Apply ethical principles in selecting strategies and designing interventions

2.3.12   Comply with legal standards in selecting strategies and designing interventions

2.4 Develop a plan for the delivery of health education/promotion

2.4.1   Use theories and/or models to guide the delivery plan

2.4.2   Identify the resources involved in the delivery of health education/promotion

2.4.3   Organize health education/promotion into a logical sequence

2.4.4   Develop a timeline for the delivery of health education/promotion

2.4.5   Develop marketing plan to deliver health program

2.4.6   Select methods and/or channels for reaching priority populations

2.4.7   Analyze the opportunity for integrating health education/promotion into other programs

2.4.8*   Develop a process for integrating health education/promotion into other programs when needed

2.4.9   Assess the sustainability of the delivery plan

2.4.10   Design and conduct pilot study of health education/promotion plan

2.5 Address factors that influence implementation of health education/promotion

2.5.1   Identify and analyze factors that foster or hinder implementation

2.5.2   Develop plans and processes to overcome potential barriers to implementation

Area III: Implement Health Education/Promotion

3.1 Coordinate logistics necessary to implement plan

3.1.1   Create an environment conducive to learning

3.1.2   Develop materials to implement plan

3.1.3   Secure resources to implement plan

3.1.4   Arrange for needed services to implement plan

3.1.5   Apply ethical principles to the implementation process

3.1.6   Comply with legal standards that apply to implementation

3.2 Train staff members and volunteers involved in implementation of health education/promotion

3.2.1*   Develop training objectives

3.2.2   Recruit individuals needed for implementation

3.2.3*   Identify training needs of individuals involved in implementation

3.2.4*   Develop training using best practices

3.2.5*   Implement training

3.2.6*   Provide support and technical assistance to those implementing the plan

3.2.7*   Evaluate training

3.2.8*   Use evaluation findings to plan/modify future training

3.3 Implement health education/promotion plan

3.3.1   Collect baseline data

3.3.2*   Apply theories and/or models of implementation

3.3.3   Assess readiness for implementation

3.3.4   Apply principles of diversity and cultural competence in implementing health education/promotion plan

3.3.5   Implement marketing plan

3.3.6   Deliver health education/promotion as designed

3.3.7   Use a variety of strategies to deliver plan

3.4 Monitor implementation of health education/promotion

3.4.1   Monitor progress in accordance with timeline

3.4.2   Assess progress in achieving objectives

3.4.3   Ensure plan is implemented consistently

3.4.4   Modify plan when needed

3.4.5   Monitor use of resources

3.4.6   Evaluate sustainability of implementation

3.4.7   Ensure compliance with legal standards

3.4.8   Monitor adherence to ethical principles in the implementation of health education/promotion

Area IV: Conduct Evaluation and Research Related to Health Education/Promotion

4.1 Develop evaluation plan for health education/promotion

4.1.1*   Determine the purpose and goals of evaluation

4.1.2*   Develop questions to be answered by the evaluation

4.1.3*   Create a logic model to guide the evaluation process

4.1.4*   Adapt/modify a logic model to guide the evaluation process

4.1.5*   Assess needed and available resources to conduct evaluation

4.1.6*   Determine the types of data (for example, qualitative, quantitative) to be collected

4.1.7*   Select a model for evaluation

4.1.8*   Develop data collection procedures for evaluation

4.1.9** Develop data analysis plan for evaluation

4.1.10* Apply ethical principles to the evaluation process

4.2 Develop a research plan for health education/promotion

4.2.1**   Create statement of purpose

4.2.2**   Assess feasibility of conducting research

4.2.3**   Conduct search for related literature

4.2.4**   Analyze and synthesize information found in the literature

4.2.5**   Develop research questions and/or hypotheses

4.2.6**   Assess the merits and limitations of qualitative and quantitative data collection

4.2.7**   Select research design to address the research questions

4.2.8**   Determine suitability of existing data collection instruments

4.2.9**   Identify research participants

4.2.10** Develop sampling plan to select participants

4.2.11** Develop data collection procedures for research

4.2.12** Develop data analysis plan for research

4.2.13** Develop a plan for non-respondent follow-up

4.2.14** Apply ethical principles to the research process

4.3 Select, adapt and/or create instruments to collect data

4.3.1**   Identify existing data collection instruments

4.3.2**   Adapt/modify existing data collection instruments

4.3.3**   Create new data collection instruments

4.3.4   Identify useable items from existing instruments

4.3.5   Adapt/modify existing items

4.3.6**   Create new items to be used in data collection

4.3.7**   Pilot test data collection instrument

4.3.8**   Establish validity of data collection instruments

4.3.9** Ensure that data collection instruments generate reliable data

4.3.10** Ensure fairness of data collection instruments (for example, reduce bias, use language appropriate to priority population)

4.4 Collect and manage data

4.4.1** Train data collectors involved in evaluation and/or research

4.4.2** Collect data based on the evaluation or research plan

4.4.3 Monitor and manage data collection

4.4.4 Use available technology to collect, monitor and manage data

4.4.5 Comply with laws and regulations when collecting, storing, and protecting participant data

4.5 Analyze data

4.5.1** Prepare data for analysis

4.5.2* Analyze data using qualitative methods

4.5.3** Analyze data using descriptive statistical methods

4.5.4** Analyze data using inferential statistical methods

4.5.5** Use technology to analyze data

4.6 Interpret results

4.6.1** Synthesize the analyzed data

4.6.2** Explain how the results address the questions and/or hypotheses

4.6.3** Compare findings to results from other studies or evaluations

4.6.4** Propose possible explanations of findings

4.6.5** Identify limitations of findings

4.6.6** Address delimitations as they relate to findings

4.6.7** Draw conclusions based on findings

4.6.8** Develop recommendations based on findings

4.7 Apply findings

4.7.1 Communicate findings to priority populations, partners, and stakeholders

4.7.2 Solicit feedback from priority populations, partners, and stakeholders

4.7.3 Evaluate feasibility of implementing recommendations

4.7.4 Incorporate findings into program improvement and refinement

4.7.5** Disseminate findings using a variety of methods

Area V: Administer and Manage Health Education/ Promotion

5.1 Manage financial resources for health education/promotion programs

5.1.1* Develop financial plan

5.1.2* Evaluate financial needs and resources

5.1.3* Identify internal and/or external funding sources

5.1.4*   Prepare budget requests

5.1.5*   Develop program budgets

5.1.6*   Manage program budgets

5.1.7*   Conduct cost analysis for programs

5.1.8*   Prepare budget reports

5.1.9*   Monitor financial plan

5.1.10*   Create requests for funding proposals

5.1.11*   Write grant proposals

5.1.12*   Conduct reviews of funding proposals

5.1.13*   Apply ethical principles when managing financial resources

5.2 Manage technology resources

5.2.1   Assess technology needs to support health education/promotion

5.2.2   Use technology to collect, store and retrieve program management data

5.2.3   Apply ethical principles in managing technology resources

5.2.4   Evaluate emerging technologies for applicability to health education/promotion

5.3 Manage relationships with partners and other stakeholders

5.3.1   Assess capacity of partners and other stakeholders to meet program goals

5.3.2*   Facilitate discussions with partners and other stakeholders regarding program resource needs

5.3.3   Create agreements (for example, memoranda of understanding) with partners and other stakeholders

5.3.4   Monitor relationships with partners and other stakeholders

5.3.5*   Elicit feedback from partners and other stakeholders

5.3.6   Evaluate relationships with partners and other stakeholders

5.4 Gain acceptance and support for health education/promotion programs

5.4.1   Demonstrate how programs align with organizational structure, mission, and goals

5.4.2   Identify evidence to justify programs

5.4.3   Create a rationale to gain or maintain program support

5.4.4   Use various communication strategies to present rationale

5.5 Demonstrate leadership

5.5.1*   Facilitate efforts to achieve organizational mission

5.5.2   Analyze an organization's culture to determine the extent to which it supports health education/promotion

5.5.3   Develop strategies to reinforce or change organizational culture to support health education/promotion

5.5.4*   Facilitate needed changes to organizational culture

5.5.5*   Conduct strategic planning

5.5.6*   Implement strategic plan

5.5.7*   Monitor strategic plan

5.5.8   Conduct program quality assurance/process improvement

5.5.9   Comply with existing laws and regulations

5.5.10   Adhere to ethical principles of the profession

5.6 Manage human resources for health education/promotion programs

5.6.1*   Assess staffing needs

5.6.2*   Develop job descriptions

5.6.3*   Apply human resource policies consistent with laws and regulations

5.6.4*   Evaluate qualifications of staff members and volunteers needed for program

5.6.5   Recruit staff members and volunteers for programs

5.6.6*   Determine staff member and volunteer professional development needs

5.6.7*   Develop strategies to enhance staff member and volunteer professional development

5.6.8*   Implement strategies to enhance the professional development of staff members and volunteers

5.6.9*   Develop and implement strategies to retain staff members and volunteers

5.6.10* Employ conflict resolution techniques

5.6.11* Facilitate team development

5.6.12* Evaluate performance of staff members and volunteers

5.6.13* Monitor performance and/or compliance of funding recipients

5.6.14* Apply ethical principles when managing human resources

Area VI: Serve as a Health Education/Promotion Resource Person

6.1 Obtain and disseminate health-related information

6.1.1   Assess needs for health-related information

6.1.2   Identify valid information resources

6.1.3   Evaluate resource materials for accuracy, relevance, and timeliness

6.1.4   Adapt information for consumer

6.1.5   Convey health-related information to consumer

6.2 Train others to use health education/promotion skills

6.2.1*   Assess training needs of potential participants

6.2.2*   Develop a plan for conducting training

6.2.3*   Identify resources needed to conduct training

6.2.4*   Implement planned training

6.2.5*   Conduct formative and summative evaluations of training

6.2.6*   Use evaluative feedback to create future trainings

6.3 Provide advice and consultation on health education/promotion issues

6.3.1*   Assess and prioritize requests for advice/consultation

6.3.2*   Establish advisory/consultative relationships

6.3.3*   Provide expert assistance and guidance

6.3.4*   Evaluate the effectiveness of the expert assistance provided

6.3.5*   Apply ethical principles in consultative relationships

Area VII: Communicate, Promote, and Advocate for Health, Health Education/Promotion, and the Profession

7.1 Identify, develop, and deliver messages using a variety of communication strategies, methods, and techniques

7.1.1   Create messages using communication theories and/or models

7.1.2   Identify level of literacy of intended audience

7.1.3   Tailor messages for intended audience

7.1.4*   Pilot test messages and delivery methods

7.1.5*   Revise messages based on pilot feedback

7.1.6   Assess and select methods and technologies used to deliver messages

7.1.7   Deliver messages using media and communication strategies

7.1.8   Evaluate the impact of the delivered messages

7.2 Engage in advocacy for health and health education/promotion

7.2.1   Identify current and emerging issues requiring advocacy

7.2.2   Engage stakeholders in advocacy initiatives

7.2.3   Access resources (for example, financial, personnel, information, data) related to identified advocacy needs

7.2.4   Develop advocacy plans in compliance with local, state, and/or federal policies and procedures

7.2.5   Use strategies that advance advocacy goals

7.2.6   Implement advocacy plans

7.2.7   Evaluate advocacy efforts

7.2.8   Comply with organizational policies related to participating in advocacy

7.2.9   Lead advocacy initiatives related to health

7.3 Influence policy and/or systems change to promote health and health education

7.3.1   Assess the impact of existing and proposed policies on health

7.3.2   Assess the impact of existing and proposed policies on health education

7.3.3   Assess the impact of existing systems on health

7.3.4   Project the impact of proposed systems changes on health education

7.3.5   Use evidence-based findings in policy analysis

7.3.6*   Develop policies to promote health using evidence-based findings

7.3.7*   Identify factors that influence decision-makers

7.3.8*   Use policy advocacy techniques to influence decision-makers

7.3.9   Use media advocacy techniques to influence decision-makers

7.3.10   Engage in legislative advocacy

7.4 Promote the health education profession

7.4.1   Explain the major responsibilities of the health education specialist

7.4.2   Explain the role of professional organizations in advancing the profession

7.4.3   Explain the benefits of participating in professional organizations

7.4.4   Advocate for professional development of health education specialists

7.4.5   Advocate for the profession

7.4.6   Explain the history of the profession and its current and future implications for professional practice

7.4.7   Explain the role of credentialing (for example, individual, program) in the promotion of the profession

7.4.8   Develop and implement a professional development plan

7.4.9**   Serve as a mentor to others in the profession

7.4.10** Develop materials that contribute to the professional literature

7.4.11** Engage in service to advance the profession

Source: A competency-based framework for health education specialists—2015. Whitehall, PA: National Commission for Health Education Credentialing, Inc. (NCHEC) and the Society for Public Health Education (SOPHE). Reprinted by permission of the National Commission for Health Education Credentialing, Inc. (NCHEC) and the Society for Public Health Education (SOPHE).

accountability in a partnership arrangement, when each organization performs its work as previously arranged.

accounting the process of recording and summarizing transactions and interpreting their affects on the program budget (Fallon & Zgodzinski, 2012).

accuracy standards "ensure that the evaluation produces findings that are considered correct" (CDC, 1999c, p. 29); a standard of evaluation.

action research see *participatory research.*

action stage a stage of change in which a person has changed overt behavior for less than six months.

active participants those who take part in most group activities.

activities the intervention or strategies component of a logic model.

act of commission doing something you should not be doing.

act of omission not doing something you should be doing.

adjourning last stage of team development "in which teams complete their work and disband, if designed to do so" (Gomez-Mejia & Balkin, 2012, p. 391).

adjustment the process whereby planners make necessary changes to the program or its implementation based on feedback from participants and partners.

Administrative and Policy Assessment part of the fourth phase of PRECEDE-PROCEED, "an analysis of the policies, resources, and circumstances prevailing in an organizational situation to facilitate or hinder the development of the health program" (Green & Kreuter, 2005, p. G–1).

Advanced level 1-health education specialist "The practice level of a health education specialist with a minimum of a baccalaureate degree with professioinal preparation in the field of health education plus various combinations of degree (baccalaureate or master's) and years of experience" (NCHEC & SOPHE, 2015, p. 89).

Advanced level 2-health education specialist "The practice level of a health education specialist with a minimum of a doctoral degree in the field of health education, irrespective of years of experience" (NCHEC & SOPHE, 2015, p. 89).

advisory board see *planning committee.*

alpha level the level of statistical significance (usually set at 0.01 or 0.05).

alternative hypothesis the hypothesis that holds there is a difference between groups, treatments, or interventions.

analysis of variance (ANOVA) a statistical test used to study group differences when the dependent variables involved represent interval or ratio data.

anonymity exists when there is no link between personal information and the person's identity.

approaches refers to formative, process, and summative evaluation and suggests these types of evaluation are clearly distinct.

attitude objective those that describe the desired attitude of those in the priority population.

attitude toward the behavior "the degree to which performance of the behavior is positively or negatively valued" (Ajzen, 2006).

audit "review and confirmation that financial reports are accurate and that standard accounting procedures were used to prepare the reports" (Johnson & Breckon, 2007, p. 288).

aversive stimulus unpleasant consequence of a behavior.

awareness objective those that describe of what those in the priority population will become aware.

barriers things that keep people from obtaining the product or adopting a behavior.

baseline data data collected prior to program implementation to serve as a comparison with data collected during the program, or more typically, with data collected at the completion of a program.

basic priority rating (BPR) a model used to prioritize needs assessment data.

behavior change theories those that help to explain how behavior change takes place.

behavioral capability the knowledge and skills necessary to perform a behavior.

behavioral economics a method of analysis that applies psychological insights into economic decision making.

behavioral objective an impact objective that describes the action or behavior in which the priority population will engage.

beneficence doing good.

benefits value or outcome the priority population receives as a result of obtaining the product.

best experiences interventions from prior or existing programs of others that have not gone through the critical research and evaluation studies and thus fall short of best practice criteria but nonetheless show promise in being effective.

best practices "recommendations for an intervention, based on critical review of multiple research and evaluation studies that substantiate the efficacy of the intervention in the populations and circumstances in which the studies were done, if not its effectiveness in other populations and situations where it might be implemented" (Green & Kreuter, 2005, p. G–1).

best processes original intervention strategies that the planners create on their own based on their knowledge and skills of good planning processes.

bias a preference that inhibits impartiality.

bivariate data analysis analysis of two variables.

blind an evaluation wherein participants do not know if they belong to the experimental group or control group.

bottom up see *grassroots*.

BPR model 2. 0 an updated version of the basic priority rating (see *basic priority rating*).

budget a statement of the estimated revenues and expenditures with an itemized listing of the nature of each.

budget narrative a statement that explains the need for the costs in a budget and how the costs were estimated.

built environment "generally refers to an interdisciplinary area of focus that describes the design, construction, management, and land use of human-made surroundings as an interrelated whole, as well as their relationship to human activities over time" (Coupland et al., 2011, p. 6).

canned program one that has been developed by an outside group and includes the basic components and materials necessary to implement it.

capacity the individual, organizational, and community resources that enable a community to take action.

capacity building activities that enhance the resources of individuals, organizations, and communities to improve their effectiveness in taking action.

categorical funds those that are earmarked or dedicated to support programs aimed at a specific health problem or determinant (i.e., risk factor).

census everyone in a population.

CHANGE tool a program planning model created by the Centers for Disease Contol and Prevention to aid in the design and delivery of health community intiatives.

chi-square a statistical test that measures the association between two nominal and/or ordinal variables.

citizen initiated see *grassroots*.

cluster sampling a probability sample that selects participants from a sampling frame as groups not individuals.

coalition "a formal alliance of organizations that come together to work for a common goal" (Butterfoss, 2007, p. 30).

cognitive pretesting the process of "an interviewer asking the respondent about how she or he went about answering the survey question or completing a self-completion questionnaire" (Collins, 2003, p. 234).

collective efficacy the people's shared belief in their collective ability to act to produce specific changes.

communication channel route through which a message is delivered to a priority population.

community "a collective body of individuals identified by common characteristics such as geography, interests, experiences, concerns, or values" (Joint Committee on Health Education and Promotion Terminology, 2012, p. S10).

community advocacy a process in which the people of a community become involved in the institutions and decisions that will impact their lives.

community building "an orientation to practice focused on community, rather than a strategic framework or approach, and on building capacities, not fixing problems" (Minkler, 2012, p. 10).

community capacity "community characteristics affecting its ability to identify, mobilize, and address problems" (Minkler & Wallerstein, 2012, p. 45).

community context the general characteristics and circumstances that define a community.

community development a "process designed to create conditions of economic and social progress for the whole community with its active participation and fullest possible reliance on the community's initiative" (United Nations, 1955, p. 6).

community empowerment when community members control decision making.

community forum a process that brings people from the priority population to discuss problems and needs.

community organizing "the process by which community groups are helped to identify common problems or change targets, mobilize resources, and develop and implement strategies to reach their collective goals" (Minkler & Wallerstein, 2012, p. 37).

community participation bottom-up, grassroots mobilization of citizens for the purpose of undertaking activities to improve the condition of something in the community.

community readiness "the degree to which a community is willing and prepared to take action on an issue" (Tri-Ethnic Center for Prevention Research at Colorado State University, 2014, p. 4).

comparison group as part of a summative evaluation or research study, a nonequivalent group (not randomly selected) that does not receive the treatment or program but is compared with the experimental group.

Competency Update Project (CUP) a six-year, multiphase process carried out by the health education profession in order to reverify the role of the entry-level health educator and to distinguish it from the role of the advanced-level health educator.

competition alternative choices for filling a need; programs or products that send messages that conflict with the behaviors program planners are promoting.

concepts primary elements or the building blocks of a theory (Glanz et al., 2008b).

concurrent validity a form of criterion validity in which a new instrument and an established valid instrument that measure the same characteristics are given to the same population and the new instrument correlates positively with the established instrument.

conditions a major component of an objective that describes when or how the outcome will be observed.

confidentiality exists when there is a link between personal information and the person's identity but that information is protected from others.

confounding variable "one that has an unpredictable or unexpected impact on the dependent variable" (Cottrell & McKenzie, 2011, p. 324).

construct a concept developed, created, or adopted for use with a specific theory (Kerlinger, 1986).

construct validity "the degree to which a measure correlates with other measures it is theoretically expected to correlate with" (Valente, 2002, p. 161).

consumer-based a process that incorporates the wants, needs, and preferences of the priority population directly into interventions and implementation.

consumer orientation a dedicated effort to understand a priority population prior to developing an intervention and then keeping this knowledge at the center of all program planning decisions.

contemplation stage a stage of change in which a person intends to take action in the next six months.

content validity the "assessment of the correspondence between the items composing the instrument and the content domain from which the items were selected" (DiIorio, 2005, p. 213).

contest a challenge between two individuals/groups in which the object is to try to outperform the competitor.

context assesses the presence of any confounding factors.

contingencies what happens if the objectives in a behavior change contract are either met or not met.

continuum theory one that identifies variables that influence action and combine them into a prediction equation (Weinstein et al., 1998).

contract an agreement between two or more parties that outlines the future behavior of those parties.

control group as part of a summative evaluation or research study, a randomly selected group of individuals, similar to the experimental group that does not receive the treatment or program but is compared with the experimental group.

convergent validity "the extent to which two measures that purport to be measuring the same topic correlate (that is, converge)" (Bowling, 2005, p. 12).

correlation represents the strength and direction of relationships between two variables.

cost-benefit analysis (CBA) measures dollars spent on a program versus dollars saved or gained.

cost-effectiveness analysis (CEA) measures dollars spent on a program versus the impact achieved.

cost-identification analysis compares interventions to determine which is least expensive in the context of impact achieved.

criterion a major component of an objective that describes how much change will occur.

criterion-related validity the "extent to which data generated from a measurement instrument are correlated with the data generated from a measure (criterion) of the phenomenon being studied, usually an individual's behavior or performance" (Cottrell & McKenzie, 2011, p. 322).

critical path method (CPM) similar to PERT (see *PERT*) but focuses on total time to complete the tasks and the critical dependent tasks.

cultural audit an evaluation of the assumptions, values, normative philosophies, and cultural characteristics of an organization in order to determine whether they support or hinder that organization's central mission (Business Dictionary, 2015b).

cultural competence "a developmental process defined as a set of values, principles, behaviors, attitudes, and policies that enable health professionals to work effectively across racial, ethnic and linguistically diverse populations" (Joint Committee on Health Education and Promotion Terminology, 2012, p. 16).

culturally competent see *cultural competence*.

culturally sensitive relevant and acceptable within the cultural framework.

culture the "patterned ways of thought and behavior that characterize a social group, which are learned through socialization processes and persist through time" (Coreil, Bryant, & Henderson, 2001, p. 29).

curriculum "a planned set of lessons or courses designed to lead to competence in an area of study" (Gilbert et al., 2015, p. 437).

data management the process of organizing, coding, and cleaning data in a useable format for the purpose of analysis and reporting.

decision makers those who have the authority to approve a plan (e.g., administrator of an organization, governing board, chief executive officer).

decisional balance refers to the pros and cons of behavioral change.

deductive method applying a generally accepted principle to an individual case.

Delphi technique a "group process that generates a consensus through a series of questionnaires" (Gilmore, 2012, p. 82).

dependent variable an outcome variable or end result indicator in an evaluation or study.

descriptive statistics data used to organize, summarize, and describe characteristics of a group.

designs forms of different types of summative evaluation.

diffusion theory explains a pattern for how innovations (e.g., products) are adopted in a population.

direct cost the portion of cost that is directly expended in providing a product or service (VentureLine, 2015)

direct reinforcement consequence given in a specific situation to increase a behavior.

disability "often defined on the basis of specific activities of daily living, work and other functions essential to full participation in community-based living" (USDHHS, 2005, p. 4).

discriminant validity "requires that the construct should not correlate with dissimilar (discriminant) variables" (Bowling, 2005, p. 12).

disincentive consequence for not acting in a certain way; also used as a means to discourage the consumer from purchasing a product or behaving in a certain way.

doers those who are willing to take on work to complete a task.

dose the number of program units delivered.

double blind study an evaluation wherein neither participants nor those implementing the program know which group is experimental and which group is the control.

early adopters in diffusion theory, the second group of people to adopt the innovation; often comprised of opinion leaders.

early majority in diffusion theory, the people who are interested in the innovation, but will need external motivation to become involved.

ecological framework see *socio-ecological approach*.

educational and ecological assessment the third phase of PRECEDE-PROCEED wherein planners identify predisposing, reinforcing, and enabling factors that contribute to problems identified in earlier phases of the model.

effectiveness in evaluation, a measure usually associated with the outcomes of a program—that is, did the program result in changes in awareness, knowledge, attitudes, skills, or especially behavior, and did the program result in improved health status (e.g., less mortality, morbidity, and disability).

efficacy expectations people's competency feelings.

elaboration amount of cognitive processing people put into receiving messages.

emotional-coping responses dealing with sources of anxiety that surround a behavior.

empowerment "[s]ocial action process for people to gain mastery over their lives and the lives of their communities" (Minkler & Wallerstein, 2012, p. 45).

enabling factor "any characteristic of the environment that facilitates action and any skill or resource required to attain a specific behavior" (Green & Kreuter, 2005, p. G-3).

Entry-level health education specialist "The practice level of a health education specialist with a minimum of a baccalaureate degree with professioinal preparation in the field of health education" (NCHEC & SOPHE, 2015, p. 89).

environmental objective an impact objective that describes how the environments (e.g., economic, emotional, physical, political, service, social) around the priority population will change.

epidemiological assessment the second phase of PRECEDE-PROCEED, wherein planners identify specific health goals or problems that contribute to the social goals or problems identified in Phase 1; and "the identification of etiological factors, or determinants of health in the genetics, behavioral patterns, and environment of the population" (Green & Kreuter, 2005, pp. 11–12).

epidemiology "[t]he study of the occurrence and distribution of health-related events, states and processes in specific populations, including the study of determinants influencing such processes, and the application of this knowledge to control relevant health problems" (Porta, 2014, p. 95).

equivalence reliability focuses on whether different forms of the same instrument when measuring the same participants will produce similar results.

ethical issues situations where competing values are at play and program planners need to make a judgment about what is the most appropriate course of action.

evaluation the process of determining the value or worth of a health promotion program or any of its components based on predetermined criteria or standards of success identified by stakeholders.

evaluation approach see *approaches*.

evaluation consultant an external evaluator.

evaluation design see *designs*.

evidence a body of data that can be used to make decisions about planning.

Evidence-Based Planning Framework for Public Health a seven-phase model for evidence-based program planning.

evidence-based practice process of systematically finding, appraising, and using evidence as the basis for decision making when planning a health promotion program (Cottrell & McKenzie, 2011).

exchange process of the marketer providing a product and its benefits to the consumer in trade for the consumer paying a price.

executive participants core group who are committed to resolution of the concern.

expectancies values people place on an expected outcome.

expectations anticipation of certain outcomes from a certain behavior.

expenditure a cost incurred while planning, implementing, or evaluating a program.

experimental design random assignment to experimental and control groups with measurement of both groups.

experimental group as part of a summative evaluation or research study, a group of individuals that receives the treatment or intervention.

external audit one conducted by an independent qualified accountant usually just once a year (Businessdictionary.com, 2011a).

external evaluation evaluation conducted by an individual or organization not affiliated with the organization conducting the program.

external personnel individuals from outside the planning agency/organization or the priority population.

external validity extent to which the program can be expected to produce similar effects in other populations.

face validity if, on the face, a measure appears to measure what it is supposed to measure (McDermott & Sarvela, 1999).

feasibility standards "ensure that the evaluation is viable and pragmatic" (CDC, 1999a, p. 27); a standard of evaluation.

fidelity ensures that programs are implemented either as intended or as per protocol.

field study the most strenuous form of pilot testing in which people from the priority population assess the process being tested in a setting that is just like or closely represents the setting in which the program will be implemented.

financial management "the process of developing and using systems to ensure that funds are spent for the purposes for which they have been appropriated" (Klingner et al., 2010, p. 88).

fiscal accountability "refers to the need for sound accounting, careful documentation of expenses, and tracking or revenues" (Issel, 2014, p. 340).

fiscal year (or **funding year** or **FY**) 12 months of financial transactions typically running from either January 1st to December 31st or July 1st to June 30th.

flex time a system in which employees can vary their work schedule to meet their personal needs.

flexibility in terms of program planning, a process that is adapted to the needs of stakeholders.

fluidity in terms of program planning, a process that is sequential and logical in nature.

focus group an "exploratory process that is used for generating hypotheses, uncovering attitudes and opinions, and acquiring and testing new ideas" (Gilmore 2012, p. 118).

formative evaluation "any combination of measurements obtained and judgments made before or during the implementation of materials, methods, activities, or programs to control, assure or improve the quality of performance or delivery" (Green & Lewis, 1986, p. 362).

formative research a process that identifies differences among subgroups within a population, identifies a subgroup, determines the wants and needs of the subgroup, and identifies factors that influence its behavior, including benefits, barriers, and readiness to change (Bryant, 1998).

forming first stage of team development "which brings the team members together so they can get acquainted and discuss their expectations" (Gomez-Mejia & Balkin, 2012, p. 390).

Framework a shortened name for the *A Competency-Based Framework for Health Education Specialists—2015* (NCHEC & SOPHE, 2015).

full-time equivalent (FTE) a unit of measurement that is calculated by dividing the average number of hours a person works by the average number of hours worked by a full-time employee.

functionality in terms of program planning, an assurance that the outcome of planning is improved health conditions, not just the production of a program plan.

Gantt chart a program management charting method that provides a graphical illustration of the time frame for tasks to be completed and what has been completed to date.

gatekeepers those who control, both formally and informally, the political climate of a community.

generalizability extent to which a program can be expected to produce similar effects in other populations.

Generalized Model a program planning model that consists of five steps plus the quasi-step of pre-planning.

GINA (Genetic Information Nondiscrimination Act of 2008) (Public Law 110–233) amends portions of HIPAA by treating genetic information as protected health information, prohibits discrimination in health coverage and employment based on genetic information.

gifts sums of money or nonmonetary items that are given voluntarily without compensation.

goal a broad statement that describes the expected outcome of the program.

grant an award of financial assistance, the principal purpose of which is to transfer a thing of value from the grantor to a recipient to carry out a specific purpose.

grantsmanship the ability to write grant proposals that are funded.

grassroots the creation of "political movement" in which those within the community are responsible for the organizing.

grassroots participation "[b]ottom-up efforts of people taking collective actions on their own behalf, and they involve the use of a sophisticated blend of confrontation and cooperation in order to achieve their ends" (Perlman, 1978, p. 65).

Guide to Community Preventive Services (Community Guide) the Website that includes the Community Preventive Services Task Force's findings and the systematic reviews on which they are based.

hard money an ongoing source of funding that is part of the operating budget.

health advocacy "the processes by which the actions of individuals or groups attempt to bring about social and/or organizational change on behalf of a particular health goal, program, interest, or population" (Joint Committee on Terminology, 2012, p. S17).

health assessments (HAs) include instruments known as health risk appraisals/assessments (HRAs), health status assessments (HSAs), various lifestyle-specific assessment instruments, and wellness and behavioral/habit inventories (SPMBoD, 1999).

health behavior behaviors that impact a person's health.

health communication "the study and use of communication strategies to inform and influence individual and community decisions that affect health" (USDHHS, 2015a, para. 1).

health education "[a]ny combination of planned learning experiences using evidence-based practices and/or sound theories that provide the opportunity to acquire knowledge, attitudes, and skills needed to adopt and maintain healthy behaviors" (Joint Committee on Health Education and Promotion Terminology, 2012, p. S17).

health education specialist "[a]n individual who has met, at a minimum, baccalaureate-level required health education academic preparation qualifications, who serves in a variety of settings, and is able to use appropriate educational strategies and methods to facilitate the development of policies, procedures, interventions, and systems conducive to the health of individuals, groups, and communities" (Joint Committee on Health Education and Promotion Terminology, 2012, p. S18).

health impact assessment "a combination of procedures, methods, and tools by which a policy, program, or project may be judged as to its potential effects on the health of a population, and the distribution of those effects within the population" (ECHP, 1999).

HIPAA (Health Insurance Portability and Accountability Act of 1996) (Public Law 104–191) sets national standards that health plans, health care clearinghouses, and health care providers who conduct certain health care transactions electronically must implement to protect and guard against the misuse of individually identifiable health information.

health literacy "the capacity to obtain, process, and understand basic health information and services to make appropriate health decisions" (USDHHS, 2015b, para. 1).

health numeracy "the degree to which individuals have the capacity to access, process, interpret, communicate, and act on numerical, quantitative, graphical, biostatistical, and probabilistic health information needed to make effective health decisions" (Golbeck et al., 2005, p. 375).

health promotion "any planned combination of educational, political, environmental, regulatory, or organizational mechanisms that support actions and conditions of living conducive to the health of individuals, groups, and communities" (Joint Committee on Terminology, 2012, p. S19).

Healthy Communities Model a planning model that came from a movement that began in the 1980s with assistance from the World Health Organization to mobilize and empower partnerships within cities and communities to enhance health and well-being.

Healthy People U. S. government publication that brought together much of what was known about the relationship of personal health behavior and health status.

Healthy Plan-It a six-phase planning model developed by the Centers for Disease Control and Prevention in 2000 to strengthen in-country management training capacity in the health sector of developing countries.

impact evaluation "the immediate observable effects of a program leading to the intended outcomes of a program; intermediate outcomes" (Green & Lewis, 1986, p. 363).

impact objectives a category of objectives comprised of learning (i.e., awareness, knowledge, attitudes, and skills), behavioral, and environmental objectives.

implementation the "act of converting planning, goals, and objectives into action through administrative structure, management activities, policies, procedures, regulations, and organizational actions of new programs" (Timmreck, 1997, p. 328).

implementation science the study of how evidence-based interventions can be applied to sustain improvements to population health (Lobb & Colditz, 2013)

incentive reward for achieving a goal; also used as a means to entice the consumer to purchase the product or adopt a behavior.

inclusion ensures that the right partners are involved with a program.

independent variable a variable that is manipulated, selected, or measured by the evaluator that causes or exerts some influence on the dependent variable.

indirect cost the portion of cost that is indirectly expended in providing a product or service (VentureLine, 2015)

inductive method individual cases are studied to formulate a general principle.

inferential statistics data used to determine relationships and causality in order to make generalizations or inferences about a population based on findings from a sample.

influencers those who control resources to facilitate the planning and implementation of a program.

informed consent includes: (1) making the participants fully aware of the relevant information about the program (2) making sure the participants comprehend the information provided; and (3) obtaining the participants voluntary agreement, free of coercion and undue influence, to participate.

in-house materials educational materials developed by the program planners.

in-kind contributions nonmonetary gifts.

innovators in diffusion theory, the very first people to adopt the innovation.

inputs in a logic model, the resources that are used to plan, implement, and evaluate a program.

institutional review board (IRB) group of individuals with authority to grant or deny permission to conduct evaluation or research; it serves to safeguard the rights, privacy, health, and well-being of those involved in the research.

institutionalized imbedded in the organization so that it becomes sustained and durable.

instrumentation a "collective term that describes all measurement instruments used" (Cottrell & McKenzie, 2011, p. 326).

intention an "indication of a person's readiness to perform a given behavior, and it is considered to be the immediate antecedent of behavior" (Ajzen, 2006).

interaction can be defined in one of two ways: (1) in planning—the degree to which practitioners effectively work and communicate with program participants; (2) in evaluation—when participants in the control or comparison group interact and learn from the experimental group.

interactive contact methods data collection methods wherein those collecting the data interact with those from whom the data are being collected.

internal audit a frequent and ongoing audit conducted by an employee of the organization not responsible for the accounting practices (BusinessDictionary.com, 2011a).

internal consistency the intercorrelations among individual items on the instrument, that is, whether all items on the instrument are measuring part of the total area.

internal evaluation evaluation conducted by one or more individuals employed by, or in some other way affiliated with, the organization conducting the program.

internal personnel individuals from within the planning agency/organization or from within the priority population.

internal validity degree to which change that was measured can be attributed to the program under investigation.

inter-rater reliability rater reliability using two or more raters.

interval level measures measurement form that puts data into categories that are mutually exclusive, exhaustive, and rank ordered; furthermore, the distance between categories can be measured and there is no absolute zero.

intervention are the planned actions that are designed to prevent disease or injury or promote health in the priority population.

intervention alignment part of the fourth phase of PRECEDE-PROCEDE wherein planners match appropriate strategies and interventions with projected changes and outcomes identified in earlier phases (Green & Kreuter, 2005).

Intervention Mapping Model a six-phase program planning model guided by diagrams and matrices that incorporate outputs of the assessment process with relevant theory to help develop appropriate interventions for priority populations.

intra-rater reliability rater reliability that is established by a single rater.

justification provides assurance that programs are supported by key stakeholders.

key informants individuals with unique knowledge about a topic.

knowledge objective an impact objective that describes the information those in the priority population will learn.

laggards in diffusion theory, people who are not very interested in innovation and would be the last to adopt it.

lapse a single slip back to an old behavior while attempting a behavior change.

late majority in diffusion theory, the people who are interested in the innovation but are more skeptical and need external motivation to become involved.

learning objectives a sub-category of impact objectives composed of four levels: awareness, knowledge, attitudes, and skills.

lesson the amount of material that can be presented during a single educational encounter.

lesson plan the written outline of a lesson.

level of significance see *alpha level.*

levels of measurement a hierarchy of four measurement levels: nominal, ordinal, interval, and ratio.

likelihood of taking recommended preventive health action weighing the threat of disease against the difference between benefits and barriers.

literacy "the ability to use printed and written information to function in society, to achieve one's goals, and to develop one's knowledge and potential" (White & Dillow, 2005, p. 4).

literature the articles, books, and other documents that explain the past and current knowledge about a particular topic.

locus of control perception of the center of control over reinforcement.

logic model "a systematic and visual way to present and share your understanding of the relationships among the resources you have to operate your program, the activities you plan, and the changes or results you hope to achieve" (WKKF, 2004, p. 1).

macro practice methods of professional change that deal with issues beyond the individual, family, and small group level.

maintenance stage a stage of change in which a person has changed overt behavior for more than six months.

management "the process of working with and through others to achieve organizational or program objectives in an efficient and ethical manner" (Shi & Johnson, 2014, p. 658).

MAP-IT Model a planning guide or model used to assist communities in adapting *Healthy People 2020.*

MAPP Model Mobilizing for Action through Planning and Partnerships—a six-phase program planning model developed by the National Association of County and City Health Officials in 2001.

mapping the visual representation of data by geography or location, linking information to a place (Kirschenbaum & Russ, 2005).

mapping community capacity a process of identifying community assets.

market "the set of all people who have an actual or potential interest in a product or service" (Kotler & Clarke, 1987, p. 108).

marketing a "set of processes for creating, communicating, and delivering value to customers" (American Marketing Association, 2007).

marketing mix combination of the product, price, place, and promotion.

mean the arithmetic average of all scores in data analysis.

measurement the process of applying numerical or narrative data from an instrument or other data-yielding tools to objects, events, or people (Windsor, 2015).

measurement instrument the item used to measure the variables.

measures of central tendency forms of univariate data analysis involving the mean, median, and mode.

measures of spread or variation how spread out the scores are in the data set.

median the midpoint of all scores in data analysis.

memorandum of agreement (MOA) see *memorandum of understanding.*

memorandum of understanding (MOU) "a document that describes the general principles of an agreement between parties, but does not amount to a substantive contract" (Dictionary. com, 2015).

mission statement a short narrative that describes the purpose and focus of a program.

mode the score or response that occurs most frequently in data analysis.

model "is a composite, a mixture of ideas or concepts taken from any number of theories and used together" (Hayden, 2014, p. 2).

motivational interviewing "is a collaborative, person-centered form of guiding to elicit and strengthen motivation for change (Miller & Rollnick, 2009, p. 137)

multiple regression a statistical test that explores the relationships between multiple independent variables and one dependent variable.

multiplicity refers to the number of components or activities that make up an intervention.

multivariate data analysis analysis of more than two variables.

need the "difference between the present situation and a more desirable one" (Gilmore, 2012, p. 8).

needs assessment the process of identifying, analyzing, and prioritizing the needs of a priority population.

negative punishment removing a positive reinforcer to decrease a behavior.

negative reinforcement removing a negative reinforcer or aversive stimulus to increase a behavior.

negligence failing to act as a reasonable (prudent) person would.

networking interaction among individuals in order to share information.

news hook event that the media would want to cover.

no contact methods data collection methods wherein those collecting the data have no contact with those from whom the data are collected.

nominal group process a highly structured process in which a few knowledgeable representatives (5 to 7) are asked to qualify and quantify specific needs.

nominal level measures measurement form that puts data into categories that are mutually exclusive and exhaustive.

nonexperimental design use of pretest and posttest comparisons, or posttest analysis only, without a control group or comparison group.

nonmaleficence not causing harm.

non-parametric test a statistical test that does not depends upon assumptions about the parameters of the population distribution(s) from which the data were drawn.

nonprobability sample a sample in which all members of a survey population do not have an equal and known probability of being selected.

nonproportional stratified random sample a stratified random sample in which the sampling units are selected so that there is equal representation from the strata.

norming third stage of team development "characterized by resolution of conflict and agreement over team goals and values" (Gomez-Mejia & Balkin, 2012, p. 390).

null hypothesis the hypothesis that holds there is no difference between two groups, treatments, or interventions.

numeracy the ability to understand and work with numbers; quantitative literacy.

objectives precise statements of intended outcome (Gilbert, Sawyer, & McNeill, 2015).

observation "notice taken of an indicator" (Green & Lewis, 1986, p. 363).

obtrusive observation when people are aware they are being measured, assessed, or tested.

occasional participants those who become involved on an irregular basis and usually only when major decisions are made.

opinion leaders those who are well respected in a community and can accurately represent the views of the priority population.

ordinal level measures measurement form that put data into categories that are mutually exclusive, exhaustive, and rank ordered.

organizational culture the formal and informal policies of an organization that express the organization's values.

outcome a major component of an objective that describes what will change as a result of the program; also the intended results in a logic model.

outcome evaluation focuses on "an ultimate goal or product of a program or treatment, generally measured in the health field by mortality or morbidity data in a population, vital measures, symptoms, signs, or physiological indicators on individuals" (Green & Lewis, 1986, p. 364).

outcome expectations value placed on expected outcomes.

outcome objective an objective that describes the change in health status, social benefits, risk factors, or quality of life of the priority population.

outputs the direct results of the program activities or interventions in a logic model.

ownership a feeling that is derived from participating in the development of a program.

parallel (or **equivalent** or **alternate**) **forms** see *equivalence reliability.*

parametric test a statistical test that depends upon assumptions about the parameters of the population distribution(s) from which the data were drawn.

participation and relevance "community organizing that 'starts where the people are' and engages community members as equals" (Minkler & Wallerstein, 2012, p. 45).

participatory data collection members of the priority population participate in data collection.

participatory research has been "defined as systematic inquiry, with the collaboration of those affected by the issue being studied, for the purposes of education and of taking action or effecting change" (Mercer et al., 2008, p. 409).

partnering the association of two more entities working together on a project of common interest.

peer education a process wherein individuals are educated by others who have similar characteristics or standing as themselves.

penetration rate number in the priority population exposed or reached.

perceived barriers costs that must be overcome in order to follow a health recommendation.

perceived behavioral control perceived ease or difficulty of performing the behavior.

perceived benefits belief that a certain action could improve one's health.

perceived seriousness/severity belief that if a disease or condition were contracted it could be serious.

perceived susceptibility belief that one is vulnerable to a certain disease or condition.

perceived threat belief that one is vulnerable to a serious health problem or to the sequelae of that illness or condition.

performing fourth stage of team development "characterized by a focus on the performance of the tasks delegated to the team" (Gomez-Mejia & Balkin, 2012, p. 391).

phased in implementation of a program by limiting the number of people able to start the program at any given time.

photovoice those in the priority population are provided with cameras and skills training, then use the cameras to convey their own images of the community's problems and strengths.

pilot testing a set of procedures used to try out various processes during program development using a small group of participants prior to implementation.

place where the priority population has access to the product or where they may engage in the desired behavior.

PATCH an acronym for a planning process called Planned Approach to Community Health.

planning committee group of individuals who are responsible for creating a program and then overseeing its implementation and evaluation.

planning models those used for planning, implementing, and evaluating programs.

planning parameters the boundaries in which the planning committee must work when planning, implementing, and evaluating the program.

planning team see *planning committee.*

population as it relates to sampling, those in the universe specified by time or place.

population-based approach planning processes used with large populations.

positive punishment adding something to a situation that decreases a behavior.

positive reinforcement a consequence of a behavior that is enjoyable or makes a person feel good.

posttest testing components of a program, service, or product with the priority population after the completion of a program.

potential building blocks located resources originating outside the neighborhood and controlled by people outside.

PRECEDE-PROCEED Model (Predisposing, Reinforcing, Enabling Constructs in Ecological Diagnosis and Evaluation—Policy, Regulatory, and Organizational Constructs in Educational and Environmental Development) a widely known and robust eight-phase program planning model.

precontemplation stage a stage of change in which a person has no intentions to take action in the next six months.

predictive validity a form of criterion validity in which the measurement used will be correlated with another measurement of the same phenomenon at another time.

predisposing factor "any characteristic of a person or population that motivates behavior prior to the occurrence of the behavior" (Green & Kreuter, 2005, p. G-6).

pre-experimental design see *nonexperimental design.*

preliminary review a form of pilot testing in which colleagues of planners review a process being tested.

preparation stage a stage of change in which a person intends to take action in the next 30 days and has taken some behavioral steps in this decision.

pre-pilot a form of pilot testing in which five or six people from the priority population assess the process being tested.

pre-planning a process carried out prior to the formal planning process that allows a core group of people to gather answers to key planning questions.

pretest testing components of a program, service, or product with the priority population prior to implementation.

pretesting can be defined in one of two ways: (1) getting feedback from the priority population on products, messages, and materials before launching a social marketing campaign, and (2) collecting baseline data prior to program implementation that will be compared with posttest data to measure the effectiveness of programs.

price what the priority population gives up to obtain the product and its associated benefits.

primary building blocks assets located in the neighborhood and largely under the control of those who live in the neighborhood.

primary data original data collected by the planners.

primary prevention measures that forestall the onset of illness or injury during the prepathogenesis period.

priority population the people for whom the program is intended.

probability sample a sample in which all in the survey population have an equal and known probability of being selected.

process evaluation "is used to monitor and document program implementation and can aid in understanding the relationship between specific program elements and program outcomes" (Saunders, Evans, & Joshi, 2005, p. 134).

process objective an objective that expresses the tasks or activities to be carried out by the program planners.

processes of change a construct of the transtheoretical model that describes the covert and overt activities that people use to progress through the stages of change (Prochaska et al., 2008).

product something (e.g., goods, services, events, experiences, information, ideas, or behaviors) that fulfills a need customers have and provides a benefit they value; obtained for a price in the exchange.

profit margin the percent of financial gain after all the expenses are paid.

PERT acronym for Program Evaluation and Review Technique; a program management charting method that provides a graphical illustration of the time frame for tasks to be completed that includes three estimates of time—optimistic, pessimistic, and probabilistic.

program kickoff see *program launch*.

program launch the first day of program implementation.

program monitoring involves the ongoing collection and analysis of data and other information to determine if the program is operating as planned.

program ownership a feeling by those in the priority population that the program in part belongs to them.

program rollout see *program launch*.

program significance measures the meaningfulness of a program (based on stakeholder preferences) regardless of statistical significance.

promotion marketing communication strategy for letting a priority population know about a product and how to obtain or purchase it.

proportional stratified random sample a stratified random sample in which the sampling units are selected in the same proportion that the strata exist in the survey population.

proposal a formal written request for funding.

propriety standards "ensure that the evaluation is ethical" (CDC, 1999a, p. 27); a standard of evaluation.

proxy measure an outcome measure that provides evidence that a behavior has occurred.

prudent acting as a reasonable person would act in a given situation.

psychometric qualities an instrument's validity, reliability, and fairness.

public domain available for anyone to use without permission.

punishment any event that follows a behavior which decreases the probability that the same behavior will be repeated in the future.

qualitative data information presented in narrative form used in evaluation to provide detailed summaries or descriptions of observations, interactions, or verbal accounts (e.g., data from focus groups, in-depth interviews).

qualitative measures are "data collected with the use of narrative and observational approaches to understand individuals' knowledge, perceptions, attitudes and behaviors" (Harris, 2010 p. 208).

qualitative method an inductive method that produces narrative data.

quality in evaluation, a measure usually associated with how a program is implemented and what can be done to improve program delivery.

quantitative data information expressed in numerical terms that can be compared on scales.

quantitative measures "are numerical data collected to understand individuals' knowledge, understanding, perceptions, and behavior" (Harris, 2010, p. 208).

quantitative method a deductive method that produces numeric data.

quasi-experimental design use of a treatment group and a nonequivalent (nonrandomized) comparison group with measurement of both groups.

random selection a method of selecting participants in which all in the survey population have an equal chance or known probability of being selected.

random-digit dialing (RDD) a method of selecting participants using random combinations of numbers to call telephone numbers.

range the difference between the highest and lowest scores in data analysis.

rater (or observer) reliability associated with the consistent measurement (or rating) of an observed event by the same or different individuals (or judges or raters) (McDermott & Sarvela, 1999).

ratio level measures measurement form that puts data into categories that are mutually exclusive, exhaustive, and rank ordered; furthermore, the distance between categories can be measured and there is an absolute zero.

reach portion of the priority population that has an opportunity to participate in a program.

recidivism slipping back to an old behavior after attempting a behavior change.

reciprocal determinism behavior changes that result from the interaction between the person and the environment.

recruitment making those in the priority population aware of a program.

reforming a phase of team development when the team may continue on by refocusing its efforts on other tasks or problems.

reinforcement any event that follows a behavior which increases the probability that the same behavior will be repeated in the future (Skinner, 1953).

reinforcing factor "any reward or punishment following or anticipated as a consequence of a behavior, serving to strengthen the motivation for the behavior after it occurs" (Green & Kreuter, 2005, p. G–7).

relapse breakdown or failure in a person's attempt to change or modify a behavior (Marlatt & George, 1998).

relapse prevention a self-control program to help individuals to anticipate and cope with the problem of relapse in the behavior change process (Marlatt & George, 1998).

reliability "an empirical estimate of the extent to which an instrument produces the same result (measure or score), if applied two or more times" (Windsor, 2015, p. 196).

request for application (RFA) a formal statement that invites grant or cooperative agreement applications for a specific task.

request for proposal (RFP) a call made by funding agencies to alert individuals and organizations that it will receive and review grant proposals.

resources the "human, fiscal, and technical assets available" (Johnson & Breckon, 2007, p. 296) to plan, implement, and evaluate a program.

response ensuring that an adequate number of people participate in a program.

return on investment (ROI) "measures the costs of a program (i.e., the investment) versus the financial return realized by that program" (Cavallo, 2006, p. 1).

Role Delineation Project a comprehensive process that led to the creation of the responsibilities and competencies of the entry-level health educator.

sample a part of the whole.

sampling the process of selecting a sample.

sampling frame a list or quasi-list of all sampling units.

sampling unit an element or set of elements considered for selection as part of a sample (Babbie, 1992); for example, an individual, organization, or geographical area.

satisfaction approval after participation.

scope the breadth and depth of the material covered in a curriculum.

secondary building blocks assets located in the neighborhood but largely controlled by people outside.

secondary data those data that have been collected by someone else and are available for use by the planners.

secondary prevention measures that lead to early diagnosis and prompt treatment of a disease, illness, or injury to limit disability, impairment, or dependency and prevent more severe pathogenesis.

seed dollars funds designated to start up a new program or project.

segmentation process of identifying groups of consumers that share similar characteristics and will respond in a like way to a marketing strategy.

segmenting the act of segmentation.

self-assessments a process wherein an individual assesses himself or herself.

self-control gaining control over one's own behavior through monitoring and adjusting it.

self-efficacy people's confidence in their ability to perform a certain behavior or task.

self-regulation see *self-control*.

self-reinforcement reinforcing oneself for a behavior performed in an appropriate manner.

self-report when individuals or groups answer questions about themselves.

sensitivity "the ability of the test to identify correctly all screened individuals who actually have the disease [problem]" (Friis & Sellers, 2009, p. 422).

sequence order in which the content of a curriculum is presented.

significant other one who has an important relationship (e.g., friend, family member, partner, spouse) with another.

simple random sample (SRS) most basic process for selecting a random sample.

single-step survey a means of gathering data in which collectors obtain the data from individuals or groups with a single contact.

skill development objective an impact objective that describes the skill those in a priority population will be able to perform.

sliding-scale fee a fee structure based on one's ability to pay.

SMART Model (Social Marketing Assessment and Response Tool) a seven-phase social marketing planning model developed in 1998.

SMART objectives ones that are specific, measurable, achievable, realistic, and time-phased (CDC, 2003).

social assessment the first phase of PRECEDE-PROCEED wherein planners seek to subjectively define the quality of life (problems and priorities) of those in the priority population.

social capital "the processes and conditions among people and organizations that lead to their accomplishing a goal of mutual social benefit, usually characterized by interrelated consucts of trust, cooperation, civic engagement, and reciprocity, reinforced by networking" (Last, 2007, p. 347)

social context "is the sociocultural forces that shape people's day-to-day experiences and that directly and indirectly affect health and behavior (Burke et al., 2009, p. 56S).

social marketing the use of marketing principles to design programs that facilitate voluntary behavior change for the purpose of improved personal or societal well-being.

social math "the practice of translating statistics and other data so they become interesting to the journalist, and meaningful to the audience" (Dorfman et al., 2004, p. 112).

social media (or **interactive media**) any type media that uses the Internet and other technologies to enhance social interaction for shaing and discussing infomation.

social network "web of social relationships and the structural characteristics of that web" (IOM, 2001, p. 7).

social support a network of individuals that provides assistance or encouragement to a person who is engaging in a new behavior.

socio-ecological approach (or **ecological prespective**) recognizing that human beavior shapes and is shaped by multiple levels of influence.

soft money a source of funding that is not an ongoing part of an operating budget.

speakers' bureau a service offered by various groups with experts who are willing to present information to others.

specificity "the ability of the test to identify only nondiseased individuals who actually do not have the disease" (Friis & Sellers, 2009, p. 424).

stability reliability (test-retest reliability) estimate of consistency over a period of time (Crocker & Algina, 1986)

stage a step in the change process.

stage theory a theory composed of an ordered set of categories into which people can be classified, and for which factors could be identified that could induce movement from one category to the next (Weinstein & Sandman, 2002a).

stakeholders any person, community, or organization with a vested interest in a health program, usually decision makers, program partners, or clients.

standards of evaluation utility, feasibility, propriety, and accuracy (*see* definitions for each term in other parts of the glossary).

statistical significance "is a statement regarding the likelihood that observed variable values happened by chance" (Sharma & Petosa, 2014, p. 281).

steering committee see *planning committee*.

storming second stage of team development "in which team members voice differences about team goals and procedures" (Gomez-Mejia & Balkin, 2012, p. 390).

strata in terms of sampling, subgroups of the survey population.

strategy a general plan of action for affecting a health problem; it may encompass several activities (CDC, 2003).

stratified random sample a probability sample that first divides the survey population into strata and then randomly selects participants from each strata.

subjective norm "the perceived social pressure to engage or not to engage in a behavior" (Ajzen, 2006).

SAM (suitability assessment of materials) an instrument that can be used to determine the suitability of educational of materials.

summative evaluation "any combination of measurements and judgments that permit conclusions to be drawn about impact, outcome or benefits of a program or method" (Green & Lewis, 1986, p. 366).

support ensures that programs have appropriate built-in reinforcement components to assist participants with the expected level of involvement and/or behavior change.

supporting participants those who are seldom involved but help to swell the ranks of a program and may contribute in nonactive ways or through financial contributions.

survey population in terms of sampling, those in the universe specified by time or place, and who are accessible.

SWOT (Strengths, Weaknesses, Opportunities, and Threats) an approach to planning that minimizes planning time and moves quickly to action steps by assessing internal strengths and weaknesses as well as external opportunities and threats, usually displayed in a 2×2 matrix.

systematic sample a probability sample that selects participants from a sampling frame by taking every Nth person after a random start.

tailoring "any combination of information or change strategies intended to reach one specific person, based upon characteristics that are unique to that person, related to the outcome of interest, and have been derived from an individual assessment" (Kreuter & Skinner, 2000, p. 1).

task development time line a program management charting method that provides a graphical illustration of the time frame for tasks to be completed.

task force "a self-contained group of 'doers' that is not ongoing. It is convened for a narrow purpose over a defined timeframe at the request of another body or committee" (Butterfoss, 2013, p. 7).

team "a small group of people with complementary skills who are committed to a common purpose, a set of performance goals, and an approach for which they hold themselves mutually accountable" (Gomez-Mejia & Balkin, 2012, p. 384).

technical assistance (or **technical support** or **capacity building assistance**) a relationship in which individuals with specific knowledge and skills share them, via advice and training, with those who need them.

technical resources (or **other resources**) includes all other resources besides human or financial.

temptation "the intensity of urges to engage in a specific behavior when in difficult situations" (Prochaska et al., 2008, p. 102).

termination a stage of change in which a person who has changed a behavior has zero temptation to return to the old behavior.

tertiary prevention measure aimed at rehabilitation following significant pathogenesis.

test–retest reliability see *stability reliability*.

theory "a set of interrelated concepts, definitions, and propositions that presents a *systematic* view of events or situations by specifying relations among variables in order to *explain* and *predict* the events of the situations" (Glanz et al., 2008b, p. 26).

three Fs of program planning fluidity, flexibility, and functionality (*see* definitions for each term in other parts of the glossary).

treatment see *intervention*.

triple blind study an evaluation wherein neither the participants, nor those implementing the program, nor the evaluators, know which group is experimental and which group is the control.

t-test a statistical test involving interval or ratio data that assesses whether the means of two groups are statistically different from each other.

Type I error rejecting the null hypothesis when it is actually true.

Type II error failing to reject the null hypothesis when it is, in fact, not true.

Type III error failure to implement the health education intervention properly (Basch et al., 1985).

unit plan "an orderly, self-contained collection of activities educationally designed to meet a set of objectives" (Gilbert et al., 2015, p. 202).

univariate data analysis analysis of one variable.

universe as it relates to sampling, all those unspecific by time and place.

unobtrusive observation when people are not aware they are being measured, assessed, or tested.

utility standards "ensure that the information needs of evaluation users are satisfied" (CDC, 1999a, p. 27); a standard of evaluation.

validity whether an instrument correctly measures what it is intended to measure.

variable a construct, characteristic, or attribute that can be measured or observed.

vendors those who sell their products to program planners.

vicarious reinforcement observation of another being reinforced.

vision statement a description of where a program will be in the future.

volunteers those who serve an organization or cause without pay or compensation.

walk-through an observation completed by walking through an area at various times on different days looking for indicators of health.

windshield tour an observation completed by driving through an area at various times on different days looking for indicators of health.

REFERENCES

Abroms, L. C., & Maibach, E. W. (2008). The effectiveness of mass communication to change public behavior. *Annual Review of Public Health, 28,* 219–234.

Airhihenbuwa, C. O., Cottrell, R. R., Adeyanju, M., Auld, M. E., Lysoby, L., & Smith, B. J. (2005). The national health educator competencies update project: Celebrating a milestone and recommending next steps for the profession. *American Journal of Health Education, 36*(6), 361–370.

Aitaoto, N., Tsark, J., & Braun, K. L. (2009). Sustainability of the pacific diabetes today coalitions. *Preventing Chronic Disease, 6*(4), 1–8. Retrieved July 16, 2015, from http://www.cdc.gov/pcd/issues/2009/oct/08_0181.htm

Ajzen, I. (1988). *Attitudes, personality, and behavior.* Chicago: Dorsey Press.

Ajzen, I. (2006). *Theory of planned behavior.* Retrieved June 9, 2015, from http://www.people.umass.edu/aizen/tpb.html

Alexander, G. (1999). Health risk appraisal. In G. C. Hyner, K. W. Peterson, J. W. Travis, J. E. Dewey, J. J. Foerster, & E. M. Framer (Eds.), *SPM handbook of health assessment tools* (pp. 5–8). Pittsburgh, PA: Society of Prospective Medicine.

Allen, J., & Hunnicutt, D. (2007) A new way of thinking: Examining strategies for gaining leadership support for health promotion. *Absolute Advantage, 6*(2), 14–17. Retrieved March 19, 2011, from http://www.welcoa.org/freeresources/index.php?category=8

Allen, R. S., Phillips, M. A., Whitehead, D., Crowther, M. R., & Prentice-Dunn, S. (2009). Living well with living wills: Application of protection motivation theory to living will execution among older adults. *Clinical Gerontologist, 32,* 44–59.

Alvarez, C. M., Dickson, P. R., & Hunter, G. K. (2014). The four faces of the Hispanic consumer: An acculturation-based segmentation. *Journal of Business Research, 67*(2), 108–115.

American Association for Health Education (AAHE), National Commission for Health Education Credentialing, Inc. (NCHEC), & Society for Public Health Education (SOPHE). (1999). *A competency-based framework for graduate-level health educators.* Reston, VA: Authors.

American Cancer Society (ACS). (2009). *Workplace Solutions: Creating a culture of health.* Retrieved May 13, 2011, from http://www.cancer.org/aboutus/drlensblog/post/2009/06/23/workplace-solutions-creating-a-culture-of-health.aspx

American Cancer Society (ACS). (2015). *Learn about cancer.* Retrieved May 23, 2015, from http://www.cancer.org/cancer/index.

American College of Sports Medicine (ACSM). (2014). *ACSM's guidelines for exercise testing and prescription* (9th ed.). Philadelphia, PA: Lippincott, Williams, & Wilkins.

American Congress of Obstetricians and Gynecologists (ACOG). (2009). *Exercise during pregnancy and the postpartum period.* Retrieved July 31, 2015, from http://www.acog.org/Resources-And-Publications/Committee-Opinions/Committee-on-Obstetric-Practice/Exercise-During-Pregnancy-and-the-Postpartum-Period.

American Psychological Association (APA). (2015). *PsycINFO.*®Retrieved May 21, 2015, from http://www.apa.org/pubs/databases/psycinfo/index.aspx

Ammary-Risch, N. J., Zambon, A., & Brown, K. M. (2010). Communicating health information effectively. In C. I. Fertman, & D. D. Allensworth (Eds.), *Health promotion programs: Theory to practice* (pp. 203–231). San Francisco: Jossey-Bass.

Andreasen, A. R. (1995). *Marketing social change. Changing behavior to promote health, social development, and the environment.* San Francisco: Jossey-Bass.

Angus, K., Cairns, G., Purves, R., Bryce, S., MacDonald, L., & Gordon, R. (2013). *Systematic literature review to examine the evidence for the effectiveness of interventions that use theories and models of behavior change: Towards the prevention and control of communicable diseases.* Stockholm, Sweden: European Centre for Disease Prevention and Control. Retrieved June 13, 2015, from http://ecdc.europa.eu/en/publications/Publications/health-communication-behaviour-change-literature-review.pdf

Anspaugh, D. J., Dignan, M. B., & Anspaugh, S. L. (2000). *Developing health promotion programs.* Boston, MA: McGraw-Hill.

Arkin, E. B. (1990). Opportunities for improving the nation's health through collaboration with the mass media. *Public Health Reports, 105*(3), 219–223.

Asharf, N. (2013, April). Rx: Human nature—How behavioral economics is promoting better health around the world. *Harvard Business Review,* 1–7.

Auld, M. E., Radius, S. M., Galer-Unti, R., Hinman, J. M., Gotsch, A. R., & Mail, P. D. (2011). Distinguishing between health education and health information dissemination. *American Journal of Public Health, 101*(3), 390–391.

Babbie, E. (1992). *The practice of social research* (6th ed.) Belmont, CA: Wadsworth Publishing Company.

Bagozzi, R. P. (1975). Marketing as exchange. *Journal of Marketing, 39,* 32–39.

Baker, E. A., Brownson, R. C., Dreisinger, M., McIntosh, L. D., & Karamehic-Muratovic, A. (2009). Examining the role of training in evidence-based public health: A qualitative study. *Health Promotion Practice, 10*(3), 342–348.

Bandura, A. (1977). *Social learning theory.* Englewood Cliffs, NJ: Prentice Hall.

Bandura, A. (1982). Self-efficacy: Mechanism in human agency. *American Pyschologist, 37*(2), 122–147.

Bandura, A. (1986). *Social foundations of thought and action.* Englewood Cliffs, NJ: Prentice Hall.

Bandura, A. (1991). Social learning theory of self-regulation. *Organizational behavior and human decision making, 50,* 248–287.

Bandura, A. (1997). *Self-efficacy: The exercise of control.* New York, NY: W. H. Freeman.

Bandura, A. (2001). Social cognitive theory: An agentic perspective. *Annual Review of Psychology, 52,* 1–26.

Baranowski, T. (1985). Methodologic issues in self-report of health behavior. *Journal of School Health, 55*(5), 179–182.

Baranowski, T., Perry, C. L., & Parcel, G. S. (2002). How individuals, environments, and health behavior interact. In K. Glanz, B. K. Rimer, & F. M. Lewis (Eds.), *Health behavior and health education: Theory, research, and practice* (3rd ed., pp. 165–184). San Francisco, CA: Jossey-Bass.

Baric, L. (1993). The settings approach—Implications for policy and strategy. *Journal of the Institute of Health Education, 31,* 17–24.

Barnes, J. A. (1954). Class and committees in a Norwegian island parish. *Human Relations, 7,* 39–58.

Barnes, M. D., Neiger, B. L., & Thackeray, R. (2003). Health communication. In R. J. Bensley & J. Brookins-Fisher (Eds.), *Community health education methods* (2nd ed., pp. 51–82). Boston, MA: Jones & Bartlett.

Barnett, K. (2012). Best practices for community health needs assessment and implementation strategy: A review of scientific methods, current practices, and future potential. *Report of proceedings from a public forum and interviews of experts convened by the Centers for Disease Control and Prevention.* Oakland, CA: The Public Health Insitute. Retrieved May 22, 2015, from http://www.phi.org/uploads/application /files/dz9vh55o3bb2x56lcrzyel83fwfu3mvu24 oqqvn5z6qaeiw2u4.pdf

Bartholomew, L. K., Parcel, G. S., Kok, G., Gottlieb, N. H., & Fernandez, M. E. (2011). *Planning health promotion programs: An intervention mapping approach* (3rd ed.). San Francisco, CA: Jossey-Bass.

Bartol, K. M., & Martin, D. C. (1991). *Management.* New York, NY: McGraw-Hill.

Basch, C. E., Sliepcevich, E. M., Gold, R. S., Duncan, D. F., & Kolbe, L. J. (1985). Avoiding Type III errors in health education program evaluations: A case study. *Health Education Quarterly, 12*(3), 315–331.

Bates, I. J., & Winder, A. E. (1984). *Introduction to health education.* Palo Alto, CA: Mayfield.

Beck, A. T., Steer, R. A., & Carbin, M. G. (1988). Psychometric properties of the Beck Depression Inventory: Twenty-five years of evaluation. *Clinical Psychology Review, 8*(1), 77–100.

Becker, M. H. (Ed.). (1974). The health belief model and personal health behavior. *Health Education Monographs, 2* (entire issue).

Becker, M. H., Drachman, R. H., & Kirscht, J. P. (1974). A new approach to explaining sick-role behavior in low income populations. *American Journal of Public Health, 64*(March), 205–216.

Becker, S. J. (2015). Direct-to-consumer marketing: A complementary approach to traditional dissemination and implementation efforts for mental health and substance abuse interventions. *Clinical Psychology: Science and Practice, 22*(1), 85–100.

Behrens, R. (1983). *Work-site health promotion: Some questions and answers to help you get started.* Washington, DC: Office of Disease Prevention and Health Promotion.

Belch, G. E., & Belch, M. A. (2015). *Advertising and promotion. An integrated marketing communications perspective* (10th ed.). New York: McGraw-Hill Irwin Education.

Bennett, G. G., & Glasgow, R. E. (2009). The delivery of public health interventions via the Internet: Actualizing their potential. *Annual Review of Public Health, 30,* 273–392.

Bensley, L. B. (2009). Using theory and ethics to guide method selection and application. In R. J. Bensley & J. Brookins-Fisher (Eds.) *Community health education methods: A practical guide* (3rd ed., pp. 3–30.). Sudbury, MA: Jones & Bartlett.

Beyer, K. M. M., & Rushton, G. (2009). Mapping cancer for community engagement. *Preventing Chronic Disease, 6*(1), A03.

Bhatt, S. (2006, December 13). Taxi stand provides place for tipsy to get cabs. *Seattle Times*.

Binkley, C., & Johnson, K. (2013). Application of the Precede-Proceed planning model in designing an oral health strategy. *Journal of Theory and Practice of Dental Public Health, 1*(3). Retrieved June 10, 2015, from http://www.ncbi.nlm.nih.gov/pmc/articles/PMC4199385/

Block, L. E. (2008). Health policy: What it is and how it works. In C. Harrington, & C. L. Estes (Eds.), *Health policy: Crisis and reform in the U.S. health care delivery system* (5th ed., pp. 4–14). Sudbury, MA: Jones & Bartlett.

Blumberg, S. J., & Luke, J. V. (2010). *Wireless substitution: Early release of estimates from the National Health Interview Survey, January–June 2014*. National Center for Health Statistics. Retrieved May 20, 2015, from: http://www.cdc.gov/nchs/data/nhis/earlyrelease/wireless201412.pdf.

Blumberg, S. J., & Luke, J. V. (2010). *Wireless substitution: Early release of estimates from the National Health Interview Survey, January–June 2010*. National Center for Health Statistics. Retrieved March 30, 2011, from: http://www.cdc.gov/nchs/nhis.htm.

Blumberg, S. J., Luke, J. V., Ganesh, N., Davern, M. E., Boudreaux, M. H., & Soderberg, K. (2011). Wireless substitution: State-level estimates from the National Health Interview Survey, January 2007–June 2010. *National Health Statistics Report, 39*, 1–28.

Bockarjova, M., & Steg, L. (2014). Can protection motivation theory predict pro-environmental behavior? Explaining the adoption of electric vehicles in the Netherlands. *Global Environmental Change 28*, 276–288.

Boeka, A., Prentice-Dunn, S., & Lokken, K. (2010). Psychosocial predictors of weight loss and intentions to comply with post-surgical guidelines following bariatric surgery. *Psychology, Health, and Medicine, 15*, 188–197.

Borg, W. R. & Gall, M. D. (1989). *Educational research: An introduction* (5th ed.). New York, NY: Longman.

Boston Univerity School of Public Health. (2013). *Behavior change models*. Retrieved on June 15, 2015, from http://sphweb.bumc.bu.edu/otlt/MPH-Modules/SB/SB721-Models/SB721-Models.html

Bowling, A. (2005). *Measuring health: A review of quality of life measurement scales* (3rd ed.). New York, NY: Open University Press.

Bradshaw, T., Lovell, K., Bee, P., & Campbell, M. (2010). The development and evaluation of a complex health education intervention for adults with a diagnosis of schizophrenia. *Journal of Psychiatric and Mental Health Nursing, 17*(6), 473–486.

Brager, G., Specht, H., & Torczyner, J. L. (1987). *Community organizing*. New York: Columbia University Press.

Braithwaite, R. L., Murphy, F., Lythcott, N., & Blumenthal, D. S. (1989). Community organization and development for health promotion within an urban black community: A conceptual model. *Health Education, 20*(5), 56–60.

Breen, M. (1999). Researching grants on the Internet. *Community Health Center Management,* March/April, 29.

Brennan Ramirez, L. K., Baker, E. A., & Metzler, M. (2008). *Promoting health equity: A resource to help communities address social determinants of health*. Atlanta: Centers for Disease Control and Prevention. Retrieved May 19, 2015, from http://www.cdc.gov/nccdphp/dch/programs/healthycommunitiesprogram/tools/pdf/SDOH-workbook.pdf

Breslow, L. (1999). From disease prevention to health promotion. *Journal of the American Medical Association, 281*(11), 1030–1033.

Bronfenbrenner, U. (1979). *The ecology of human development*. Cambridge, MA: Harvard University Press.

Brown, L. D., Feinberg, M. E., & Greenberg, M. T. (2012). Measuring coalition functioning: Refining constructs through factor analysis. *Health Education & Behavior, 39*(4), 486–497.

Brown-Connolly, N. E., Concha, J. B., & English, J. (2014). Mobile health is worth it! Economic benefit and impact on health of a population-based mobile screening program in New Mexico. *Telemedicine and e-Health, 20*(1), 18–23.

Brown-Johnson, C. G., England, L. J., Glantz, S. A., & Ling, P. M. (2014). Tobacco industry marketing to low socioeconomic status women in the USA. *Tobacco Control*. Advance online publication. doi:10.1136/tobaccocontrol-2014-051602

Brownson, R. C., Baker, E. A., Leet, T. L., Gillespie, K. N., & True, W. R. (2011). *Evidence-based public health* (2nd ed.). New York, NY: Oxford University Press.

Brownson, R. C., Chriqui, J. F., & Stamatakis, K. A. (2009). Understanding evidence-based public health policy. *American Journal of Public Health, 99*(9), 1576–1583.

Brownson, R. C., Diez Roux, A. V., Swartz, K. (2014). Commentary: Generating rigorous evidence for public health: The need for new thinking to improve research and practice. *Annual Review of Public Health, 35*, 1–7.

Brownson, R. C., Fielding, J. E., & Maylahn, C. M. (2009). Evidence-based public health: A fundamental concept for public health practice. *Annual Review of Public Health, 30*, 175–201.

Brownson, R. C., Haire-Joshu, D., & Luke, D. A. (2006). Shaping the context of health: A review of environmental and policy approaches in the prevention of chronic diseases. *Annual Review of Public Health, 27,* 341–370.

Bryan, R. L., Kreuter, M. W., & Brownson, R. C. (2009). Integrating adult learning principles into training for public health practice. *Health Promotion Practice, 10*(4), 557–563.

Bryant, C. (1998, June). *Social marketing: A tool for excellence.* Eighth annual conference on social marketing in public health. Clearwater Beach, FL.

Bryant, C., Forthofer, M., McCormack-Brown, K., Landis, D., & McDermott, R. J. (2000). Community-based prevention marketing: The next steps in disseminating behavior change. *American Journal of Health Behavior, 24*(1), 61–68.

Buckner, A., Ndjakani, Y., Banks, B. & Blumenthal, D. (2010). Using service-learning to teach community health: The Morehouse School of Medicine community health course. *Academic Medicine, 85*(10), 1645–1651.

Bui, L., Mullan, B., & McCaffrey, K. (2013). Protection motivation theory and physical activity in the general population: A systematic literature review. *Pyschology, Health & Medicine, 18*(5), 522–542.

Burke, N. J., Joseph, G., Pasick, R. J., & Barker, J. C. (2009). Theorizing social context: Rethinking behavioral theory. *Health Education & Behavior, 36*(Suppl. 1), 55S–70S.

BusinessDictionary.com (2015a). *Audit, external audit, internal audit.* Retrieved July 29, 2015, from http://www.businessdictionary.com/definition/audit.html

BusinessDictionary.com (2015b). *Cultural audit.* Retrieved July 2, 2015, from http://www.business dictionary.com/definition/cultural-audit.html

Butterfoss, F. D. (2007). *Coalitions and partnerships in community health.* San Francisco: Jossey-Bass.

Butterfoss, F. D. (2009). Building and sustaining coalitions. In R. J. Bensley & J. Brookins-Fisher (Eds.), *Community health education methods: A practical guide* (3rd ed., pp. 299–331). Sudbury, MA: Jones & Bartlett.

Butterfoss, F. D. (2013). *Ignite! Getting your community coalition "fired up" for change.* Bloomington, IN: AuthorHouse.

Butterfoss, F. D., & Kegler, M. C. (2012). A coalition model for community action. In M. Minkler (Ed.), *Community organizing and community building for health and welfare* (3rd ed., pp. 309–328). New Brunswick, NJ: Rutgers University Press.

Capwell, E. M., Butterfoss, F., & Francisco, V. T. (2000). Why evaluate? *Health Promotion Practice, 1*(1), 15–20.

Catalani, C., & Minkler, M. (2010). Photovoice: A review of the literature in health and public health. *Health Education & Behavior, 37*(3) 424–451.

Cavallo, D. (2006). Using return on investment analysis to evaluate health promotion programs: Challenges and opportunities. *Health Promotion Economics, 1*(3), 1–4. Retrieved May 13, 2015, from http://www.rti.org/

Centers for Disease Control and Prevention. U.S. Department of Health and Human Services. (n.d.a). *Planned approach to community health: Guide for local coordinator.*

Centers for Disease Control and Prevention. (n.d.b). Summary of the Internal Revenue Service's April 5, 2013, notce of proposed rule making on community health needs assessments for charitable hospitals. Retrieved May 19, 2015 from http://www.cdc.gov /phlp/docs/summary-irs-rule.pdfAtlanta, GA: Author. Retrieved July 27, 2015, from http://www. lgreen.net/patch.pdf

Centers for Disease Control and Prevention. (1999a). Framework for program evaluation in public health. *Morbidity and Mortality Weekly Report, 48*(RR-11), 1–40.

Centers for Disease Control and Prevention. (1999b). Ten great public health achievements—United States, 1900–1999. *Morbidity and Mortality Weekly Report, 48*(12), 241–243.

Centers for Disease Control and Prevention. (2000). *Healthy plan-it: A tool for planning and managing public health programs. Sustainable Management Development Program.* Atlanta, GA: Author.

Centers for Disease Control and Prevention. (2001). *Ten Great Public Health Achievements in the 20th Century.* Retrieved May 8, 2015, from http://www .cdc.gov/about/history/tengpha.htm

Centers for Disease Control and Prevention. (2003). *CDCynergy 3.0: Your guide effective health communication* (CD ROM Version 3.0). Atlanta, GA: Author.

Centers for Disease Control and Prevention. (2006). *What is GIS?* Retrieved May 22, 2015, from http:// www.cdc.gov/gis/whatis.htm

Centers for Disease Control and Prevention. (2008a). Data collection methods for program evaluation: Focus groups. *Evaluation Briefs,* No. 13. Retrieved on May 21, 2015, from http:// www.cdc.gov/HealthyYouth/evaluation/pdf/ brief13.pdf

Centers for Disease Control and Prevention. (2008b). Integrating the strategic plan, logic model, and work plan. *Evaluation Briefs,* No. 5. Retrieved on July 29, 2015, from http://www.cdc.gov/ HealthyYouth/evaluation/pdf/brief5.pdf

Centers for Disease Control and Prevention (CDC). (2009a). *Simply put.* Retrieved August 25, 2015, from http://www.cdc.gov/healthliteracy/pdf /Simply_Put.pdf

Centers for Disease Control and Prevention. (2009b). Writing SMART objectives. *Evaluation Briefs,* No. 3b. Retrieved on June 2, 2015, from http://www.cdc.gov/HealthyYouth/evaluation/ pdf/brief3b.pdf

Centers for Disease Control and Prevention (2010a). *Community health assessment and group evaluation action guide: Building a foundation of knowledge to prioritize community needs.* Atlanta: U.S. Department of Health and Human Services.

Centers for Disease Control and Prevention (CDC). (2010b). *Logic model.* Retrieved July 28, 2015, from http://www.cdc.gov/nccdphp/dnpao/hwi/programdesign/logic_model.htm

Centers for Disease Control and Prevention (CDC). (2011a). *Gateway to health communication & social marketing practice.* Retrieved June 22, 2015, from http://www.cdc.gov/HealthCommunication/HealthBasics/WhatIsHC.html

Centers for Disease Control and Prevention (CDC). (2011b). *The health communicator's social media toolkit.* Retrieved June 24, 2015, from http://www.cdc.gov/healthcommunication/ToolsTemplates/SocialMediaToolkit_BM.pdf

Centers for Disease Control and Prevention. (2011c). *Introduction to program evaluation for public health programs: A self-study guide.* Retrieved July 28, 2015, from: http://www.cdc.gov/eval/guide/cdcevalmanual.pdf

Centers for Disease Control and Prevention (CDC). (2012a). *CDC's guide to writing for social media.* Retrieved June 24, 2015, from http://www.cdc.gov/socialmedia/Tools/guidelines/pdf/GuidetoWritingforSocialMedia.pdf

Centers for Disease Control and Prevention (CDC). (2012b). *National diabetes prevention program.* Retrieved May 13, 2015, from http://www.cdc.gov/diabetes/prevention/newsroom/overview.htm

Centers for Disease Control and Prevention (CDC). (2013). *Health Education Curriculum Anaysis Tool (HECAT).* Retrieved July 20, 2015, from http://www.cdc.gov/HealthyYouth/HECAT/

Centers for Disease Control and Prevention (CDC). (2014a). *2014 national diabetes statistics report.* Retrieved May 13, 2015, from http://www.cdc.gov/diabetes/data/statistics/2014StatisticsReport.html

Centers for Disease Control and Prevention (CDC). (2014b). *Social media at CDC: Data & metrics.* Retrieved June 22, 2015, from http://www.cdc.gov/SocialMedia/Data/index.html

Centers for Disease Control and Prevention (CDC). (2014c). *Workplace health promotion.* Retrieved March 20, 2011, from http://www.cdc.gov/workplacehealthpromotion/

Centers for Disease Control and Prevention (CDC). (2015a). *Behavioral Risk Factor Surveillence System.* Retrieved September 3, 2015, from http://www.cdc.gov/brfss/

Centers for Disease Control and Prevention (CDC). (2015b). *Chronic disease overview.* Retrieved May 9, 2015, from http://www.cdc.gov/chronicdisease/overview/index.htm.

Centers for Disease Control and Prevention (CDC). (2015c). *The Guide to community preventive services.* Retrieved May 14, 2015, from http://www.thecommunityguide.org/index.html

Centers for Disease Control and Prevention (CDC). (2015d). *Health impact assessment.* Retrieved May 23, 2015, from http://www.cdc.gov/healthyplaces/hia.htm

Centers for Disease Control and Prevention. (2015e). *Life Expectancy.* Retrieved May 9, 2015, from http://www.cdc.gov/nchs/fastats/life-expectancy.htm

Centers for Disease Control and Prevention (CDC). (2015f). *Public health economics and tools.* Retrieved May 13, 2015, from http://www.cdc.gov/stltpublichealth/pheconomics/

Centers for Disease Control and Prevention (CDC). (2015g). *Smoking & tobacco use: Fast facts.* Retrieved May 13, 2015, from http://www.cdc.gov/tobacco/data_statistics/fact_sheets/fast_facts/

Centers for Medicare & Medicaid Services. (2015a). *FAQS about Afforable Care Act implementation (part XXV).* Retrieved May 24, 2015, from https://www.cms.gov/CCIIO/Resources/Fact-Sheets-and-FAQs/Downloads/Tri-agency-Wellness-FAQS-4-16-15pdf-AdobeAcrobat-Pro.pdf

Centers for Medicare & Medicaid Services. (2015b). *National health expenditures 2013 highlights.* Retrieved May 24, 2015, from http://www.cms.gov/Research-Statistics-Data-and-Systems/Statistics-Trends-and Rports/NationalHealthExpendData/downloads/highlights.pdf

Central Intelligence Agency (CIA). (2015). *The world factbook.* Retrieved May 9, 2015, from https://www.cia.gov/library/publications/resources/the-world-factbook/

Chambers, D. A. & Kerner, J. F. (2007, March 27). Closing the gap between discovery and delievery. Prresented at the Dissemination and Implementsation Research Workshop: Harnessing Science to Maximize Health. Rockville, MD,: National Institutes for Health. Retrieved May 14, 2015, from http://cancercontrol.cancer.gov/IS/dissemination_implement_rw.html

Champion, V. L., & Skinner, C. S (2008). *The health belief model.* In K. Glanz, B. K. Rimer, & K. Viswanath (Eds.), *Health behavior and health education: Theory, research, and practice* (4th ed., pp. 45–65). San Francisco: Jossey-Bass.

Chang, S. J., Choi, S., Kim, S-A., & Song, M. (2014). Intervention strategies based on information-motivation-behavioral skills model for health behavior change: A ststematic review. *Asian Nursing Research, 8*(3), 172–181.

Chaplin, J. P., & Krawiec, T. S. (1979). *Systems and theories of psychology* (4th ed.). New York: Holt, Rinehart & Winston.

Chapman, L. S. (1997). Securing support from top management. *The Art of Health Promotion, 1*(2), 1–7.

Chapman, L. S. (2003). Biometric screening in health promotion: Is it really as important as we think? *The Art of Health Promotion, 7*(2), 1–12.

Chapman, L. S. (2005). Incentives: An introduction and story–Part I. *Absolute Advantage, 4*(7), 1–46. Retrieved March 19, 2011, from http://www.welcoa.org/freesources/pdf/index.php?category=8

Chapman, L. S. (2006). Planning wellness: Getting off to a good start–Part I. *Absolute Advantage, 5*(4), 1–87. Retrieved March 19, 2011, from http://www.welcoa.org/freesources/pdf/index.php?category=8

Chapman, L. S. (2009). Building a sustainable administrative infrastructure for worksite wellness programs. *The Art of Health Promotion, 24*(12), 1–11.

Chapman, L. S. (2012). Meta-evaluation of worksite health promotion economic return studies. *The Art of Health Promotion, March/April*, 1–11.

Chapman, L. S., Lesch, N., & Baun, M. P. (2007). The role of health and wellness coaching in worksite health promotion. *American Journal of Health Promotion, 21*(6), suppl. 1–10.

Chapman, L. S., Whitehead, D., & Connors, M. C. (2008). The changing role of incentives in health promotion and wellness. *The Art of Health Promotion, 23*(11), 1–12.

Checkoway, B. (1989). Community participation for health promotion: Prescription for public policy. *Wellness Perspectives: Research, Theory and Practice, 6*(1), 18–26.

Chen, H. T. (2015). *Theory-driven evaluation and the integrated evaluation perspective* (2nd ed.). Thousand Oaks, CA: Sage Publications, Inc.

Clark, N. M., Friedman, A. R., & Lachance, L. L. (2006). *Summing it up: Collective lessons from the experience of seven coalitions, 7*(2), 149S–152S.

Clark, N. M., Janz, N. K., Dodge, J. A., & Sharpe, P. A. (1992). Self-regulation of health behavior: The "take PRIDE" program. *Health Education Quarterly, 19*(3), 341–354.

Cleary, M. J., & Neiger, B. L. (1998). *The certified health education specialist: A self-study guide for professional competency* (3rd ed.). Allentown, PA: National Commission for Health Education Credentialing.

Clow, K. E., & Baack, D. (2014). *Integrated advertising, promotion and marketing communications* (6th ed.). Upper Saddle River, NJ: Pearson.

Coalition of National Health Education Organizations (CNHEO). (n.d.). *Code of ethics for the health education profession.* Retrieved July 31, 2015, from http://cnheo.org/ethics.html

Cohen, J. (1960). A coefficient of agreement for nominal scales. *Educational and Psychological Measurement, 20*(1), 37–46.

Cohen, J. T., Neumann, P. J., & Weinstein, M. C. (2008). Does preventive care save money? Health economics and the presidential candidates. *The New England Journal of Medicine, 358*(7), 661–663.

Cole, R., & Horacek, T. (2009). Applying Precede-Proceed to develop an intuitive eating nondieting approach to weight management pilot program. *Journal of Nutrition Education and Behavior, 41*(2), 120–126.

Collins, D. (2003). Pretesting survey instruments: An overview of cognitive methods. *Quality of Life Research, 12*(3), 229–238.

Community Preventive Services Task Force (2006 & 2007). *Assessment of health risks with feedback to change emoployees' health.* Retrieved May 21, 2015, from http://www.thecommunityguide.org/worksite/ahrf.html

Cook, T. D., & Campbell, D. T. (1979). *Quasi-experimentation: Design and analysis issues for field settings.* Boston: Houghton Mifflin.

Cottrell, R. R., Girvan, J. T., McKenzie, J. F., & Seabert, D. M. (2015). *Principles and foundations of health promotion and education* (6th ed.). San Francisco: Pearson.

Cottrell, R. R., & McKenzie, J. F. (2011). *Health promotion and education research methods: Using the five-chapter thesis/dissertation model* (2nd ed.). Sudbury, MA: Jones & Bartlett.

Coupland, K. Rikhy, S. Hill, K., & McNeil, D. (2011). *State of evidence: The built environment and health 2011–2015.* Alberta, Canada: Public Health Innovation and Decision Support, Population, & Public Health, Alberta Health Services.

Courtney, A. (2004). Using community-based prevention marketing to promote physical activity among teens. *Social Marketing Quarterly, 10*, 3-4, 58–61.

Cowdery, J. E., Wang, M. Q., Eddy, J. M., & Trucks, J. K. (1995). A theory-driven health promotion program in a university setting. *Journal of Health Education, 26*(4), 248–250.

Cozby, P. C. (1985). *Methods in behavioral research* (3rd ed.). Palo Alto, CA: Mayfield.

Craig, C. L., Marshall, A. A., Sjöström, M., Bauman, A. E. Booth, M. L., Ainsworth, B. E., Pratt, M., Ekelund, U., Yngve, A., Sallis, J. F., & Oja, P. (2003).

International physical activity questionnaire: 12-country reliability and validity. *Medicine & Science in Sports & Exercise, 35*(8), 1381–95

Creswell, J. W. (2002). Educational research: Planning, conducting and evaluating quantitative and qualitative research. Merrill Prentice Hall: Upper Saddle River, NJ.

Crocker, L., & Algina, J. (1986). *Introduction to classical and modern test theory.* Orlando, FL: Holt, Rinehart and Winston,

Crosby, R. A., Kegler, M. C., & DiClemente, R. J. (2009). Theory in health promotion practice and research. In R. J. DiClemente, R. A. Crosby, & M. C. Kegler (Eds.), *Emerging theories in health promotion practice and research* (2nd ed., pp. 4–17). San Francisco: Jossey-Bass.

Crosby, R. A., Salazar, L. E., & DiClemente, R. J. (2013). How theory informs health promotion and public health practice. In R. J. DiClemente, L. E., Salazar, & R. A. Crosby, *Health behavior theory for public health: Principles, foundations, and applications* (pp. 27–44). Burlington, MA: Jones & Bartlett Learning.

Cummings, C., Gordon, J. R., & Marlatt, G. A. (1980). Relapse: Prevention and prediction. In W. R. Miller (Ed.), *Addictive behaviors* (pp. 291–322). Oxford, U.K.: Pergamon Press.

Dane, F. C. (1990). Research methods. Pacific Grove, CA: Brooks/Cole Publishing Company.

Datta, J., & Petticrew, M. (2013). Challenges to evaluating complex interventions: A content analysis of published papers. *BMC Public Health, 13,* 568. doi:10.1186/1471-2458-13-568

Davidson, A. (2015). *Social determinats of health: A comparative approach.* Ontario, Canada: Oxford University Press.

Davis, P. C., & Rankin, L. L. (2006). Guidelines for making existing health education programs more culturally appropriate. *American Journal of Health Education, 37*(4), 250–252.

Dedhia, R. C., Smith, K. J., Weissfeld, J. L., Saul, M. I., Lee, S. C., Myers, E. N., & Johnson, J. T. (2011). Cost-identification analysis of total laryngectomy: An itemized approach to hospital costs. *Otolaryngology Head Neck Surgery, 144*(2), 220–224.

Deeds, S. G. (1992). *The health education specialist: Self-study for professional competence.* Los Alamitos, CA: Loose Canon.

Della, L. J., DeJoy, D. M., Goetzel, R. Z., Ozminkowski, R. J., & Wilson, M. G. (2008). Assessing management support for worksite health promotion: Psychometric analysis of the leading by example (LBE) instrument. *American Journal of Health Promotion, 22*(5), 359–367.

Della, L. J., DeJoy, D. M., Mitchell, S. G., Goetzel, R. Z., Roemer, E. C., & Wilson, M. G. (2010). Management support of workplace health promotion. Field test of the leading by example tool. *American Journal of Health Promotion, 25*(2), 138–146.

Dessler, G. (2012). *Fundamentals of human resource management* (2nd ed.). Boston: Prentice Hall.

Devito-Staub, G. (2014). *Constructing a cardiac health risk profile: Building the foundation for a community cardiac wellness program for the city of Twinsburg, Ohio.* Retrieved June 10, 2015, from http://www.usfa.fema.gov/pdf/efop/efo48512.pdf

DiClemente, R. J., Crosby, R. A., & Kegler, M. (2009). *Emerging theories in health promotion practice and research* (2nd ed.). San Francisco: Jossey-Bass.

DiClemente, R. J., Salazar, L. E., & Crosby, R. A. (2013). *Health behavior theory for public health: Principles, foundations, and applications.* Burlington, MA: Jones & Bartlett Learning.

Dictionary.com. (2015). *Memorandum of understanding.* Retrieved July 20, 2015, from http://dictionary.reference.com/browse/memorandum%20of%20understanding?&o=100074&s=t

Dietrich, T., Rundle-Thiele, S., Leo, C., & Connor, J. (2015). One size (never) fits all: Segment differences observed following a school-based alcohol social marketing program. *Journal of School Health, 85*(4), 251–259.

Dignan, M. B. (1995). *Measurement and evaluation of health education* (3rd ed.). Springfield, IL: Charles C. Thomas.

DiIorio, C. K. (2005). *Measurement in health behavior.* San Francisco, CA: Jossey-Bass.

Dishman, R. K., Sallis, J. F., & Orenstein, D. R. (1985). The determinants of physical activity and exercise. *Public Health Reports, 100*(2), 158–171.

Doak, C. C., Doak, L. G., & Root, J. H. (1996). *Teaching patients with low literacy skills* (2nd ed.). Philadelphia, PA: J. B. Lippincott.

Doll, L. S., Bonzo, S. E., Mercy, J. A., & Sleet, D. A. (Eds.). (2007). *Handbook of injury and violence prevention.* New York, NY: Springer.

Dorfman, L., Woodruff, K., Herbert, K., & Ervice, J. (2004). *Making the case for early care and education: A message development guide for advocates.* Berkeley, CA: Berkeley Media Studies Group. Retrieved March 28, 2011, from http://www.bmsg.org/documents/YellowBookrev.pdf.

Downey, L. H., Ireson, C. L., & Scutchfield, F. D. (2009). The use of photovoice as a method of facilitating deliberation. *Health Promotion Practice, 10*(3), 419–427.

Drum, C. E., Peterson, J. J., Culley, C., Krahn, G., Heller, T., Kimpton, T., McCubbin, J., Rimmer, J., Seekins, T., Suzuki, R., & White, G. W. (2009). Guidelines and criteria for the implementation of community-based health promotion programs for individuals with disabilities. *American Journal of Health Promotion, 24*(2), 93–101.

Dunn, W. N. (1994). *Public policy analysis: An introduction*. Englewood Cliffs, NJ: Prentice Hall.

Edberg, M. (2015). *Essentials of health behavior: Social and behavioral theory in public health* (2nd ed.). Burlington, MA: Jones & Bartlett Learning.

Edwards, P. J., Robersts, I, Clarke, M. J. Diguiseppi, C., Wentz, R., Kwan, I Cooper, R, Felix, L. M., & Pratap, S. (2009). Methods to increase response to postal and electronic questions. *Cochrane Database Systematic Review, July 8*(3), MR000008.

Edwards, R. W., Jumper-Thurman, P., Plested, B. A., Oetting, E. R., & Swanson, L. (2000). Community readiness: Research to practice. *Journal of Community Psychology, 28*(3), 291–307.

Eng, E., & Blanchard, L. (1990–91). Action-oriented community diagnosis: A health education tool. *International Quarterly of Community Health Education, 11*(2), 96–97.

Erfurt, J. C., Foote, A., Heirich, M. A., & Gregg, W. (1990). Improving participation in worksite wellness: Comparing health education classes, a menu approach, and follow-up counseling. *American Journal of Health Promotion, 4*(4), 270–278.

Erickson, W., Lee, C., & von Schrader, S. (2015). *Disability statistics from the 2013 American Community Survey (ACS)*. Ithaca, NY: Cornell University Employment and Disability Institute (EDI). Retrieved July 31, 2015, from http://www.disabilitystatistics.org

Estrada, C., Martin-Hryniewicz, M., Peek, B. T., Collins, C., & Byrd, J. C. (2004). Literacy and numeracy skills and anticoagulation control. *American Journal of Medical Science, 328*, 88–93.

Fallon, L. F., & Zgodzinski, E. J. (2012). *Essentials of public health management* (3rd ed.). Sudbury, MA: Jones & Bartlett Learning.

Fernander, A. F., Rayens, M. K., Adkins, S., & Hahn, E. J. (2014). Local smoke-freee public policies, quitline call rate, and smoking status in Kentucky. *American Journal of Health Promotion, 29*(2), 123–126.

Fernandez, M., Gonzales, A., Tortolero-Luna, G., Partida, S., & Bartholomew, L. (2005). Using intervention mapping to develop a breast and cervical cancer screening program for Hispanic farmworkers: Cultivando la salud. *Health Promotion Practice, 6*(4), 394–404.

Fertman, C. I., Spiller, K. A., & Mickalide, A. D. (2010). Developing and increasing program funding. In C. I. Fertman & D. Allenworth (Eds.), *Health promotion programs: From theory to practice* (pp. 233–255). San Francisco: Jossey-Bass.

Fink, A. (2015). *Evaluation fundamentals: Insights into program effectiveness, quality and value* (3rd ed.). Thousand Oaks, CA: Sage Publications, Inc.

Fishbein, M. (Ed.) (1967). *Readings in attitudes theory measurement*. New York, NY: John Wiley & Sons.

Fishbein, M., & Ajzen, I. (1975). *Belief, attitude, intention and behavior: An introduction to theory and research.* Reading, MA: Addison-Wesley.

Fisher, J. D., & Fisher, W. A. (1992). Changing AIDS risk behavior. *Psychological Bulletin, 111*, 455–474.

Fisher, J. D., Fisher, W. A., & Shuper, P. A. (2009). The informational-motivation-behavioral skills model of HIV preventive behavior. In R. J. DiClemente, R. A. Crosby, & M. C. Kegler (Eds.), *Emerging theories in health promotion practice and research* (2nd ed., pp. 21–63). San Francisco: Jossey-Bass.

Fitzpatrick, J. L., Sanders, J. R., & Worthen, B. R. (2004). *Program evaluation: Alternative approaches and practical guidelines* (3rd ed.). Boston, MA: Pearson.

Flint's Youth Violence Prevention Center (FYVPC). (2006). *Photovoice*. Flint, MI: Author. Retrieved April 2, 2011, from http://www.sph.umich.edu/yvpc/projects/photovoice/

Flores, L. M., Davis, R., & Culross, P. (2007). Community health: A critical approach to addressing chronic diseases. *Preventing Chronic Diseases, 4*(4). Retrieved August 25, 2015, from http://www.cdc.gov/pcd/issues/2007/oct/toc.htm

Floyd, D. L., Prentice-Dunn, S., & Rogers, R. W. (2000). A meta-analysis of research on protection motivation theory. *Journal of Applied Social Psychology, 30*, 407–429.

Forthofer, M. S., & Bryant, C. A. (2000). Using audience-segmentation techniques to tailor health behavior change strategies. *American Journal of Health Behavior, 24*(1), 36–43.

Frankish, C. J., Lovato, C. Y., & Shannon, W. J. (1998). Models, theories, and principles of health promotion with multicultural populations. In R. M. Huff & M. V. Kline (Eds.), *Promoting health in multicultural populations* (pp. 41–72). Thousand Oaks, CA: Sage.

French, S. A., Jeffery, R. W., & Oliphant, J. A. (1994). Facility access and self-reward as methods to promote physical activity among healthy sedentary adults. *American Journal of Health Promotion, 8*(4), 257–259, 262.

Frieden, T. R. (2010). A framework for public health action: The health impact pyramid. *American Journal of Public Health, 100*(4), 590–595.

Friedman, A. L., Bozniak, A., Ford, J., Hill, A., Olson, K., Ledsky, R., . . . & Brookmeyer, K. (2014). Reaching youth with sexually transmitted disease testing building on successes, challenges, and lessons learned from local get yourself tested campaigns. *Social Marketing Quarterly, 20*(2), 116–138.

Friis, R. H., & Sellers, T. A. (2009). *Epidemiology for public health practice*. Sudbury, MA: Jones & Bartlett.

Furlong, N., Lovelace, E., & Lovelace, K. (2000). *Research methods and statistics: An integrated approach.* Belmont, CA: Wadsworth/Thompson Learning.

Gaesser, G. A., Angadi, S. S., & Sawyer, B. J. (2011). Exercise and diet, independent of weight loss, improve cardiometaboloc risk profile in overweight and obese individuals. *The Physician and Sportsmedicine, 39*(2), 87–97.

Gagne, R. (1985). *The conditions of learning* (4th ed.). New York, NY: Holt, Rinehart, Winston.

Galer-Unti, R. A., Tappe, M. K., & Lachenmayr, S. (2004). Advocacy 101: Getting started in health education advocacy. *Health Promotion Practice, 5*(3), 280–288.

Gambatese, J. A. (2008). Research issues in prevention through design. *Journal of Safety Research, 39*, 153–158.

Garvin, C. D., & Cox, F. M. (2001). A history of community organizing since the Civil War with special reference to oppressed communities." In J. Rothman, J. L. Erlich, & J. E. Tropman (Eds.) *Strategies of Community Intervention* (5th ed.). Itasca, IL: Peacock, 65–100.

Gaston, A., & Prapavessis, H. (2012). Using combined protection motivation theory and health action process approach intervention to promote exercise during pregnancy. *Journal of Behavioral Medicine, 34*, 173–184.

George, D., & Mallery, P. (2003). *SPSS for Windows step by step: A simple guide and reference.* Boston: Allyn & Bacon.

Getha-Taylor, H. (2008). Identifying collaborative competencies. *Review of Public Personnel Administration, 28*(2), 103–119.

Gilbert, G. G., Sawyer, R. G., & McNeill, E. B. (2015). *Health education: Creating strategies for school and community health* (4th ed.). Burlington, MA: Jones & Bartlett Learning.

Giles, W., Holmes-Chavez, A, & Collins, J. (2009). Cultivating healthy communities: The CDC perspective. *Health Promotion Practice 10*(2), 86S-87S.

Gilmore, G. D. (2012). *Needs and capacity assessment strategies for health education and health promotion* (4th ed.). Burlington, MA: Jones & Bartlett Learning.

Gittell, R., & Vidal, A. (1998). *Community organizing: Building social capital as a development strategy.* Thousand Oaks, CA: Sage.

Glanz, K. (n.d.). Social and behavioral theories. In Office of Behavior & Social Science Research, National Institutes of Health, Department of Health and Human Services, *e-Source: The authority on behavioral & social science research* (Ch. 5). Retrieved July 21, 2015, from http://www.esourceresearch.org/tabid/724/default.aspx

Glanz, K., & Bishop, D. B. (2010). The role of behavioral science theory in the development and implementation of public health interventions. *Annual Review of Public Health, 31,* 399–418.

Glanz, K., & Rimer, B. K. (1995). *Theory at a glance: A guide for health promotion practice* (NIH Pub. No. 95–3896). Washington, DC: National Cancer Institute.

Glanz, K., Rimer, B. K., & Viswanath, K. (Eds.). (2008a). *Health behavior and health education: Theory, research, and practice* (4th ed.). San Francisco: Jossey-Bass.

Glanz, K., Rimer, B. K., & Viswanath, K. (2008b). Theory, research, and practice in health behavior and health education. In K. Glanz, B. K. Rimer, & K. Viswanath (Eds.), *Health behavior and health education: Theory, research, and practice* (4th ed., pp. 23–40). San Francisco: Jossey-Bass.

Glasgow, R. E. (2002). Evaluation of theory-based interventions: The RE-AIM model. In K. Glanz, B. K. Rimer, & F. M. Lewis (Eds.), *Health behavior and health education: Theory research, and practice* (3rd ed., pp. 530–544). San Francisco, CA: Jossey-Bass.

Glasgow, R. E., Vogt, T. M., & Boles, S. M. (1999). Evaluating the public health impact of health promotion interventions: The RE-AIM framework. *American Journal of Public Health, 89*(9), 1322–1327.

Goetzel, R. Z., & Ozminkowski, R. J. (2008). The health and cost benefits of worksite health-promotion programs. *Annual Review of Public Health, 29,* 303–323.

Goetzel, R. Z., Tabrizi, M. J., Roemer, E. C., Smith, K. J., & Kent, K. (2013). A review of recent organizational health assessments. *The Art of Health Promotion, 27*(5), TAHP-1–10.

Golaszewski, T., Allen, J., & Edington, D. (2008). Working together to create supportive environments in worksite health promotion. *The Art of Health Promotion, 22*(14), 1–11.

Golbeck, A. L., Ahlers-Schmidt, C. R., Paschal, A. M., & Dismuke, S. E., (2005). A definition and operational framework for health numeracy. *American Journal of Preventive Medicine, 29,* 375–376.

Goldman, K. D. (1998). Promoting new ideas on the job: Practical theory-based strategies. *The Health Educator, 30*(1), 49–52.

Goldman, K. D., & Schmalz, K. J. (2006). Logic models: The picture worth ten thousand words. *Health Promotion Practice, 7*(1), 8–12.

Goldsmith, M. (2006). Ethics in health education: Issues, concerns, and future directions. *The Health Education Monograph Series, 23*(1), 33–37.

Goldstein, M. G., DePue, J., Kazura, A., & Niaura, R. (1998). Models for provider-patient interaction: Applications to health behavior change. In S. A. Shumaker, E. B. Schron, J. K. Ockene, & W. L. McBee (Eds.), *The handbook of health behavior change* (2nd ed., pp. 85–113). New York: Springer.

Goldstein, S. M. (1997). Community coalitions: A self-assessment tool. *American Journal of Health Promotion, 11*(6), 430–435.

Gomez-Mejia, L. R., & Balkin, D. B. (2012). *Management: People, performance, change.* Boston: Prentice Hall.

Goode, A. D., Winkler, E. A. H., Lawler, S. P., Reeves, M. M., Owen, N., & Eakin, E. G. (2011). A telephone-delivered physical activity and dietary intervention for type-2 diabestes and hypertension: Does intervention influence outcomes? *American Journal of Health Promotion, 25*(4), 257–263.

Goodhard, F. W., Hsu, J., Baek, J. H., Coleman, A., Maresca, F., & Miller, M. (2006). A view through a different lens: Photovoice as a tool for student advocacy. *Journal of American College Health, 55,* 53–56.

Goodlad, J. I., & Su Z. (1992). Organization and the curriculum. In P. W. Jackson (Ed.). *Handbook of research in the curriculum* (pp. 327–344). New York, NY: Macmillan.

Goodman, R. M., McLeroy, K. R., Steckler, A. B., & Hoyle, R. H. (1993). Development of level of institutionalization scales for health promotion programs. *Health Education Quarterly, 20*(2), 161–178.

Goodman, R. M., Speers, M. A., McLeroy, K., Fawcett, S., Kegler, M., Parker, E., Smith, S. R., Sterling, T. D., & Wallerstein, N. (1998). Identifying and defining the dimensions of community capacity to provide a basis for measurement. *Health Education and Behavior, 25*(3), 258–278.

Goodman, R. M., & Steckler, A. (1989). A model for the institutionalization of health promotion programs. *Family and Community Health, 11*(4), 63–78.

Goodson, P. (2010). *Theory in health promotion research and practice: Thinking outside the box.* Sudbury, MA: Jones & Bartlett.

Goodwin, A., Kirley, B., Sandt, L., Hall, W., Thomas, L., O'Brien, N., & Summerlin, D. (2013). *Countermeasures that work: A highway safety countermeasures guide for State Highway Safety Offices.* 7th edition. (Report No. DOT HS 811 727). Washington, DC: National Highway Traffic Safety Administration.

Graff, R. (2013). Using a geographic information system to improve childhood lead-screening efforts. *Preventing Chronic Disease, 10,* 120273.

Grant Central Station, (n.d.). *Writing a budget narrative.* Retrieved July 22, 2015, from http://grant-central-station.com/articles/33/

Grattan, Jr., B. J. & Connolly-Schoonen, J. (2012). Addressing weight loss recidivism: A clinical focus on metabolic rate and pyschological aspects of obesity. *International Scholarly Research Notices: Obesity, 2012,* 5 pages. Retrieved on June 17, 2015, from http://www.hindawi.com/journals/isrn/2012/567530/

Green, L. W. (1989, March). *The health promotion program of the Henry J. Kaiser Family Foundation.* Paper presented at a public lecture at Mankato State University, Mankato, MN.

Green, L. W. (1999). Health education's contributions to public health in the twentieth century: A glimpse through health promotion's rear-view mirror. In J. E. Fielding, L.B. Lave, & B. Starfield (Eds.), *Annual review of public health* (pp. 67–88). Palo Alto, CA: Annual Reviews.

Green, L. W., & Fielding J. E. (2011). The U.S. healthy people initiative: Its genesis and its sustainability. *Annual Review of Public Health, 32,* 451–470.

Green, L. W., & Kreuter, M. W. (1999). *Health promotion planning: An educational and ecological approach* (3rd ed.). Mountain View, CA: Mayfield.

Green, L. W., & Kreuter, M. W. (2005). *Health program planning: An educational and ecological approach* (4th ed.). Boston, MA: McGraw-Hill.

Green, L. W., & Lewis, F. M. (1986). *Measurement and evaluation in health education and health promotion.* Palo Alto, CA: Mayfield.

Grier, S., & Bryant, C. A. (2005). Social marketing in public health. *Annual Review of Public Health, 26,* 313–339.

Grudzien, L. (2009). *New interim final GINA regulations affect wellness programs.* Retrieved July 9, 2015, from http://larrygrudzien.com/benefits_attorney/new-interim-final-gina-regulations-affect-wellness programs/

Grunbaum, J. A., Gingiss, P., Orpinas, P., Batey, L. S., & Parcel, G. S (1995). A comprehensive approach to school health program needs assessment. *Journal of School Health, 65*(2), 54–59.

Gurley, L. (2007, April). *Assessing progress on the nation's health promotion agenda: Healthy People 2010.* Presentation at a public lecture at Ball State University, Muncie, IN.

Guyer, M. (1999). Grants: Finding a funding source. *Grant Source* (pp. 1–3). Columbus, OH: Office of the Auditor, State of Ohio.

Hall, C. L. (1943). *Principles of behavior.* New York: Appleton-Century-Crofts.

Hancock, T., & Minkler, M. (2012). Community health assessment or healthy community assessment: Whose community? Whose health? Whose assessment? In M. Minkler (Ed.). *Community organizing and community building for health and welfare* (3rd ed., pp. 153–170). New Brunswick, NJ: Rutgers University Press.

Hanlon, J. J. (1954). The design of public health programs for underdeveloped countries. *Public Health Reports, 69,* 1028–1032.

Harris, J. H. (2001). Selecting the right vendor for your health promotion program. *Absolute Advantage, 1*(4), 4–5.

Harris, J. H., McKenzie, J. F., & Zuti, W. B. (1986). How to select the right vendor for your company's health promotion program. *Fitness in Business, 1*(October), pp. 53–56.

Harris, J. R., Hannon, P. A., Beresford, S. A. A., Linnan, L. A. & McLellan, D. L. (2014). Health promotion in smaller worplaces in the United States. *Annual Review of Public Health, 35*, 327–342.

Harris, M. J. (2010). *Evaluating public and community health programs.* San Francisco: Jossey-Bass.

Hartman, J. M., Forsen, J. W., Wallace, M. S., & Neely, J. G. (2002). Tutorials in clinical research: Part IV—Recognizing and controlling bias. *Laryngosscope, 112*, 23–31.

Haveman, R. H. (2010). Principles to guide the development of population health incentives. *Preventing chronic disease, 7*(5), 1–5. Retrieved July 9, 2015, from http://www.cdc.gov/pcd/issues/2010/sep/10_0044.htm.

Hayden, J. (2014). *Introduction to health behavior theory* (2nd ed.). Burlington, MA: Jones & Bartlett Learning.

Hayes-Constant, T., Winkler, J., Bishop, A., & Taboada-Palomino, L. (2014). Perilous uncertainty: Situating women's breast health seeking in Northern Peru. *Qualitative Health Research, 24*(6), 811–823.

Hawe, P. (2015). Lessons from complex interventions to improve health. *Annual Review of Public Health, 36*, 307–323.

Health Enhancement Research Organization. (2014). *HERO employee health management best practices scorecard.* Retrieved May 24, 2015, from http://hero-health.org/scorecard/

Heaney, C. A., & Israel, B. A. (2008). Social networks and social support. In K. Glanz, B. K. Rimer, & K. Viswanath (Eds.), *Health behavior and health education: Theory, research, and practice* (4th ed., pp. 189–210). San Francisco: Jossey-Bass.

Helitzer, D., Willging, C., Hathorn, G., & Benally, J. (2009). Using logic models in a community-based agricultural injury prevention project. *Public Health Reports, 124*(Suppl. 1), 63–73.

Hergenrather, K. C., Rhodes, S. D., & Bardhoshi, G. (2009). Photovoice as community-based participatory research: A qualitative review. *American Journal of Health Behavior, 33*(6), 686–698.

Hershey, J. (2011). *Implementing MAPP in the New River Valley, Virginia: A planning partnership approach to improve the community's health and quality of life through mobilized partnerships and strategic action.* (Thesis). Retrieved June 10, 2015, from http://scholar.lib.vt.edu/theses/available/etd-04082011-012806/unrestricted/Hershey_JH_D2011_f1.pdf.

Hether, H. J. (2014). Dialogic communication in the health care context: A case study of Kaiser Permanente's social media practices. *Public Relations Review, 40*(5), 856–858.

Hitt, M. A., Black, J. S., & Porter, L. W. (2012). *Management* (3rd ed.). Boston: Prentice Hall.

Hopkins, K. D., Stanley, J. C., & Hopkins, B. R. (1990). *Educational and psychological measurement and evaluation* (7th ed.). Englewood Cliffs, NJ: Prentice Hall.

Howlett, B., Rogo, E. J., & Shelton, T. G. (2014). *Evidence-based practice for health professionals: An interprofessional approach.* Burlington, MA: Jones & Bartlett Learning.

Hunnicutt, D. (2001). *A dynamic incentive campaign … Step-by-step: Walking your way to wellness.* Retrieved May 17, 2007, from http://www.welcoa.org/freeresources/pdf/stepbystep_ic.pdf

Hunnicutt, D. (2007). The power of planning. *Absolute Advantage, 6*(7), 5–11. Retrieved March 19, 2011, from http://www.welcoa.org/freeresources/index.php?category=8

Hunnicutt, D. (2008a). *Guilty until proven innocent.* WELCOA's *Absolute Advantage, 7*(7), 10–19. Retrieved April 2, 2011, from http://www.welcoa.org/freeresources/index.php?category=8

Hunnicutt, D. (2008b). *The benefits of conducting a personal health assessment.* WELCOA's *Absolute Advantage, 7*(7), 2–9. Retrieved April 2, 2011, from http://www.welcoa.org/freeresources/index.php?category=8

Hunnicutt, D. (2009). *Creating a culture of wellness: A WELCOA quick-inventory.* Retrieved July 2, 2015, from https://www.welcoa.org/?s=WELCOA+Quick+Inventory&c=site

Hunnicutt, D., & Jahn, M. (2011). *Making the case for worksite wellness programs.* Retrieved March 23, 2011, from http://www.welcoa.org/freeresources/index.php?category=8

Hunnicutt, D., & Leffelman, B. (2006). WELCOA's 7 benchmarks of success. *Absolute Advantage, 6*(1), 2–29. Retrieved March 19, 2011, from http://www.welcoa.org/freeresources/index.php?category=8

Hurlburt, R. T. (2003). *Comprehending behavioral statistics* (3rd ed.). Belmont, CA: Wadsworth/ Thomson Learning.

Institute of Medicine (IOM). (2001). *Health and behavior: The interplay of biological, behavioral, and societal influences.* Washington, DC: National Academy Press.

Institute of Medicine (IOM). (2003). *The future of the public's health in the 21st century.* Washington, DC: National Academy Press.

Institute of Medicine (IOM). (2005). *Does the built environment influence physical activity? Examining the evidence.* Washington, DC: National Academy Press.

Israel, B. A., Checkoway, B., Schulz, A., & Zimmerman, M. (1994). Health education and community empowerment: Conceptualizing and measuring perceptions of individual, organizational, and community control. *Health Education Quarterly, 21*(2), 149–170.

Issel, L. M. (2014). *Health program planning and evaluation: A practical, systematic approach for community health* (3rd ed.). SBurlington, MA: Jones & Bartlett Learning.

Iton, A. (2014). *2014 commencement keynote by Anthony Iton, MD, JD, MPH'97*. University of California, Berkeley. Retrieved May 22, 2015, from http://sph.berkeley.edu/sites/default/files/Iton_keynote_5-18-14_v2.pdf

Jacobs, J. A., Dodson, E. A., Baker, E. A., Deshpande, A. D., & Brownson, R. C. (2010). Barriers to evidence-based decision making in public health: A national survey of chronic disease practitioners. *Public Health Reports, 125*(5), 736–742.

Jacobsen, D., Eggen, P., & Kauchak, D. (1989). *Methods for teaching: A skills approach* (3rd ed.). Columbus, OH: Merrill.

Janz, N. K., & Becker, M. H. (1984). The health belief model: A decade later. *Health Education Quarterly, 11*(1), 1–47.

Janz, N. K., Champion, V. L., & Strecher, V. J. (2002). The health belief model. In K. Glanz, B. K. Rimer, & F. M. Lewis (Eds.), *Health behavior and health education: Theory, research, and practice* (3rd ed., pp. 45–66). San Francisco, CA: Jossey-Bass.

John, R., Kerby, D. S., & Landers, P. S. (2004). A market segmentation approach to nutrition education among low-income individuals. *Social Marketing Quarterly, 10*, 3–4, 24–38.

Johnson, G., Scholes, K., & Sexty, R. W. (1989). *Exploring strategic management.* Scarborough, Ontario: Prentice Hall.

Johnson, J. A., & Breckon, D. J. (2007). *Managing health education and health promotion programs: Leadership skills for the 21st century* (2nd ed.). Sudbury, MA: Jones & Bartlett.

Joint Committee on Health Education and Promotion Terminology. (2012). Report of the 2011 Joint Committee on Health Education and Promotion Terminology. *American Journal of Health Education 43*(2), S1–19.

Jones, C. J., Smith, H., & Llewwllyn, C. (2014). Evaluating the effectiveness of health belief model interventions in improving adherence: A systematic *review. Health Psychology Review, 8*(3), 253–269.

Jones-Webb, R., Nelson, T., McKee, P., & Toomey, T. (2014). An implementation model to increase the effectiveness of alcohol control policies. *American Journal of Health Promotion, 28*(5), 328–335.

Kaiser Family Foundation (KFF). (2015). *State health facts.* Retrieved May 24, 2015, from http://kff.org/statedata/

Karwalajtys, T., Kaczorowski, J., Chambers, L. W., Hall, H., McDonough, B., Dolovich, L., Sebaldt, R., Lohfeld, L., & Hutchinson, B. (2013.) Community mobilization, participation, and blood pressure status in a cardiovascular health awareness program in Ontario. *American Journal of Health Promotion, 27*(4), 252–261.

Kawachi, I., Subramanian, S. V. & Kim, D. (2008). *Social capital and health.* New York, NY: Springer Science and Business Media.

Kegler, M. C., & Swan, D. W. (2011). An initial attempt at operationalizing and testing the community coalition action theory. *Health Education & Behavior, 38*(3), 261–270.

Kerlinger, F. N. (1986). *Foundations of behavioral research* (3rd ed.). Austin, TX: Holt, Rinehart, & Winston.

King, A. C., Goldberg, J. H., Salmon, J., Owen, N., Dunstan, D., Weber, D., Doyle, C., & Robinson, T. N. (2010). Indentifying subgroups of U.S. adults at risk for prolonged television viewing to inform program development. *American Journal of Preventive Medicine, 38*(1), 17–26.

King, D. E., Mainous, A. G., Carnemolla, M., & Everett, C. J. (2009). Adherence to health lifestyle habits in U.S. adults, 1988–2006. *The American Journal of Medicine, 122*, 528–534.

Kinzie, M. B. (2005). Instructional design strategies for health behavior change. *Patient Education and Counseling, 56*, 3–15.

Kirsch, I. S., Jungeblut, A., Jenkins, L., & Kolstad, A. (1993). *Adult literacy in America: A first look at the findings of the National Adult Literacy Survey* (NCES 93275). Washington, DC: U.S. Department of Education.

Kirschenbaum, J., & Corburn, J. (2012). Community mapping and digital technology. In M. Minkler (Ed.). *Community organizing and community building for health and welfare* (3rd ed., pp. 444–448). New Brunswick, NJ: Rutgers University Press.

Kline, M. V., & Huff, R. M. (1999). Tips for the practitioner. In R. M. Huff & M. V. Kline (Eds.), *Promoting health in multicultural populations* (pp. 103–111). Thousand Oaks, CA: Sage.

Klingner, D. E., Nalbandian, J., & Llorens, J. (2010). *Public personnel management: Contexts and strategies* (6th ed.). New York: Longman.

Kochanek, K. D., Murphy, S. L., Xu, J., & Arias, E (2014). Mortality in the United States, 2013. *NCHS*

Data Brief, No. 178. Hyattsville, MD: National Center for Health Statistics.

Koelen, M., Vaandragger, L., & Colomer, C. (2001). Health promotion research: Dilemmas and challenges. *Journal of Epidemiology and Community Health, 55*(4), 257–262.

Kotler, P., & Clarke, R. N. (1987). *Marketing for health care organizations*. Englewood Cliffs, NJ: Prentice Hall.

Kotler, P., & Keller, K. L. (2016). *A framework for marketing management* (6th ed.) Upper Saddle River, NJ: Pearson.

Kotler, P., & Zaltman, G. (1971). Social marketing: An approach to planned social change. *Journal of Marketing, 35*, 3–12.

Krahn G. (2003). Changing concepts in health, wellness and disability. Institute on Disability and Development (Ed.). *Proceedings of Changing Concepts of Health and Disability: State of the Science Conference and Policy Forum 2003*. Portland: Oregon Health and Science University.

Kramer, L., Schwartz, P., Cheadle, A., Borton, J. E., Wright, M., Chase, C., & Lindley, C. (2010). Promoting policy and environmental change using photovoice in the Kaiser Permanente community health initiative. *Health Promotion Practice, 11*(3), 332–339.

Krefetz, D. G., Steer, R. A., Gulab, N. A., & Beck, A. T. (2002). Convergent validity of the Beck Depression Inventory-II with the Reynolds Adolescent Depression Scale in psychiatric inpatients. *Journal of Personality Assessment,78*(3), 451–460.

Kreps, G. L., Barnes, M. D., Neiger, B. L., & Thackeray, R. (2009). Health communication. In Robert J. Bensley & J. Brookins-Fisher (Eds.) *Community health education methods: A practical guide* (3rd ed., pp. 73–102). Sudbury, MA: Jones & Bartlett.

Kretzmann, J. P., & McKnight, J. L. (1993). Introduction from *Building communities from inside out: A path toward finding and mobilizing a community's assets*. Retrieved July 16, 2015, from http://www.ipr.northwestern.edu/publications/books/

Kreuter, M. W., & Skinner, C. S. (2000). What's in a name? *Health Education Research, Theory, and Practice, 15*(1), 1–4.

Kreuter, M. W., Farrell, D., Olevitch, L., & Brennan, L. (1999). *Tailoring health messages: Customizing communication with computer technology*. Mahwah, NJ: Erlbaum.

Kutner, M., Greenberg, E., Jin, Y., & Paulsen, C. (2006). *The health literacy of America's adults: Results from the 2003 National Assessment of Adult Literacy* (NCES 2006-483). Washington, DC: National Center for Education Statistics, U.S. Department of Education.

Laine, J., Kuvaja-Kollner, V., Pietila, E., Koivuneva, M., Valtonen, H., & Kankaanpaa, E. (2014.) Cost-effectiveness of population-level physical activity interventions: A systematic review. *American Journal of Health Promotion, 29*(2), 71–80.

Lalonde, M. (1974). *A new perspective on the health of Canadians: A working document*. Ottawa, ON: Minister of Health.

Lambert, C. (2006, March-April). The marketplace of perceptions. *Harvard Magazine*, 50–57, 93–95.

Lancaster, B., & Kreuter, M. (2002). Planned approach to community health (PATCH). In L. Breslow (Ed.). *Encyclopedia of public health*. Farmington Hills, MI: Gale Cengage. Retrieved July 22, 2015, from http://www.encyclopedia.com/doc/1G2-3404000652.html

Lando, J., Williams, S. M., Sturgis, S., & Williams, B. (2006). A logic model for the integration of mental health into chronic disease prevention and health promotion. *Preventing Chronic Disease, 3*(2), 1–5. Retrieved July 28, 2015, from http://www.cdc.gov/pcd/issues/2006/apr/05_0215.htm

Last, J. M. (Ed.). (2007). *A Dictionary of Public Health* (4th ed.). New York, NY: Oxford University Press.

Lee, N. R. & Kotler, P. A. (2016). *Social Marketing: Changing Behaviors For Good*. (5th ed). Thousand Oaks, CA: Sage.

Leedy, P. D. (1993). *Practical Research: Planning and Design* (5th ed.). New York, NY: Macmillan.

Lefebvre, R. C. (2006). Partnerships for social marketing programs: An example from the National Bone Health Campaign. *Social Marketing Quarterly, 12*(1), 41–54.

Leventhal, H., & Cleary, P. D. (1980). The smoking problem: A review of the research and theory in behavioral risk modification. *Psychological Bulletin, 88*(2), 370–405.

Lewin, K. (1935). *A dynamic theory of personality*. New York: McGraw-Hill.

Lewin, K. (1936). *Principles of topological psychology*. New York: McGraw-Hill.

Lewin, K., Dembo, T., Festinger, L., & Sears, P. S. (1944). Level of aspiration. In J. Hunt (Ed.), *Personality and the behavior disorders* (pp. 333–378). New York: Ronald Press.

Li, C., & Bernoff, J. (2008). *Groundswell: Winning in a world transformed by social technologies*. Boston: Harvard Business Press.

Liang, B. A., & Mackey, T. (2011). Direct-to-consumer advertising with interactive Internet media: Global regulation and public health issues. *JAMA, 305*(8), 824–825.

Lindenberger, J. H., & Bryant, C. A., (2000). Promoting breastfeeding in the WIC program: A social marketing case study. *American Journal Health Behavior, 24*(1), 53–60.

Lindsey, L. L. M., Hamner, H. C., Prue, C. E., Flores, A. L., Valencia, D., Correra-Sierra, E., & Kopfman, J. E. (2007). Understanding optimal nutrition among women of childbearing age in the United States and Puerto Rico: Employing formative research to lay the foundation for National Birth Defects Prevention Campaigns. *Journal of Health Communication: International Perspectives, 12*(8), 733–757.

Lobb, R., & Colditz, G. A. (2013). Implementation science and its application to population health. *Annual Review of Public Health, 34*, 235–251.

Lobo, R., Petrich, M., & Burns, S. K. (2014). Supporting health promotion practitioners to undertake evaluation for program development. *BMC Public Health, 14*, 1315. doi:10.1186/1471-2458-14-1315

Lovelace, K. A., Bibeau, D. L., Donnell, B. M., Johnson, H. H., Glascoff, M. A., & Tyler, E. (2009). Public health educators participation in teams: Implications for preparation and practice. *Health Promotion Practice, 10*(3), 428–435.

Lucan, S. C., Hillier, A., Schechter, C. B., & Glanz, K. (2014). Objective and self-reported factors associated with food-environment perceptions and fruit-and-vegetable consumption: A multilevel analysis. *Preventing Chronic Disease, 11*, 130324.

Luquis, R. R. (2014). Culturally appropriate communication. In M. A. Pérez & R. R. Luquis, (Eds.), *Cultural competence in health education and health promotion* (2nd ed.) pp. 193–216). San Francisco: Jossey-Bass.

Luquis, R. R., & Pérez, M. A. (2003). Achieving cultural competence: The challenges for health educators. *American Journal of Health Education, 34*(3), 131–138.

Luquis, R., Pérez, M., & Young, K. (2006). Cultural competence development in health education professional preparation programs. *American Journal of Health Education, 37*(4), 233–241.

Luszczynska, A., & Sutton, S. (2005). Attitudes and expectations. In J. Kerr, R. Weitkunat, & M. Moretti (Eds.), *ABC of behavior change: A guide to successful disease prevention and health promotion* (pp. 71–84). Edinburgh: Elsevier.

Lynch, M., Squiers, L., Lewis, M. A., Moultrie, R., Kish-Doto, J., Boudewyns, V., . . . & Mitchell, E. W. (2014). Understanding women's preconception health goals: Audience segmentation strategies for a preconception health campaign. *Social Marketing Quarterly, 20*(3), 148–164.

MacAskill, S., Stead, M., MacKintosh, A. M., & Hastings, G. (2002). "You cannae just take cigarettes away from somebody and no' gie them something back"; Can social marketing help solve the problem of low-income smoking? *Social Marketing Quarterly, 8*(1), 19–34.

Maibach, E. W., Leiserowitz, A., Roser-Renouf, C., & Mertz, C. K. (2011). Identifying like-minded audiences for global warming public engagement campaigns: An audience segmentation analysis and tool development. *PLoS ONE, 6*(3), e17571. Doi:10.1371/journal.pone.0017571

Marcarin, S. (Ed.). (1995). *Cumulative index to nursing & allied health literature: CINAHL.* Volume 40, Part A. Glendale, CA.

Marlatt, G. A. (1982). Relapse prevention: A self-control program for treatment of addictive behaviors. In R. B. Sturat (Ed.), *Adherence, compliance, and generalization in behavioral medicine* (pp. 329–377). New York: Brunner/Mazel.

Marlatt, G. A., & George, W. H. (1998). Relapse prevention and the maintenance of optimal health. In S. A. Shumaker, E. B. Schron, J. K. Ockene, & W. L. McBee (Eds.), *The handbook of health behavior change* (2nd ed., pp. 33–58). New York: Springer.

Martinez-Cossio, N. (2008). Developing culturally appropriate needs assessment and planning, implementation, and evaluation for health education and health promotion programs. In M. A. Pérez & R. R. Luquis, R. (Eds.), *Cultural competence in health education and health promotion* (pp. 125–145). San Francisco: Jossey-Bass.

Mausner, J. S., & Kramer, S. (1985). *Epidemiology— An introductory text* (2nd ed.). Philadelphia, PA: W. B. Saunders.

Mazloomymahmoodabad, S., Masoudy, G., Fallahzadeh, H., & Jalili, Z. (2014). Education based on Precede-Proceed on quality of life in elders. *Global Journal of Health Science, 6*(6), 178–184.

McAlister, A. L., Perry, C. L., & Parcel, G. S. (2008). How individual, environments, and health behaviors interact: Social cognitive theory. In K. Glanz, B. K. Rimer, & K. Viswanath (Eds.), *Health behavior and health education: Theory, research, and practice* (4th ed., pp. 169–188). San Francisco: Jossey-Bass.

McCaul, K. D., Bakdash, M. B., Geoboy, M. J., Gerbert, B., & Tedesco, L. A. (1990). Promoting self-protective health behaviors in dentistry. *Annals of Behavioral Medicine, 12*, 156–160.

McClendon, B. T., & Prentice-Dunn, S. (2001). Reducing skin cancer risk: An intervention based upon protection motivation theory. *Journal of Health Psychology, 6*(3), 321–328.

McDade-Montez, E., Cvengros, J., & Christensen, A. (2005). Personality and individual differences. In J. Kerr, R. Weitkunat, & M. Moretti (Eds.), *ABC of behavior change: A guide to successful disease prevention and health promotion* (pp. 57–70). Edinburgh: Elsevier.

McDermott, R. J., & Sarvela, P. D. (1999). *Health education evaluation and measurement: A practitioner's perspective* (2nd ed.). New York: WCB/McGraw-Hill.

McDonald, M., & Wilson, H. (2011). *Marketing Plans* (7th ed.). United Kingdom: Wiley.

McEachan, R., Lawton, R., Jackson, C., Conner, M., & Lunt, J. (2008). Evidence, theory and context: Using intervention mapping to develop a worksite physical activity intervention. *BMC Public Health*, doi:10.1186/1471-2458-8-326.

McGinnis, J. M., Williams-Russo, P., & Knickman, J.R. (2002). The case for more active policy attention to health promotion. *Health Affairs, 21*(2), 78–93.

McKenzie, J. F. (1986). Cost-benefit and cost-effectiveness as a part of evaluation of health promotion programs. *The Eta Sigma Gamman, 18*(2), 10–16.

McKenzie, J. F. (1988). Twelve steps in developing a schoolsite health education/promotion program for faculty and staff. *The Journal of School Health, 58*(4), 149–153.

McKenzie, J. F., & Pinger, R. R. (2015). *An introduction to community and public health* (8th ed.). Burlington, MA: Jones & Bartlett Learning.

McKenzie, J. F., Wood, M. L., Kotecki, J. E., Clark, J. K., & Brey, R. A. (1999). Establishing content validity: Using qualitative and quantitative steps. *American Journal of Health Behavior, 23*(4), 311–318.

McKleroy, V. S., Galbraith, J. S., Cummings, B., Jones, P., Harshbarger, C., Collins, C., Gelaude, D., Carey, J. W., & ADAPT Team. (2006). Adapting evidence-based behavioral interventions for new settings and target populations. *AIDS Education and Prevention, 19*(Suppl. A), 59–73.

McKnight, J. L., & Kretzmann, J. P. (2005). Mapping community capacity. In M. Minkler (Ed.), *Community organizing and community building for health* (pp. 158–172). New Brunswick, NJ: Rutgers University Press.

McKnight, J. L., & Kretzmann, J. P. (2012). Mapping community capacity. In M. Minkler (Ed.), *Community organizing and community building for health and welfare* (pp. 171–186). New Brunswick, NJ: Rutgers University Press.

McLeroy, K. R., Bibeau, D., Steckler, A., & Glanz, K. (1988). An ecological perspective on health promotion programs. *Health Education Quarterly, 15*, 351–377.

Mendy, V. L., Perryman, B., Hawkins, J, & Dove, C. (2014). Planning for the strategic recruitment of barbershops for blood pressure screening and referral in the Mississippi delta region. *Preventing Chronic Disease,11*, 140179.

Mercer, S. L., Green, L. W., Cargo, M., Potter, M. A., Daniel, M., Olds, R. S., & Reed-Gross, E. (2008). Reliability-tested guidelines for assessing participatory research projects. In M. Minkler & N. Wallerstein (Eds.). *Community-based participatory research for health: From process to outcomes* (2nd ed.) (pp. 407–418). San Francisco, CA: Jossey-Bass.

Miller, M. (2009). *A community organizer's tale: People and power in San Francisco.* Berkeley, CA: Heyday Books.

Miller, T., & Hendrie, D. (2008). *Substance abuse prevention dollars and cents: A cost-benefit analysis,* DHHS Pub. No. (SMA) 07-4298. Rockville, MD: Center for Substance Abuse Prevention.

Miller, W. R. (1983). Motivational interviewing with problem drinkers. *Behavioural Psychotherapy, 11*(2), 147–172.

Miller, W. R., & Rollnick, S. (2009). Ten things that motivational interviewing is not. *Behavioural and Cognitive Psychotherapy, 37*, 129–140.

Mindell, J. S., Boltong, A., & Forde, I. (2008). A review of health impact assessment frameworks. *Public Health, 122*, 1177–1187.

Minelli, M. J., & Breckon, D. J. (2009). *Community health education: Settings, roles, and skills* (5th ed.). Sudbury, MA: Jones & Bartlett.

Minkler, M. (2012). Introduction to community organizing and community building. In M. Minkler (Ed.). *Community organizing and community building for health and welfare* (3rd ed., pp. 5–26). New Brunswick, NJ: Rutgers University Press.

Minkler, M., & Wallerstein, N. (2012). Improving health through community organization and community building: Perspectives from health education and social work. In M. Minkler (Ed.). *Community organizing and community building for health and welfare* (3rd ed., pp. 37–58). New Brunswick, NJ: Rutgers University Press.

Minkler, M., Wallerstein, N., & Wilson, N. (2008). Improving health through community organization and community building. In K. Glanz, B. K. Rimer, & K. Viswanath (Eds.), *Health behavior and health education: Theory, research, and practice* (4th ed., pp. 287–312). San Francisco: Jossey-Bass.

Mishoe, S. C. (2008). Consumer health care information on the Internet: Does the public benefit? *Respiratory Care, 53*(10), 1285–1286.

Mokdad, A. H., Marks, J. S., Stroup, D. F., & Gerberding, J. L. (2004). Actual causes of death, in the United States, 2000. *Journal of the American Medical Association, 291*(10), 1238–1245.

Mokdad, A. H., Marks, J. S., Stroup, D. F., & Gerberding, J. L. (2005). Correction: Actual causes of death in the United States, 2000. *Journal of the American Medical Association, 293*(3), 293–294.

Monaghan, P. F., Bryant, C. A., Baldwin, J. A., Zhu, Y., Ibrahimou, B., Lind, J. D., Contreras, R. B., Tovar, A., Moreno, T., & McDermott, R. J. (2008). Using community-based prevention marketing to improve farm worker safety. *Social Marketing Quarterly, 14*(4), 71–87.

Mondros, J. B., & Wilson, S. M. (1994). *Organizing for power and empowerment.* New York: Columbia Press.

Montaño, D. E., & Kasprzyk, D. (2008). Theory of reasoned action, theory of planned behavior, and the integrated behavioral model. In K. Glanz, B. K. Rimer, & K. Viswanath (Eds.), *Health behavior and health education: Theory, research, and practice* (4th ed., pp. 67–96). San Francisco: Jossey-Bass.

Muir Gray, J. A. (1997). *Evidenced-based healthcare: How to make health policy and management decisions.* Edinburgh, Scotland & New York, NY: Churchill Livingstone

Munro, S., & Lewin, S., Swart, T, & Volmink, J. (2007). A review of health behavior theories: How useful are these for developing interventions to promote long-term medication adherence for TB and HIV/AIDS? *BMC Public Health, 7,* 104.

National Association of County and City Health Officials (NACCHO). (n.d.). *Community health assessment & improvement processes.* Washington, DC: Author. Retrieved May 23, 2015, from http://www.naccho.org/topics/infrastructure/CHAIP/upload/CHA-and-CHIP-Processes-JJE.pdf

National Association of County and City Health Officials (NACCHO). (2001). *Mobilizing for action through planning and partnerships (MAPP).* Washington, DC: Author.

National Business Group on Health. (2015). WISCORE®. Retrieved May 24, 2015, from https://www.businessgrouphealth.org/scorecard_v6/index.cfm?event=logon.landing

National Cancer Institute (NCI). (n.d.). *Making health communication programs work* (NIH Pub. No. 04-5145). Retrieved May 21, 2015, from http://www.cancer.gov/publications/health-communication/pink-book.pdf

National Center for Chronic Disease Prevention and Health Promotion (NCCDPHP), Centers for Disease Prevention and Control. (n.d.). *Evaluation guide: Writing SMART objectives.* Retrieved June 2, 2015, from http://www.cdc.gov/dhdsp/programs/spha/evaluation_guides/docs/smart_objectives.pdf

National Center for Health Statistics (NCHS). (2015). *Health, United States, 2014: With special feature on adults Aged 55–64.* Hyattsville, MD: Author.

National Center for Injury Prevention and Control (NCIPC). (2008; revised 2010). *Adding Power to Our Voices: A Framing Guide for Communicating About Injury.* Atlanta: Author. Retrieved May 14, 2015, from http://www.cdc.gov/injury/pdfs/cdcframingguide-a.pdf

National Commission for Health Education Credentialing, Inc. (NCHEC). (1985). *A framework for the development of competency-based curricula for entry-level health educators.* New York, NY: Author.

National Commission for Health Education Credentialing, Inc. (NCHEC). (1996). *A competency-based framework for professional development of certified health education specialists.* New York: Author.

National Commission for Health Education Credentialing, Inc. (NCHEC). (2015). *Overview.* Retrieved May 11, 2015, from http://www.nchec.org/overview

National Commission for Health Education Credentialing (NCHEC), & Society for Public Health Education (SOPHE). (2015). *A competency-based framework for health education specialists—2015.* Whitehall, PA: Author.

National Commission for Health Education Credentialing, (NCHEC), Society for Public Health Education (SOPHE), & American Association for Health Education (AAHE). (2006). *A competency-based framework for health educators.* Whitehall, PA: Author.

National Commission for Health Education Credentialing (NCHEC), Society for Public Health Education (SOPHE), & American Association for Health Education (AAHE). (2010). *A competency-based framework for health education specialists—2010.* Whitehall, PA: Author.

National Commission for the Protection of Human Subjects of Biomedical and Behavioral Research. (1979). *The Belmont Report: Ethical Principles and Guidelines for the Protection of Human Subject Research.* Retrieved September 22, 2015, from http://www.hhs.gov/ohrp/humansubjects/guidance/belmont.html

National Highway Traffic Safety Administration (NHTSA). (2015). *Traffic safety facts.* Retrieved May 19, 2015, from http://www-nrd.nhtsa.dot.gov/Pubs/812151.pdf

National Research Council of the National Academies. (2011). *Improving health in the United States: The role of health impact assessment.* Washington, DC: The National Academies Press.

National Task Force on the Preparation and Practice of Health Educators, Inc. (1985). *A framework for the development of competency-based curricula for entry-level health educators.* New York: Author.

Neiger, B. L., & Thackeray, R. (1998). *Social marketing: Making public health sense.* Paper presented at the annual meeting of the Utah Public Health Association, Provo, UT.

Neiger, B. L., & Thackeray, R. (2002). Application of the SMART Model in two successful social marketing campaigns. *American Journal of Health Education, 33,* 291–293.

Neiger, B. L., Thackeray, R., Barnes, M. D., & McKenzie, J. F. (2003). Positioning social marketing as a planning process for health education. *American Journal of Health Studies, 18*(2/3), 75–80.

Neiger, B. L., Thackeray, R., & Fagen, M. C. (2011). Basic priority rating model 2.0: Current applications for priority setting in health promotion practice. *Health Promotion Practice, 12*(2), 166–171.

Neiger, B. L., Thackeray, R., Merrill, R. M., Miner, K. M., Larsen, L., & Chalkley, C. M. (2001). The impact of social marketing on fruit and vegetable consumption and physical activity among public health employees at the Utah Department of Health. *Social Marketing Quarterly, 7*, 9–28.

Net.MBA (2002–2010). *CPM-critical path method.* Retrieved July 29, 2015, from http://netmba.com /operations/project/cpm/

Neutens, J. J., & Rubinson, L. (2014). *Research techniques for health sciences* (5th ed.). Boston, MA: Pearson.

Newcomer, K. E., & Wirtz, P. W. (2004). Using statistics in evaluation. In J. S. Wholey, H. P. Hatry, & K. E. Newcomer (Eds.), *Handbook of practical program evaluation* (2nd ed., pp. 439–478). San Francisco, CA: Jossey-Bass.

Norwood, S. L. (2000). *Research strategies for advanced practice nurses.* Upper Saddle River, NJ: Prentice Hall.

Nutbeam, D., & Harris, E. (1999). *Theory in a nutshell: A guide to health promotion theory.* Sydney, Australia: McGraw-Hill.

Nye, R. D. (1979). *What is B. F. Skinner really saying?* Englewood Cliffs, NJ: Prentice Hall.

Nye, R. D. (1992). *The legacy of B. F. Skinner: Concepts and perspectives, controversies, and misunderstandings.* Pacific Grove, CA: Brooks/Cole.

O'Donnell, M. P. (2014). Editor's notes: What is the ROI of workplace health promotion? The answer just got simpler by making the question more complicated. *American Journal of Health Promotion, 28*(6), iv–v.

Office of Minority Health (OMH). (2013). *The National CLAS) standards.* Retrieved July 20, 2015, from http://www.minorityhealth.hhs.gov/omh/browse .aspx?lvl=2&lvlid=53

Offiong, C., Oji, V., Bunyan, W., Lewis, J., Moore, C., & Olusanya, O. (2011). The role of colleges and schools of pharmacy in the advent of Healthy People 2020. *American Journal of Pharmaceutical Education, 75*(3), 56.

Oliver, T. R. (2006). The politics of public health policy. *Annual Review of Public Health, 27,* 195–233.

Ornstein, A. C., & Hunkins, F. P. (1998). *Curriculum: Foundations, principals, and issues* (3rd ed.). Boston, MA: Allyn & Bacon.

Osborn, C. Y., & Egede, L. E. (2010). Validation of an information-motivation-behavioral skills model of diabetes self-care (IMB-DSC). *Patient Education & Counseling, 79*(1), 49–54.

Pagels, A., Hylander, B., & Alvarsson, M. (2015). A multi-dimensional support program for patients with diabetic kidney disease. *Journal of Renal Care*, Advance online publication. doi:10.1111/jorc.12114.

Painter, J. F., Borba, C. P. C., Hynes, M., Mays, D., & Glanz, K. (2008). The use of theory in health behavior research from 2000 to 2005: A systematic review. *Annals of Behavioral Medicine, 35*, 358–362.

Panagiotou, G. (2003). Bringing SWOT into focus. *Business Strategy Review 14*(2), 8–10.

Parcel, G. S. (1983). Theoretical models for application in school health education research. *Health Education, 15*(4), 39–49.

Parcel, G. S. (1995). Diffusion research: The smart choices project. *Health Education Research: Theory and Practice, 10*(3), 279–281.

Parcel, G. S., & Baranowski, T. (1981). Social learning theory and health education. *Health Education, 12*(3), 14–18.

Parkinson, R. S., & Associates. (1982). *Managing health promotion in the workplace: Guidelines for implementation and evaluation.* Palo Alto, CA: Mayfield.

Pasick, R. J., D'Onofrio, C. N., & Otero-Sabogal, R. (1996). Similarities and differences across cultures: Questions to inform a third generation for health promotion research. *Health Education, 23*(Suppl.), S142–S161.

Patton, M. Q. (1988). *How to use qualitative methods in evaluation.* Newbury Park, CA: Sage.

Patton, R. P., Corry, J. M., Gettman, L. R., & Graff, J. S. (1986). *Implementing health/fitness programs.* Champaign, IL: Human Kinetics.

Pavlov, I. (1927). *Conditional reflexes.* Oxford: Oxford University Press.

The Pell Institute for the Study of Opportunity in Highert Education. (2015). *Using a logic model.* Retrieved July 28, 2015, from http://toolkit.pellinstitute.org /evaluation-guide/plan-budget/using-a-logic-model/

Pellmar, T. C., Brandt, Jr., E. N., & Baird, M. (2002). Health and behavior: The interplay of biological, behavioral, and social influences: Summary of an Institute of Medicine Report. *American Journal of Health Promotion, 16*(4), 206–219.

Pérez, M. A., & Luquis, R. R. (Eds.). (2014). *Cultural competence in health education and health promotion* (2nd ed.). San Francisco: Jossey-Bass.

Perlman, J. (1978). Grassroots participation from neighborhood to nation. In S. Langton (Ed.), *Citizen participation in America* (pp. 65–79). Lexington, MA: Lexington Books.

Perrin, K. M. (2015). *Principles of evaluation and research for health care programs.* Burlington, MA: Jones and Bartlett Learning.

Pescatello, L. S., Murphy, D., Vollono, J., Lynch, E., Bernene, J., & Costanzo, D. (2001). The cardiovascular health impact of an incentive worksite health promotion program. *American Journal of Health Promotion, 16*(1), 16–20.

Petersen, D. J., & Alexander, G. R. (2001). *Needs assessment in public health: A practical guide for students and professionals.* New York, NY: Kluwer Academic/Plenum.

Petty, R. E., Barden, J., & Wheeler, S. C. (2009). The elaboration likelihood model of persuasion: Developing health promotions for sustained behavioral change. In R. J. DiClemente, R. A. Crosby, & M. C. Kegler (Eds.), *Emerging theories in health promotion practice and research* (2nd ed., pp. 185–214). San Francisco: Jossey-Bass.

Petty, R. E., & Briñol, P. (2012). The elaboration likelihood model. In P. A. M. Van Lange, A. W. Kruglanski, & E. T. Higgins (Eds.), *Handbook of theories of social psychology* (pp. 224–245). Thousand Oaks, CA: Sage Publications, Inc.

Petty, R. E., Wheeler, S. C., & Bizer, G. Y. (1999). Is there one persuasion process or more? Lumping versus splitting in attitude change theories. *Psychology Inquiry, 10,* 156–163.

Pew Research Center. (2014). *Health fact sheet.* Retrieved May 20, 2015, from http://www.pewinternet.org/fact-sheets/health-fact-sheet/

Picarella, R. (2015). Successful partnerships in employee wellness—A focus on integration and achieving best-in-class outcomes: Expert interview of Dr. Terry Paul. Omaha, NE: Wellness Council of America. Retrieved May 17, 2015, from https://www.welcoa.org/resources/expert-interview-paul-terry/

Pickett, G. E., & Hanlon, J. J. (1990). *Public health: Administration and practice* (9th ed.). St. Louis, MO: Mosby-Year Book.

Poland, B., Krupa, G., & McCall, D. (2009). Settings for health promotion: An analytic framework to guide intervention design and implementation. *Health Promotion Practice, 10*(4), 505–516.

Poole, K., Kumpfer, K., & Pett, M. (2001). The impact of an incentive-based worksite health promotion program on modifiable health risk factors. *American Journal of Health Promotion, 16*(1), 21–26.

Porta, M. (Ed.). (2014). *A dictionary of epidemiology* (6th ed.). New York, NY: Oxford University Press.

Prentice-Dunn, S., McMath, B. F., & Cramer, R. J. (2009). Protection motivation theory and stages of change in sun protective behavior. *Journal of Health Psychology, 14,* 297–305.

Prentice-Dunn, S., & Rogers, R. W. (1986). Protection motivation theory and preventive health: Beyond the health belief model. *Health Education Research: Theory and Practice, 1*(3), 153–161.

Prevention Institute. (2011). *Collaboration multiplier.* Retrieved May 17, 2015, from http://www.preventioninstitute.org/component/jlibrary/article/id-44/127.html

Prochaska, J. O. (1979). *Systems of psychotherapy: A transtheoretical analysis.* Homewood, IL: Dorsey Press.

Prochaska, J. O., DiClemente, C. C., & Norcross, J. C. (1992). In search of how people change: Applications to addictive behaviors. *American Psychologist, 47*(9), 1102–1114.

Prochaska, J. O., Johnson, S., & Lee, P. (1998). The transtheoretical model of behavior change. In S. A. Shumaker, E. B. Schron, J. K. Ockene, & W. L. McBee (Eds.), *The handbook of health behavior change* (2nd ed., pp. 59–84). New York: Springer.

Prochaska, J. O, Redding, C. A., & Evers, K. E. (2008). The transtheoretical model and stages of change. In K. Glanz, B. K. Rimer, & K. Viswanath (Eds.), *Health behavior and health education: Theory, research, and practice* (4th ed., pp. 97–121). San Francisco: Jossey-Bass.

Prochaska, J. O., Redding, C. A., Harlow, L. L., Rossi, J. S., & Velicer, W. F. (1994). The transtheoretical model of change and HIV prevention: A review. *Health Education Quarterly, 21*(4), 471–486.

Public Health Accreditation Board. (2013a). *Public Health Accreditation Board standards and measures, version 1.5.* Retrieved May 19, 2015, from http://www.phaboard.org/wp-content/uploads/SM-Version-1.5-Board-adopted-FINAL-01-24-2014.docx.pdf

Public Health Accreditation Board. (2013b). *Public health department accreditation background.* Retrieved May 19, 2015, from http://www.phaboard.org/about-phab/public-health-accreditation-background/

Putman, R. D. (1995). Bowling alone: America's declining social capital. *Journal of Democracy, 6*(1), 65–78.

Raju, J. D., Soni, A., Aziz, N., Tiemstra, J. D., & Hasnain, M. (2012). A patient-centered telephone intervention using the asthma action plan. *Family Medicine, 44*(5), 348–350.

Ramaprasad, J. (2005). Warning signals, wind speeds and what next: A pilot project for disaster preparedness among residents of central Vietnam's lagoons. *Social Marketing Quarterly, 11*(2), 41–53.

Redding, C. A., Rossi, J. S., Rossi, S. R., Velicer, W. F., & Prochaska, J. O. (1999). Health behavior models. In G. C. Hyner, K. W. Peterson, J. W. Travis, J. E. Dewey, J. J. Foerster, & E. M. Framer (Eds.), *SPM handbook of health assessment tools* (pp. 83–93). Pittsburgh, PA: Society of Prospective Medicine.

Reeves, M. J., & Rafferty, A. P. (2005). Healthy lifestyle characteristics among adults in the United States, 2000. *Archives of Internal Medicine, 165,* 854–857.

Richards, T. B., Berkowitz, Z., Thomas, C. C., Foster, S. L., Gardner, A., King, J. B., Ledford, K., & Royalty, J (2010.) Choropleth map design for cancer incidence, part 2. *Preventing Chronic Disease, 7*(1), A2.

Riedel, J., & Calao, R. (2014). Change is hard: The promise of behavioral economics. *American Journal of Health Promotion, 28*(6), TAHP-8-TAHP-11.

Riegelman, R. (2014). *Public health 101: Healthy people-health populations* (2nd ed.). Sudbury, MA: Jones & Bartlett Learning.

Rimer, B. K., & Glanz, K. (2005). *Theory at a glance: A guide for health promotion practice* (2nd ed.). (NIH Pub. No. 05-3896). Washington, DC: National Cancer Institute.

Robbins, L. C., & Hall, J. H. (1970). *How to practice prospective medicine.* Indianapolis, IN: Methodist Hospital of Indiana.

Robinson, K. L., Driedger, M. S., Elliott, S. J., & Eyles, J. (2006). Understanding facilitators of and barriers to health promotion practice. *Health Promotion Practice, 7*(4), 467-476.

Robison, J. (1998). To reward?... or not to reward?: Questioning the wisdom of using external reinforcement on health promotion programs. *American Journal of Health Promotion, 13*(1), 1-3.

Rogers, E. M. (1962). *Diffusion of innovations.* New York: Free Press of Glencoe.

Rogers, E. M. (2003). *Diffusion of innovations* (5th ed.). New York, NY: Free Press.

Rogers, R. W. (1975). A protection motivation theory of fear appeals and attitude change. *Journal of Psychology, 91*, 93-114.

Rogers, R. W. (1983). Cognitive and physiological processes in fear-based attitude change: A revised theory of protection motivation. In J. Cacioppo & R. Petty (Eds.), *Social psychophysiology: A sourcebook* (pp. 153-176). New York: Guilford.

Rogers, R. W. (1984). Changing health-related attitudes and behaviors: The role of preventative health psychology. In J. H. Harvey, J. E. Maddux, R. P. McGlynn, & C. D. Stoltenberg (Eds.), *Social perception in clinical and counseling psychology* (vol. 2, pp. 91-112). Lubbock: Texas Tech University Press.

Rogers, R. W., & Prentice-Dunn, S. (1997). Protection motivation theory. In D. Gochman (Ed.), *Handbook of health behavior research. Vol. 1: Determinants of health behavior: Personal and social* (pp.113-132). New York: Plenum.

Rosati, M. J., Cupp, P. K., Chookhare, W, Miller, B. A., Byrnes, H. F.... Atwood, K.A. (2012). Successful implementation of Thai family matters: Strategies and implications. *Health Promotion Practice, 13*(3), 355-363.

Rosenstock, I. M. (1966). Why people use health services. *Milbank Memorial Fund Quarterly, 44*, 94-124.

Rosenstock, I. M. (1990). The health belief model: Explaining health behavior through expectancies. In K. Glanz, f. M. Lewis, & B. K. Rimer (Eds.). *Health behaviour and health education* (pp. 39-62). San Francisco: Josey-Bass.

Rosenstock, I. M., Strecher, V. J., & Becker, M. H. (1988). Social learning theory and the health belief model. *Health Education Quarterly, 15*(2), 175-183.

Ross, H. S., & Mico, P. R. (1980). *Theory and practice in health education.* Palo Alto, CA: Mayfield.

Ross, M. G. (1967). *Community organization: Theory, principles, and practice.* New York: Harper & Row.

Rothman, J. (2001). Approaches to community intervention. In J. Rothman, J. L. Erlich, & J. E. Tropman, (Eds.), *Strategies of Community Intervention* (6th ed., pp. 27-64). Itasca, IL: Peacock.

Rothman, J. (2007). Multi modes of intervention at the macro level. *Journal of Community Practice, 15*(4), 11-40.

Rothman, J., & Tropman, J. E. (1987). Models of community organization and macro practice perspectives: Their mixing and phasing. In F. M. Cox, J. L. Erlich, J. Rothman, & J. E. Tropman (Eds.), *Strategies of community organization: Macro practice* (pp. 3-26). Itasca, IL: Peacock.

Rothschild, M. L. (1999). Carrots, sticks, and promises: A conceptual framework for the management of public health and social issue behaviors. *Journal of Marketing, 63*, 24-37.

Rothschild, M. L., Mastin, B., & Miller, T. W. (2006). Reducing alcohol-impaired driving crashes through the use of social marketing. *Accident Analysis and Prevention, 38*(6), 1218-1230.

Rotter, J. B. (1954). *Social learning and clinical psychology.* New York: Prentice Hall.

Rowe, A., McClelland, A., & Billingham, K. (2001). *Community health needs assessment: An introductory guide for the family health nurse in Europe.* Copenhagen, Denmark: World Health Organization.

Rubak, S., Sandbaek, A., Lauritzen, T., & Christensen, B. (2005). Motivational interviewing: A systematic review and meta-anlysis. *The British Journal of General Practice, 55*(513), 305-312.

Ruberto, R. A., & Brissette, I. F. (2014). Geographic access to diabetes prevention program sites: New York State Department of Health. *Preventing Chronic Disease, 11*, 130400.

Runyan, C. W., & Frire, K. E. (2007). Developing interventions when there is little science. In L. S. Doll, S. E. Bonzo, J. A. Mercy, & D. A. Sleet (Eds.), *Handbook of injury and violence prevention* (pp. 411-431). New York, NY: Springer.

Ryan, M., Chapman, L. S., & Rink, M. J. (2008). Planning worksite health promotion programs: Models, methods, and design implications. *The Art of Health Promotion, 22*(16), 1–12.

Salleh, N., Hussein, R., Mohamed, N., Karim, N. S. A., Ahlan, A. R., & Aditiawarman, U. (2012). Examining informational disclosure behavior on social network sites using protection motivation theory, trust and risk. *Journal of Internet Social Networking & Virtual Communities,* 11 pages.

Sallis, J. F., Owen, N., & Fisher, E. B. (2008). Ecological models of health behavior. In K. Glanz, B. K. Rimer, & K. Viswanath (Eds.), *Health behavior and health education: Theory, research, and practice* (4th ed., pp. 465–485). San Francisco: Jossey-Bass.

Samson, A. (Ed.) (2014). *The behavioral economics guide 2014.* Retrieved July 17, 2015, from http://www.behavioral economics.com

Samueli Institute. (2015). *Optimal healing environments assessment.* Retrieved May 24, 2015, from https://www.samueliinstitute.org/for-hospitals-and-health-care/ohe-services

Sauber-Schatz, E. K., West, B. A., & Bergen, G. (2014). Vital signs: Restraint use and motor vehicle occupant death rates among children aged 0–12 years—United States, 2002–2011. *Morbidity and Mortality Weekly Report, 63*(5), 113–118.

Saunders, R. P., Evans, M. H., & Joshi, P. (2005). Developing a process-evaluation plan for assessing health promotion program implementation: A how-to guide. *Health Promotion Practice, 6*(2), 134–147.

Schaafsma, D., Stoffelen, J., Kok, G., & Curfs, L. (2012). Exploring the development of existing sex education programs for people with intellectual disabilities: An intervention mapping approach. *Journal of Applied Research in Intellectual Disabilities, 26*(2), 157–166.

Schiavo, R. (2014). *Health communication: From theory to practice* (2nd ed.). San Francisco, CA: Jossey-Bass.

Schmid, K. L., Rivers, S. E., Latimer, A. E., & Salovey, P. (2008). Targeting or tailoring: maximizing resources to create effective health communications. *Marketing Health Services, 28*(1), 32–37.

Schmitz, C. C., & Parsons, B. A. (1999). Everything you wanted to know about logic models but were afraid to ask. *Insites.* Retrieved July 28, 2015, from http://www.insites.org/evaluations-and-resources/other-evaluation-and-planning-resources

Schultz, P. W., Colehour, J., Vohr, J., Bonn, L., Bullock, A., & Sadler, A. (2015). Using Social Marketing to Spur Residential Adoption of ENERGY STAR®-Certified LED Lighting. *Social Marketing Quarterly, 21*(2), 61–78.

Selig, S., Tropiano, E., & Greene-Moton, E. (2006). Teaching cultural competence to reduce health disparities. *Health Promotion Practice, 7*(3), 247S–255S.

Serxner, S. A. (2013). A different approach to population health and behavior change: Moving from incentives to motivation-based approach. *American Journal of Health Promotion, 27*(4), TAHP 4–7.

Sharma, M. (2012). Information-motivation-behavior skills (IMB) model: Need for utilization in alcohol and drug education. *Journal of Alcohol & Drug Education, 56*(1), 3–7.

Sharma, M., & Petosa, R. L. (2014). *Measurement and evaluation for health educators.* Burlington, MA: Jones & Bartlett Learning.

Sharma, M., & Romas, J. A. (2012). *Theoretical foundations of health education and health promotion.* Burlington, MA: Jones & Bartlett Learning.

Shea, S., & Basch, C. E. (1990). A review of five major community-based cardiovascular disease prevention programs: Part I, rationale, design and theoretical framework. *American Journal of Health Promotion, 4*(3), 203–213.

Sherrill, W. W., Crew, L., Mayo, R. M., Mayo, W. F., Rogers, B. L., & Haynes, D. F. (2005). Educational and health services innovation to improve care for rural Hispanic communities in the U.S. *Education for Health, 18*(3), 356–367.

Shi, L., & Johnson, A. (2014). *Novick & Morrow's public health administration: Principles for population-based management* (3rd ed.). Burlington, MA: Jones & Bartlett Learning.

Siegel, S., & Castellan Jr, N. J. (1988). *Nonparametric statistics for the behavioral sciences.* New York: McGraw-Hill.

Simons-Morton, B., McLeroy, K. R., & Wendel, M. L. (2012). *Behavior theory in health promotion practice and research.* Burlington, MA: Jones & Bartlett Learning.

Simpson, V. L., Hyner, G. C., & Anderson, J. G. (2013). Lifestyle behavior change and repeat health risk appraisal participation: A structural equation modeling approach. *American Journal of Health Promotion, 28*(2), 128–135.

Skinner, B. F. (1953). *Science and human behavior.* New York: Free Press.

Slater, M. D., Kelly, K. J., & Thackeray, R. (2006). Segmentation on a shoestring: Health audience segmentation in limited-budget and local social marketing interventions. *Health Promotion Practice, 7,* 170–173.

Sleet, D. A. (2015 April). *Injuries—An enormous public health problem.* Presentation at the annual meeting of the Society for Public Health Education in Portland, OR.

Sleet, D. A., & Cole, S. L. (2010). Leadership for change and sustainability. In C. I. Fertman & D. Allenworth (Eds.), *Health promotion programs: From theory to practice* (pp. 291–310). San Francisco: Jossey-Bass.

Snow, L. (2001). *The organization of hope: A workbook for rural asset-based community development.* Evanston, IL: Institute for Policy Research, Northwestern University.

Soet, J. E., & Basch, C. E. (1997). The telephone as a communication medium for health education. *Health Education & Behavior, 24*(6), 759–772.

Solomon, D. D. (1987). Evaluating community programs. In F. M. Cox, J. L. Erlich, J. Rolhman, & J. E. Tropman (Eds.), *Strategies of community organization: Macro practices* (pp. 366–368). Itasca, IL: Peacock.

Spaulding, D. T. (2014). *Program evaluation in practice: Core concepts and examples for discussion and analysis* (2nd ed.). San Francisco, CA: Jossey-Bass.

Spencer, L., Adams, T. B., Malone, S., Roy, L., & Yost, E. (2006). Applying the transtheoretical model to exercise: A systematic and comprehensive review of the literature. *Health Promotion Practice, 7*(4), 428–443.

SPM Board of Directors (SPMBoD). (1999). Ethics guidelines for the development and use of health assessments. In G. C. Hyner, K. W. Peterson, J. W. Travis, J. E. Dewey, J.J. Foerster, & E. M. Framer (Eds.), *SPM handbook of health assessment tools* (p. xxiii). Pittsburgh, PA: Society of Prospective Medicine.

Stacy, R. D. (1987). Instrument evaluation guides for survey research in health education and health promotion. *Health Education, 18*(5), 65–67.

State Health Access Data Assistance Center (SHADAC). (2009). *The impact of wireless-only households on state surveys of health insurance coverage* (Issue Brief #15). Minneapolis: University of Minnesota. Retrieved May 20, 2015, from http://www.rwjf.org/content/dam/farm/reports/issue_briefs/2009/rwjf37483

Staples, L. (2012). Selecting and "cutting" the issue. In M. Minkler (Ed.). *Community organizing and community building for health and welfare* (3rd ed., pp. 187–214). New Brunswick, NJ: Rutgers University Press.

Staten, L. K., Birnbaum, A. S., Jobe, J. B., & Elder, J. P. (2006). A typology of middle school girls: Audience segmentation related to physical activity. *Health Education Behavior, 33*(1), 66–80.

Steckler, A., Goodman, R. M., McLeroy, K. R., Davis, S., & Koch, G. (1992). Measuring the diffusion of innovative health promotion programs. *American Journal of Health Promotion, 6*(3), 214–224.

Steckler, A., & Linnan, L. (Eds.). (2002). *Process evaluation for public health interventions and research.* San Francisco, CA: Jossey-Bass.

Steckler, A., McLeroy, K. R., Goodman, R. M., Bird, S. T., & McCormick, L. (1992). Toward integrating qualitative and quantitative methods: An introduction. *Health Education Quarterly, 19*(1), 1–8.

Stevens, S. S. (1946). On the theory of scales of measurement. *Science, 103*, 677–680.

Stewart-Brown, S. (2006). *What is the evidence on school health promotion in improving health or preventing disease and, specifically, what is the effectiveness of the health promoting schools approach?* Copenhagen: WHO Regional Office for Europe. Retrieved March 26, 2011, from http://www.euro.who.int/document/e88185.pdf

Strecher, V. J., DeVellis, B. M., Becker, M. H., & Rosenstock, I. M. (1986). The role of self-efficacy in achieving health behavior change. *Health Education Quarterly, 13*(1), 73–91.

Strecher, V. J., & Rosenstock, I. M. (1997). The health belief model. In K. Glanz, F. M. Lewis, & B. K. Rimer (Eds.), *Health behavior and health education: Theory, research, and practice* (pp. 41–59). San Francisco: Jossey-Bass.

Streiner, D. L., Norman, G. R., & Cairney, J. (2015). *Health meansurement scales: A practical guide to their development and use* (5th ed.). Oxford, United Kingdom, Oxfor University Press.

STEPS Centre. (2015). *Photovoice.* Retrieved May 21, 2015, from http://steps-centre.org/methods/pathways-methods/vignettes/photovoice/?referralDomain=

Strycker, L. A., Foster, L. S., Pettigrew, L., Donnelly-Perry, J., Jordan, S., & Glasgow, R. E. (1997). Steering committee enhancements on health promotion program delivery. *American Journal of Health Promotion, 11*(6), 437–440.

Substance Abuse and Mental Health Services Administration (SAMHSA). (1999). Motivational interviewing as a counseling style. In *SAMHSA/Center for Substance Abuse Treatment: Treatment Improvement Protocols* (Chapter 3). Rockville, MD: Author. Retrieved June 23, 2015, from http://www.ncbi.nlm.nih.gov/books/NBK64964/

Substance Abuse and Mental Health Services Administration (SAMHSA). (2015). *Motivational interviewing.* Retrieved August 24, 2015, from http://nrepp.samhsa.gov/ViewIntervention.aspx?id=346

Suggs, L. S., & McIntyre, C. (2009). Are we there yet? An examination of online tailored health communication. *Health Education & Behavior, 36*(2), 278–288.

Sullivan, L.M. (2008). *Essentials of biostatistics in public health.* Sudbury, MA: Jones & Bartlett.

Sutton, S. (n.d.). *Health behavior constructs: Theory, measurement, & research—Stages.* National Cancer Institute. Retrieved on June 15, 2015, from http://cancercontrol.cancer.gov/Brp/constructs/stages/index.html

Szreter, S. & Woolcock, M. (2004) Health by association? Social capital, social theory, and the political economy of public health. *International Journal of Epidemiology, 33*(4), 650–67.

Taylor, L., & Quigley, R. (2002). *Health impact assessment: A review of reviews.* London: NHS, Health Development Agency. Retrieved May 23, 2015, from http://www.who.int/hia/evidence/en/hia_review.pdf

Taylor, S. M., Elliott, S., & Riley, B. (1998). Heart health promotion: Predisposition, capacity and implementation in Ontario public health units, 1994–1996. *Canadian Journal of Public Health, 6,* 410–414.

TechTarget. (2007–2015a). *Gantt chart.* Retrieved July 29, 2015, from http://searchsoftwarequality.techtarget.com/definition/Gantt-chart

TechTarget. (2007–2015b). *PERT-chart.* Retrieved July 29, 2015, from http://searchsoftwarequality.techtarget.com/definition/PERT-chart

Terry, P. E. (2012). Do health health professionals have the wherewithal to change organizational cultures? *American Journal of Health Promotion, 26*(6), TAHP 10–12.

Terry, P. E. (2014). Case study: How can this organization's culture support employee health? *American Journal of Health Promotion, 28*(3), TAHP 11–12.

Terry, P. E., & Anderson, D. R. (2011). Finding common ground in the use of financial incentives for employee health management: A call for progress-based approach. *American Journal of Health Promotion, 26*(1), ev–evii.

Terry, P. E., Seaverson, E. L. D., Grossmeier, J., & Anderson, D. R. (2011). Effectiveness of a worksite telephone-based weight management program. *American Journal of Health Promotion, 25*(3), 186–189.

Tervalon, M., & Garcia, J. (1998). Cultural humility versus cultural competence: A critical distinction in defining physician training outcomes in multicultural education. *Journal of Health Care for the Poor and Underserved, 9*(2), 117–125.

Teufel-Shone, N. I., & Williams, S. (2010). Focus groups in small communities. *Preventing Chronic Disease, 7*(3), A67. Retrieved on May 21, 2015, from http://www.cdc.gov/pcd/issues/2010/May/pdf/09_0164.pdf

Thackeray, R., & Bennion, S. R. (2009). *Social media matters: Expanding your reach and effectiveness in social marketing.* Paper presented at the Social Marketing and Public Health Conference, Tampa, FL.

Thackeray, R., Fulkerson, K. N., & Neiger, B. L. (2012). Defining the product in social marketing: An analysis of published research from 1999–2009. *A Journal of Non-Profit and Public Sector Marketing, 23*(2).

Thackeray, R., & Hunter, M. (2010). Empowering youth: Use of technology in advocacy to affect social change. *Journal of Computer-Mediated Communication, 15,* 575–591.

Thackeray, R., & McCormack Brown, K. (2005). Social marketing's unique contribution to health promotion practice. *Health Promotion Practice, 6*(4), 365–368.

Thackeray, R., & Neiger, B. L. (2009). A multidirectional communication model: Implications for social marketing practice. *Health Promotion Practice, 10,* 2, 171–175.

Thackeray, R., Neiger, B. L., Hanson, C. L., & McKenzie, J. F. (2008). Enhancing promotional strategies within social marketing programs: Use of Web 2.0 social media. *Health Promotion Practice, 9*(4), 338–343.

Thackeray, R., Neiger, B. L., & Keller, H. (2012). Integrating social media and social marketing: A four-step process. *Health Promotion Practice, 13*(2), 165–168.

Thorndike, E. L. (1898). Animal intelligence: An experimental study of the associative processes in animals. *Psychological Monographs, 2*(8).

Timmreck, T. C. (1997). *Health services cyclopedic dictionary* (3rd ed.). Boston, MA: Jones & Bartlett.

Timmreck, T. C. (2003). *Planning, program development, and evaluation* (2nd ed.). Boston, MA: Jones & Bartlett.

Tomioka, M., & Braun, K. L. (2013). Implementing evidence-based programs: A four-step protocol for assuring replication with fidelity. *Health Promotion Practice, 14*(6), 850–858.

Trickett, E. J. (2011). Community-based participatory research as worldview or instrumental strategy: Is it lost in translational research? *American Journal of Public Health, 101*(8), 1353–1355.

Tri-Ethnic Center for Prevention, Colorado State University (2014). *Community readiness for community change* (2nd ed.). Retrieved on June 17, 2015, from http://triethniccenter.colostate.edu/docs/CR_Handbook_2014.pdf

Trust for America's Health (TFAH). (2009). *Prevention for a healthier America: Investments in disease prevention yield significant savings, stronger communities.* Retrieved May 13, 2015, from http://healthyamericans.org/reports/prevention08/Prevention08.pdf

Tuckman, B. W. (1965). Developmental sequence in small groups. *Psychological Bulletin, 63,* 384–399.

Tuckman, B. W. (2001). Developmental sequence in small groups. *Group Facilitation: A Research and Applications Journal, 3*, 66–81.

Tuckman, B. W., & Jensen, M. A. C. (1977). Stages of small group development revisited. *Group and Organizational Studies, 2*, 419–427.

Turnock, B. J. (2012). *Public health: What it is and how it works* (5th ed.). Burlington, MA: Jones & Bartlett Learning.

Ueda, Y., Sobue, T., Morimoto, A., Egawa-Takata, T., Hashizume, C., Kishida, H., ... & Kimura, T. (2015). Evaluation of a free-coupon program for cervical cancer screening among the young: A nationally funded program conducted by a local government in Japan. *Journal of Epidemiology, 25*(1), 50.

United Nations. (1955). *Social progress through community development.* New York: Author.

U.S. Census Bureau (USCB). (2010). *Men and women wait longer to marry.* Retrieved May 29, 2011, from http://www.census.gov/newsroom/releases /archives/families_households/cb10-174.html

U.S. Department of Agriculture (USDA). (n.d.). Principles of motivational interviewing. Retrieved on June 23, 2015, from http://www.nal.usda.gov /wicworks/WIC_Learning_Online/support/job _aids/MI.pdf

U.S. Department of Education (USDE), National Center for Education Statistics (NCES). (n.d.). *National assessment of adult literacy.* Retrieved June 24, 2015, from http://nces.ed.gov/naal/

U.S. Department of Health, Education, and Welfare (USDHEW), Public Health Service. (1979). *Healthy people: The surgeon general's report on health promotion and disease prevention* (Publication No. 79-55071). Washington, DC: Author.

U.S. Department of Health and Human Services. (1980). *Promoting health/preventing disease: Objectives for the nation.* Washington, DC: U.S. Government Printing Office.

U.S. Department of Health and Human Services. (1990). *Healthy People 2000: National health promotion disease prevention objectives* (DHHS Publication No. [PHS] 90–50212). Washington, DC: U.S. Government Printing Office.

U.S. Department of Health and Human Services (USDHHS). (2000). *Healthy People 2010* (CD-ROM Version). Washington, DC: Author.

U.S. Department of Health and Human Services (USDHHS). (2001). *Youth violence: A report of the Surgeon General.* Washington, DC: Author. Retrieved July 31, 2015, from http://www.ncbi .nlm.nih.gov/books/NBK44294/

U.S. Department of Health and Human Services. (2003). *Prevention makes common"cents."*

Retrieved March 24, 2007, from http://aspe.hhs. gov/health/prevention/

U.S. Department of Health and Human Services (USDHHS). (2005). *The surgeon general's call to action to improve the heath and wellness of persons with disabilities.* Washington, DC: Author. Retrieved July 29, 2015, from http://www.ncbi.nlm.nih.gov /books/NBK44667/

U.S. Department of Health and Human Services. (2007). *HP 2010 midcourse review: Appendix C: Technical appendix.* Retrieved June 3, 2015, from http://www.healthypeople.gov/2010/data /midcourse/html/default.htm

U.S. Department of Health and Human Services. (2009). *Secretary's advisory committee on national health promotion and disease prevention objectives for 2020-Minutes: Twelfth meeting May 15, 2019.* Retrieved June 3, 2015, from http://www.healthypeople.gov/2020 /minutes-twelfth-meeting-may-15-2009/page/3/0

U.S. Department of Health and Human Services (USDHHS). (2010). *National action plan to improve health literacy.* Retrieved June 24, 2015, from http:// www.health.gov/communication/hlactionplan/

U.S. Department of Health and Human Services (USDHHS). (2015a). *Health communication.* Retrieved June 24, 2015, from http://health.gov /communication/resources/

U.S. Department of Health and Human Services (USDHHS). (2015b). *Health literacy.* Retrieved June 24, 2015, from http://health.gov /communication/literacy/

U.S. Department of Health and Human Services (USDHHS). (2015c). *Healthy People 2020.* Retrieved May 9, 2015, from http://www.healthypeople.gov/

U.S. Department of Health and Human Services (USDHHS). (2015d). *MAP-IT: A guide to using Healthy People 2020 in your community.* Retrieved June 10, 2015, from http://www.healthypeople .gov/2020/tools-and-resources/Program-Planning

U.S. Department of Health and Human Services (USDHHS). (2015e). *Regulations.* Retrieved July 31, 2015, from http://www.hhs.gov/ohrp /humansubjects/index.html

U.S. Department of Health and Human Services (USDHHS), Centers for Disease Control and Prevention. (n.d.). *Planned approach to community health: Guide for local coordinator.* Atlanta: Author.

U.S. Department of Health and Human Services (USDHHS), Office of Civil Rights (OCR). (n.d.). *Health information privacy.* Retrieved May 21, 2015, from http://www.hhs.gov/ocr/privacy

U.S. Deaprtment of Justice (USDJ). (n.d.). *Getting started: Types of evaluation activities, program monitoring.* Retrieved July 29, 2015, from https:// www.bja.gov/evaluation/guide/gs2.htm

U.S. Department of Labor (USDOL). (n.d). *Fact sheet: The Affordable Care Act and wellness programs.* Retrieved July 9, 2015, from http://www.dol.gov/ebsa/newsroom/fswellnessprogram.html

U.S. Department of Labor (USDOL). (n.d). *Summary of the major laws of the Department of Labor.* Retrieved July 29, 2015, from http://www.dol.gov/opa/aboutdol/lawsprog.htm

U.S. Department of Labor (USDOL), Bureau of Labor Statistics (BLS). (2015). *21-1091 health educators.* Retrieved May 11, 2015, from http://www.bls.gov/oes/current/oes211091.htm

U.S. National Library of Medicine (NLM). (2015). *Fact sheet MEDLINE®.* Retrieved May 21, 2015, from http://www.nlm.nih.gov/pubs/factsheets/medline.html

U.S. National Library of Medicine (NLM). (n.d). *PubMed.* Retrieved May 22, 2015, from http://www.ncbi.nlm.nih.gov/pubmed

University of Kansas. (2014). *Chapter 3, Section 20: Implementing photovoice in your community.* Retrieved May 21, 2015, from http://ctb.ku.edu/en/table-of-contents/assessment/assessing-community-needs-and-resources/photovoice/main

University of Kansas. (2015a). *Chapter 2, Section 1: Developing a logic model or theory of change.* Retrieved July 28, 2015, from http://ctb.ku.edu/en/table-of-contents/overview/models-for-community-health-and-development/logic-model-development/main

University of Kansas. (2015b). *Chapter 42, Section 5: Writing a grant.* Retrieved September 23, 2015, from http://ctb.ku.edu/en/table-of-contents/finances/grants-and-financial-resources/writing-a-grant/main

University of Nevada, Reno, Cooperative Extension (UNRCE). (2003). *Community leaders guide.* Retrieved July 17, 2015, from http://www.unce.unr.edu/publications/files/cd/2001/eb0103.pdf

University of Rhode Island, Cancer Prevention Research Center. (2015). *Transtheoretical model.* Retrieved June 13, 2015 from http://web.uri.edu/cprc/transtheoretical-model/

University of Wisconsin Population Health Institute. (2015). *County health rankings & roadmap.* Retrieved May 24, 2015, from http://www.countyhealthrankings.org/

Utah Department of Health (2011). *The truth campaign: Marketing resources. Tobacco Prevention and Control Program.* Retrieved October 1, 2015, from: http://www.tobaccofreeutah.org/pdfs/TRUTHeval.pdf

Valente, T. W. (2002). *Evaluating health promotion programs.* New York, NY: Oxford University Press.

Valente, T. W. (2010). *Social networks and health: Models, methods, and applications.* New York, NY: Oxford University Press.

van Dam, R. M., Li, T., Spiegelman, D., Franco, O. H., & Hu, F. B. (2008). Combined impact of lifestyle factors on mortality: Prospective cohort study of U.S. women. *British Medical Journal, 337,* a1440.

Van Der Wagen, L., & Carlos, B. R. (2005). *Event management: For tourism, cultural, business, and sporting events.* Upper Saddle River, NJ: Pearson Prentice Hall.

Vaughn, E. J., & Krenz, V. D. (2014). Planning, implementing, and evaluating culturally appropriate programs. In M. A. Pérez & R. R. Luquis (Eds.), *Cultural competence in health education and health promotion* (2nd ed.) (pp. 171–192). San Francisco, CA: Jossey-Bass

VentureLine. (2015). *Glossary.* Retrieved on July 21, 2015, from https://www.ventureline.com/

Vogele, C. (2005). Education. In J. Kerr, R. Weikunat, & M. Moretti (Eds.), *ABC of behavior change: A guide to successful disease prevention and health promotion* (pp. 271–287). Edinburgh: Elsevier Churchill Livingstone.

Voogt, C., Poelen, E., Kleinjan, M., Lemmers, L., & Engels, R. (2014). The development of a web-based brief alcohol intervention in reducing heavy drinking among college students: An intervention mapping approach. *Health Promotion International, 29*(4), 669–679.

Wallerstein, N. (1987). Empowerment education: Freire's ideas applied to youth. *Youth Policy, 9,* 11–15.

Wallston, K. A. (1992). Hocus-pocus, the focus isn't strictly on locus: Rotter's social learning theory modified for health. *Cognitive Therapy and Research, 16,* 183–199.

Wallston, K. A. (1994). Theoretically based strategies for health behavior change. In M. P. O'Donnell & J. S. Harris (Eds.), *Health promotion in the workplace* (2nd ed., pp. 185–203). Albany, NY: Delmar.

Wallston, K. A. (2007). Multidimensional health locus of control (MHLC) scales. Retrieved on June 16, 2007, from http://www.nursing.vanderbilt.edu/faculty/kwallston/mhlcscales.htm

Wallston, K. A., Stein, M. J., & Smith. K. A. (1994). Form C of MHLC scales: A condition-specific measure of locus of control. *Journal of Personality Assessment, 63,* 534–553.

Wallston, K. A., Wallston, B. S., & DeVellis, R. (1978). Development of the multidimensional health locus of control (MHLC) scales. *Health Education Monographs, 6,* 160–170.

Walsh, D. C., Rudd, R. E., Moeykens, B. A., & Moloney, T. W. (1993). Social marketing for public health. *Health Affairs, 12,* 104–119.

Walter, C. (2005). Community building practice. In M. Minkler (Ed.), *Community organizing and community building for health* (2nd ed., pp. 66–78). New Brunswick, NJ: Rutgers University Press.

Wang, C. C., & Burris, M. A. (1994). Empowerment through photovoice: Portraits of participation. *Health Education Quarterly, 21*(2), 171–186.

Wang, C. C., & Burris, M. A. (1997). Photovoice: Concept, methodology, and use for participatory needs assessment. *Health Education and Behavior, 24*(3), 369–387.

Wang, C. C., Morrel-Samuels, S., Hutchinson, P. M., Bell, L., & Pestronk, R. M. (2004). Flint photovoice: Community building among youths, adults, and policymakers. *American Journal of Public Health, 94*(6), 911–913.

Wang, C. C., Yi, W. K., Tao, Z. W., & Carovano, K. (1998). Photovoice as a participatory health promotion strategy. *Health Promotion International, 13*(1), 75–87.

Warren, M. R. (1963). *The community in America.* Chicago, IL: Rand McNally.

Warren, M. R., Thompson, J. P., & Saegert, S. (2001). The role of social capital in combating poverty. In S. Saegert, J. P. Thompson, & M. R. Warren (Eds.), *Social capital and poor communities* (pp. 1–28). New York: Sage Foundation.

Washington University Prevention Research Center. (2015). *Evidence based public health course.* Retrieved June 10, 2015, from http://prcstl.wustl.edu/training/Pages/EBPH-Course-Information.aspx

Washtenaw County Public Health (WCPH). (2009). *Youth photovoice: Implementation toolkit.* Ann Arbor, MI: Author

Watson, J. B. (1925). *Behaviorism.* New York: Norton.

Wayman, J., Beal, T., Thackeray, R., & McCormack Brown, K. (2007). Competition. Friend or foe? *Health Promotion Practice, 8*(2), 134–139.

Weinstein, N. D. (1988). The precaution adoption process. *Health Psychology, 7*, 355–386.

Weinstein, N. D., & Rothman, A. J., & Sutton, S. R. (1998). Stage theories of health behavior: Conceptual and methodological issues. *Health Psychology, 17*, 290–299.

Weinstein, N. D., & Sandman, P. M. (1992). A model of the precaution adoption process: Evidence from home radon testing. *Health Psychology, 11*, 170–180.

Weinstein, N. D., & Sandman, P. M. (2002a). The precaution adoption process model. In K. Glanz, B. K. Rimer, & F. M. Lewis (Eds.), *Health behavior and health education: Theory, research, and practice* (3rd ed., pp. 121–143). San Francisco, CA: Jossey-Bass.

Weinstein, N. D., & Sandman, P. M. (2002b). The precaution adoption process model and its application. In R. J. DiClemente, R. A. Crosby, & M. C. Kegler (Eds.), *Emerging theories in health promotion practice and research: Strategies for improving public health* (pp. 16–39). San Francisco, CA: Jossey-Bass.

Weinstein, N. D., Sandman, P. M., & Blalock, S. J. (2008). The precaution adoption process model. In K. Glanz, B. K. Rimer, & K. Viswanath (Eds.), *Health behavior and health education: Theory, research, and practice* (4th ed., pp. 123–147). San Francisco: Jossey-Bass.

Weiss, C. H. (1984). Increasing the likelihood of influencing decisions. In L. Rutman (Ed.), *Evaluation research methods: A basic guide* (2nd ed., pp. 159–190). Beverly Hills, CA: Sage.

Weiss, C. H. (1998). *Evaluation* (2nd ed.). Upper Saddle River, NJ: Prentice-Hall.

White, S., & Dillow, S. (2005). *Key concepts and features of the 2003 National Assessment of Adult Literacy* (NCES 2006-471). Washington, DC: National Center for Education Statistics, U.S. Department of Education.

Whittingham, J., Ruiter, R. A., Zimbile, F., & Kok, G. (2008). Experimental pretesting of public health campaigns: A case study. *Journal of Health Communication, 13*, 216–229.

Wiecha, J. L., Hannon, C., & Meyer, K. (2013). A toolkit to promote fidelity to health promotion interventions in afterschool programs. *Health Promotion Practice, 14*(3), 370–379.

Wilbur, C. (1983). Live for life—The Johnson & Johnson program. *Preventive Medicine, 12*(5), 672–681.

Willard-Grace, R., Chen, E. H., Hessler, D., DeVore, D., Prado, C., Bodenheimer, T., & Thom, D. H. (2015). Health coaching by medical assistants to improve control of diabetes, hypertension, hyperlipidemia in low-income patients: A randomized controlled trial. *Annals of Family Medicine, 13*(2), 130–138.

Wilson, M. G. (1990). Factors associated with, issues related to, and suggestions for increasing participation in workplace health promotion programs. *Health Values, 14*(4), 29–36.

Windsor, R. A. (2015). *Evaluation of health promotion, health education, and disease prevention programs* (5th ed.). New York, NY: Oxford University Press.

W. K. Kellogg Foundation (WKKF). (2004). *Logic model development guide.* Battle Creek, MI: Author.

Woods, N. K., Watson-Thompson, J., Schober, D. J., Markt, B., & Fawcett, S. (2014). An empirical case study of the effects of training and technical assistance on community coalition functioning and sustainability. *Health Promotion Practice, 15*(5), 739–749.

World Health Organization (WHO). (2001). *Community health needs assessment.* Retrieved May 19 2015, from http://www.euro.who.int/__data/assets/pdf_file/0018/102249/E73494.pdf

World Health Organization (WHO). (2009). *Milestones in health promotion: Statements from global conferences.* Retrieved August 25, 2015, from http://www.who.int/healthpromotion/Milestones_Health_Promotion_05022010.pdf

World Health Organization (WHO). (2015). *Health impact assessment: Why use HIA?* Retrieved May 23, 2015, from http://www.who.int/hia/about/why/en/

Wright, P. A. (Ed.). (1994). *Technical assistance bulletin: A key step in developing prevention materials is to obtain expert and gatekeepers' reviews.* Bethesda, MD: Center for Substance Abuse Prevention (CSAP) Communications Team.

Wu, C. S. T., Wong, H. T., Chou, L. Y., To, B. P. W., Lee, W. L., & Loke, A. Y. (2014). Correlates of protective motivation theory (PMT) to adolescent drug use intention. *International Journal of Environmental Research and Public Health, 11*, 671–684.

Wurzbach, M. E. (Ed.). (2002). *Community health education and promotion: A guide to program design and evaluation* (2nd ed.). Gaithersburg, MD: Aspen.

Yamane, T. (1973). *Statistics: An introductory analysis* (3rd ed.). New York, NY: Harper & Row.

Zimmerman, F. J. (2009). Using behavioral economics to promote physical *activity. Preventive Medicine, 49*, 289–291.

COVER

Edhar Shvets/Shutterstock

CHAPTER 1

p. 2 Based on Miniño, Xu, & Kochanek (2010). Mokdad, Marks, Stroup, & Greberding (2004, 2005); p. 3 Green 1999, p.69. Green, L. W. (1999). Health education's contributions to public health in the twentieth century: A glimpse through health promotion's rear-view mirror. In J. E. Fielding, L.B. Lave, & B. Starfield (Eds.), Annual review of public health (pp. 67–88). Palo Alto, CA: Annual Reviews; p. 4 Breslow 1999, p. 1031. Breslow, L. (1999). From disease prevention to health promotion. Journal of the American Medical Association, 281(11), 1030–1033; p. 4 American Journal of Health Education, Report of the 2011 Joint Committee on Health Education and Promotion Terminology, p 13; p. 5 Pearson Education; p. 9 U.S. Department of Labor Bureau of Labor Statistics (BLS), (Standard Occupation Classification [SOC] 21-1091), Paragraph 1, 2015; p. 11 Adapted from Public Health: Administration and Practice. George E. Pickett and John J. Hanlon. Copyright © 1990 by McGraw Hill Education; p. 12 Pearson Education.

CHAPTER 2

p. 19 Art of Health Promotion. L. S. Chapman. Copyright © 1997 by The American Journal of Health Promotion. Reproduced with permission. p. 20 Pearson Education; p. 21 Pearson Education; p. 22 Adapted from ACS (2009). CDC (2010c). and Chapman (1997); p. 24 McGinnis and colleagues (2002). McGinnis, J. M., Williams-Russo, P., & Knickman, J.R. (2002). The case for more active policy attention to health promotion. Health Affairs, 21(2), 78–93; p. 25 Pearson Education; p. 27 Pearson Education; p. 28 TM Toole, J Gambatese; The trajectories of prevention through design in construction. Journal of Safety Research, 39(2) pp. 225–230; p. 28 Pearson Education; p. 30 (WHO, 2014, para. 4); pp. 31–32 Guide to Community Preventive Services. Reducing tobacco use and secondhand smoke exposure: comprehensive tobacco control programs. www.thecommunityguide.org/tobacco/comprehensive.html. Last updated: 11/13/2014; p. 35 Pearson Education.

CHAPTER 3

p. 42 Pearson Education; p. 45 Achieving Healthier Communities through MAPP: A User's Handbook. Copyright © 2009 by the National Association of County and City Health Officials. Reprinted with permission; p. 49 Adapted from Health Promotion Planning. Lawrence W. Green and Marshall W. Kreuter. Copyright © 2005 by McGraw-Hill.

CHAPTER 4

p. 68 Brennan Ramirez et al, 2008, p. 54. Brennan Ramirez, L. K., Baker, E. A., & Metzler, M. (2008). Promoting Health Equity: A Resource to Help Communities Address Social Determinants of Health. Atlanta: Centers for Disease Control and Prevention. Retrieved March 29,2011, from http://www.cdc.gov/nccdphp/dach/chaps; p. 74 U.S. Department of Health and Human Services, Centers for Disease Control and Prevention (no date), p. A3–12; p. 87 Pearson Education; p. 89 Adapted from Deeds (1992) and Marcarin (1995); p. 90 Pearson Education; p. 95 Neiger, Thackeray, & Fagen, 2011, p. 166, 168. S.Neiger, B. L., Thackeray, R., & Fagen, M. C. (2011). Basic priority rating model 2.0: Current applications for priority setting in health promotion practice. Health Promotion Practice, 12(2), 166–171. © 2011 Sage Publications; p. 97 Green L, Kreuter M. (1999). Health promotion planning: An educational and ecological approach. 3rd edition. Mountain View, CA: Mayfield Publishing Company; p. 101 Based on (WHO, 2015, para. 1).

CHAPTER 5

p. 110 Pearson Education; p. 122 Pearson Education; p. 123 Pearson Education; p. 127 Pearson Education.

CHAPTER 7

p. 152 Nutbeam and Harris 1999. Nutbeam, D., & Harris, E. (1999). Theory in a nutshell: A guide to health promotion theory. Sydney, Australia: McGraw-Hill; p. 153 Pearson Education; p. 158 Pearson Education; p. 160 Pearson Education; p. 161 Theory of Planned Behavior Diagram. Icek Ajzen. Copyright © 2006 by Icek Ajzen. Reprinted with permission; p. 162 Theory of Planned Behavior Diagram. Icek Ajzen. Copyright © 2006 by Icek Ajzen. Reprinted with permission; p. 162 Champion, V.L., & Skinner, C.S. (2008). The health belief model. In Glanz K, Rimer BK, Viswanath K, Eds. (4th ed). Health Behavior and Health Education: Theory, Research, and Practice. San Francisco: Jossey-Bass. pp. 45-65. (graph on p48); p. 163 Pearson Education; p. 164 Prentice-Dunn and Rogers 1986, p. 156. Prentice-Dunn, S., & Rogers, R. W. (1986). Protection motivation theory and preventive; p. 167 "Changing AIDS-Risk Behavior." J. D. and W. A. Fisher from Psychological Bulletin 111(3). Copyright © 1992 by the American Psychological Association.; p. 171 "Models for Provider-Patient Interaction: Applications to Health Behavior Change." M. G. Goldstein from The Handbook of Health Behavior Change by Sally Shumaker. Reproduced with permission of Springer Publishing Company, Incorporated via Copyright Clearance Center; p. 172 Prochaska et al., 2008, 103. Prochaska, J. O, Redding, C. A., & Evers, K. E. (2008). The transtheoretical model and stages of change. In K. Glanz, B. K. Rimer, & K. Viswanath

477

(Eds.), Health behavior and health education: Theory, research, and practice (4th ed., pp. 97–121). San Francisco: Jossey-Bass; p. 173 Surgical versus Nonsurgical Therapy for Lumbar Spinal Stenosis; James N. Weinstein, D.O., M.S., Tor D. Tosteson, Sc.D., Jon D. Lurie, M.D., M.S., Anna N.A. Tosteson, Sc.D., Emily Blood, M.S., Brett Hanscom, M.S., Harry Herkowitz, M.D., Frank Cammisa, M.D., Todd Albert, M.D., Scott D. Boden, M.D., Alan Hilibrand, M.D., Harley Goldberg, D.O., Sigurd Berven, M.D., and Howard An, M.D. for the SPORT Investigators. New England Journal of Medicine, 2008; 358:794-810 February 21, 2008. © 2008 Massachusetts Medical Society; p. 174 Pearson Education; p. 175 Based on: Health Behavior and Health Education: Theory, Research, and Practice, by Karen Glanz, Barbara K. Rimer, and K. Viswanath. Copyright © 2008 by John Wiley & Sons, Inc.; p. 178 Glanz and Rimer 1995 p. 15. Glanz, K., & Rimer, B. K. (1995). Theory at a glance: A guide for health promotion practice (NIH Pub. No. 95–3896). Washington, DC: National Cancer Institute; p. 181 Edberg, 2007, p.59. Edberg, M. (2007). Essentials of health behavior: Social and behavioral theory in public health. Sudbury, MA: Jones & Bartlett; p. 182 Based on Introduction to Health Behavior Theory. by J. Hayden. Copyright © 2014 by Jones & Bartlett Learning; p. health: Beyond the health belief model. Health Education Research: Theory and Practice, 1(3), 153–161. Oxford University Press; p. 183 Pearson Education; p. 185 "Community readiness: Research to practice." Ruth W. Edwards, Pamela Jumper-Thurman, Barbara A. Plested, Eugene R. Oetting, Louis Swanson, in Journal of Community Psychology 28(3). Copyright © 2000 by John Wiley & Sons, Inc; p. 186 "Community readiness: Research to practice." Ruth W. Edwards, Pamela Jumper-Thurman, Barbara A. Plested, Eugene R. Oetting, Louis Swanson, in Journal of Community Psychology 28(3). Copyright © 2000 by John Wiley & Sons, Inc.

CHAPTER 8

p. 195 Thackeray, R., & Neiger, B. L. (2009). A multidirectional communication model: Implications for social marketing practice. Health Promotion Practice, 10(2), 171–175. © 2009 Sage Publications; p. 198 Adapted from United States Department of Agriculture (n.d.); p. 200 Pearson Education; p. 200 Adult Literacy in America: A First Look at the Findings of the National Adult Literacy Survey; Kirsch, Jungeblut, Jenkins, & Kolstad. U.S. Department of Education Office of Educational Research and Improvement; p. 201 White & Dillow (2005). White, S., & Dillow, S. (2005). Key concepts and features of the 2003 National Assessment of Adult Literacy (NCES 2006-471). Washington, DC: National Center for Education Statistics, U.S. Department of Education; p. 205 Pearson Education; p. 206 Pearson Education; p. 216 Pearson Education; p. 222 © 2009 Larry Grudzien, Attorney at Law. All Right Reserved; p. 226 McKleroy et al. 2006. McKleroy, V. S., Galbraith, J. S., Cummings, B., Jones, P., Harshbarger, C., Collins, C., Gelaude, D., Carey, J. W., & ADAPT Team. (2006). Adapting evidence-based behavioral interventions for new settings and target populations. AIDS Education and Prevention, 19(Suppl. A), 59–73; p. 228 Pearson Education; p. 231 Pearson Education.

CHAPTER 9

p. 238 An Introduction to Community & Public Health, James F. McKenzie, Robert R. Pinger, © 2015 Jones & Bartlett Learning; p. 241 Minkler, M., & Wallerstein, N. (2012). Improving health through community organization and community building: Perspectives from health education and social work. In M. Minkler (Ed.). Community organizing and community building for health and welfare

(3rd ed., p. 44). New Brunswick, NJ: Rutgers University Press; p. 242 Minkler, Meredith and Nina Wallerstein. "Figure 3.1: Community Organization and Community—Building Typology" in Community Organizing and Community Building for Health and Welfare. Copyright © 2012 by Meredith Minkler. Reprinted by permission of Rutgers University Press; p. 243 Pearson Education; p. 247 Butterfoss, 2007, p. 30. Butterfoss, F. D. (2007). Coalitions and partnerships in community health. San Francisco: Jossey-Bass; p. 250 Kretzman, John P. and John L. McKnight. "Figure 10.1: Neighborhood Needs Map", "Mapping Community Capacity" in Community Organizing and Community Building for Health and Welfare. Copyright © 2012 by Meredith Minkler. Reprinted by permission of Rutgers University Press; p. 251 Kretzman, John P. and John L. McKnight. "Figure 10.2: Neighborhood Assets Map", "Mapping Community Capacity" in Community Organizing and Community Building for Health and Welfare. Copyright © 2012 by Meredith Minkler. Reprinted by permission of Rutgers University Press.

CHAPTER 10

p. 265 Adapted from: "How to Select the Right Vendor for Your Company's Selecting Health Promotion Program." J. H. Harris, J. F. McKenzie, and W. B. Zuti, from Fitness in Business 1. Copyright © 1986 by American School Health Association.; p. 266 Pearson Education; p. 270 Pearson Education; p. 272 Teaching Patients with Low Literacy Skills, 2nd Edition. C. C. Doak, L. G. Doak, & J. H. Root. Copyright © 1996 by J. B. Lippincott Company. Reprinted with permission of the authors; p. 283 Pearson Education; p. 286 Pearson Education.

CHAPTER 11

p. 295 Pearson Education; p. 298 Pearson Education; p. 301 Adapted from Lynch, Squires, Lewis, Moultrie, Kish-Doto, Boudewyns, et al, 2014; p. 309 Staten LK, Birnbaum AS, Jobe JB, Elder JP. A typology of middle school girls: Audience segmentation related to physical activity. Health Education & Behavior. 2006;33:66–80; p. 313 Pearson Education.

CHAPTER 12

p. 321 Pearson Education; p. 324 Pearson Education; p. 323 Pearson Education; p. 325 Pearson Education; p. 326 Pearson Education; p. 331 Pearson Education; p. 334 United States Department of Justice.

CHAPTER 13

p. 356 CDC (1999c), p. 4.

CHAPTER 14

p. 367 Pearson Education; p. 370 Adapted from Steckler & Linnan (2002); and Saunders, Evans, & Joshi (2005); p. 372 Pearson Education; p. 379 Pearson Education; p. 380 Pearson Education; p. 380 Pearson Education.

CHAPTER 15

p. 395 Fitzpatrick, J. L., Sanders, J. R., & Worthen, B. R. (2004). Program Evaluation: Alternative Approaches and Practical Guidelines (3rd ed.). United States, Pearson; p. 396 Wurzback, Mary Ellen, Ed. (2002) Community Health Education and Practice (2e) United States, Jones & Bartlett Learning; p. 399 Weiss, C. (1984). Increasing the likelihood of influencing decisions. In L. Rutman (Ed.), Evaluation research methods: A basic guide (pp. 159–190). Beverly Hills, CA: Sage.